ESSENTIALS OF

Cardiac Radiology and Imaging

Charles B. Higgins, M.D.

Professor and Vice Chairman of Radiology
Chief, Magnetic Resonance Imaging
University of California, San Francisco
School of Medicine
San Francisco, California

With 12 Contributors

J. B. Lippincott Company   Philadelphia
New York   London   Hagerstown

Sponsoring Editor: Charles McCormick, Jr.
Production Manager: Robert D. Bartleson
Production: P. M. Gordon Associates
Compositor: Compset, Inc.
Printer/Binder: Halliday Lithographic Co.

1 3 5 6 4 2

Library of Congress Cataloging-in-Publication Data

Higgins, Charles B.
    Essentials of cardiac radiology and imaging / by Charles
  B. Higgins ; with 12 contributors.
        p.   cm.
    ISBN 0–397–51107–8
      1. Heart—Imaging.   2. Heart—Diseases—Diagnosis.
    I. Title. [DNLM: 1. Cardiovascular Diseases—diagnosis.
    2. Cardiovascular Diseases—radiography.
    3. Echocardiography—methods.   4. Magnetic Resonance—
    methods.   WG 141 H636e]
    RC683.5.I42H54   1992
    616.1′20754—dc20
    DNLM/DLC
    for Library of Congress   91–36634
                                                              CIP

The authors and publisher have exerted every effort to ensure
that drug selection and dosage set forth in this text are in accord
with current recommendations and practice at the time of publication. However, in view of ongoing research, changes in gov-
ernment regulations, and the constant flow of information relating to drug therapy and drug reactions, the reader is urged
to check the package insert for each drug for any change in
indications and dosage and for added warnings and precau-
tions. This is particularly important when the recommended
agent is a new or infrequently employed drug.

This book is dedicated to my parents and to Sally

Contributors

Elias H. Botvinick, M.D.
Professor of Medicine and Radiology
University of California, San Francisco
School of Medicine
San Francisco, California

Michael W. Dae, M.D.
Associate Professor of Radiology and Medicine
University of California, San Francisco
School of Medicine
San Francisco, California

Bernard G. Fish, M.D.
Assistant Professor of Pediatrics
Pediatric Cardiology
New York Medical College
Medical Director
Pediatric Echocardiography Laboratory
West Chester County Medical Center
Valhalla, New York

Mark A. Greenberg, M.D.
Director of Cardiac Catheterization Laboratory
Montefiore Medical Center
Associate Professor of Medicine
Albert Einstein College of Medicine
Bronx, New York

Christian E. Hardy, M.D.
Chief of Cardiology
Director of Cardiac Catheterization Laboratory
Director of Electrophysiology
Children's Hospital
Oakland, California

Robert S. Hattner, M.D.
Associate Professor of Radiology
Senior Attending Nuclear Physician
University of California, San Francisco
School of Medicine
San Francisco, California

Charles B. Higgins, M.D.
Professor and Vice Chairman of Radiology
Chief, Magnetic Resonance Imaging
University of California, San Francisco
School of Medicine
San Francisco, California

Ronald B. Himelman, M.D.
Cardiology Attending
Desert Hospital
Palm Springs, California

Jeffrey S. Klein, M.D.
Assistant Professor of Radiology
Attending Radiologist
University of California, San Francisco
School of Medicine
San Francisco, California

J. William O'Connell, M.S.
Department of Radiology
University of California, San Francisco
School of Medicine
San Francisco, California

Douglas A. Ortendahl, Ph.D.
Associate Professor of Physics
Department of Radiology
University of California, San Francisco
School of Medicine
San Francisco, California

Hugo Spindola-Franco, M.D.
Professor of Radiology
Albert Einstein College of Medicine of
  Yeshiva University
Director, Cardiac Radiology
Department of Radiology
Montefiore Medical Center
Bronx, New York

James G. Sullivan, R.D.C.S., A.S.
Cardiovascular Technologist
Grossmont College
Senior Cardiovascular Technologist
Children's Hospital
Oakland, California

Preface

This book is intended to instruct readers in the essentials of the several imaging techniques used for the evaluation of cardiovascular disease. It is not designed to be an encyclopedic rendition of the enormous amount of information and literature on this topic.

The impetus to prepare the volume has come from the numerous trainees in Radiology and Cardiology with whom I have worked during the past fifteen years. They have requested and even urged me to provide a book with the basic facts of cardiovascular radiography and angiography. Several of the chapters are elaborations on a series of lectures and demonstration sessions that I have given each year during this time. I have tried to stress a systematic approach to the interpretation of imaging studies. The systems presented in the chapters are not necessarily unique or even robust in regard to the vicissitudes of the disease processes. However, the student must use a system or risk being lost in an enormous morass of facts.

A guiding principle in the designation of chapters and in the length of the book is the practical consideration that residents and fellows have so much material to study that they will be unable to expend more than a month in reading a book on this topic. It seems appropriate that a book dealing with the essentials of a discipline should conform to the time duration of rotations designated for the topic. Consequently, this book was designed so that most of it can be read during a one-month rotation.

In the preparation of this book, I have been assisted by several colleagues. Their contributions are greatly appreciated. I also wish to express my gratitude for the care and skill of Shirley Semigran and Elizabeth Ruyle in preparing the book.

C.B.H.

Contents

Chapter 1

Radiography of Acquired Heart Disease

Charles B. Higgins

The thoracic radiograph is one of the earliest points of departure in the evaluation of heart disease. It may provide the first indication that cardiac disease is present, but more frequently is used to determine the severity of known or suspected disease. The severity of some cardiac diseases is readily reflected on the thoracic radiograph, while other significant diseases cause little or no alteration in the pulmonary vessels or cardiac silhouette. Consequently, the thoracic radiograph may have only limited value in the assessment of some diseases, while in others it may serve as one of the most sensitive and reliable gauges of the course of the disease. The propensity of various cardiac diseases to cause substantial cardiomegaly serves as the major dividing line in our system for cataloging acquired heart disease.

Approach to the Chest X-ray in Acquired Heart Disease

A systematic approach is directed toward dissection of the pertinent findings from the radiograph and, with each finding, toward narrowing the array of diagnostic considerations. A free-floating approach relies upon the chance that an overall "gestalt" will whisper the correct diagnosis to you. This faulty approach may cause the physician to ignore salient features of the cardiovascular anatomy.

A five-step systematic approach permits the orderly examination of the thoracic radiograph, and at each step it is possible to narrow the diagnostic possibilities (Figs. 1-1 and 1-2). A radiographic classification of acquired heart disease is used in association with this five-step examination (Fig. 1-2, Table 1-1).

The five steps in the examination of the thoracic radiograph in patients with suspected cardiac disease are

1. Thoracic musculoskeletal structures.
2. Pulmonary vascularity.
3. Overall heart size.
4. Specific chamber enlargement.
5. Great arteries (ascending aorta, aortic knob, main pulmonary arterial segment).

Thoracic Musculoskeletal Structures

Examination of the thoracic wall discloses evidence of prior operations, such as rib or sternal deformities or sternal wire sutures. Sternal deformities such as pectus may serve as a clue to cardiac lesions associated with it, such as Marfan's syndrome, and mitral valve prolapse; or the deformity may be responsible for a cardiac murmur or even symptoms caused by cardiac compression. Narrow anteroposterior diameter of the thorax can be caused by a straight thoracic spine (straightback syndrome) or pectus excavatum. A narrow anteroposterior diameter is defined as a distance between sternum and anterior border of the vertebral body that measures less than 8 cm and a ratio of the transverse diameter (determined by frontal view) to the anteroposterior diameter (determined by lateral view) exceeding 2.75.[1] The anteroposterior diameter is the maximum diameter from the undersurface of the sternum to the anterior border of the vertebral body.

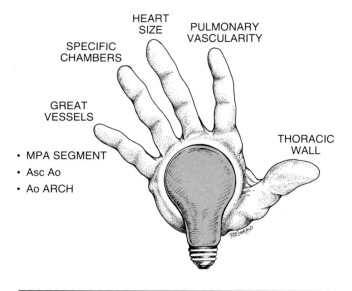

SPECIFIC
CHAMBERS

HEART
SIZE

PULMONARY
VASCULARITY

GREAT
VESSELS

THORACIC
WALL

• MPA SEGMENT
• Asc Ao
• Ao ARCH

Figure 1-1. Five-step approach to analysis of the thoracic radiograph in cardiac disease.

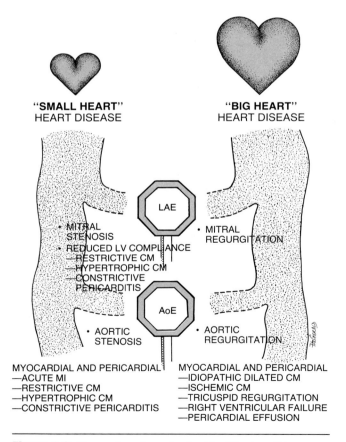

"SMALL HEART"
HEART DISEASE

"BIG HEART"
HEART DISEASE

LAE

AoE

• MITRAL
STENOSIS
• REDUCED LV COMPLIANCE
—RESTRICTIVE CM
—HYPERTROPHIC CM
—CONSTRICTIVE
PERICARDITIS

• MITRAL
REGURGITATION

• AORTIC
STENOSIS

• AORTIC
REGURGITATION

MYOCARDIAL AND PERICARDIAL
—ACUTE MI
—RESTRICTIVE CM
—HYPERTROPHIC CM
—CONSTRICTIVE PERICARDITIS

MYOCARDIAL AND PERICARDIAL
—IDIOPATHIC DILATED CM
—ISCHEMIC CM
—TRICUSPID REGURGITATION
—RIGHT VENTRICULAR FAILURE
—PERICARDIAL EFFUSION

Figure 1-2. Diagnostic pathway for the identification of the hemodynamically predominant cardiac lesion. Signposts gleaned from the thoracic radiograph guide the analysis.

Table 1-1

Radiographic Classification of Acquired Heart Disease

Small Heart (C/T < 0.55)	Large Heart (C/T > 0.55)
Aortic stenosis	Aortic regurgitation
Arterial hypertension	Mitral regurgitation
Mitral stenosis	Tricuspid regurgitation
Acute myocardial infarction	High output states
Hypertrophic cardiomyopathy	Congestive cardiomyopathy
Restrictive cardiomyopathy	Ischemic cardiomyopathy
Constrictive pericarditis	Pericardial effusion
	Paracardiac mass

Pulmonary Vascularity

There are three steps in assessing pulmonary vascularity: the type of abnormality (pulmonary arterial overcirculation vs. pulmonary venous hypertension); the severity of the pulmonary vascular abnormality; and determination of the symmetry, asymmetry, or even focal nature of the abnormality. In patients with acquired heart disease the type of abnormality is usually pulmonary venous hypertension (PVH). The major signs of PVH are equal or larger diameter of the upper compared to the lower lobe vessels; loss of prominence or clear visualization of the right lower lobe pulmonary artery; prominence of the interstitial markings, especially the appearance of Kerley a and b lines; indistinctness of the pulmonary vascular margins and/or hilar vessels; loss of the right hilar angle; and alveolar filling (Figs. 1-3, 1-4, 1-5). After repeated episodes of pulmonary edema in longstanding cases of mitral valve disease, permanent interstitial lines or ossific nodules may appear (Fig. 1-4*D*). Ossific nodules are small foci of bony metaplasia that only appear in the lungs after multiple episodes of edema and chronic pulmonary venous hypertension. Foci of hemosiderin may form fibrotic nodules in patients with multiple episodes of edema as well as those who have had multiple episodes of pulmonary hemorrhage.

The severity of pulmonary venous hypertension can be gauged by the signs observed. The radiographic severity of PVH can be divided into three grades of severity: grade I (redistribution of pulmonary blood volume); grade II (interstitial pulmonary edema); grade III (alveolar pulmonary edema) (Table 1-2). The pulmonary venous pressure (or mean left atrial wedge pressure) associated with edema varies depending upon whether the cardiac dysfunction is acute or chronic (Table 1-3). The venous pressure in chronic disease is approximately 5 mm Hg greater for each grade of PVH than in acute disease.

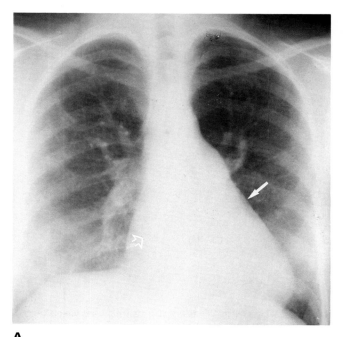

A

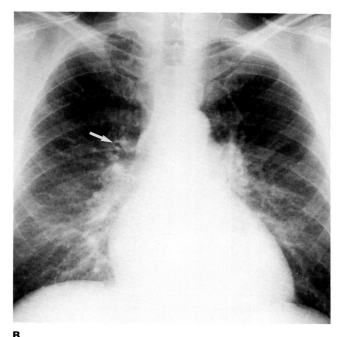

B

Figure 1-3. *A:* Pulmonary venous hypertension, grade I, in mitral valve disease. Radiograph in mitral regurgitation demonstrates redistribution of pulmonary blood flow (upper lobe vessels larger than lower lobe vessels) indicating grade I pulmonary venous hypertension. There is mild cardiomegaly and a slight convexity along the upper left cardiac border, indicating left atrial enlargement (*arrow*). There is a right retrocardiac density (*open arrow*) indicative of left atrial enlargement. *B:* Radiograph demonstrates indistinctness of the right inferior pulmonary artery, which is one of the early signs of pulmonary venous hypertension. There is also peribronchial cuffing (*arrow*).

Asymmetric PVH. Asymmetric distribution of pulmonary venous hypertension or pulmonary edema raises a number of diagnostic possibilities (Table 1-4, Fig. 1-6). The most frequent cause of such asymmetry is probably gravitational (see Fig. 1-6G); patients with heart disease frequently sleep lying on their right side because of consciousness of the prominent left-sided pulsation (prominent point of maximum impulse in the presence of cardiomegaly). The next most frequent cause is underlying lung disease such as chronic obstructive pulmonary disease, which obliterates portions of the pulmonary vascular bed. Edema or pulmonary venous distension appears in the normal or less severely abnormal portions of the lungs. Unilateral pulmonary edema may occur contralateral to an occluded or severely stenotic pulmonary artery. Such unilateral edema might appear contralateral to a pulmonary embolism, or a pulmonary arterial stenosis caused by congenital anomalies (branch pulmonary arterial stenosis, proximal interruption or agenesis of a pulmonary artery) or acquired diseases (bronchogenic carcinoma, Takayasu's arteritis, fibrosing mediastinitis [see Fig. 1-6D,E], mediastinal tu-

mors). Unilateral edema can infrequently be caused by unilateral obstruction of pulmonary veins due to mediastinal or lung tumors, primary and secondary tumors of the heart and pericardium, mediastinal fibrosis, and complications of the Mustard procedure and other procedures used in congenital heart disease (see Fig. 1-6). Finally, pulmonary edema induced by reinflation of a collapsed lung or after thoracentesis must be considered.

Pulmonary edema may occur in the absence of underlying cardiac disease. Such noncardiogenic edema is usually due to damage to the "alveolar-capillary membrane," causing a leak of fluid into the lung at normal or near normal pulmonary venous pressure and capillary oncotic pressure. A partial list of the many settings in which this occurs is shown in Table 1-5.

Overall Heart Size

Acquired heart disease can be divided into two groups, depending upon the presence or absence of substantial cardiomegaly. One group is named "small heart heart

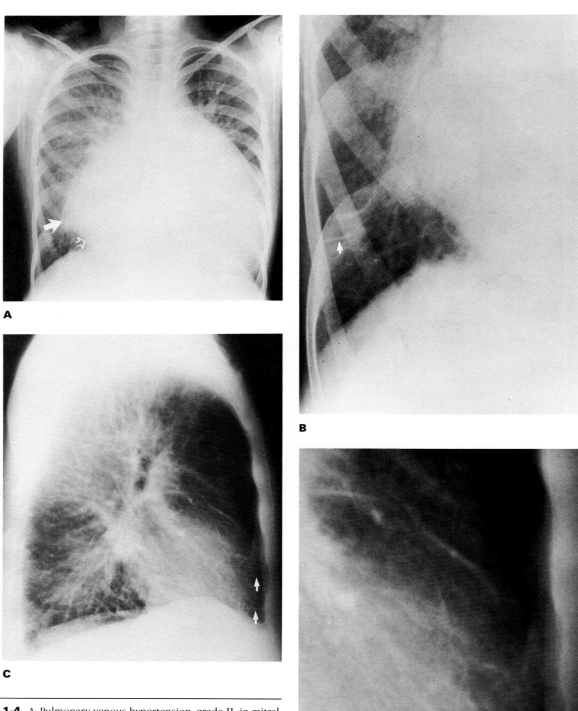

Figure 1-4. *A:* Pulmonary venous hypertension, grade II, in mitral stenosis and regurgitation. Radiography demonstrates interstitial pulmonary edema (Kerley B line), indicating grade II pulmonary venous hypertension. Note horizontal linear densities near the right costophrenic angle. Upper lobe vessels are prominent. There is cardiomegaly and gigantic left atrial enlargement. The right border of the left atrium (*arrow*) extends further to the right than the right atrial border (*open arrow*). *B:* Magnified view of the right costophrenic angle in same patient depicts the Kerley B lines (*arrow*). *C:* Lateral radiograph in a patient with interstitial pulmonary edema demonstrates the prominent interstitial lines in lungs, especially in the lower lobes and the retrosternal region. *D:* Magnified view of retrosternal region of the same radiograph as *C* shows the Kerley B lines in the retrosternal region (*arrows*).

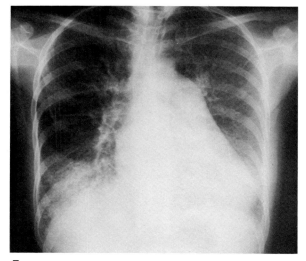

E

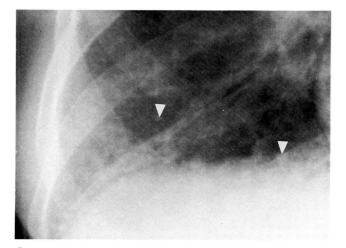

G

F

Figure 1-4 (*continued*). *E:* Interstitial pulmonary edema in a patient with mitral stenosis. Note the Kerley B line at the right costophrenic angle. Enlargement of the main pulmonary artery indicates pulmonary arterial hypertension. *F:* Ossific nodules (*arrowhead*) are evident in the lower lobes in a patient with mitral stenosis who has suffered multiple episodes of pulmonary edema. *G:* Magnified view of left costophrenic region of the same patient as *F.* Note the ossific nodules (*arrowhead*).

disease." The "small heart heart disease" is associated with a normal heart size or only mild cardiomegaly. For the sake of our discussion, we arbitrarily set a cardiothoracic (CT) ratio of less than 0.55 as consistent with this group of lesions. Obviously, the choice of 0.55 is somewhat arbitrary. The CT ratio is calculated using the convention of measuring the thoracic diameter as the distance from the inner margin of the ribs at the level of the dome of the right hemidiaphragm and the cardiac diameter as the horizontal distance between the most rightward and most leftward margins of the cardiac shadow (Fig. 1-7). The second group is called "big heart heart disease" and is characterized by substantial cardiomegaly (CT ratio > 0.5).

The pathophysiologic factors associated with "small

heart heart disease" are pressure overload and/or reduced ventricular compliance. The pathophysiologic factors associated with "big heart heart disease" are volume overload and myocardial failure. Pericardial effusion also is included in this group.

The cardiac lesions included in the two groups are listed in Table 1-1. The major pressure overload types of acquired lesions are aortic and mitral stenosis and hypertension. The major volume overload types of acquired lesions are aortic, mitral and tricuspid regurgitation and high output states. Cardiac disease that causes reduced left ventricular compliance or resistances to full expansion of the ventricles are acute myocardial infarction, hy-

(*Text continues on page 9*)

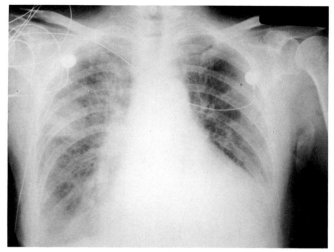

A

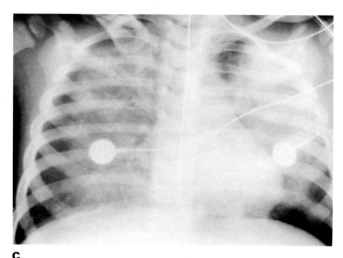

C

B

Figure 1-5. *A:* Alveolar pulmonary edema (grade III pulmonary venous hypertension). Confluent alveolar filling is evident in the right lung. *B:* Magnified view of right lung shows the alveolar filling process and obscuration of vessels in the right lung. *C:* Generalized pulmonary edema in a child who has suffered near-drowning. Alveolar filling is shown in both lungs.

Table 1-2

Signs of PVH: Grades of Severity

Grade I: Vascular Redistribution
Equal upper and lower lobe vessels
Larger upper lobe vessels

Grade II: Interstitial Edema
Kerley A and/or B lines
Increased prominence of "interstitial markings"
Peribronchial cuffing
Loss of the hilar angle
Enlargement and indistinctness of hila
Subpleural edema (increased thickness of pleura)
Loss of visibility of much of the descending branch of the right pulmonary artery

Grade III
Confluent acinar shadows (pulmonary alveolar edema)
Perihilar alveolar filling
Lower lobe or more generalized alveolar filling

Table 1-3

Correlates of LA Pressure (Mean)* and PVH

		Acute Disease (Myocardial Infarction)	Chronic Disease (Mitral Stenosis)
Grade I	PVH	12–19 mm Hg	15–25 mm Hg
Grade II	PVH	20–25 mm Hg	25–30 mm Hg
Grade III	PVH	>25 mm Hg	>30 mm Hg

LA mean pressure is usually inferred from the mean pulmonary wedge pressure.

Correlation between LA pressure and radiographic signs of pulmonary edema is only fair due to phase lag between rapid pressure changes and slower changes in radiographic alterations.[5]

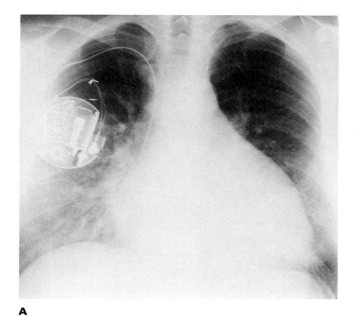

A

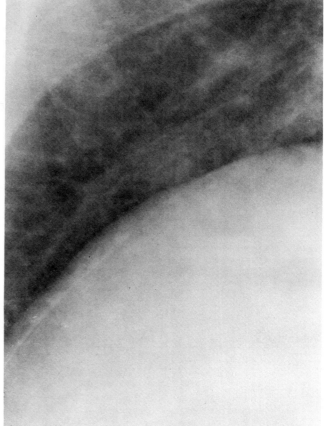

B

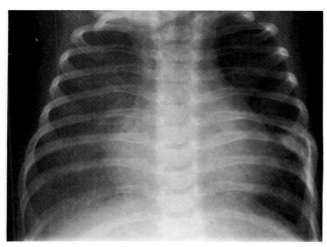

C

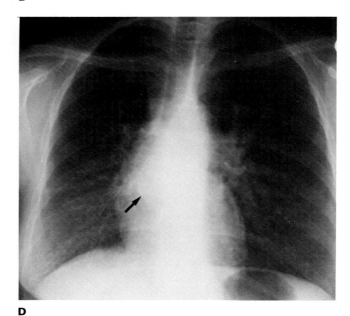

D

Figure 1-6. *A:* Asymmetric pulmonary edema. Unilateral pulmonary edema in a patient with a metastatic tumor selectively obstructing the right pulmonary veins. Note the increased density of the right lower lung field. *B:* Magnified view demonstrates the prominent interstitial lines (interstitial edema) and indistinct vessels of the right lower lobe. *C:* Unilateral pulmonary edema of right lung in a patient after Mustard procedure for transposition of great arteries. Intra-atrial baffle has caused obstruction to the entrance of right pulmonary veins. *D:* Interstitial pulmonary edema of right lung produced by fibrosing mediastinitis (histoplasmosis) causing obstruction of right pulmonary veins. The mediastinum is shifted rightward owing to decreased volume of right lung, and a subcarinal mass is evident (*arrow*). (*continued*)

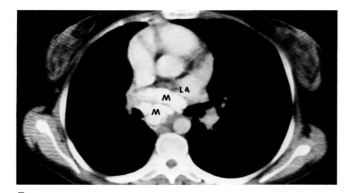

E

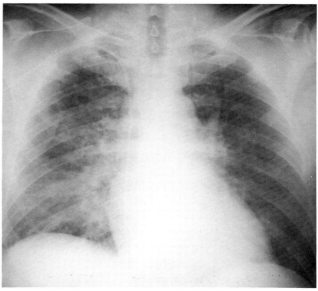

F

Figure 1-6 (*continued*). *E:* CT scan in same patient as *D* shows a calcified mass (M) of fibrous tissue posterior to and impinging upon the left atrium (LA). *F:* Asymmetric pulmonary edema due to gravitation; the patient persistently reclined on the right side.

Table 1-4

Unilateral Pulmonary Edema

1. Gravitational
2. Chronic lung disease (emphysema)
3. Unilateral pulmonary arterial obstruction
   a. Thromboembolic disease
   b. Extrinsic obstruction of pulmonary artery
      Lung Ca; thoracic aortic aneurysm; mediastinal fibrosis
4. Unilateral pulmonary venous obstruction
   a. Left atrial tumor
   b. Mediastinal tumor encasing pulmonary veins
   c. Mediastinal fibrosis
5. Re-expansion pulmonary edema
      Post pneumothorax; post thorocentesis

Table 1-5

Noncardiogenic Pulmonary Edema

1. Drowning
2. Asphyxia
3. Upper airway obstruction
4. High altitude
5. Increased intracranial pressure
6. Re-expansion pulmonary edema
7. Noxious gases
      Smoke inhalation
      Nitrous dioxide (silo filler's disease)
      Sulfur dioxide
      Others
8. Drugs
      Aspirin
      Valium, librium, barbiturates, heroin
      Cocaine, methadone
9. Poisons
      Parathion
10. Blood transfusion reaction
11. Contrast media reaction
12. Adult respiratory distress syndrome

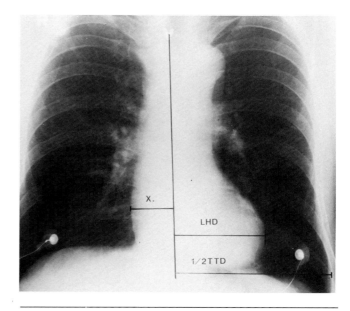

Figure 1-7. Measurement of cardiac dimensions. Cardiac dimension is measured as the maximum dimension of the heart (X + LHD) and the thoracic dimension is the maximum dimension of the thorax as defined by the distance between the inner aspects of the ribs. The distance from the middle of the spine to the inner aspect of the rib is half of the transthoracic dimension (½TTD). (LHD, left heart dimension.)

pertrophic cardiomyopathy, restrictive cardiomyopathy, and constrictive pericardial disease.

Specific Chamber Enlargement

It is not until the fourth step in the examination of the chest x-ray that attention should be directed toward determining specific chamber enlargement. A critical observation is the identification of left atrial enlargement. It is also necessary to determine which ventricle is enlarged or whether both ventricles are enlarged. It is sometimes not possible to clearly determine the type of ventricular enlargement on the thoracic radiograph. The several radiographic signs observed with enlargement of each of the cardiac chambers are given below.

Left Atrial Enlargement

1. Right retrocardiac double density. Distance from the middle of the double density (lateral border of left atrium to the middle of the left bronchus is less than 7 cm in greater than 90% of normal subjects and greater than 7 cm in 90% of patients with left atrial enlargement, proven by echocardiography (Figs. 1-8, 1-9). In cases of severe left atrial enlargement, the left atrial border may ex-

tend further to the right than the right atrial border (Fig. 1-10).
2. Enlargement of the left atrial appendage. This is seen as a bulge along the left cardiac border just beneath the main pulmonary artery segment (Figs. 1-11, 1-12). Using the left bronchus as an orientation point, the bulge above it is the main pulmonary artery segment, while the bulge at the level of and/or just below the left bronchus is the left atrial appendage.
3. Spreading of the carina and/or elevation of the left bronchus (Fig. 1-13).
4. Horizontal orientation of the distal portion of the left bronchus.
5. Posterior displacement of the left upper lobe bronchus (Fig. 1-14). On the lateral radiograph, the circular shadow of the right upper lobe and left bronchi are located along a vertical line drawn through the middle of the trachea. Left atrial enlargement causes displacement of the left bronchus posterior to this line and beyond the plane of the trachea.
6. Filling of the clear space between the top of the left atrium and the left bronchus on the right posterior (left anterior) oblique view. However, the cardiac x-ray series (posteroanterior [PA], lateral and both obliques) is seldom used now

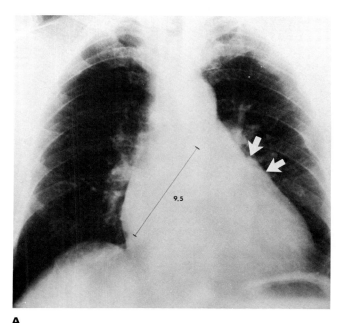

A

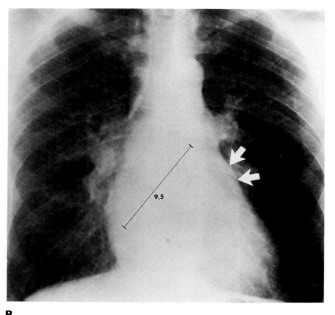

B

Figure 1-8. *A:* Rheumatic mitral regurgitation. Left atrial double density is used for the diagnosis of left atrial enlargement. The left atrial dimension is the length of a line from the middle of the double density to the medial border of the left bronchus. Note the prominent bulge on the left upper cardiac border, which indicates left atrial appendage enlargement (*arrows*). *B:* Mitral stenosis. Radiograph shows interstitial pulmonary edema, especially in right lower lobe. There is left atrial enlargement as indicated by left atrial dimension (9.5 cm) and enlarged left atrial appendage (*arrows*).

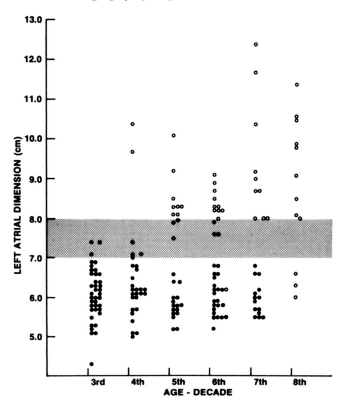

Figure 1-9. Graph shows left atrial dimensions in normal subjects and patients with left atrial enlargement at various decades of age. Closed dots represent patients with normal left atrial size, defined by echocardiography. Open dots show those with left atrial enlargement. A left atrial dimension of less than 7 cm is considered normal at most decades. A dimension greater than 8 cm indicates left atrial enlargement. A transition zone exists between 7 and 8 cm. (Reproduced with permission from Higgins CB, Reinke RT, Jones WE, et al. Left atrial dimension on the frontal thoracic radiograph: a method for assessing left atrial enlargement. Am J Radiol 1978;130:251.)

for determining specific chamber enlargement, since it has been replaced with the echocardiogram.

Right Atrial Enlargement

1. Lateral bulging of the right heart border on the PA radiograph (Fig. 1-15).
2. Prominent convexity of the right heart border on the left anterior oblique view (Fig. 1-16).
3. Elongation of the right heart border on the PA view. A rough rule is that a length of the right atrial border exceeding 50% of the mediastinal cardiovascular shadow is a sign of substantial right atrial enlargement (Fig. 1-17).

Left Ventricular Enlargement

1. On the PA view, leftward and downward displacement of the cardiac apex. The vector of enlargement of the left ventricle is leftward and

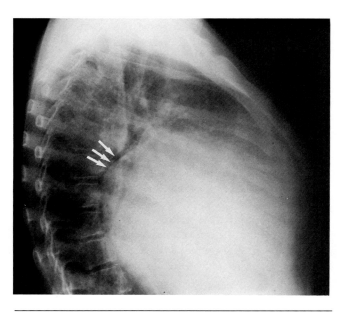

Figure 1-10. Mitral regurgitation and stenosis with giant left atrium. Lateral view shows posterior displacement of the left bronchus (*arrows*) by the enlarged left atrium.

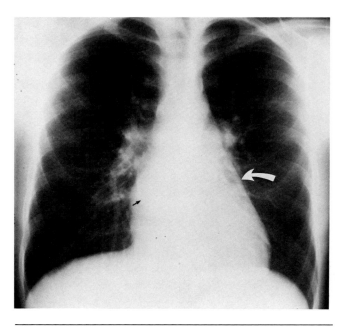

Figure 1-11. Mitral stenosis causing mild left atrial enlargement. Subtle convexity along upper left cardiac border is caused by enlargement of left atrial appendage (*curved arrow*). Note right retrocardiac double density (*small arrow*).

downward compared to the vector of right ventricular enlargement, which is leftward only or perhaps leftward plus upward (Figs. 1-18, 1-19).
2. On the lateral view, the posterior border of the heart is displaced posteriorly. The Hoffman–Rigler sign is measured 2.0 cm above the intersec-

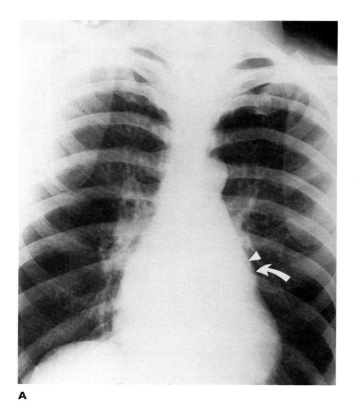

A

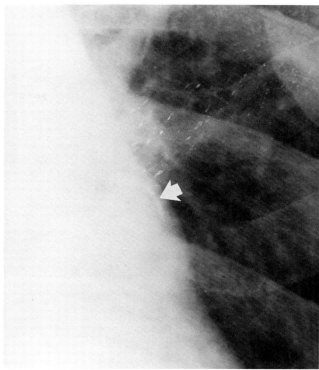

B

Figure 1-12. *A:* Mitral stenosis causing moderate enlargement of left atrium and appendage (*curved arrow*). Wall of appendage is calcified (*arrowhead*). *B:* Enlargement of *A* shows curvilinear calcification (*arrow*) of the appendage.

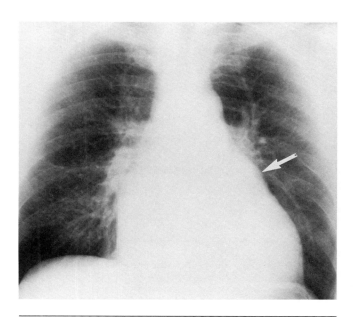

Figure 1-13. Mitral stenosis and regurgitation causing marked enlargement of left atrium and appendage (*arrow*).

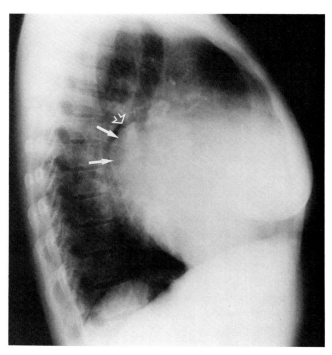

Figure 1-14. Lateral thoracic radiograph shows posterior displacement of the left bronchus (*open arrow*) by a massively enlarged left atrium. *Closed arrows* indicate the posterior wall of the left atrium.

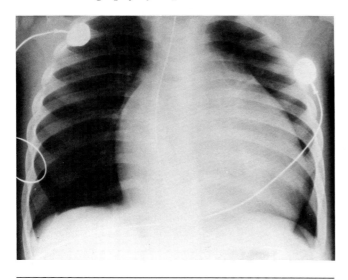

Figure 1-15. Tricuspid regurgitation. Severe right atrial enlargement is evident by the elongation of the right atrial shadow. The length of the right atrial border exceeds 60% of the height of the mediastinal cardiovascular structures (top of the arch).

tion of the diaphragm and the inferior vena cava[3] (Fig. 1-20). A positive measurement for left ventricular (LV) enlargement is a posterior border of the heart extending more than 1.8 cm behind the inferior vena caval shadow at this level.

Right Ventricular Enlargement

1. On the PA view, the left border of the heart is enlarged directly laterally or laterally and slightly superiorly (Fig. 1-19*B*). In some instances this may cause the apex to be displaced superiorly ("upward tipped apex") (Fig. 1-21), and in the extreme form causes the "boot shape" (Fig. 1-22).
2. On the lateral view, the retrosternal space is encroached upon by the enlarged RV (Fig. 1-23). Right ventricular (RV) enlargement is inferred by contact of the right heart border over greater

(*Text continues on page 15*)

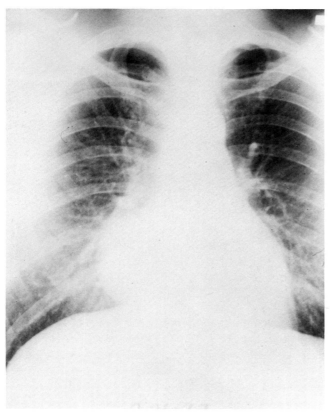

A

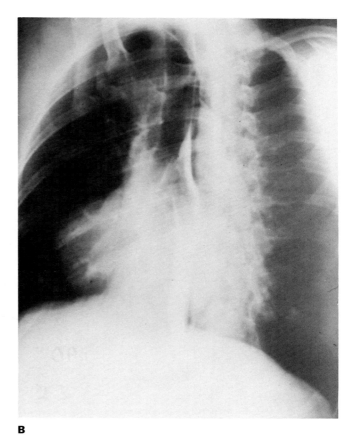

B

Figure 1-16. Idiopathic dilatation of the right atrium. Frontal (*A*) and RAO views (*B*) demonstrate the prominent right atrial border. Note the prominent anterior convexity on the RAO view, which is a definite sign of right atrial enlargement. Idiopathic dilatation of the right atrium is a rare entity in which there is substantial right atrial enlargement in the absence of tricuspid valve disease or right ventricular abnormality.

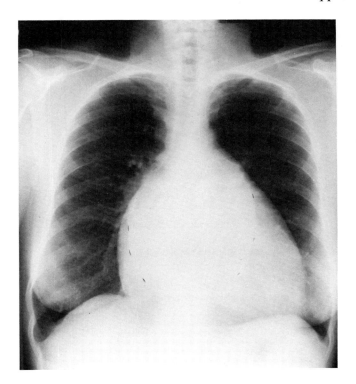

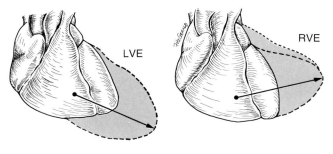

Figure 1-17. Mitral and tricuspid regurgitation. Frontal radiograph shows prominent double densities on both sides of the spine due to marked left atrial enlargement (interrupted curved lines). Right atrial enlargement is shown by the elongation of the right-sided convexity. Prominent upper left cardiac border is caused by dilatation of the right ventricular outflow region.

Figure 1-18. The vector of enlargement for the left and right ventricles. For left ventricular enlargement (LVE), the vector is directed leftward and caudal. For right ventricular enlargement (RVE), the vector is directed leftward or leftward and slightly cranial.

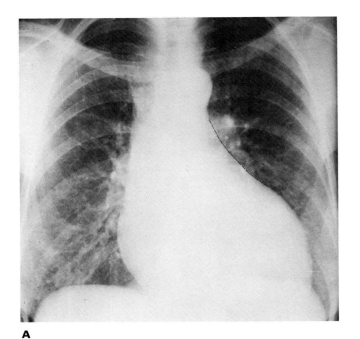

A

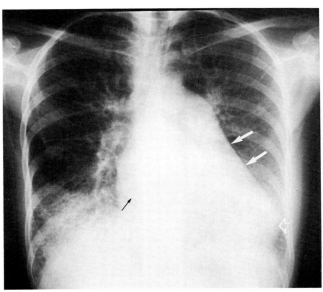

B

Figure 1-19. *A:* Aortic regurgitation. The ventricular contour is enlarged along a left inferolateral vector, causing the apex to droop over the left hemidiaphragm. Concavity along upper left cardiac border (*broken line*) indicates that the right ventricle is not enlarged. *B:* Mitral stenosis with pulmonary arterial hypertension and pulmonary edema. Cardiomegaly is caused by right ventricular enlargement. The vector of enlargement of the ventricle is directly lateral, indicating right ventricular enlargement. Most lateral portion of the apex is located above the diaphragm (*open arrow*). There is interstitial pulmonary edema (note Kerley B lines at right costophrenic angle), left atrial enlargement indicated by double density (*small arrow*), and pulmonary arterial enlargement. There is fullness of the upper left cardiac border caused by enlargement of right ventricular outflow region (*arrows*).

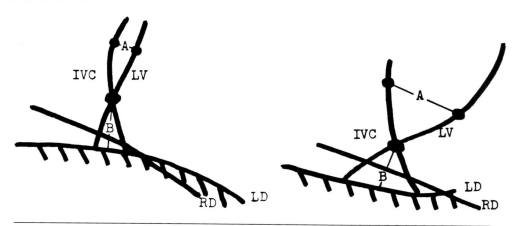

Figure 1-20. *Left*: Hoffman–Rigler measurement for a normal heart. The measurement is done on the lateral radiograph. Diagram of the inferior cardiac border as found on the lateral radiograph. *B* is the distance from the left diaphragm (LD) to the point of crossing of the inferior vena cava (IVC) and the posterior border of the left ventricle (LV). *A* is the distance from the IVC to the left heart border at a distance of 2 cm cranial to point *A*. The normal value for distance *A* is less than 1.5 cm and for distance *B* is greater than 1 cm. *Right*: Hoffman–Rigler measurement in the presence of left ventricular enlargement. In comparison to the normal heart, a value for *A* exceeding 2 cm and a value *B* less than 1 cm indicates left ventricular enlargement. (Reproduced from Hoffman RB, Rigler RG: Evaluation of left ventricular enlargement in the lateral projection of the chest. Radiology 1965;85:93–100, with permission of the Radiological Society of North America.)

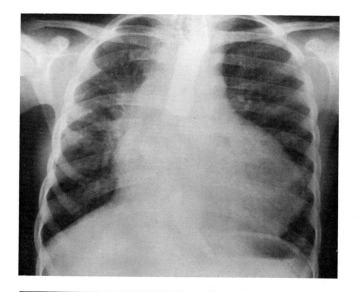

Figure 1-21. Tetralogy of Fallot after right systemic-pulmonary shunt. Substantial right ventricular enlargement is evident. The vector of enlargement of the ventricular mass is leftward and slightly cranial, causing uplifting of the apex in relation to the diaphragm.

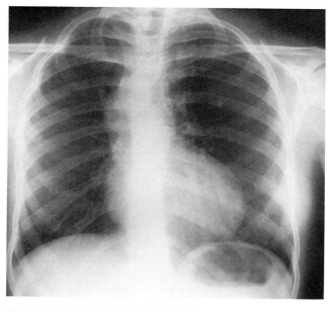

Figure 1-22. Boot-shaped heart. Right ventricular enlargement causing severe uplifting of the cardiac apex.

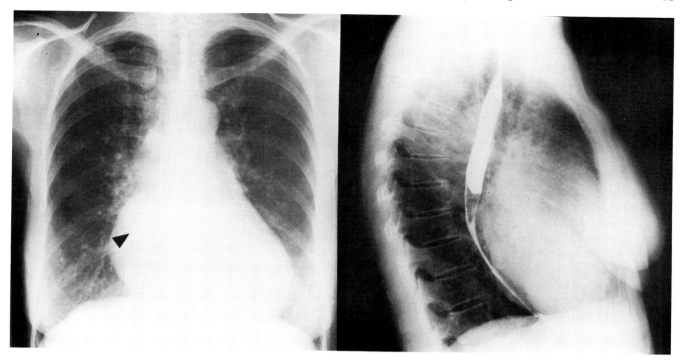

Figure 1-23. Mitral stenosis. Frontal (*left*) and lateral (*right*) thoracic radiographs of a patient with mitral stenosis demonstrate left atrial and right ventricular enlargement. Grade I PVH is indicated by cephalic redistribution of pulmonary blood flow. Note the small diameter of the lower lobe vessels. Signs of left atrial enlargement include right retrocardiac double density on frontal view (*arrowhead*) and displacement with compression upon the esophageal barium column on lateral view. Right ventricular enlargement is indicated by lateral displacement of the ventricular margin (apex uplifted) on the frontal view and encroachment of anterior border of the heart into the retrosternal space on the lateral view. The anterior border of the heart makes contact with the sternum for more than 40% of the sternal length.

than one-third of the sternal length. A prominent convexity to the anterior border rather than the usual straight surface is an early sign of RV enlargement.

3. On the right anterior oblique (RAO) view, the right (anterior) border of the heart shows a prominent convexity in the presence of RV enlargement (see Fig. 1-16).

Signposts for Cardiac Valvular Lesions

A signpost gives directions along the road. The signposts on the thoracic radiograph also give direction; they direct attention to a certain cardiac valve.

There are three signposts:

1. Left atrial enlargement.
2. Ascending aortic enlargement.
3. Right atrial enlargement.

These are the most useful signs that point specifically to

1. Mitral valve (left atrium).
2. Aortic valve (ascending aorta).
3. Tricuspid valve (right atrium).

Using our classification system ("big heart vs. small heart heart disease") and applying the signpost, we can analyze the thoracic radiograph in accordance with the flow diagram shown in Figure 1-2. Obviously, this schema works well for diseases causing typical alterations in the chest x-ray. Of course, a specific cardiac lesion does not always cause typical features because of other associated abnormalities or because the lesion is very mild or has been present for insufficient time to alter the cardiac morphology to a degree that is discernible on the thoracic radiograph.

The schema can be briefly described by considering the chest x-ray that shows a normal heart size or mild cardiomegaly in a patient with significant heart disease. This means that the lesion likely causes pressure overload (hypertension, aortic stenosis or mitral stenosis) or reduced LV compliance. If the left atrial signpost is present, then attention is directed to the mitral valve (Fig. 1-24). The diagnosis should be either mitral valvular stenosis or resistance to left atrial emptying. Diseases that significantly reduce LV compliance (and increase LV diastolic pressure) cause resistance to left atrial emptying and thereby induce left atrial enlargement. Several diseases that may reduce LV compliance are hypertrophic cardiomyopathy, restrictive cardiomyopathy, and constrictive pericardial disease. Acute myocardial infarction may also reduce LV compliance but usually this has not been present for a sufficient time to cause left atrial enlargement. Left ventricular hypertrophy from any cause can reduce LV compliance if it is sufficiently severe.

If the ascending aorta is enlarged, then this signpost points to the aortic valve, indicating aortic stenosis (Fig.

1-25). Systemic hypertension can produce a similar appearance, although it usually causes enlargement of the entire thoracic aorta rather than the ascending aorta alone. If no signposts are present, then the diagnosis is unlikely to be a valvular lesion. The absence of signposts should direct attention to a disease directly afflicting the myocardium or pericardium, such as acute myocardial infarction, hypertrophic cardiomyopathy, restrictive cardiomyopathy, or constrictive pericardial disease. However, even these diseases can sometimes induce left atrial enlargement, as stated above.

The schema for a patient with substantial cardiomegaly proceeds along a similar path. The "big heart" suggests that there is either a volume overload lesion (valvular regurgitation) or myocardial failure or pericardial effusion. High output states are certainly a volume overload and can cause substantial cardiomegaly, but sometimes they cause only mild cardiomegaly. If left atrial enlargement is noted, then the signpost points to

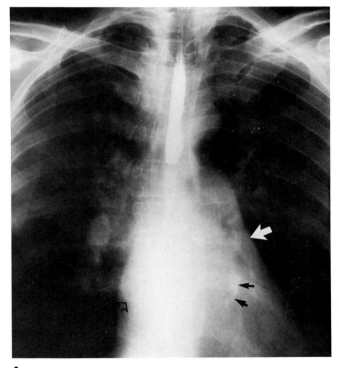

A

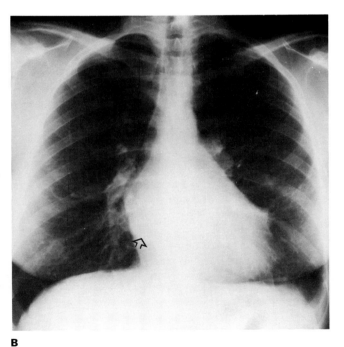

B

Figure 1-24. *A:* Mitral stenosis. Frontal radiograph (overpenetrated) demonstrates the retrocardiac double density (*open arrow*), enlargement of left atrial appendage (*arrow*) and main pulmonary arterial segment. The main pulmonary arterial segment is located above the left bronchus and the appendage is situated below the bronchus. The ascending aorta appears small, which is typical in cases of isolated mitral valve disease. Note the calcification in the mitral valve (*small arrows*). Double density shows that the left atrial enlargement is mild. *B:* Mitral stenosis. Frontal radiograph is well penetrated to demonstrate the double density (*open arrow*). Double density is longer and extends farther to the right than the radiography in *A,* indicating a greater degree of enlargement of the left atrium. Prominence of the left atrial appendage is not present because it was amputated during closed commissurotomy. The ascending aorta is small, consistent with isolated mitral valve disease.

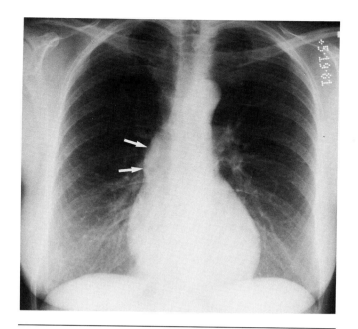

Figure 1-25. Aortic stenosis. Frontal radiograph shows normal cardiac size and normal pulmonary vascularity. The sole abnormality in this 40-year-old subject is enlargement of the ascending aorta (*arrows*). The shadow of the posterior aortic arch is normal.

mitral regurgitation (see Fig. 1-17). If the ascending aorta is enlarged in "big heart" heart disease, then this signpost points to aortic regurgitation (Fig. 1-26). If the right atrium is enlarged, then this signpost points to tricuspid regurgitation (see Fig. 1-15). Acquired pulmonic regurgitation is rare, except as a consequence of operation for right ventricular outflow obstruction, and is not considered in this schema. If no signposts are present then the favored diagnostic considerations are congestive (dilated) cardiomyopathy or pericardial effusion.

Signs of Pulmonary Venous Hypertension

Enlarged Upper Lobe Vessels

The initial sign of PVH is dilatation of the upper lobe veins so that they approximate the diameter of the lower lobe vessels. This equalization of vascular diameter indicates mild pulmonary venous hypertension. Pulmonary venous hypertension is defined by a mean left atrial or pulmonary venous pressure exceeding 12 mm Hg. Further elevation of pulmonary venous pressure causes in-

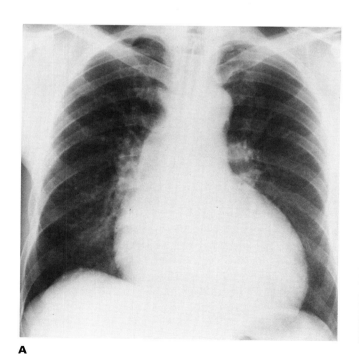

A

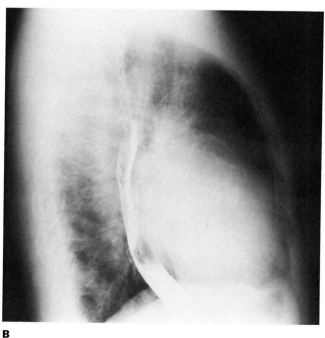

B

Figure 1-26. Aortic regurgitation. Frontal (*A*) and lateral (*B*) radiographs show marked cardiomegaly with displacement of ventricular contour laterally and caudally, indicating left ventricular enlargement. The ascending aorta and contour of posterior aortic arch are enlarged. Lateral view shows posterior displacement of the ventricular contour and a normal retrocardiac space.

creasing dilatation of the upper lobe vessels and eventually reduction of diameter of the lower lobe vessels. Veins in the first interspace with a diameter exceeding 3 mm suggest pulmonary venous hypertension or a left-to-right shunt. The size of the lower lobe vessels distinguishes the two; they also are enlarged in shunt lesions. This reversal of the normal gradient in blood flow from apex to base of the lung is called *redistribution of pulmonary blood flow* or *pulmonary vascular cephalization.* A readily recognizable sign of redistribution is a relatively small diameter, or even nonvisibility, of the descending branch of the right pulmonary artery.

When redistribution is the only sign of PVH, it is considered to be grade I. The mean left atrial pressure associated with grade I PVH is related to the chronicity of PVH. Upper lobe vessel dilatation is abrupt and prominent when the pressure rise is acute, as in patients with acute myocardial infarction. Chronic elevation of pulmonary venous pressure, as in patients with congestive cardiomyopathy, may exist without any discernible enlargement of upper lobe vessels. The relationship between signs of PVH and mean left atrial pressure in acute and chronic disease is shown in Table 1-3. The relationship is neither close nor exact owing to a lag between the elevation of pressure and the onset of the radiographic signs. Moreover, upper lobe vessel enlargement may not appear in patients with pulmonary parenchymal disease in the upper lobe, such as tuberculosis and other granulomatous diseases, pneumoconiosis, emphysema, and giant bullous disease. Likewise, parenchymal disease in the lower lobe can render the upper lobe vessels relatively prominent.

Enlargement of the central portion of the upper lobe pulmonary veins may cause increased prominence of the hila with elevation of pulmonary venous pressure. Such venous enlargement causes loss of the acute angle formed by the crossing of the shadow of the upper lobe vein and the inferior pulmonary artery in the right hilum (loss of right hilar angle).[4] This finding is most readily identified by comparing sequential radiographs.

Interstitial Lines and Fluid

The presence of interstitial lines is the essential diagnostic sign of grade II PVH. Interstitial lines can represent several pathologies, including fluid (pulmonary edema), hemosiderin (pulmonary hemosiderosis), fibrosis, and tumor cells (lymphangitic carcinoma) in the interstitial space and interstitial lymphatics. Prominent interstitial lines can be caused by a current episode of pulmonary edema or may represent fibrosis resulting from prior episodes of pulmonary edema. Interstitial edema precedes alveolar edema. Both ensue when hydrostatic pressure exceeds colloid osmotic pressure and the capacity of pul-

monary lymphatic channels to transport excessive fluid from the interstitium. Pulmonary interstitial lymphatic channels dilate in this situation and consequently their increased diameter contributes to the prominence of the interstitial markings. Deposition of radiodense hemosiderin in the interstitial space is a consequence of previous episodes of pulmonary edema and may also contribute to prominence of the interstitial lines. The radiographs of most patients with mean pulmonary venous pressure exceeding 20 mm Hg show signs of interstitial pulmonary edema.

Fluid in the interstitial space produces radiographic signs by obscuring the usual sharp interface between intrapulmonary vessels and air spaces; thickening the rim of interstitial tissue surrounding vessels; and rendering interlobular septa and intrapulmonary lymphatic channels visible. Consequently, the signs of interstitial edema are indistinctness of pulmonary vessels, especially in the lower lobes (see Fig. 1-4); loss of visibility of the descending branch of the right pulmonary artery (see Figs. 1-4, 1-5); indistinctness of the hilar margins (see Figs. 1-4, 1-5); Kerley B lines (see Fig. 1-4); Kerley A lines; and thickening of the pleural line, especially at the costophrenic angles (see Fig. 1-4).

The most prominent vessel on the frontal thoracic radiograph is the descending branch of the right pulmonary artery. This vessel can usually be readily visualized from the lower hilum and continuing into its branches extending to the diaphragm. A useful sign of interstitial edema is loss of clear visibility of the vessel a few centimeters beyond the hilum. Likewise, interstitial fluid diminishes the contrast between lung and hilar vessels, causing hilar indistinctness (hilar haze). Distension of the central portion of the pulmonary veins, especially the upper lobe veins, enlarges the hila. So, hilar enlargement and indistinctness may be evident when comparing radiographs in a patient who has experienced a change in pulmonary venous pressure.

Kerley B lines (basal septal lines) are short horizontal lines of variable thickness that usually make contact with the pleural surface. They are most frequently identified at the costophrenic angles (see Fig. 1-4), but may also be seen in the retrosternal space on the lateral view (see Fig. 1-4D). The Kerley B line is an interlobular septum distended by fluid in acute edema but sometimes made visible by fibrosis or hemosiderin deposition as a consequence of prior episodes of pulmonary edema. The Kerley B line usually disappears after reduction of pulmonary venous pressure. However, a phase lag is recognized between the time at which venous pressure rises or declines and the flux of fluid into and out of the interstitial space.[5,6] A closer relationship exists between the presence of interstitial lines and measurement of extravascular lung water than the level of pulmonary venous pressure. Kerley A lines are diagonal lines up to 3 to 4 cm in length, located in the middle and center portions of the lungs and radiating from the hilar or left atrial region. The Kerley A lines represent distension of the perilymphatic channels anastomosing between the peripheral and central pulmonary lymphatic networks. A lobular pattern of the interlobular septa may be observed in the lower lung zones, and is apparently caused by intersecting septa oriented *en face* to the frontal radiograph.

Subpleural Edema and Pleural Effusion

Thickening of the pleural line represents subpleural edema. This is fluid collecting beneath the visceral pleura of the lung in an interstitial tissue plane continuous with the interlobular septa. Sequential thoracic radiographs can be compared to detect thickening of the pleural line at the costophrenic angle coincident with elevated pulmonary venous pressure. Fluid in the space also contributes to increased thickness of the major and minor fissures in this setting. Thickening of the pleural line is one of the earliest and most frequent signs of PVH on the portable film obtained within the first day after the onset of acute myocardial infarction.[7]

Pleural effusions are common in patients with PVH. These effusions initially obscure the costophrenic angle and thicken the major and minor fissures. Although they certainly occur in left-sided failure, they are frequent and large in right-sided failure or combined elevation in right and left ventricular end-diastolic pressures. Pleural effusion caused by cardiac disease is alleged to be initially, and sometimes only, a right-sided effusion. Although right-sided pleural effusion may be more common than isolated left effusion in heart disease, isolated left effusions are sometimes observed. Preferential right pleural effusion in heart disease is likely caused by the preference of patients with heart disease to sleep on their right side because of consciousness of prominent pulsation of their enlarged hearts when lying on their left side.

Alveolar Edema

Alveolar edema is indicated by the appearance of acinar confluent shadow. Alveolar filling becomes evident initially in the perihilar regions and lower lung fields (see Fig. 1-5). Alveolar edema generally ensues when pulmonary venous pressure exceeds 25 mm Hg in acute processes and exceeds 30 mm Hg in chronic diseases. Signs of interstitial and alveolar edema frequently coexist. Pulmonary edema frequently shows gravitational distribution, causing it to be more severe or only evident in the right lung when patients preferentially lie or sleep on their left sides. Atypical distribution of alveolar edema may be caused by underlying lung disease such as emphysema and pulmonary thromboembolic disease. Alveolar edema may change or disappear rapidly in response to changes in hemodynamic states. However, sometimes there is a considerable lag between the decline in pulmonary venous pressure and the resolution of alveolar edema owing to phase lag caused by fluid fluxes between intra-alveolar and vascular spaces.[5]

Ossific and Siderotic Nodules

Hemosiderin deposition in the lungs of sufficient quantity causes permanent prominence of interstitial markings and septal lines. The lower lung fields may also be diffusely mottled. These changes may not be appreciably altered with changes in hemodynamic status.

Ossific nodules may be caused by chronic PVH and repeated episodes of alveolar pulmonary edema. They are infrequently observed today and are usually observed in patients with chronic mitral stenosis with suspected episodes of pulmonary edema (see Fig. 1-4F,G). Ossific nodules represent heterotopic bone formation caused by development of intra-alveolar edema. These nodules are very dense and rounded and are located in the lower lobes. The uniform size, lower lobe distribution, and association with mitral valve disease distinguish them from the multiple pulmonary calcification observed in histoplasmosis and varicella pneumonia.

Radiographic Features of Specific Cardiac Lesions

Aortic Stenosis

Aortic stenosis is a pressure overload lesion for which the compensatory mechanism is concentric left ventricular hypertrophy. Concentric left ventricular hypertrophy causes a slight reduction in the volume of the left ventricular chamber but causes little increase in overall cardiac size. Consequently, aortic stenosis, for much of its natural history, is a disease that is clearly "small heart heart disease." There is little or no cardiac enlargement. The so-called left ventricular configuration of the cardiac contour is relatively nonspecific and sometimes an imaginary perception of those attempting to recognize an abnormality in the cardiac contour in this relatively radiographically silent lesion. The pulmonary vascularity is also generally normal for much of the course of aortic stenosis. However, in the decompensated phase of aortic stenosis there may be evidence of pulmonary venous hypertension due to LV failure, and occasionally, when left ventricular hypertrophy has reduced LV compliance considerably, there may also be signs of pulmonary venous hypertension even when the left ventricle has not failed.

Enlargement of the ascending aorta is present in nearly all patients with aortic stenosis. It should be noted that aortic stenosis enlarges only the ascending aorta and leaves the aortic knob and descending aorta normal in size (Figs. 1-25, 1-27) while aortic regurgitation enlarges the entire thoracic aorta. The ascending aorta and the aortic arch are usually prominent in patients with aortic regurgitation (see Fig. 1-26). Calcification of the aortic valve is also a sign of aortic stenosis, but is observed on the radiograph in only a minority of patients with this disease (see Fig. 1-27). There is a relationship between the density of the calcification of the aortic valve that is observed on fluoroscopy and the severity of the gradient across the aortic valve.[8] Enlargement of the aorta in older patients may provide no insight into the diagnosis of aortic valve disease, since atherosclerotic and other degenerative changes of the aorta, such as arteriomegaly, are more common than aortic valve disease in elderly patients.

The chest radiograph is not very useful in assessing the severity of aortic stenosis. Since the severity of aortic stenosis is frequently reflected in the severity of left ventricular hypertrophy or the severity of the increase in left ventricular wall thickness, modalities which depict both the endocardial and epicardial surface of the left ventricle are optimal for determining the severity of a left ventricular hypertrophy. In this regard, both echocardiography and electrocardiographically gated magnetic resonance imaging display the endocardial and epicardial borders and can be used to define the severity of left ventricular hypertrophy and quantitate left ventricular mass. These techniques, therefore, are effective in assessing the severity of aortic stenosis. The degree of enlargement of the ascending aorta bears no relationship to the severity of the gradient across the aortic valve. Indeed, enlargement of the ascending aorta to substantial degrees may occur as a consequence of the eccentric jet across a nonstenotic bicuspid valve. Since aortic stenosis in its compensated form causes little or no increase in pulmonary venous pressure, the signs of pulmonary venous hypertension cannot be used to assess the severity of aortic stenosis. A recognizably calcified aortic valve on the chest radiograph is usually a sign of significant aortic stenosis, but it is a relatively insensitive sign. Late in the natural history of aortic stenosis there may be left ventricular failure with left ventricular dilatation and signs of pulmonary venous hypertension.

The three major etiologies of aortic stenosis are (1) congenital aortic stenosis; (2) degeneration of a bicuspid or even a tricuspid aortic valve; and (3) rheumatic heart disease. The congenitally stenotic aortic valve is usually unicuspid or bicuspid. Aortic stenosis from a degenerat-

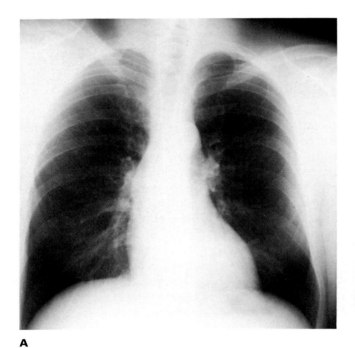

A

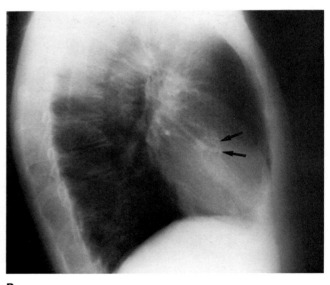

B

Figure 1-27. Aortic stenosis with calcification in 43-year-old man. Frontal radiograph (*A*) shows a nearly normal appearance except for enlargement of the ascending aorta. Lateral view (*B*) demonstrates heavy calcification (*arrows*) of the aortic valve. Note that the calcification is anterior to a line passing from the lower border of the right pulmonary artery to the intersection of the diaphragm and sternum. Valvular calcification posterior to this line is assigned to the mitral valve.

ed bicuspid aortic valve usually presents in the fourth or fifth decade, whereas aortic stenosis caused by degeneration of a tricuspid valve usually presents in the sixth or seventh decade or even later. The degree (extent or density) of calcification of the aortic valve in the elderly may not be closely related to the severity of stenosis. Aortic valve disease is a cause of calcification of the ascending aorta in elderly patients.[9]

Hypertension

Hypertensive heart disease is a pressure overload lesion and consequently is associated with a normal heart size for much of the compensated phase of this disease. The severity or even the presence of left ventricular hypertrophy cannot be reliably determined from the thoracic radiograph. As discussed above, the severity of left ventricular hypertrophy can be defined from other noninvasive studies such as echocardiography and magnetic resonance imaging.

The characteristic radiographic features of hypertensive heart disease are normal pulmonary vascularity, normal heart size, frequently no chamber enlargement, and a prominent thoracic aorta. The only abnormality on the radiograph that indicates the presence of this disease is enlargement of the thoracic aorta (Fig. 1-28). In this instance the ascending aorta is usually not as prominently enlarged as in aortic stenosis, but in addition there is enlargement of the aortic knob and the descending aorta. In older patients with hypertension there is frequently substantial tortuosity of the thoracic aorta as well.

In the patient with chronic renal disease and hypertension, the thoracic radiograph may also show evidence of hypervolemia and there may be some degree of left ventricular and cardiac enlargement.

Mitral Stenosis

The features of a thoracic radiograph are frequently quite diagnostic for mitral stenosis (Figs. 1-3, 1-4, 1-13, 1-23, 1-24, 1-29, 1-30, 1-31). Likewise, the radiograph provides considerable insight into the severity of mitral stenosis.

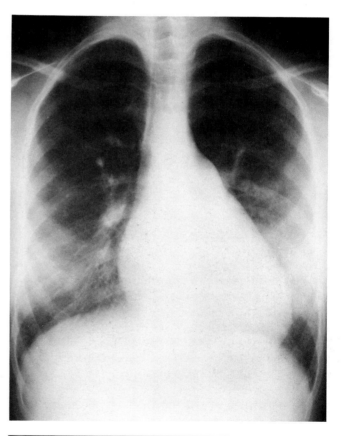

Figure 1-29. Mitral stenosis with pulmonary venous hypertension and pulmonary arterial hypertension (PAH). Frontal view shows retrocardiac double density due to left atrial enlargement and prominent left atrial appendage. Grade II PVH is indicated by obscuration of the lower lobe vascularity, especially the distal portion of the right inferior pulmonary artery and prominent interstitial marking at the right costophrenic angle. Enlargement of the main pulmonary artery segment indicates PAH.

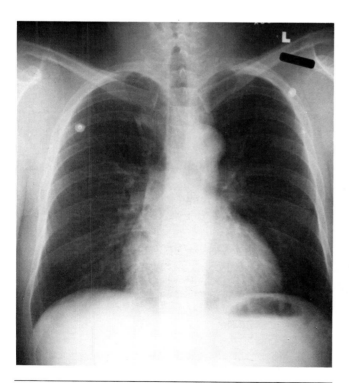

Figure 1-28. Systemic hypertension. Frontal view shows borderline cardiomegaly and prominence of the entire thoracic aorta.

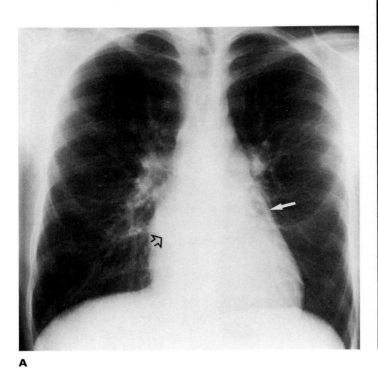

A

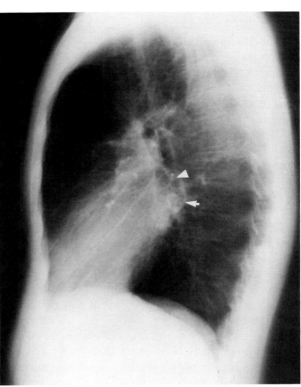

B

Figure 1-30. Mild mitral stenosis. Frontal (*A*) and lateral (*B*) radiographs. Mild pulmonary venous hypertension is indicated by equalization of the diameter of upper and lower lobe vessels. A small retrocardiac density (*open arrow*) and subtle focal evagination of upper left cardiac border (*arrow*) indicate mild enlargement of body and appendage of left atrium. Normal cardiac size with a small ascending aorta is evident. Lateral view shows posterior extension of left atrial region (*arrow*) and posterior displacement of left bronchus (*arrowhead*).

Although mitral stenosis is a pressure overload lesion that causes little increase in overall heart size during the early phase of the disease, it does produce characteristic enlargement of the left atrium and the left atrial appendage and produces signs of pulmonary venous hypertension.

The chest radiograph demonstrates evidence of pulmonary venous hypertension in nearly all patients with significant mitral stenosis. In some patients there may be only equalization of the caliber of the blood vessels in the upper and lower lobe regions when the disease is mild, whereas in others there may be intermittent pulmonary edema. The overall heart size is normal but there is a signpost for this diagnosis: enlargement of the left atrium. This signpost points to the mitral valve as the causative lesion and indicates the diagnosis of mitral stenosis. There is usually enlargement of the atrial appendage, especially in patients in whom stenosis is caused by rheumatic heart disease.[10] This is the majority of patients. The left ventricle is usually not enlarged. The right ven-

tricle may be either mildly or very substantially enlarged, depending upon the severity of pulmonary arterial hypertension (see Fig. 1-31).

Enlargement of the heart in a patient with known mitral stenosis is sometimes encountered. The enlargement is usually due to right heart dilatation. The responsible mechanism is either pulmonary arterial hypertension or rheumatic involvement of the tricuspid valve, causing tricuspid regurgitation. When the right ventricle and other right-sided chambers are substantially enlarged, one can expect to see enlargement of the main pulmonary artery in patients in whom the right-sided enlargement is caused by secondary pulmonary arterial hypertension (see Fig. 1-31). When right-sided chambers are enlarged but the main pulmonary artery is normal in size, then one must suspect a right-sided cardiac lesion, usually tricuspid regurgitation, as the cause of the enlargement. When the left ventricle is enlarged in a patient with mitral stenosis, then one must consider the likelihood that there is a substantial element of mitral regur-

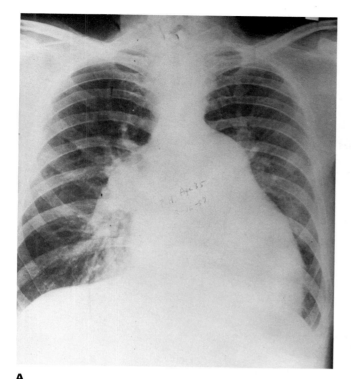

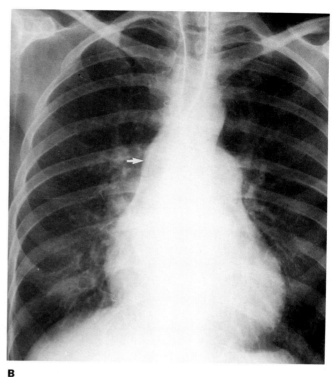

A   **B**

Figure 1-31. Two cases of severe mitral stenosis with pulmonary arterial hypertension. Cardiomegaly caused by right ventricular enlargement. *A:* Frontal radiograph displays enlarged upper lobe vessels (grade I PVH) and markedly enlarged main pulmonary artery and hilar arteries (severe PAH). The latter finding explains the presence of substantial right ventricular enlargement. *B:* Frontal radiograph shows grade II PVH with enlargement of main pulmonary arterial segment. Prominent ascending aorta (*arrow*) suggests concurrent aortic valve disease.

gitation as well as stenosis (see Fig. 1-10). When the thoracic aorta, as well as the left ventricle, is enlarged in a patient with mitral stenosis, then one must consider the additional diagnosis of aortic regurgitation. Associated enlargement of the ascending aorta can also be due to rheumatic aortic stenosis. Finally, it is possible that ventricular enlargement in a patient with mitral stenosis is due to rheumatic myocardial disease, although this is now a rare complication.

Hypertrophic Cardiomyopathy

The chest radiograph is neither specific nor sensitive for the diagnosis of hypertrophic cardiomyopathy. More than 50% of the patients with hypertrophic cardiomyopathy have a normal chest x-ray.[11] In a minority of patients there is some abnormality of the chest x-ray, which is usually relatively vague and not particularly indicative of this disease. Since some patients with hypertrophic cardiomyopathy have a reduction in left ventricular compliance, the radiograph may sometimes demonstrate pulmonary venous hypertension. The degree of pulmonary venous hypertension is usually relatively mild. The overall heart size is generally normal. In patients with reduced left ventricular compliance left atrial size may be increased. Approximately 30% of patients with symptomatic hypertrophic cardiomyopathy have associated mitral regurgitation.[11] Because of the mitral regurgitation there again is a proclivity to left atrial enlargement (Fig. 1-32). In a minority of patients the left cardiac border appears squared. This is caused by a prominent evagination on the upper left cardiac border (Fig. 1-33). This focal enlargement is a consequence of extreme enlargement of the upper or outflow portion of the ventricular septum.

The plain radiograph is relatively useless for defining the severity of hypertrophic cardiomyopathy. The severity of hypertrophic cardiomyopathy is determined with the use of echocardiography, which demonstrates the degree and distribution of the hypertrophy within the left ventricle (Fig. 1-34). Likewise, magnetic resonance imaging also provides considerable insight into the distribution of the left ventricular hypertrophy (Fig. 1-35).

In patients with the obstructive form of hyper-

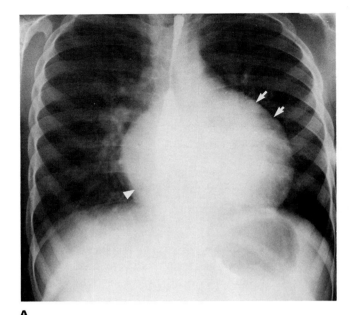

A

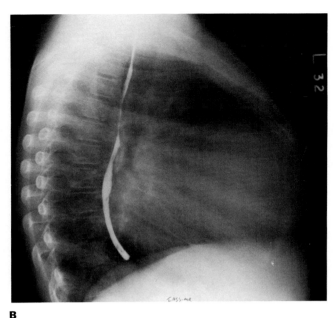

B

Figure 1-32. Hypertrophic cardiomyopathy with mitral regurgitation. Frontal (*A*) and lateral (*B*) radiographs show prominent convexity of upper left cardiac border (*arrows*) due to marked septal hypertrophy. Left atrial double density on frontal view (*arrowhead*) and posterior prominence on lateral view indicate marked left atrial enlargement caused by mitral regurgitation.

trophic cardiomyopathy, there is a systolic ejection murmur. The plain radiograph in these patients does not reveal the enlarged ascending aorta as it does in patients with aortic valvular stenosis. Consequently, in a patient with a murmur indicative of left ventricular outflow obstruction, the absence of enlargement of the ascending aorta may suggest the diagnosis of hypertrophic cardiomyopathy, obstructive form (see Fig. 1-33).

Cardiac enlargement may occur in patients with hypertrophic cardiomyopathy either due to end-stage disease with dilatation of the left ventricle or due to left atrial and left ventricular enlargement as a consequence of substantial mitral regurgitation (Fig. 1-32). Consequently, when the plain radiograph demonstrates cardiomegaly in such patients, look for the sign of left atrial enlargement in order to attempt to differentiate between these two diagnostic possibilities.

Hypertrophic cardiomyopathy may occur as part of certain syndromes, including neurofibromatosis, lentiginosis syndrome and Noonan's syndrome.

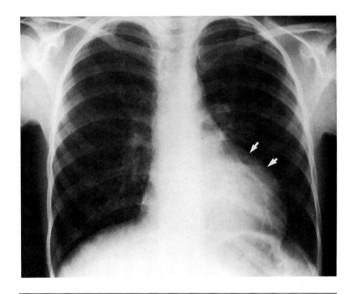

Figure 1-33. Hypertrophic cardiomyopathy. Normal cardiac size with slightly abnormal contour due to prominent convexity of upper left cardiac border (*arrows*) caused by septal hypertrophy.

Restrictive Cardiomyopathy

Restrictive cardiomyopathy is a relatively rare disease that may occur in an idiopathic form or may be the form of cardiomyopathy that is a consequence of various infiltrative diseases of the left ventricle. Types of infiltrative processes of the left ventricle that may produce restrictive cardiomyopathy include sarcoidosis, hemochromatosis, and amyloidosis.

During the early stage of restrictive cardiomyopathy the cardiac size is within normal limits. Restrictive cardio-

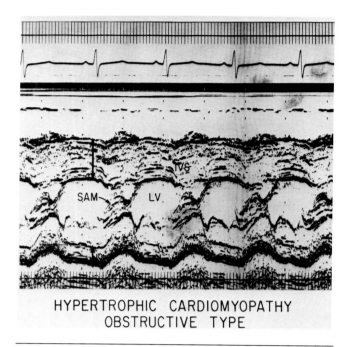

HYPERTROPHIC CARDIOMYOPATHY
OBSTRUCTIVE TYPE

Figure 1-34. M-mode echocardiogram in hypertrophic cardiomyopathy. There is asymmetrical thickening of the ventricular septum (end-diastolic thickness = 23 mm) compared to the posterior wall (end-diastolic thickness = 10 mm). R wave of ECG marks the time of end diastole. Systolic anterior motion of the anterior mitral valve leaflet is consistent with outflow obstruction of the LV. (IVS, interventricular septum; LV, left ventricle; SAM, systolic anterior motion.)

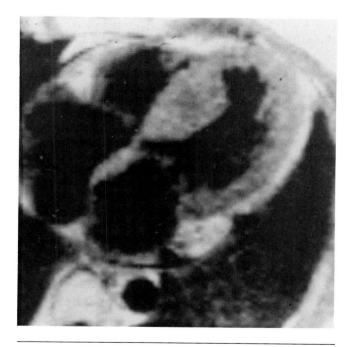

Figure 1-35. ECG gated magnetic resonance image acquired at the middle of the ventricles shows the severe asymmetric thickening of the ventricular septum compared to the normal thickness of the posterolateral wall of the LV.

myopathy has as its main physiologic deficit a reduction of LV compliance. Because of the reduced compliance, there is frequently an elevation in pulmonary venous pressure, which of course is reflected on the chest radiograph as various degrees of pulmonary venous hypertension (Fig. 1-36). Likewise, because of the reduced LV compliance, there is a rise in left atrial pressure, which may cause a left atrial enlargement to be visible on the radiograph. Because the major radiographic features of this disease are pulmonary venous hypertension and left atrial enlargement, the plain radiograph may mimic the appearance of mitral stenosis. At advanced stages of the disease there is frequently some degree of LV enlargement that, along with the left atrial enlargement, usually results in a mild to moderate cardiomegaly. However, in some patients the restrictive cardiomyopathy may progress into a stage of congestive cardiomyopathy associated with considerable cardiomegaly and LV enlargement.

The plain radiograph may provide some insight into the severity of restrictive cardiomyopathy since it reflects the degree of pulmonary venous hypertension and thereby the severity of the reduction in LV compliance. The major gauge of severity on the chest radiograph is the degree of pulmonary venous hypertension.

Acute Myocardial Infarction

The plain radiograph is obtained in the emergency room in most patients who are afflicted with an acute myocardial infarction. The initial chest x-ray or a chest x-ray within the first 24 hours after the onset of acute myocardial infarction is normal in approximately 50% of patients with initial acute myocardial infarction.[7,12] In the other 50% of patients the most frequent finding is some degree of pulmonary venous hypertension or pulmonary edema along with a normal heart size (Figs. 1-37, 1-38). The major pathogenic deficit in the early phase of acute myocardial infarction is an abrupt decrease in left ventricular compliance, which results in increase in pulmonary venous pressure. The increase in pulmonary venous pressure is reflected on the chest x-ray by varying degrees of pulmonary venous hypertension or pulmonary edema. It is unusual for the patient with a first acute myocardial infarction, even when the infarction is severe and eventually lethal, to have cardiomegaly or perceptible left ventricular enlargement.

The plain chest x-ray does provide some insight into the severity of the acute myocardial infarction. The gauge of severity is the degree of pulmonary venous hypertension. Indeed, a relationship has been shown between the degree of pulmonary venous hypertension on the plain radiograph within the first 24 hours and the percentage of early and late survival after the initial myo-

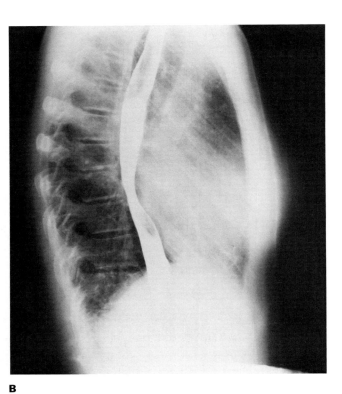

A

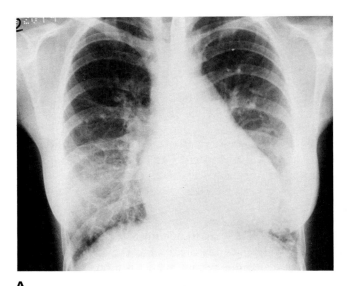

B

Figure 1-36. Restrictive cardiomyopathy. Frontal (*A*) and lateral (*B*) radiographs show interstitial pulmonary edema, left atrial and right ventricular enlargement. Note Kerley B lines and other interstitial lines along with subpleural edema in both lower lobes. Impression on esophageal barium column on lateral view indicates left atrial enlargement. Right ventricular enlargement is shown by lateral expansion of ventricular contour and encroachment upon retrosternal space.

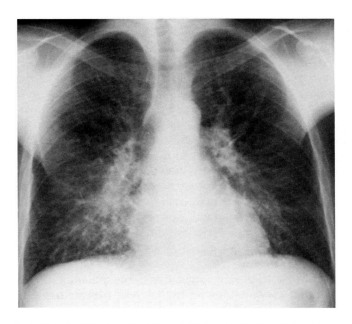

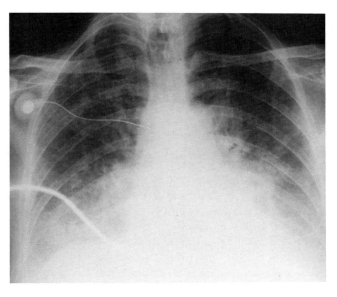

Figure 1-37. Acute myocardial infarction with interstitial pulmonary edema (grade II PVH) is indicated by Kerley B lines and prominent interstitial marking, causing obscuration of vascular margins in lower lobes. Cardiac size is normal.

Figure 1-38. Acute myocardial infarction with alveolar pulmonary edema (grade III PVH). Note alveolar filling in perihilar regions and lower lobes with normal heart size.

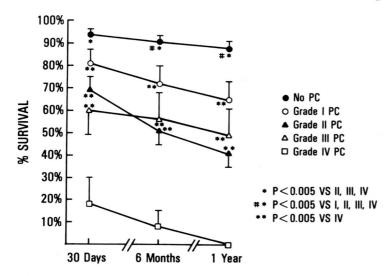

Figure 1-39. Graph demonstrates the 30-day, 6-month, and 12-month survival in relation to the severity of PVH on the initial chest x-ray of patients after acute myocardial infarction. With any degree of PVH, survival is decreased compared to patients with no PVH. (Reproduced with permission from Battler A, Karliner JS, Higgins CB, et al. The initial chest x-ray film in acute myocardial infarction: prediction of early and late mortality and survival. Circulation 1980;61:1004.)

cardial infarction (Fig. 1-39).[7] The plain radiograph may also be useful in demonstrating complications of acute myocardial infarction. These complications include cardiac rupture; pericardial effusion; LV aneurysm, both true and false; papillary muscle rupture; and intractable congestive heart failure. The majority of patients with a true aneurysm of the left ventricle demonstrate a normal chest x-ray. However, in many patients there is evidence of an abnormal cardiac configuration, especially an abnormal evagination along the mid-portion of the left cardiac border or in the region of the cardiac apex (Fig. 1-40). The abnormal contour is generally in these sites because the most frequent location of a true LV aneurysm is the anterolateral wall or the apical wall of the left ventricle. Calcification of the anterolateral region of the left ventricle is suggestive of LV aneurysm (Fig. 1-40*C*). An abnormal evagination that is localized to the posterior wall or the diaphragmatic wall of the left ventricle should raise the possibility of a false aneurysm of the left ventricle (Fig. 1-41).[15] Although only approximately 4% to 5% of true aneurysms of the left ventricle involve the upper diaphragmatic and posterior wall,[15] these are the most frequent sites for false aneurysm of the left ventricle.[14] Consequently, an abnormal contour or a double density localized to these sites should raise this diagnostic possibility. The differentiation of a false from a true aneurysm becomes important because of the known propensity of false aneurysms to be complicated by late rupture. Other plain radiographic signs of a false aneurysm are an aneurysm that is extremely large in size with prominent projection off the posterior or diaphragmatic surface of the heart (Figs. 1-41, 1-42), and an increase in the size of the aneurysm on segmental studies (Fig. 1-43). A false aneurysm is more frequently associated with occlusion of either circumflex or right coronary artery, whereas the

true aneurysm is most frequently associated with occlusion of the left anterior descending coronary artery.

Papillary muscle rupture is a dramatic event that usually induces severe and many times intractable pulmonary edema (Fig. 1-44). Partial rupture of the papillary muscle, resulting in less severe mitral regurgitation, may produce a moderate degree of mitral regurgitation and less severe or even no evidence of pulmonary edema. The dramatic plain radiographic findings in acute papillary muscle rupture are pulmonary edema with little increase in left atrial size or cardiomegaly (see Fig. 1-44). If the patient survives beyond several weeks or months, then varying degrees of left atrial enlargement and cardiomegaly may be present. Postinfarctional rupture of the ventricular septum may produce a radiographic appearance very similar to that of acute mitral regurgitation. The radiographic signs of acute ventricular septal defect include increase in the prominence of the pulmonary arteries, that is, pulmonary arterial recirculation; usually pulmonary edema; and mild degrees of cardiomegaly. Again, if the patient tolerates the episode and survives for several weeks to months, then the degree of cardiomegaly may be more considerable and there may even be signs of left atrial enlargement. Dressler's syndrome is another complication of acute myocardial infarction and occurs within the first weeks to months after an acute myocardial infarction. This is an autoimmune response to various antigens that are released during the acute myocardial infarction. This autoimmune response involves the pericardial and pleural surfaces, eventuating in pericardial and pleural effusions. Chest radiograph in this syndrome demonstrates an increase in cardiac size as a consequence of the pericardial effusion, along with evidence of unilateral or bilateral pleural effusions.

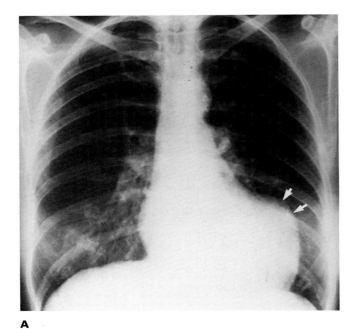

A

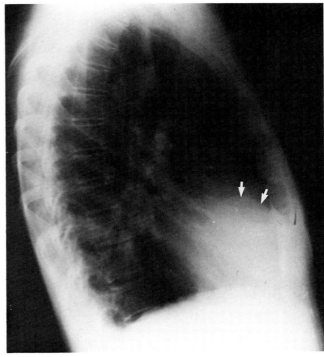

B

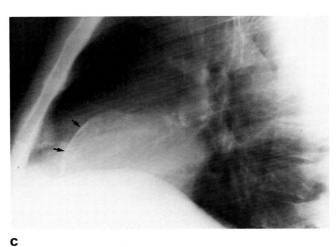

C

Figure 1-40. Left ventricular aneurysm complicating myocardial infarction. Frontal (*A*) and lateral (*B*) views. Abnormal evagination of left cardiac border (*arrows*) is typical for aneurysm involving the anterolateral and/or apical segment of the LV. Lateral view demonstrates an anterior double density (*arrows*) characteristic of an anterolateral aneurysm. *C:* Lateral radiograph in another patient demonstrates calcification (*arrows*) of a large anterolateral aneurysm of the LV.

Constrictive Pericarditis

Constrictive pericarditis is being encountered with increasing frequency. In the past the most frequent cause of constrictive pericarditis was complicated viral pericarditis. Recently, the major causes of constrictive pericarditis have been iatrogenic. The most frequent is postoperative bleeding associated with cardiac surgery, especially coronary revascularization procedures. The second most frequent is mediastinal irradiation, and the third most frequent is repeated episodes of viral pericarditis. Uremic pericardial disease may also eventuate in constrictive pericarditis, but usually this disease produces an effusive, constrictive type of pericardial disease.

The plain radiograph is usually abnormal in patients with hemodynamically significant constrictive pericarditis. Because of pericardial constriction there is restriction to left atrial emptying during diastole, with subsequent rise in left atrial and pulmonary venous pressures. The rise in pulmonary venous pressure is reflected on the chest radiograph by signs of pulmonary venous hypertension, such as redistribution and interstitial or alveolar pulmonary edema. The overall cardiac size is usually normal or there is only mild cardiomegaly. There is frequently left atrial enlargement but normal ventricular size.

The cardiac contour in a minority of patients has a pathognomonic appearance (Figs. 1-45, 1-46). This con-

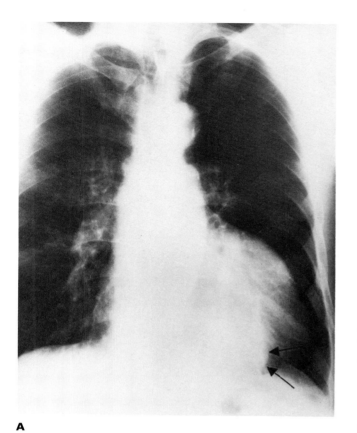
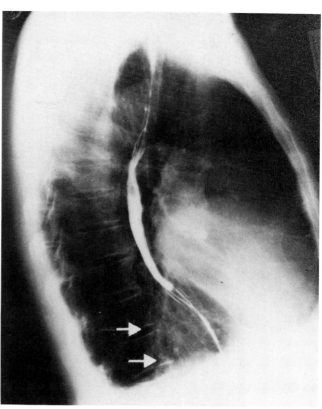

A **B**

Figure 1-41. Left ventricular false aneurysm complicating myocardial infarction. Frontal (*A*) and lateral (*B*) radiographs show left retrocardiac density (*arrows*) on frontal view and large posterior evagination (*arrows*) of LV contour on lateral view. Large size and posterior location are characteristic for false aneurysm.

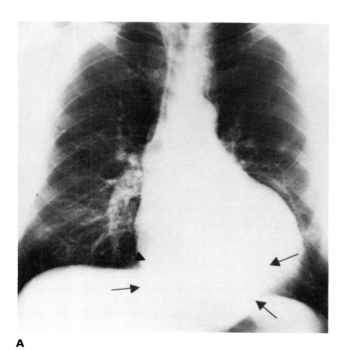
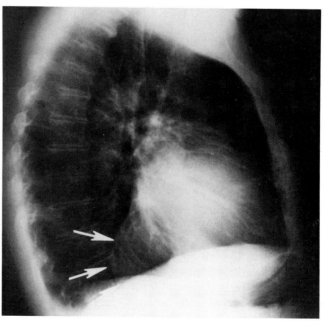

A **B**

Figure 1-42. False aneurysm of left ventricle complicating acute myocardial infarction. Frontal view (*A*) shows large retrocardiac double density (*arrows*) and cardiomegaly. Lateral view (*B*) demonstrates posterior site (*arrows*) of the large aneurysm.

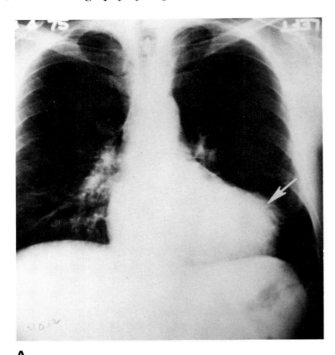

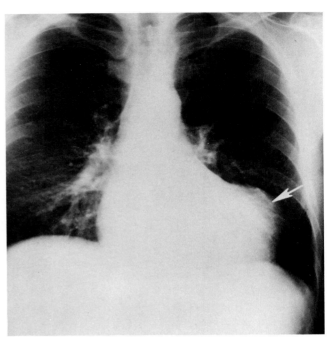

A

B

Figure 1-43. Interval enlargement of LV false aneurysm. Initial (*A*) and latter (*B*) radiographs indicate enlargement of the LV aneurysm (*arrow*) between the radiographs performed over an interval of several months.

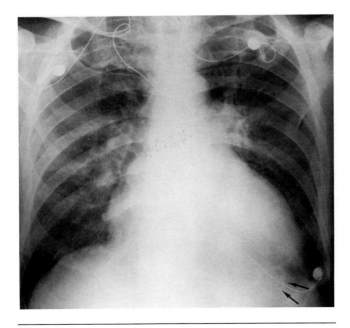

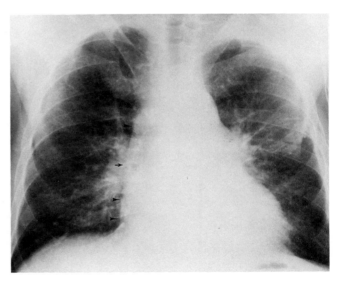

Figure 1-45. Constrictive pericarditis. Frontal radiograph shows grade I PVH and flattened right cardiac contour (*arrowheads*), which are characteristic features of constrictive pericarditis.

Figure 1-44. Mitral regurgitation complicating myocardial infarction. Perihilar pulmonary edema and cardiomegaly. Calcification (*arrows*) near apex indicates a prior infarction.

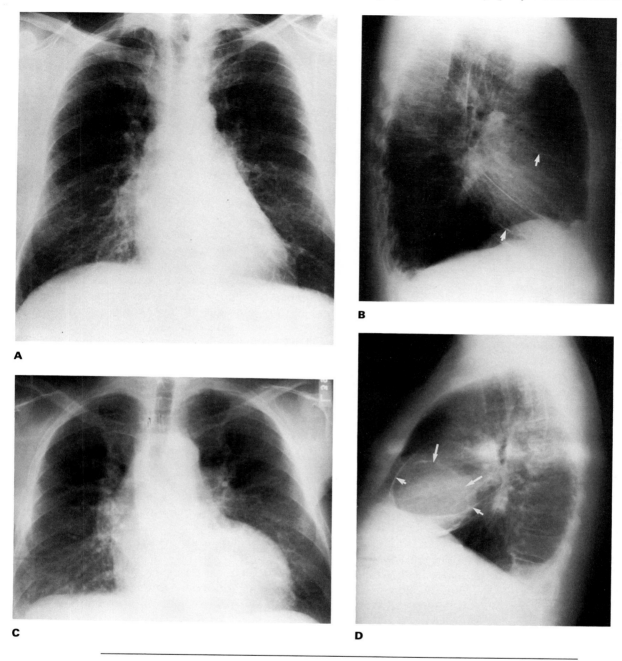

Figure 1-46. Two cases of constrictive pericarditis. Frontal (*A*) radiograph shows flattening of right cardiac contours and LV apex. Lateral (*B*) view demonstrates pericardial calcification (*arrows*). Frontal (*C*) and lateral (*D*) radiographs in another case show the flattened right heart border and pericardial calcification. Note that the calcification involves the atrioventricular (*long arrows*) and the interventricular (*short arrows*) grooves.

sists of flattening of the right heart border on the frontal radiograph and frequently flattening of the lower portion of the left cardiac border as well. Such flattening of the cardiac contours is likely a consequence of the pericardial scarring and retraction, which flattens out the normal right atrial contour. Unfortunately, this specific finding is observed in a minority of patients with constrictive peri-

carditis. Another specific finding in this disease is the presence of pericardial calcification (see Fig. 1-46). Pericardial calcification is generally most densely distributed in the grooves of the heart, such as the atrioventricular groove and the interventricular groove. The most sensitive method for detecting such calcification is computed tomography (Fig. 1-47). Failure to demonstrate pericar-

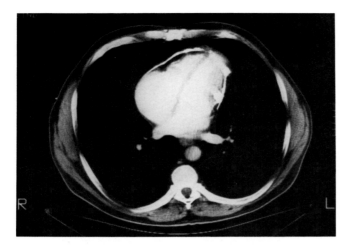

Figure 1-47. CT scan demonstrates calcification of the pericardium.

dial calcification by radiography or fluoroscopy should prompt the use of computed tomography.

Ancillary findings in significant constrictive pericarditis are pleural effusion and sometimes elevation of the hemidiaphragms as a consequence of ascites. There is frequently distention of the superior vena cava, reflecting systemic venous hypertension.

The plain radiograph provides an assessment of the severity of constrictive pericarditis by the gauge of the pulmonary venous hypertension. In some patients there may be a substantial degree of cardiomegaly as a consequence of associated pericardial effusion. Although most patients with symptomatic constrictive pericarditis do not have pericardial effusion, there is an entity referred to as *effusive constrictive pericarditis,* in which pericardial constriction exists but there is a pericardial effusion as well.[17] It has been noted at the time of cardiac catheterization that after removal of the pericardial effusion, the hemodynamics of constriction persist. This finding supports the notion that constriction of the ventricles is due to a large extent to the visceral pericardium.

"Big Heart Heart Disease"

Aortic Regurgitation

Aortic regurgitation is characterized on the plain radiograph by a substantial degree of left ventricular enlargement, which is due predominantly to left ventricular enlargement (see Figs. 1-19*A,* 1-26). A signpost pointing to the aortic valve is present in this disease, consisting of enlargement of the ascending aorta, aortic knob, and usually the descending thoracic aorta (see Fig. 1-26). As opposed to aortic stenosis, the enlargement of the thoracic

aorta involves the aortic knob as well as the ascending aorta. Consequently, "big heart heart disease" with the aortic signpost indicates aortic regurgitation.

The severity of aortic regurgitation is reflected by the plain radiograph. Since this is a volume overload lesion, the extent of the increase in volume of the heart is related to the severity and the duration of aortic regurgitation. Of course, this is only a rough association. However, several publications have demonstrated that the long-term prognosis in patients who are treated with aortic valve replacement for aortic regurgitation is influenced by the degree of cardiomegaly noted on the chest x-ray prior to operation.[18] In patients with a cardiothoracic ratio of less than 56%, there is a 5-year survival of 84% compared to the 5-year survival rate of 46% in patients with a cardiothoracic ratio of greater than 60%. For most of the course of aortic regurgitation the pulmonary vascularity is normal. This corresponds with the relatively asymptomatic nature of this disease for much of its natural history. Consequently, the presence of pulmonary venous hypertension in a patient with aortic regurgitation indicates left ventricular failure and can frequently be associated with end-stage aortic valve disease. Because the presence of pulmonary venous hypertension in a patient with aortic regurgitation is frequently associated with a dire prognosis, the signs of pulmonary venous hypertension cannot be relied upon to monitor the course and severity of this disease.

Mitral Regurgitation

The plain radiograph in mitral regurgitation shows variable degrees of pulmonary venous hypertension, cardiomegaly, left atrial enlargement, left ventricular enlargement (Figs. 1-8, 1-10, 1-48), and sometimes signs of right-sided chamber enlargement. In the presence of isolated mitral regurgitation the ascending aorta is relatively small. Consequently, recognition of prominence of the ascending aorta in a patient with isolated mitral valve disease raises the prospect of associated aortic valve disease.

The left atrial appendage is generally enlarged in patients who have a rheumatic etiology of the mitral regurgitation. On the other hand, the left atrial appendage is frequently not enlarged in patients who otherwise have left atrial enlargement when the etiology is other than rheumatic heart disease. One study has demonstrated that more than 90% of patients with a rheumatic cause of mitral regurgitation have left atrial appendage enlargement, whereas patients with nonrheumatic causes of left atrial enlargement show a frequency of enlargement of the left atrial appendage less than 10%.[10]

The severity of pulmonary venous hypertension in mitral regurgitation is generally less than in isolated mitral stenosis. Most patients with compensated mitral re-

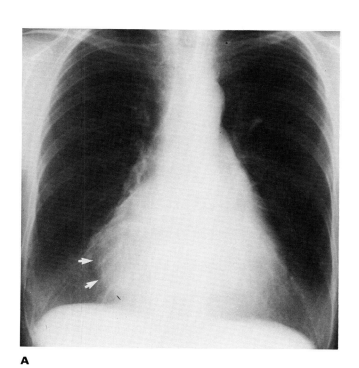

A

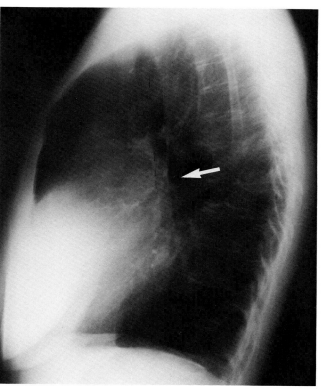

B

Figure 1-48. Mitral regurgitation, frontal (*A*) and lateral (*B*) radiographs. There is cardiomegaly and marked left atrial enlargement with pulmonary venous hypertension. The left atrium is enlarged to the extent that it forms the right heart border on frontal view (*arrows*). Posterior expansion of left atrium on lateral view also indicates substantial left atrial enlargement. The left bronchus is displaced behind the trachea (*broken black line*).

gurgitation have minimal or no signs of pulmonary venous hypertension. A practical axiom is that mitral stenosis causes pulmonary venous hypertension that is prominent compared to the degree of left atrial enlargement, whereas mitral regurgitation is associated with left atrial enlargement that is out of proportion to the expected severity of pulmonary venous hypertension. Patients with mixed mitral stenosis and mitral regurgitation may have very substantial left atrial enlargement as well as prominent signs of pulmonary venous hypertension (see Fig. 1-10). The giant left atrium can be associated with either mitral stenosis or regurgitation, but is more frequently caused by the latter. The right border of the left atrium may extend beyond the border of the right atrium rather than causing a right retrocardiac double density (see Fig. 1-10).

The plain radiograph may be useful in assessing the severity of mitral regurgitation. Because this is a volume overload lesion, the overall heart size may be a reasonable indicator of the severity of regurgitation. Likewise, the overall heart size may be of some prognostic use in patients undergoing mitral valve replacement. In general, patients with the lesser degrees of cardiomegaly demonstrate a greater 5-year survival rate after replacement of the mitral valve.

Mitral regurgitation has numerous etiologies. Indeed, numerous systemic diseases may be associated with mitral regurgitation. Whereas the most frequent cause of mitral regurgitation in past years was rheumatic heart disease, it is now clear that other etiologies are more common. The most frequent cause of mitral regurgitation at the current time is mitral valve prolapse. Other notable etiologies are postinfarctional papillary muscle dysfunction; rheumatic mitral valve disease; infectious endocarditis; rupture of the chordae tendineae as a consequence of degenerative mitral valve disease; and certain systemic diseases such as Marfan's syndrome. It should also be recognized that prominent calcification of the anulus of the mitral valve recognized on the chest x-ray (Fig. 1-49) may provide an insight into the etiology of mitral regurgitation, since this entity can be associated with significant mitral regurgitation.

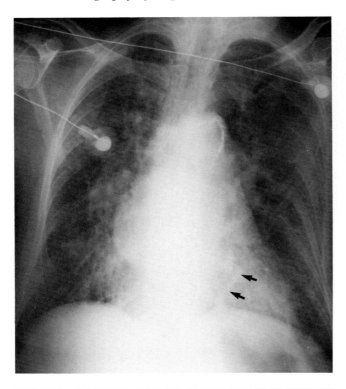

Figure 1-49. Calcification of mitral anulus (*arrows*) in patient with mitral stenosis. There is interstitial pulmonary edema and left atrial enlargement (right retrocardiac double density).

Tricuspid Regurgitation

The signs of tricuspid regurgitation on the plain radiograph may be difficult to discern. Signs of right atrial enlargement are frequently dubious and not sharply discriminated from normal. Indeed, there must be substantial right atrial enlargement before it is possible to recognize its occurrence. In general the best sign of right atrial enlargement is elongation of the right atrial border. The radiographic signs of tricuspid regurgitation are normal or perhaps reduced prominence of the pulmonary vascularity, cardiomegaly, right atrial enlargement, and occasionally signs of superior vena caval and especially inferior vena caval enlargement (Fig. 1-50).

Cardiomegaly, with the signpost of right atrial enlargement, would indicate the likely diagnosis of tricuspid regurgitation. The cardiac contour in patients with tricuspid regurgitation must be differentiated from a very similar cardiac contour occurring in subjects with congestive cardiomyopathy and pericardial effusion.

Tricuspid regurgitation is encountered more frequently in recent years because of the increasing use of recreational drugs. One of the more common complications of the use of intravenous drugs is the occurrence of bacterial endocarditis on the tricuspid valve, resulting in tricuspid regurgitation. Other causes of tricuspid re-

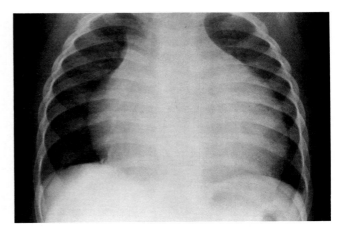

Figure 1-50. Tricuspid regurgitation. The features of this lesion are diminished pulmonary vascularity, marked cardiomegaly, and right atrial and right ventricular enlargement. Lateral displacement and elongation of the right atrial border are characteristic of right atrial enlargement.

gurgitation are rheumatic heart disease and various types of right ventricular dysplasia.

Congestive Cardiomyopathy

The radiographic appearance in congestive cardiomyopathy is relatively nonspecific. There is usually some degree of pulmonary venous hypertension and substantial cardiomegaly (Fig. 1-51). Characteristically, the cardiomegaly exists without the presence of signposts involving either the aortic, mitral, or tricuspid valve. Consequently, substantial cardiomegaly ("big heart heart disease"), without radiographic signposts, should raise the diagnostic consideration of congestive cardiomyopathy. Of course, a similar appearance can exist with pericardial effusion. At the current time, the most common cause of congestive or dilated cardiomyopathy is ischemic heart disease. However, from a strict classification point of view ischemic heart disease should not be considered part of the group of congestive cardiomyopathies. Congestive cardiomyopathy is actually defined by the International Conference on Myocardial Disease as a dilated cardiomyopathy without known etiologic identification.

The chest x-ray demonstrates pulmonary venous hypertension in many but not all patients with congestive cardiomyopathy. Indeed, even patients with a very low ejection fraction may have few signs of pulmonary venous hypertension because of chronic compensatory mechanisms within the lungs. However, when these patients are in a poorly compensated phase of the disease, then signs of persistent and fluctuating degrees of pulmonary edema are frequently recognized (Figs. 1-52, 1-53). The overall heart size in patients with congestive cardiomyopathy does bear a relationship to prognosis.[19]

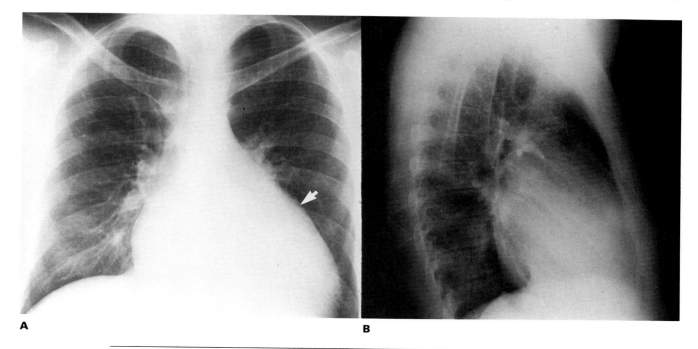

A   **B**

Figure 1-51. Congestive cardiomyopathy. Frontal (*A*) and lateral (*B*) radiographs show biventricular enlargement and mild grade I PVH. Enlargement of left ventricle is indicated by a vector of ventricular enlargement directed laterally and caudally on the frontal view and posterior displacement on the lateral view. The posterior border of the left ventricle extends several centimeters behind the shadow of the inferior vena cava. Right ventricle enlargement is indicated by prominent convexity of upper left cardiac border (right ventricular outflow tract, *arrow*) on the frontal view and filling of the retrosternal clear space on lateral view.

Pericardial Effusion

The cardiac configuration in pericardial effusion is relatively nonspecific. It has been stated that the presence of substantial cardiomegaly in the absence of signs of pulmonary venous hypertension or even reduced pulmonary blood flow, should be a clue to the presence of pericardial effusion (Fig. 1-54). This radiographic appearance is actually quite nonspecific. Similar to the appearance of congestive cardiomyopathy, the cardiac configuration is that of cardiomegaly without radiographic signpost. A specific appearance providing a diagnosis of pericardial effusion is relatively infrequent in this entity. The so-called water bottle appearance of the heart is nonspecific and difficult to recognize. The "fat pad" sign seen on the lateral radiograph does permit identification but occurs in a small minority of patients (Fig. 1-55). The varying-density sign is also sometimes present on the frontal radiograph (see Fig. 1-54). This consists of a density at the periphery of the cardiac contour less than that at the central portion of the cardiac contour. The cause of this varying density is that the x-ray beam encounters only fluid toward the periphery of the pericardial effusion, while in the center of the pericardial effusion the radiographic beam must pass through both water anteriorly and the cardiac substance more centrally.

With the frequent use of echocardiography, large pericardial effusions are being encountered less frequently. The diagnosis of pericardial effusion from radiographic signs is now a useless exercise. The presence of any degree of pericardial effusion can be easily recognized by echocardiography. Consequently, when one has any suspicion of the presence of pericardial effusion, an echocardiogram should be obtained to exclude this diagnosis. Effusions can also be readily demonstrated by computed tomography (Fig. 1-56) and magnetic resonance imaging.

There are numerous etiologies for a pericardial effusion. Some of the major considerations are infectious and autoimmune pericarditis, uremic pericarditis, congestive heart failure, pericardial metastasis, and pericardial trauma, especially from recent operation. The cardiac contour may be asymmetrically enlarged (Fig. 1-57) or show peculiar evaginations when an effusion occurs into a pericardial diverticulum where there is a loculated pericardial effusion.

Paracardiac Masses

Enlargement of the cardiac contour may not always indicate cardiac enlargement or pericardial effusion. One must also consider the less likely possibility that the en-

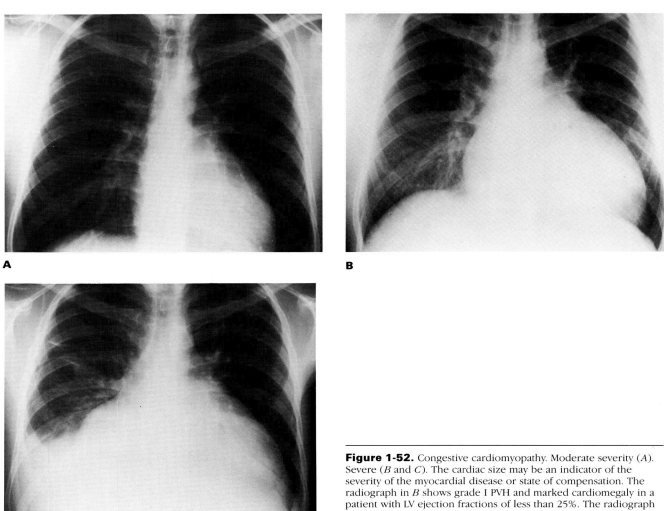

A

B

C

Figure 1-52. Congestive cardiomyopathy. Moderate severity (*A*). Severe (*B* and *C*). The cardiac size may be an indicator of the severity of the myocardial disease or state of compensation. The radiograph in *B* shows grade I PVH and marked cardiomegaly in a patient with LV ejection fractions of less than 25%. The radiograph in *C* shows end-stage disease with cardiomegaly, pericardial and pleural effusions. The patient in *A* has an ejection fraction of 35%; there is no PVH and only mild cardiomegaly.

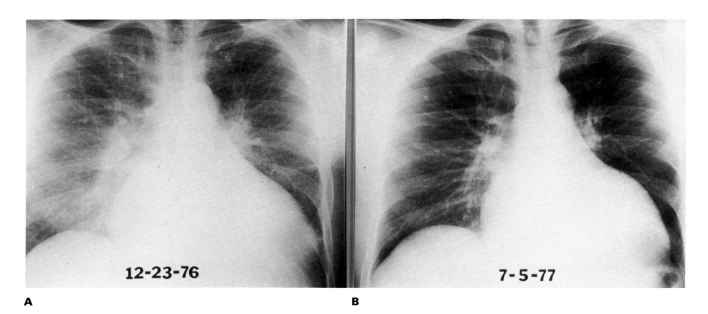

A

B

Figure 1-53. Congestive cardiomyopathy, monitoring treatment. Radiographs obtained at a time when congestive heart failure was inadequately controlled (*A*) and at a time of optimal treatment (*B*).

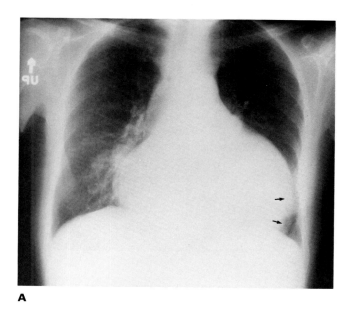

A

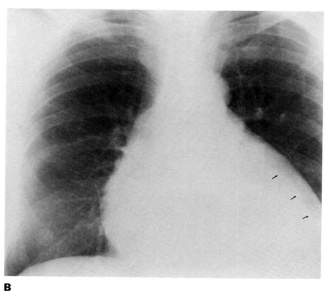

B

Figure 1-54. Pericardial effusion. *A:* varying cardiac density sign shows a transition of density near the margin of the cardiac silhouette (*arrows*). *B:* frontal radiograph in another patient shows the variable density sign, especially near apex (*arrows*).

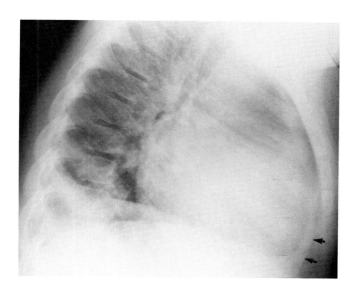

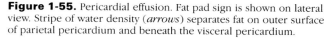

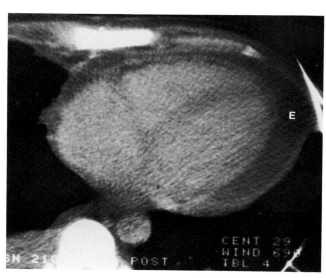

E

Figure 1-55. Pericardial effusion. Fat pad sign is shown on lateral view. Stripe of water density (*arrows*) separates fat on outer surface of parietal pericardium and beneath the visceral pericardium.

Figure 1-56. CT scan in patient with pericardial effusion. Contrast enhancement demarcates the parietal and visceral pericardium and shows the pericardial effusion (E).

largement represents a cardiac or paracardiac mass (Figs. 1-58, 1-59). Such consideration should be prompted by recognition of an unusual cardiac contour. The various causes of paracardiac masses are legion, but a few ready considerations are pericardial cysts, paracardiac tumors such as lymphoma and germinal cell tumor, cardiac tu-

mors such as rhabdomyoma, metastasis to lymph nodes within the pericardiophrenic angle, eventration or hernia of the diaphragm, neural tumors of the phrenic nerve, and various types of skeletal muscle tumors arising from the diaphragm. The diagnosis of the paracardiac mass can be readily made by computed tomography and even

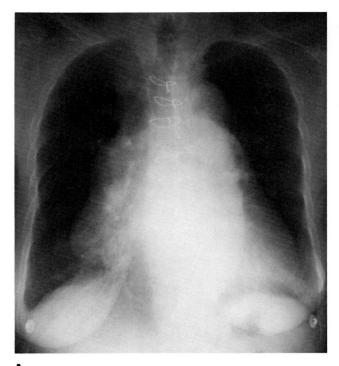

A

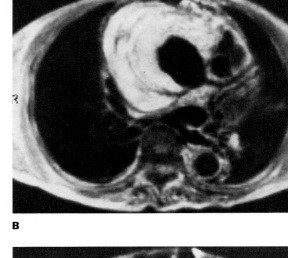

B

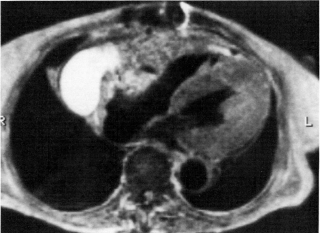

C

Figure 1-57. Asymmetric (loculated) pericardial effusion demonstrated on thoracic radiograph (*A*) and ECG gated magnetic resonance image (MRI) (*B* and *C*). Focal enlargement of cardiomediastinal shadow is shown on radiograph. The MRI (T1 weighted) shows a fluid collection with high signal intensity surrounding base of aorta and right side of pericardial space. The effusion is hemorrhage from aortotomy site after aortic valve replacement.

more precisely with gated magnetic resonance imaging (Fig. 1-59). The echocardiogram can also usually differentiate between a cardiac and noncardiac cause of the enlargement of the cardiac contour. However, because of the more narrow field of view of the echocardiogram, this is not ideal for the demonstration and evaluation of paracardiac masses.

Abnormal Cardiac Contours

Enlargement of the Main Pulmonary Arterial Segment

Enlargement of the main pulmonary artery segment is usually due to enlargement of the main pulmonary artery itself. The causes of enlargement of the main pulmonary

artery are valvular pulmonic stenosis, pulmonic regurgitation, absence of the pulmonary valve (Fig. 1-60), partial absence of the pericardium (Fig. 1-61), pulmonary arterial hypertension, idiopathic dilatation of the main pulmonary artery (Fig. 1-62), and excess pulmonary blood flow such as occurs in left-to-right shunts.

Enlargement of the main pulmonary artery segment is the main indicator of pulmonary arterial hypertension. Whenever one recognizes enlargement of the main pulmonary artery segment in a patient with no known pulmonary valvular disease the differential diagnosis of pulmonary arterial hypertension must be considered. The differential diagnosis of pulmonary hypertension should bring to mind a systematic organization of the diagnostic possibilities. There are five diagnostic categories for pulmonary arterial hypertension. These are (1) pulmonary arterial hypertension resulting from pul-

Abnormal Cardiac Contours

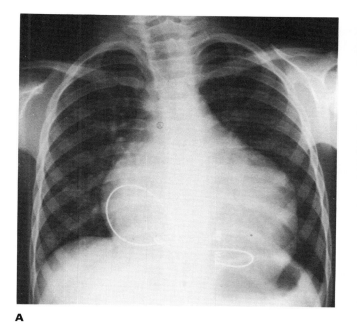

A

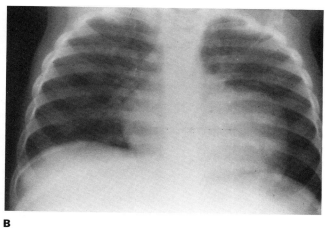

B

Figure 1-58. Cardiac tumor causing abnormal cardiac contour. Abnormal cardiac contour in both patients is due to tumor causing an abnormal evagination of upper left cardiac border. *A* shows pacing wire; complete heart block can be caused by cardiac tumors.

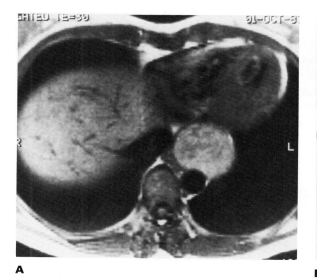

A

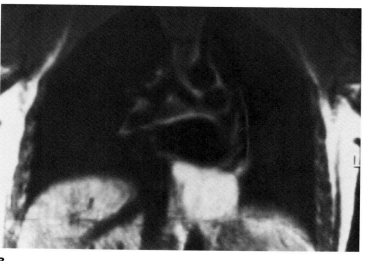

B

Figure 1-59. Transverse (*A*) and coronal (*B*) magnetic resonance images (ECG gated) demonstrate a paracardiac mass. A mass adjacent to the heart can cause an abnormal cardiac contour; the mass is immediately posterior and in contact with the left ventricular margin.

monary venous hypertension; (2) pulmonary arterial hypertension resulting from left-to-right shunts resulting in pulmonary arteriolar disease (arteriolopathy); (3) pulmonary arterial hypertension resulting from obliteration of the pulmonary vascular bed from chronic lung disease; (4) pulmonary arterial hypertension resulting from obliteration of the pulmonary vascular bed as a consequence of pulmonary embolic disease or schistosomiasis; and (5) primary pulmonary hypertension. Radiographic signs that permit the differential diagnosis of the various causes include the following:

1. Signs of pulmonary venous hypertension would indicate the likelihood that the pulmonary arterial hypertension is secondary to pulmonary venous hypertension (see Fig. 1-31).
2. Signs of chronic lung disease such as chronic obstructive pulmonary disease or interstitial lung disease would indicate this as the etiology (Fig. 1-63).
3. Asymmetric pulmonary vascularity or signs of pulmonary scarring might indicate the presence of chronic thromboembolic disease (Fig. 1-64).

4. Marked enlargement of the central pulmonary arteries or signs of enlargement of the specific cardiac chambers may indicate the presence of a previous left-to-right shunt that has resulted in the Eisenmenger's syndrome (Fig. 1-65).

Aside from these considerations in patients with enlargement of the main pulmonary arterial segment, one must also consider that this segment is enlarged for a reason other than an enlarged main pulmonary arterial segment. Tumors may not uncommonly present in this region. The lateral radiograph may demonstrate an anterior mediastinal mass, or the frontal radiograph may demonstrate the hilum overlay sign. Although the hilum overlay sign has been relied on as an indicator of a nonvascular cause of enlargement of the main pulmonary artery segment, it is now clear that this sign may not always be valid.

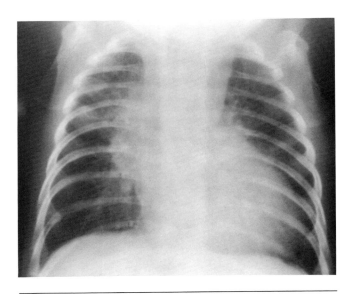

Figure 1-60. Aneurysmal dilatation of the pulmonary artery due to congenitally absent pulmonary valve. The main and right pulmonary arteries are aneurysmally dilated. This radiographic appearance is so characteristic as to be almost pathognomonic for this abnormality.

Enlargement of Left Atrial Appendage Region

An evagination ("mogul") in the region of the left atrial appendage on the frontal view should also prompt a series of differential diagnostic considerations. The left atrial appendage region is considered to be the region immediately adjacent to and below the left bronchus (Fig. 1-66). This is in contradistinction to the region of the main pulmonary artery segment, which is above the left bronchus. The two normal structures which reside within this area are the left atrial appendage and the right ventricular outflow tract; the left atrium is situated posterior to the right ventricular outflow region. The outflow portion of the ventricular septum is also located within this region. The pericardium covers the left atrial appendage and the right ventricular outflow tract in this region as in other parts of the heart. Other structures can occasionally

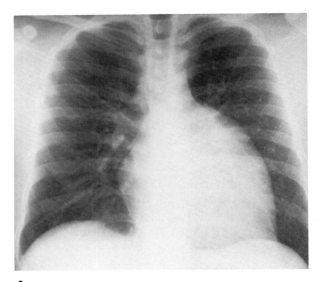

A

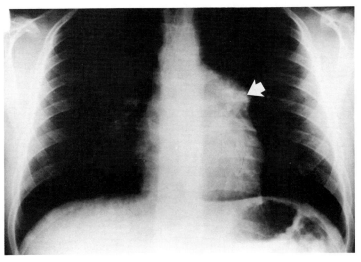

B

Figure 1-61. Complete (*A*) and partial (*B*) absence of left pericardium. Complete absence causes shift of heart to left without shift of mediastinum (note central position of trachea), and prominence convexity of upper left cardiac margin. Partial absence causes a prominent convexity (*arrow*) of the upper left cardiac margin, especially in the region of the pulmonary arterial or left atrial appendage segments.

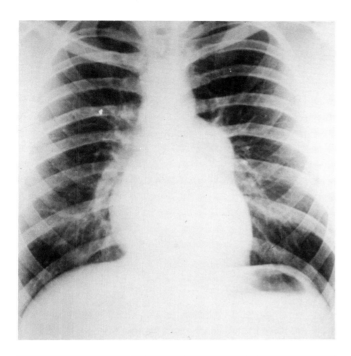

Figure 1-62. Idiopathic dilatation of pulmonary artery. Aneurysmal dilatation of the pulmonary artery without apparent cause is discernible on radiograph.

be abnormally positioned at this site. The abnormally positioned structures that can lie within this site are a juxtaposed right atrial appendage and a transposed ascending aorta with the associated inverted right ventricular outflow region.

The differential diagnoses of an evagination in this region include the following:

1. Enlargement of the left atrial appendage (Figs. 1-11, 1-12, 1-67). Enlargement of the left atrial appendage is a signature of rheumatic mitral valve disease.[10] Radiographically visible, enlargement of the left atrial appendage is usually produced by rheumatic mitral valve disease.

2. Partial or complete absence of the pericardium (see Fig. 1-61).[22,23] Partial absence of the pericardium results in a window on the left side of the pericardium through which the left atrial appendage herniates. The left atrial appendage, after herniating through the window, frequently is enlarged, producing a prominent convexity in the area of the left atrial appendage (see Fig. 1-61*B*). Complete absence of the pericardium frequently results in rotation of the heart towards the left, causing the promi-

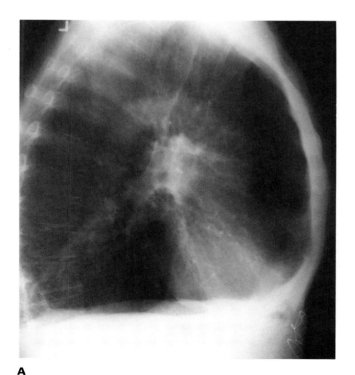

A

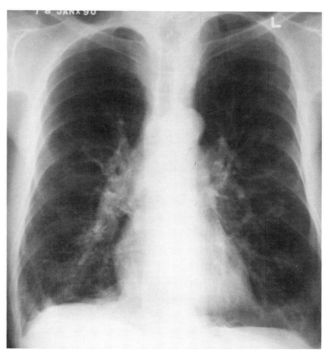

B

Figure 1-63. Pulmonary arterial hypertension due to chronic obstructive pulmonary disease. There is hyperaeration, flattened diaphragms, and markedly enlarged pulmonary arterial segments.

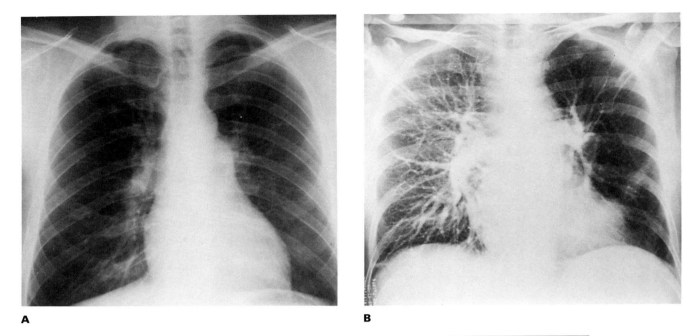

A

B

Figure 1-64. Pulmonary arterial hypertension due to chronic thromboembolic disease. Thoracic radiograph (A) shows asymmetry of blood flow (reduced in left lung) which is a clue to thromboembolism as the cause of pulmonary arterial hypertension. Arteriogram (B) demonstrates obstruction of segmental pulmonary arteries on left and filling defect in the left pulmonary artery.

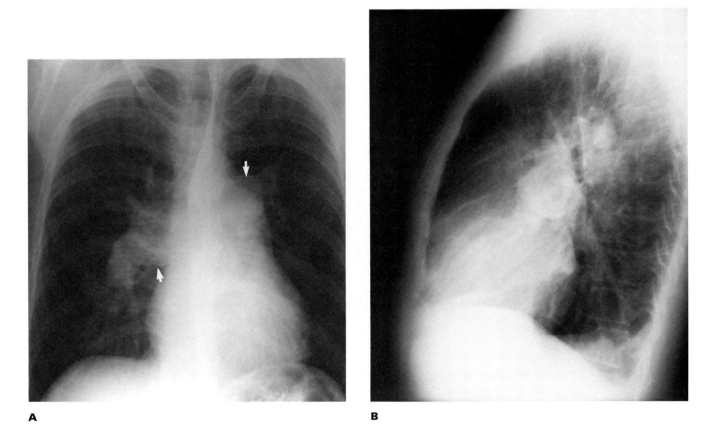

A

B

Figure 1-65. Pulmonary arterial hypertension due to Eisenmenger complex; the underlying lesion was atrial septal defect. Frontal (A) and lateral (B) views show the markedly enlarged main and right pulmonary arterial segments. There is calcification (*arrows*) in the pulmonary arteries consistent with systemic arterial pressure level in the pulmonary circulation.

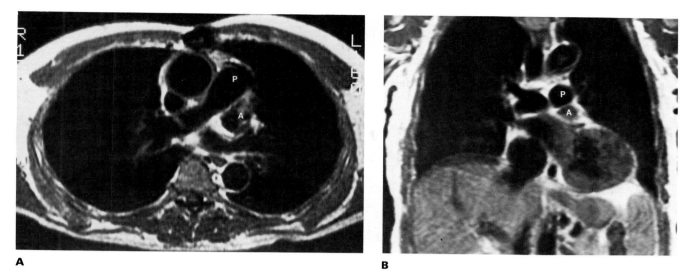

Figure 1-66. Transaxial and coronal magnetic resonance images display the anatomical relationships along the upper left cardiac border. The main and left pulmonary artery (P) have an interface with the lung in the region above the left bronchus while the left atrial appendage (A) has its interface slightly below the left bronchus. (P, pulmonary artery; A, left atrial appendage.)

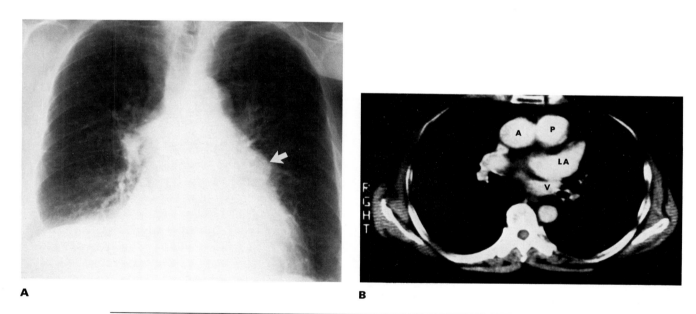

Figure 1-67. Thoracic radiograph (*A*) and CT scan (*B*) in a patient with aneurysmal dilatation of left atrial appendage (*arrow*). The marked convexity at the expected site of appendage was confirmed to be due to an extreme degree of enlargement of the left atrial appendage. (A, aorta; LA, left atrial appendage; P, pulmonary artery; V, left upper pulmonary vein.)

nence of the right ventricular outflow tract in this region (Fig. 1-61*A*).

3. Enlargement of the right ventricular outflow tract. Enlargement of the right ventricular outflow tract is usually a consequence of volume overload lesions of the right-sided cardiac chamber, such as in left-to-right shunts, or valvular pulmonic stenosis.

4. Hypertrophy of the outflow ventricular septum. Visible hypertrophy of the outflow ventricular septum is unusual, even in patients with hypertrophic cardiomyopathy. However, in some pa-

tients with the extreme forms of hypertrophic cardiomyopathy there is a prominent evagination in this region which is produced by such hypertrophy (see Fig. 1-33).

5. Levo-transposition of the great arteries. The levo-transposed ascending aorta, along with the associated inverted right ventricular outflow tract, produces an elongated convexity along the upper left cardiac border (Fig. 1-68). This appearance is almost pathognomonic of this diagnosis.

6. Juxtaposition of the atrial appendages. In this abnormality the right atrial appendage is abnormally positioned just superior to the left atrial appendage (Fig. 1-69). The combination of the two atrial appendages along the upper left cardiac border produces the prominence in this region. This entity is associated with cyanotic congenital heart disease, usually tricuspid atresia and/or transposition of the great arteries.

7. Ventricular aneurysm (see Fig. 1-40).
8. Ventricular tumor (see Fig. 1-58*B*).
9. Atrial tumor.
10. Aneurysm or pseudoaneurysm of the circumflex coronary artery.
11. Pericardial cyst or tumor.
12. Mediastinal tumor.

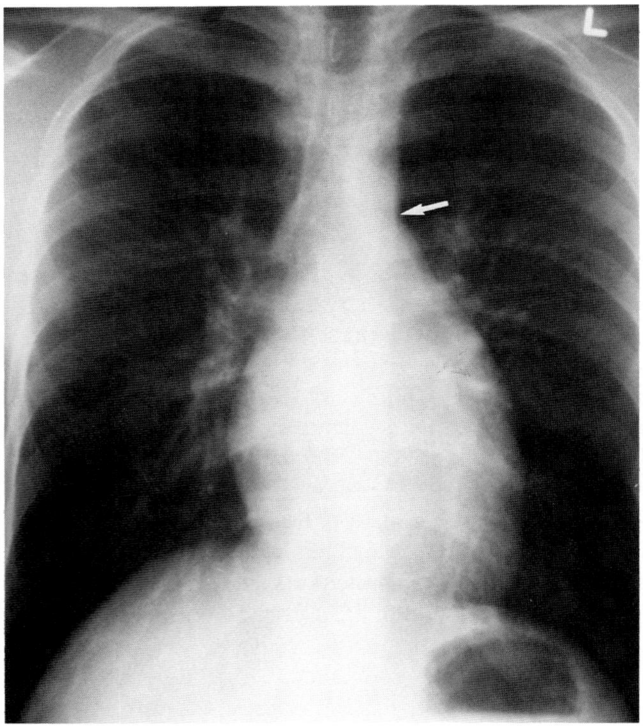

Enlargement of the Left Cardiac Border—Ventricular Region

Enlargement along the lower left cardiac border in the region of the ventricles is most frequently caused by enlargement of either the right or left ventricle. An abnormal convexity within this region can be ascribed to

1. Left ventricular aneurysm (see Figs. 1-40, 1-43).
2. Left ventricular tumor.
3. Pericardial cyst or tumor (Fig. 1-70).
4. Left ventricular diverticulum.
5. Mediastinal or lung tumor.

Enlargement of the Right Heart Contour

Enlargement of the right heart contour in the frontal view is generally ascribed to right atrial enlargement. There are a few other abnormalities that can also enlarge this

Figure 1-68. Corrected transposition (l-transposition of great arteries with inversion of ventricles, L ventricle loop). Prominent convexity of upper left cardiac border is caused by the combined contour of the ascending aorta and inverted right ventricle. Intersection of lines representing lateral margins of ascending and descending aortic segments is characteristic (*arrow*).

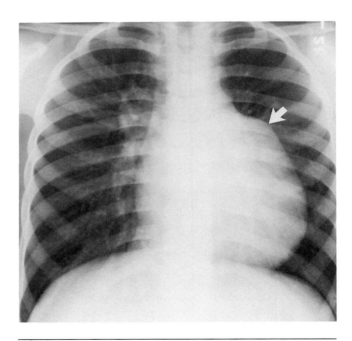

Figure 1-69. Juxtaposed right atrial appendage causes prominent convexity of upper left cardiac border (*arrow*).

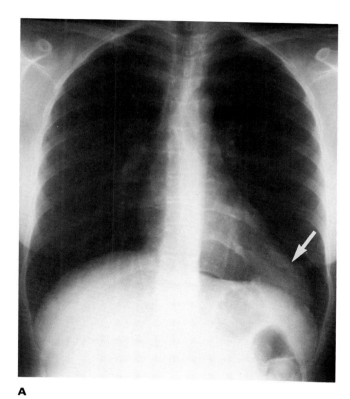

A

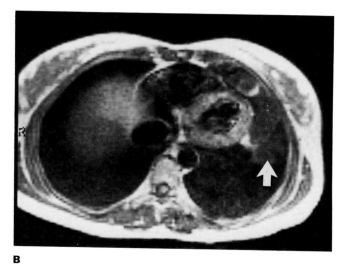

B

Figure 1-70. Thoracic radiograph (*A*) and ECG gated magnetic resonance image (*B*) in a patient with a pericardial cyst (*arrow*) adjacent to the cardiac apex. On T1-weighted MRI, fluid within the cyst produces lower signal intensity than myocardium.

contour and produce an abnormality in the contour. These include absence of the right pericardium; pericardial cyst (Figs. 1-71, 1-72); pericardial fat pad; pericardial tumor; and mediastinal tumor. Eventration of the right hemidiaphragm or right diaphragmatic hernia may also produce enlargement and an abnormality in this contour; this pathology can usually be clearly discerned on the lateral radiograph (Fig. 1-73).

Cardiac Calcification

Calcification in the central cardiovascular structures is common and is an important diagnostic sign. In a few instances, calcification of a specific shape and location is pathognomonic for a disease. The various cardiovascular calcifications include the following:

1. Coronary arterial calcification (Fig. 1-74). Coronary arterial calcification is frequently observed by fluoroscopy[24,25] or by computed tomography.[26] It must be both dense and extensive to be recognized on the thoracic radiograph. It is most frequently observed on the frontal view at a site called the *coronary arterial calcification triangle*.[24] This is a region lying just medial to the region occupied by the left atrial appendage.

When sufficiently dense and extensive to be visualized on the radiography, it is generally associated with hemodynamically insignificant coronary obstruction disease.

2. Ascending aortic calcification. This is most frequently observed on the right anterolateral margin of the ascending aorta in elderly patients, especially in the presence of aortic valve disease.[9] It is generally present in patients with leutic aortitis.

3. Mitral annular calcification (see Fig. 1-49). This is a dense C-shaped calcification in the region of the aortic valve. It may be a causative factor of mitral regurgitation. It is frequently observed in apparently normal elderly patients.

4. Aortic annular calcification. Circular calcification in the region of the aortic valve. Extension of this calcification into the region of the conducting system can produce complete heart block.

5. Valvular calcification—aortic and mitral. Calcification of the aortic valve of sufficient density and extent to be visualized on the radiograph is nearly always associated with hemodynamically important aortic stenosis (gradient > 50 mm Hg).

6. Left ventricular mural calcification. This is most frequently located in the anterolateral or apical

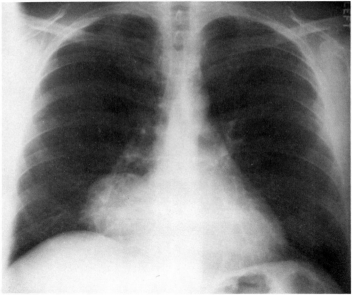

A

B

Figure 1-71. Pericardial cyst. Frontal (*A*) and lateral (*B*) radiographs in one patient demonstrate mass at right cardiodiaphragmatic angle. Lateral view shows the anterior location.

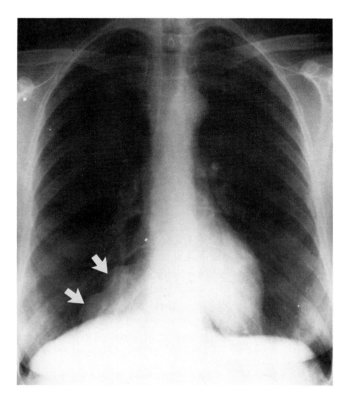

regions of the left ventricle and marks the site of a transmural myocardial infarction or aneurysm (see Fig. 1-40*C*).

7. Pericardial calcification indicates restrictive pericarditis. It is located usually in the interventricular or atrioventricular grooves of the heart (see Fig. 1-46).

8. Unusual sites of calcification may represent intracardiac tumor (left atrial myxoma), pericardial tumor (dermoid), or healed granulomas (myocardial tuberculoma). An extremely rare process of the left ventricle, Loeffler's eosinophilic fibroplasia, can cause calcification of the left ventricular wall.

Figure 1-72. Pericardial cyst. Lobulated cyst (*arrows*) along right cardiac border.

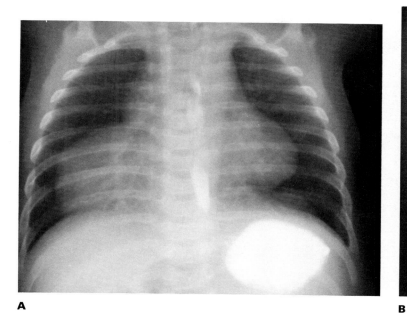

A

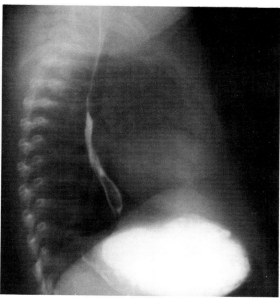

B

Figure 1-73. Right diaphragmatic eventration. Frontal (*A*) and lateral (*B*) radiographs show a mass at the right cardiodiaphragmatic angle.

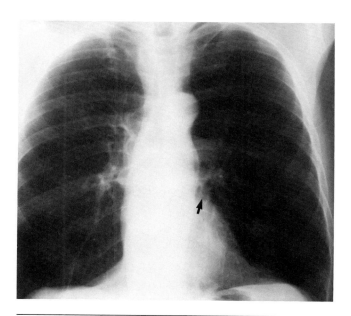

Figure 1-74. Calcification in the left anterior descending coronary artery (*arrow*). A triangular region at the base of the heart represents the most common site where coronary arterial calcification is observed on the frontal radiograph.

References

1. Datey KK, Deshmukl MM, Engeneer SD, Dalvi CB. Straight-back syndrome. Br Heart J 1964;26:614.
2. Higgins CB, Reinke RT, Jones WE, et al. Left atrial dimension on the frontal thoracic radiograph: a method for assessing left atrial enlargement. Am J Radiol 1978;130:251.
3. Hoffman RB, Rigler LG. Evaluation of left ventricular enlargement in the lateral projection of the chest. Radiology 1965;85:93.
4. Doppman JC, Lavendar JP. The hilum and the large left ventricle. Radiology 1963;80:931.
5. Kostuk WJ, Barr JW, Simon AL, et al. Correlation between the chest film and hemodynamics in acute myocardial infarction. Circulation 1973;48:624.
6. McHugh TJ, Forrester JS, Adler L, et al. Pulmonary vascular congestion in acute myocardial infarction: hemodynamic and radiographic correlations. Ann Intern Med 1972;76:29.
7. Battler A, Karliner JS, Higgins CB, et al. The initial chest x-ray film in acute myocardial infarction: prediction of early and late mortality and survival. Circulation 1980;61:1004.
8. Spindola-Franco H, Fish BG, Dachman A, et al. Recognition of bicuspid aortic valve by plain film calcification pattern. Am J Radiol 1982;139:867.
9. Higgins CB, Reinke RT. Non-syphilitic etiology of linear calcification of the ascending aorta. Radiology 1974;113:606.
10. Green CE, Kelley MJ, Higgins CB. Etiologic significance of enlargement of the left atrial appendage in adults. Radiology 1982;142:21.
11. Braunwald E, Lambrew CT, Rockoff SD, et al. Idiopathic hypertrophic subaortic stenosis. Circulation 1964;29:Suppl 4:3.
12. Higgins CB, Lipton MJ. Radiography of acute myocardial infarction. Radiol Clin North Am 1980;18:359.
13. Baron MG. Postinfarction aneurysm of the left ventricle. Circulation 1971;43:762.
14. Higgins CB, Lipton MJ, Johnson AD, et al. False aneurysm of the left ventricle. Radiology 1978;127:21.
15. Loop FD, Effler DB, Webster JS, et al. Posterior ventricular aneurysms. Etiological factors and results of surgical treatment. N Engl J Med 1973;288:257.
16. Cornell SH, Rossi NP. Roentgenographic findings in constrictive pericarditis. Am J Radiol 1968;102:301.

17. Hancock EW. Subacute effusive constrictive pericarditis. Circulation 1971;43:183.

18. Braun LO, Kincaid OW, McGoon DC. Prognosis of aortic valve replacement in relation to preoperative heart size. J Thorac Cardiovasc Surg 1973;65:381.

19. Engler R, Ray R, Higgins CB, et al. The clinical assessment and follow-up of functional capacity in patients with chronic congestive cardiomyopathy. Am J Cardiol 1982;49:1832.

20. Lane EJ, Carsky EW. Epicardial fat: lateral film analysis in normal and pericardial effusion. Radiology 1968;91:1.

21. Tehranzadeh J, Kelly MJ. The differential density sign of pericardial effusion. Radiology 1979;133:23.

22. Nasser WK, Helmer C, Tavel ME, et al. Congenital absence of left pericardium. Circulation 1970;41:469.

23. Lind TA, Pitt MJ, Groves BM, et al. The abnormal left hilum. Circulation 1975;51:183.

24. Souza AS, Bream PR, Elliott LP. Chest film detection of coronary artery calcification. The value of the CAC triangle. Radiology 1978;129:7.

25. Green CE, Kelley MJ. A renewed role for fluoroscopy in the evaluation of cardiac disease. Radiol Clin North Am 1980;18:345.

26. Agatson AS, Janowitz WR, Hildner FJ, et al. Quantification of coronary artery calcium using ultrafast computed tomography. J Am Coll Cardiol 1990;15:827.

Chapter 2

Radiography of Congenital Heart Disease

Charles B. Higgins

The radiographic diagnosis of congenital heart disease can be a confusing and difficult topic because of the myriad of congenital heart lesions that exist. Assessment of the plain radiograph can usually provide only a notion of the generic type of congenital heart lesion rather than a clear indication of specific lesions. An approach that is cognizant of the realistic insights possible from the plain radiograph must be pursued. Such an approach should be based upon the observations on the radiograph that can be made with some degree of certitude and in which there is minimal ambiguity. Such an approach should also take advantage of the clinical information upon which one can rely. The current classification system depends upon a few clinical observations and a few findings on the radiograph that can be made with reasonable reliability. As shown for acquired heart disease, the thoracic radiograph should be evaluated by a five-step approach. At each step certain critical observations should be made (Fig. 2-1).

Clinical-Radiographic Classification of Congenital Heart Disease

This classification depends upon two clinical data:

1. Cyanotic or noncyanotic.
2. Symptoms of congestive heart failure, such as dyspnea, tachypnea, tachycardia, and frequent respiratory infections.

The salient radiographic findings are:

1. Increased or decreased pulmonary arterial vascularity.
2. Cardiomegaly or nearly normal heart size.

This classification system permits most major lesions involving right-to-left or left-to-right shunts to be classified into four categories (Table 2-1). A fifth group consists of patients with primarily pulmonary venous congestion (Table 2-2). Therefore, the interpretation of the chest x-ray attempts to decide which class or category of congenital heart lesions exists. The decision upon the specific lesion is usually based upon the statistical frequency of a particular cardiac lesion within one or more groups. Based upon the clinical and radiographic findings, there are four groups of congenital heart lesions. The groups as used in this classification system are:

Group I, Left-to-Right Shunts

Criteria:
1. Noncyanotic. Sometimes symptoms of pulmonary congestion or congestive heart failure.
2. Radiographic signs of pulmonary arterial overcirculation (Fig. 2-2).

The lesions included in this group are listed in Table 2-1.

Group II, Right-to-Left Shunts with Little or No Cardiomegaly

Criteria:
1. Cyanosis.
2. Decreased or normal pulmonary arterial vascularity and little or no cardiomegaly (Fig. 2-3).

The lesions included in this group are listed in Table 2-1.

Group III, Right-to-Left Shunts with Cardiomegaly

Criteria:
1. Cyanosis.

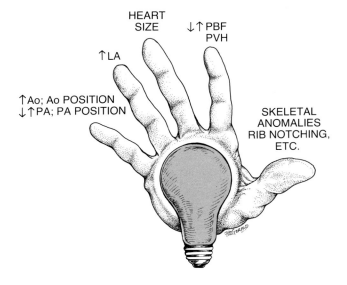

Figure 2-1. Five step approach to thoracic radiography in congenital heart disease: the enlightened hand.

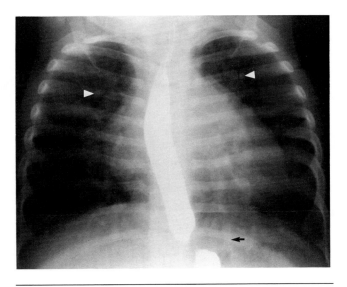

Figure 2-2. Ventricular septal defect. Pulmonary arterial overcirculation and cardiomegaly. Pulmonary arterial overcirculation is indicated by prominent hilar vessels; peripheral portion of segmental pulmonary arteries are visible behind the diaphragms (*arrow*); and prominent peripheral-en face vessels ("shunt vessels," *arrowheads*).

2. Radiographic evidence of normal or decreased pulmonary blood flow and cardiomegaly (Fig. 2-4).

The lesions included in this group are listed in Table 2-1.

Table 2-1

Classification of Shunt Lesions

Group I Lesions

Acyanotic; pulmonary arterial overcirculation
  Atrial septal defect
  Partial anomalous pulmonary venous connection
  Atrioventricular septal defect (endocardial cushion defect)
  Ventricular septal defect
  Patent ductus arteriosus
  Other aortic level shunts, i.e., ruptured sinus of Valsalva
    aneurysm; aorticopulmonary window, etc.

Group II Lesions

Cyanotic; decreased pulmonary vascularity, no cardiomegaly
  Tetralogy of Fallot
  Transposition with pulmonic stenosis and VSD
  Double outlet right ventricle with pulmonic stenosis and VSD
  Double outlet left ventricle with pulmonic stenosis and VSD
  Single ventricle (univentricular atrioventricular connection) with
    pulmonic stenosis
  Corrected transposition with pulmonic stenosis and VSD
  Pulmonic atresia with intact ventricular septum, type I
  Pulmonic stenosis with atrioventricular septal defect
  Hypoplastic right ventricle syndrome
  Some types of tricuspid atresia (large ASD and pulmonary
    stenosis or atresia)

Group III Lesions

Cyanotic; decreased pulmonary vascularity; cardiomegaly
  Ebstein's anomaly
  Pulmonary stenosis (critical) with ASD or patent foramen ovale
  Some types of tricuspid atresia (restrictive ASD)
  Pulmonary atresia with intact ventricular septum, type II
  Transient tricuspid regurgitation of the newborn

Group IV Lesions

Cyanosis; pulmonary arterial overcirculation
  Transposition of great arteries
  Truncus arteriosus
  Total anomalous pulmonary venous connection
  Tricuspid atresia
  Single ventricle (univentricular atrioventricular connection)
  Double outlet right ventricle
  Double outlet left ventricle
  Atrioventricular septal defect (complete form)
  Hypoplastic left heart syndrome
  Pulmonary arteriovenous fistula(e)

Group IV, Admixture Lesions, i.e., Both Right-to-Left and Left-to-Right Shunts

Criteria:

1. Cyanosis.
2. Radiographic evidence of increased pulmonary arterial vascularity and usually cardiomegaly (Fig. 2-5).

The lesions in this group are listed in Table 2-1.

It is frequently difficult to distinguish between normal and diminished pulmonary vascularity. However, this observation can be greatly simplified when one remembers that normal pulmonary vascularity as gleaned from

Acyanotic + Pulm $\overline{\text{Art}}$ are

ASD ① Pulmonary arterial overcirculation.

Generally 2:1 shunt must exist before pulmonary plethora
is universally present. 50-60% of pts $\bar{c}$ <2:1 shunt
have only mild or no pulmonary plethora.

Pulm edema rarely occurs in simple ASD.

② Enlargement of RA

③ Enlargement of RV

④ Enlargement of main + hilar pulm artery segments
In older pts the Right PA is especially
prominent.

⑤ Small asc AO + arch

⑥ Small SVC shadow.

Calc in Pulm arteries = Pulmonary Arterial HTN

PAPVC

Coexist $\bar{c}$ 10-15% of secundum defects + nearly
100% of sinus venosus defects.
Sites of anomalous connection to the ® ♡ are
★ ® SVC - most common
Azygous vein
RA
Coronary sinus
Ⓛ SVC
Subclavian veins
IVC. - may be above or below the diaphragm.
- Most commonly involves upper ® pulm veins.
Anomalous drainage of Ⓛ pulm veins is rare + usu to L SVC.
→

(Sinus venosus ASD
® upper pulm vein drains into SVC just above RA.)
Drainage of RLPV to IVC → Scimitar).

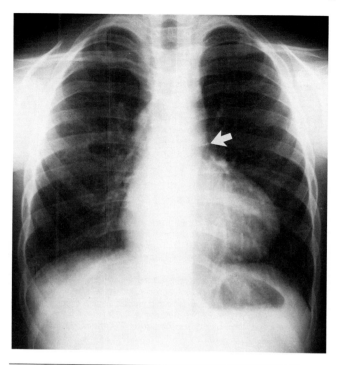

Figure 2-3. Tetralogy of Fallot. Decreased pulmonary vascularity *without* cardiomegaly. The main pulmonary arterial segment is concave (*arrow*) and the hilar vessels are small. Apex is situated high above the diaphragm and the thoracic aorta is prominent; both are features of this lesion.

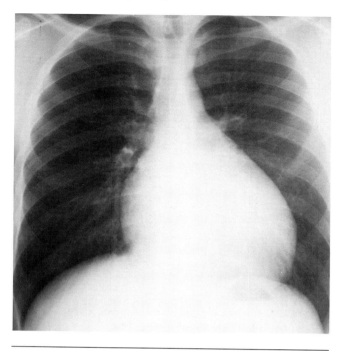

Figure 2-4. Ebstein's anomaly. Decreased pulmonary vascularity with cardiomegaly. Hilar vessels are small and segmental pulmonary arteries are hardly visible, especially in the upper lobes. Vector of enlargement of the left side of the heart is directly lateral, indicating right ventricular enlargement.

Table 2-2

Group V Lesions

Pulmonary venous hypertension (congestion)
Cardiomegaly disproportionate to pulmonary vascularity
A. Nonstructural heart disease in newborn
   Asphyxia
   Hypervolemia, hyperviscosity
      overhydration
      twin–twin transfusion
      maternal–fetal transfusion
      excess stripping of the cord
   Paroxysmal atrial tachycardia
   Heart block
   Hypoglycemia
   Hypocalcemia
   Hydrops fetalis
   Systemic hypertension
B Structural heart disease in newborn
   Hypoplastic left heart syndrome
   Total anomalous pulmonary venous connection, type III
   Coarctation of the aorta
   Critical aortic stenosis
   Endocardial fibroelastosis
   Anomalous origin of the coronary artery from the pulmonary
      artery
   Intrauterine myocarditis

the radiograph in a patient with cyanosis can be equated with decreased pulmonary vascularity. Consequently, the major observation on the radiograph in terms of pulmonary vascularity in the cyanotic patient is to determine whether the pulmonary vascularity is increased. Normal or diminished pulmonary vascularity in a patient with cyanosis indicates that the lesion produces a right-to-left shunt. Increased pulmonary vascularity in a cyanotic patient indicates that there is an admixture lesion; the cyanosis is indicative of right-to-left shunting, and increased pulmonary vascularity is a sign of left-to-right shunting.

Examination of the chest x-ray should be systematic; a five-step approach is useful (see Fig. 2-1). The first step should not be deleted, since a number of cardiac lesions are associated with skeletal abnormalities (see Table 2-3).

Groups of Congenital Heart Lesions

Group I. Group I contains all of the left-to-right shunts. Consequently, this is the group into which most of the patients with congenital heart disease will be classified. The criteria that place a patient within this category depend for the most part upon the absence of cyanosis

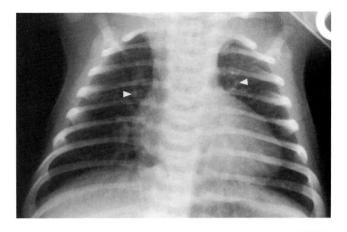

Figure 2-5. Transposition of the great arteries. Pulmonary arterial overcirculation in the presence of cyanosis. Cardiomegaly is present. Prominent hilar vessels and en face peripheral vessels ("shunt vessels," *arrowheads*).

Table 2-3

Skeletal Abnormalities and Syndromes Associated with Congenital Heart Disease

Rib notching (coarctation of aorta)
11 ribs (Down's syndrome, AVSD)
Double manubrial ossification center (Down's syndrome, AVSD)
Multiple sternal ossification centers (cyanotic heart disease)
Bulging sternum (large left-to-right shunt)
Pectus excavatum (Marfan's syndrome)
Scoliosis (Marfan's syndrome, tetralogy, and other cyanotic lesions)
Ellis–Van Creveld syndrome (common atrium)
Holt–Oram syndrome (ASD, VSD)
Turner's syndrome (coarctation)
Trisomy 18 (VSD, others)
Trisomy 13–15 (VSD, others)
Marfan's syndrome (aortic regurgitation, aortoannular ectasia, mitral valve prolapse)
Ehler's–Danlos syndrome (aortic regurgitation, aortoannular ectasia)
Osteogenesis imperfecta (aortic regurgitation)
Limb and vertebral anomalies (vacterl syndrome, VSD)

ASD, atrial septal defect; AVSD, atrioventricular septal defect (atrioventricular canal defect); VSD, ventricular septal defect.

with the subsequent demonstration on the chest radiograph of increased pulmonary arterial vascularity (Figs. 2-2, 2-6, 2-7). The degree of cardiomegaly is usually in proportion to the increase in pulmonary vascularity. The left-to-right shunts are volume overload lesions. Consequently, there is frequently cardiomegaly, and this cardiomegaly should in general be in proportion to the prominence of the pulmonary vascularity. When cardiomegaly is out of proportion to the pulmonary arterial vascularity, then one must consider a number of possibilities. One of these is that the left-to-right shunt is diminishing in size because of a decrease in the size of the ventricular septal defect. Another consideration is the coexistence of additional cardiac lesion(s), such as primary myocardial disease or coarctation of the aorta.

Two useful signposts can be used to help to distinguish among the various types of left-to-right shunts (Fig. 2-8). The first of these is the left atrium. Left atrial enlargement indicates that the predominant lesion is *not* an atrial-level shunt but rather a ventricular septal defect or a patent ductus arteriosus. The atrial septal defect and partial anomalous pulmonary venous connection lack both of the two signposts (Figs. 2-7, 2-9). The next signpost is the aortic arch. A prominent aortic arch distinguishes between patent ductus arteriosus and ventricular septal defect. The aortic arch usually has a normal dimension or is small in ventricular septal defect (Figs. 2-2, 2-6, 2-10). Patent ductus arteriosus is associated with left atrial enlargement and a prominent aortic arch (Fig. 2-11). In young infants, prominence of the aortic arch may be difficult to recognize, so this signpost may not always be available. Consequently, since a ventricular septal defect is a more common lesion, this should be the diagnosis when there is left atrial enlargement and no clearly discernible enlargement of the aortic arch. An

exception to this rule is in the premature infant, where a patent ductus arteriosus is statistically by far the most common congenital heart lesion. The radiograph of the premature infant with patent ductus arteriosus usually does not disclose signs of left atrial and aortic arch enlargement.

The plain radiograph may be useful in determining the severity and progression of left-to-right shunts. The severe volume overload with large left-to-right shunts causes pulmonary venous congestion or pulmonary edema in addition to pulmonary arterial overcirculation (see Fig. 2-10). In patients with large left-to-right shunts there should also be substantial cardiomegaly.

Group II. A lesion is included in group II when there is cyanosis and the plain radiograph demonstrates diminished or normal pulmonary vascularity and the absence of substantial cardiomegaly (Figs. 2-3, 2-12, 2-13, 2-14). The pathophysiology that produces this constellation of findings involves a nonrestrictive intracardiac shunt and severe obstruction to pulmonary blood flow. The nonrestrictive intracardiac shunt permits equalization of the pressures between two chambers, and this prevents substantial enlargement of the right ventricle. Consequently, there is usually little or no cardiomegaly. An example of the importance of the size of the intracardiac defect is in patients with tricuspid atresia. The patient with tricuspid atresia with a large atrial septal defect demonstrates little or no cardiomegaly (see Fig. 2-13A). On the other hand, the patient with tricuspid atresia with

(*Text continues on page 57*)

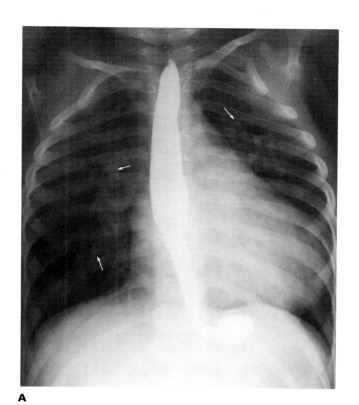

A

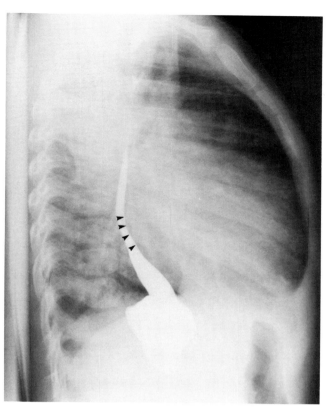

B

Figure 2-6. Ventricular septal defect. Frontal (*A*) and lateral (*B*) views. Pulmonary arterial overcirculation is evident by shunt vessels (*arrows*) and prominent hilar vessels. Heart size is increased in proportion to overcirculation. Left atrial enlargement produces impression upon and displacement of the barium-filled esophagus (*arrowheads*).

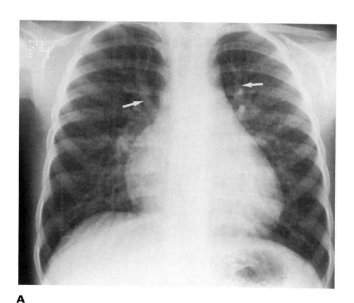

A

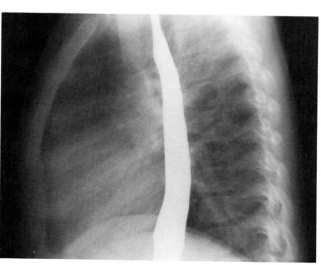

B

Figure 2-7. Atrial septal defect. Frontal (*A*) and lateral (*B*) views. Pulmonary arterial circulation shown by large hilar and segmental pulmonary arteries. Note the prominence of the segmental arteries in the upper lobes (*arrows*). The absence of left atrial enlargement indicates an atrial level shunt.

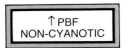

GROUP I LESIONS

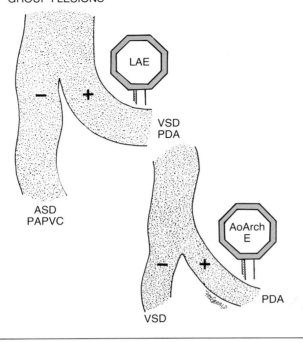

Figure 2-8. Signposts on the diagnostic pathway of left-to-right shunts.

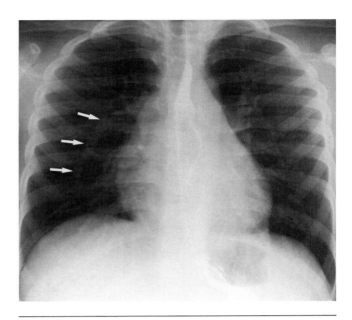

Figure 2-9. Partial anomalous pulmonary venous connection. Anomalous course of a vessel through the right pulmonary region (*arrows*).

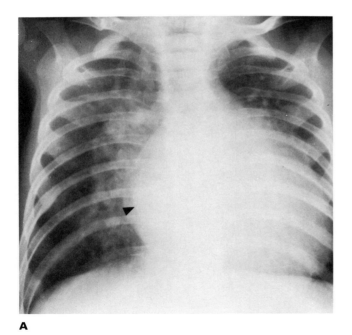

A

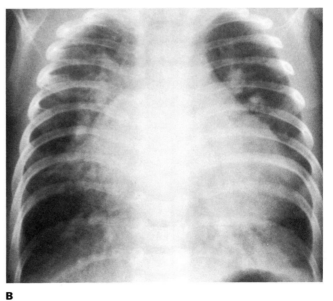

B

Figure 2-10. Ventricular septal defects. Two patients. Large volume left-to-right shunts causing interstitial pulmonary edema. Severe pulmonary atrial overcirculation and cardiomegaly. Double density (*arrowhead, A*) or increased density (*B*) in right retrocardiac region is evidence of left atrial enlargement. Indistinct hilar and segmental arteries is caused by interstitial edema.

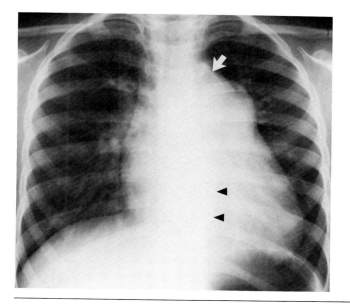

Figure 2-11. Patent ductus arteriosus. Pulmonary arterial overcirculation and cardiomegaly. The prominent aortic arch (*arrow*) and descending aorta (*arrowheads*) are diagnostic signs of patent ductus arteriosus.

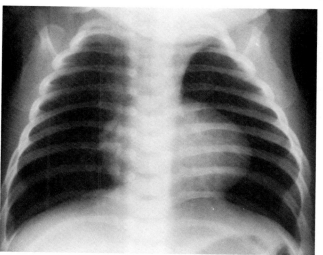

A

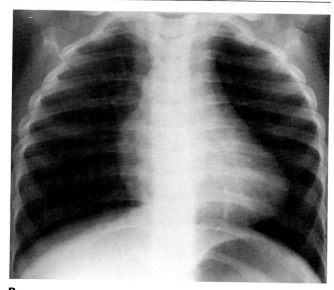

B

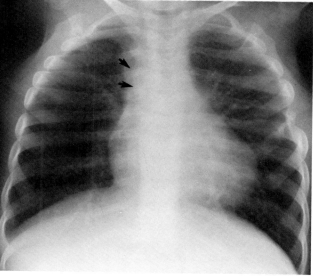

C

Figure 2-12. *A:* Single ventricle with pulmonic stenosis. Decreased pulmonary vascularity is indicated by concave main pulmonary arterial segment; there are no visible hilar arteries, and vessels within the lungs are severely attenuated. Cardiomegaly is not present. Heart size is normal for an anteroposterior view in a neonate. *B:* Transposition of great arteries with pulmonic stenosis and VSD. There is decreased vascularity and an absence of substantial cardiomegaly. *C:* Double outlet right ventricle with pulmonic stenosis (a VSD is always present in this anomaly). There is decreased vascularity and an absence of cardiomegaly. Note right aortic arch (*arrows*).

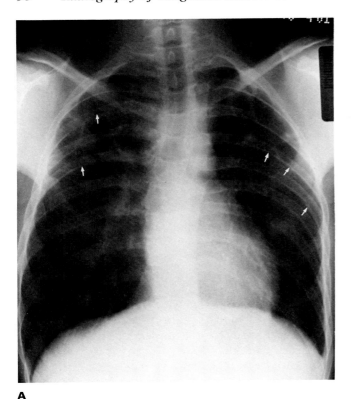

A

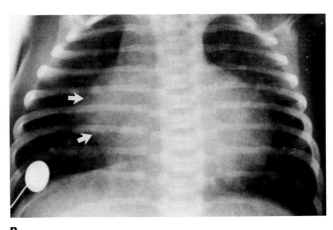

B

Figure 2-13. *A:* Tricuspid atresia with large (nonrestrictive) ASD, severe pulmonary stenosis, normal arterioventricular connections. Decreased pulmonary vascularity and no cardiomegaly. Rib notching (*arrows*) is present owing to intercostal arterial to pulmonary collaterals (a rare cause of rib notching). *B:* Tricuspid atresia with small (restrictive) ASD and large VSD. Small ASD is responsible for right atrial enlargement and thus cardiomegaly. Large VSD results in pulmonary arterial overcirculation. Right atrial enlargement is evident by the prominent lateral extension and elongation of the right border of the heart (*arrows*).

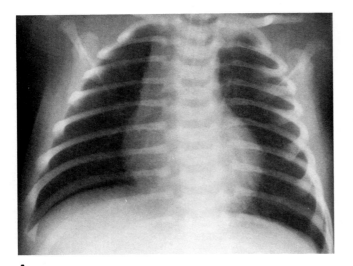

A

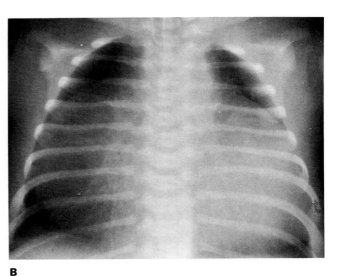

B

Figure 2-14. *A:* Pulmonary atresia with intact ventricular septum, type I. Pulmonary vascularity is decreased and cardiomegaly absent. *B:* Pulmonary atresia with intact ventricular septum, type II. Substantial tricuspid regurgitation in association with this anomaly (type II) causes right-sided chamber enlargement, especially right atrial enlargement. The "wall-to-wall" heart is usually caused by severe tricuspid regurgitation.

a restrictive atrial septal defect experiences substantial right atrial enlargement, which results in a degree of cardiomegaly (see Fig. 2-13*B*). Consequently, the lesions of the former patient would be classified in group II while those of the latter patient would be classified in group III or IV. Tricuspid atresia can be classified in group IV when there is an associated increase in pulmonary blood flow, which is caused by either a large left-to-right shunt at the ventricular septal level or the concurrence of transposition of the great vessels. Transposition of the great arteries does occur in approximately 30% of patients with tricuspid atresia.

Statistically the most common lesion in group II is tetralogy of Fallot. The remaining diagnostic considerations are, for the most part, variants of tetralogy of Fallot. Some examples of these lesions are transposition of the great arteries with severe pulmonary stenosis and ventricular septal defect (see Fig. 2-12*B*) and double-outlet right ventricle with severe pulmonic stenosis and an unrestrictive ventricular septal defect (see Fig. 2-12*C*). Table 2-1 provides a reasonably complete list of the differential diagnostic considerations in group II. It should be noted, however, that the plain radiograph infrequently permits a specific diagnosis among this myriad of lesions.

Group III. The group III lesions differ from the group II lesions by the radiographic observation of car-

diomegaly (Figs. 2-4, 2-13, 2-14, 2-15, 2-16). These patients have cyanosis, normal or decreased pulmonary vascularity, and a substantial degree of cardiomegaly. The cardiac chamber that is most often enlarged in this lesion is the right atrium. Many of the patients in this category have substantial tricuspid regurgitation, which is a major pathogenetic mechanism of the right atrial enlargement and cardiomegaly. The "wall-to-wall" heart (extension from the right to the left chest wall) should prompt the diagnostic consideration of a lesion causing tricuspid regurgitation.

There is no statistically dominant diagnostic consideration in this category. There are four or five lesions that must be considered in the differential diagnosis. These are pulmonary stenosis with an atrial septal defect or patent foramen ovale; type II pulmonary atresia with intact ventricular septum (see Fig. 2-14); tricuspid atresia with a restrictive atrial septal defect (see Fig. 2-13); and Ebstein's anomaly (see Fig. 2-15). In the infant with this constellation of findings, perhaps the most frequent diagnosis is critical pulmonic stenosis with a restrictive interatrial communication. In the older child and adult with this constellation of findings the most likely diagnosis is Ebstein's anomaly. Another unusual diagnosis in this category, which appears only in the neonatal period, is transient tricuspid regurgitation of the newborn (see Fig. 2-16). In this entity there is frequently substantial cardio-

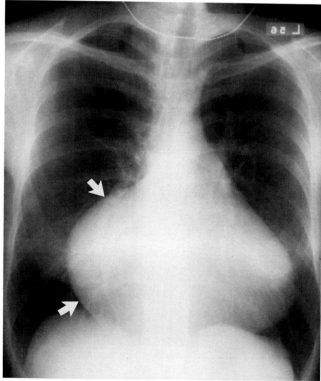

A

B

Figure 2-15. Ebstein's anomaly in infant (*A*) and in adult (*B*). Decreased pulmonary vascularity and marked cardiomegaly. Note the prominent bulging and elongation of the right heart border indicative of severe right atrial enlargement (*arrows*).

megaly, diminished pulmonary blood flow, and cyanosis within the first few days of life. However, with reduction in pulmonary vascular resistsance over time, the amount of tricuspid regurgitation decreases and the cardiomegaly resolves.

Group IV. A lesion is included in this group when the radiograph displays pulmonary arterial overcirculation in the presence of cyanosis. The heart size is usually increased. The observation of increased pulmonary vascularity in a patient with cyanosis is an incongruous finding and should immediately alert the observer to the presence of an admixture lesion rather than a strictly left-to-right shunt. An aid to remembering the major diagnoses in this category is the letter T. The most common diagnosis in this category is transposition of the great arteries, which is the most frequent cyanotic congenital heart lesion at birth (see Fig. 2-5). The other diagnostic considerations are truncus arteriosus (Fig. 2-17), total anomalous pulmonary venous connection (Fig. 2-18), tricuspid atresia (see Fig. 2-13*B*), and single ("tingle") ventricle (Fig. 2-19). Double-outlet right ventricle and double-outlet left ventricle are also considered in this category but these can be brought to mind when one thinks of transposition of the great arteries, since these lesions are essentially hybrids of the latter condition. The

lesion that is frequently forgotten in this group is multiple pulmonary arterial venous malformations. The patient with multiple pulmonary arterial venous malformations is frequently mildly or even moderately cyanotic and because of the several malformations within the lung, there is the appearance of increased pulmonary aterial vascularity.

Pulmonary Venous Congestion or Pulmonary Edema

A fifth group of congenital lesions are those that produce predominantly pulmonary venous congestion and alter the pulmonary venous vascularity rather than the pulmonary arterial vascularity. Patients with these lesions may have shunts, but inclusion in group V requires that the predominant pathophysiologic event is pulmonary venous congestion (Figs. 2-20, 2-21, Table 2-2).

The clinical features of the group V lesions are lack of cyanosis and frequently, severe symptoms of heart failure. This usually consists of dyspnea, tachypnea, and tachycardia. The salient radiographic findings are indistinctness of the pulmonary vascularity, especially in the perihilar area, or interstitial pulmonary edema (Figs. 2-20, 2-21). Another observation that places a lesion into this group is disproportionately prominent cardiomegaly

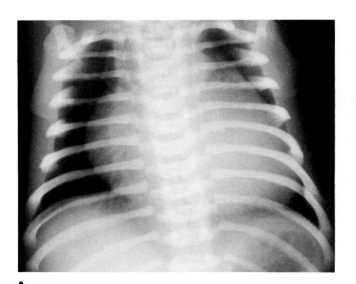

A

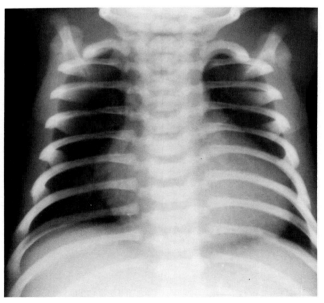

B

Figure 2-16. Transient tricuspid regurgitation of the newborn on day one (*A*) and day 7 (*B*). Pulmonary vascularity is decreased and marked cardiomegaly is present. Right atrial enlargement and cardiomegaly have diminished on the later radiograph because of resolution of tricuspid regurgitation.

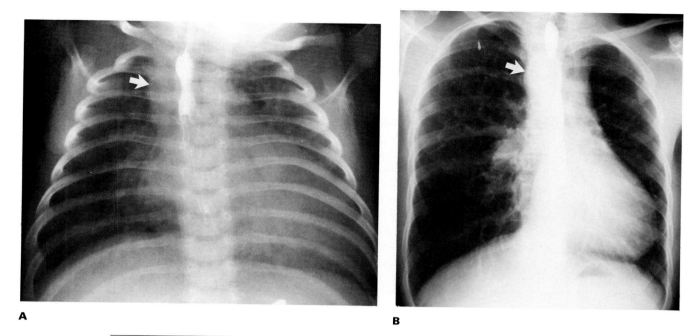

A

B

Figure 2-17. Two cases of truncus arteriosus. Pulmonary arterial overcirculation and right aortic arch (*arrow*) are characteristics of truncus arteriosus.

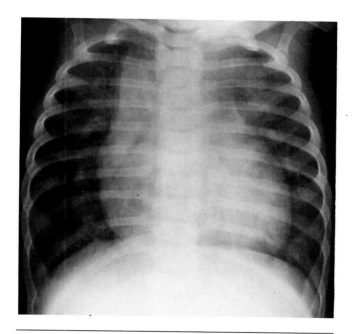

Figure 2-18. Total anomalous pulmonary venous connection, supracardiac type (type I). Pulmonary arterial overcirculation and cardiomegaly are present. Enlargement of supracardiac region is caused by enlarged left-sided vertical vein and dilated right superior vena cava; it is characteristic of this anomaly. Although evident in this case, it is *un*usual to observe this "snowman appearance" in an infant.

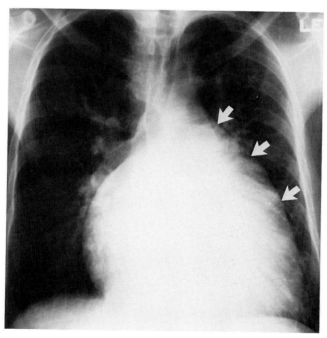

Figure 2-19. Single ventricle (univentricular atrioventricular connection) with l-TGA. Single ventricle of the left ventricular type with inverted diminutive right ventricular (RV) outlet chamber. Convexity of upper left cardiac border (*arrows*) is caused by l-transposed aorta and inverted RV outlet chamber.

in comparison to the prominence of pulmonary vascularity (Figs. 2-22, 2-23, 2-24).

The lesions included in this category are listed in Table 2-2. It should be noted that the statistical frequency of the lesions in this category are also important in deciding upon the diagnosis. Diagnosis in this category includes conditions that produce reversible stresses upon the heart of the newborn as well as structural cardiac lesions. Lesions in this category tend to present at certain times after birth, for instance, the nonstructural causes of

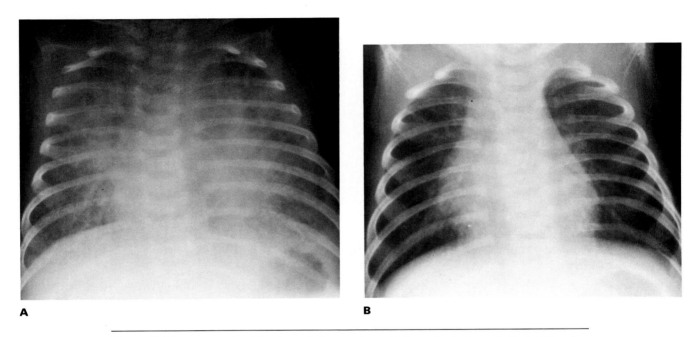

A   **B**

Figure 2-20. Paroxysmal atrial tachycardia in a newborn. Radiographs during arrhythmia (*A*) and after cardioversion (*B*). During the arrhythmia there exist severe pulmonary edema and cardiomegaly. After cardioversion, pulmonary edema is alleviated and heart size is reduced.

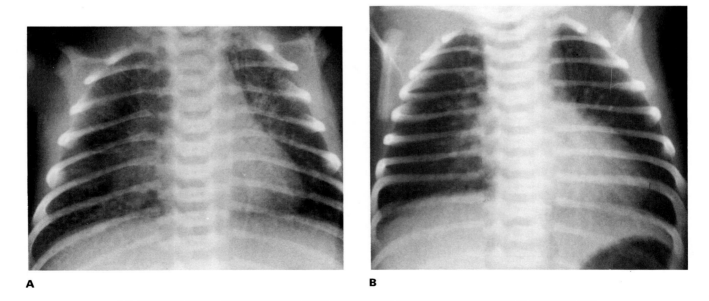

A   **B**

Figure 2-21. TAPVC, type III. Radiographs from two newborns. *A* shows interstitial pulmonary edema and normal heart size. *B* shows fluid in minor fissure and perihilar vascular indistinctness consistent with pulmonary venous hypertension (congestion) and normal heart size.

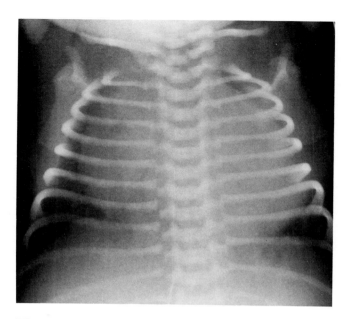

Figure 2-22. Hydrops fetalis. Cardiomegaly is disproportionately great relative to the pulmonary vascularity, which is not increased.

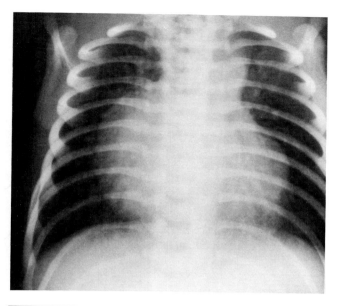

Figure 2-23. Hypoplastic left heart. Pulmonary venous congestion and edema and cardiomegaly. Prominent right atrium and ventricle are characteristic features of this lesion.

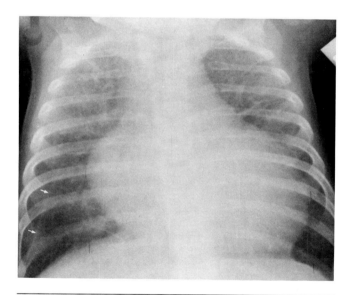

Figure 2-24. Endocardial fibrelastosis. Pulmonary edema and cardiomegaly. Indistinctness, pulmonary vessels, prominent interlobular septa and fluid in the right major (*small arrows*) and minor fissures are features of interstitial edema.

pulmonary venous congestion or edema, usually present within the first day or two of life (see Figs. 2-20, 2-22). Several abnormalities that may be encountered within the first day of life include severe anemia (hydrops fetalis), asphyxia, hypocalcemia, hypoglycemia, abnormalities of heart rate and rhythm, hypervolemia, and intrauterine myocarditis. Pulmonary venous congestion with

substantial cardiomegaly presenting in the first day or so of life is a feature of hypoplastic left heart (see Fig. 2-23). Pulmonary venous congestion with an essentially normal heart size presenting within the first day or so of life is the feature of total anomalous pulmonary venous connection, infradiaphragmatic type with obstruction (see Fig. 2-21). In the infant presenting with these features between 1 week and 3 weeks of age, statistically the most common diagnosis is coarctation of the aorta. Rib notching is not evident in infants with coarctation.

The lesions that tend to present at approximately 4 to 6 weeks of age are endocardial fibroelastosis (see Fig. 2-24) and anomalous left coronary artery (Fig. 2-25). A rare cause of the radiographic features of group V is Pompey's disease and other glycogenoses (Fig. 2-26). However, these lesions may present earlier.

Specific Lesions

Acyanotic

Atrial Septal Defect. There are four types of atrial septal defects: secundum (most frequent); primum; sinus venosus (superior and inferior vena caval locations); and coronary sinus (least frequent) (Fig. 2-27). The primum type is usually part of an atrioventricular septal defect, which in the past was called endocardial cushion defect. In addition, a patent foramen ovale exists in many children with congenital heart disease, and the

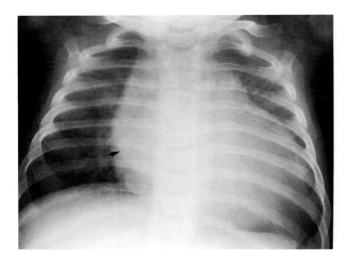

Figure 2-25. Anomalous origin of left coronary artery from the pulmonary artery. Cardiomegaly disproportionate to pulmonary vascularity in a noncyanotic infant is evident. Left atrial enlargement (right retrocardia double density, *arrow*) is caused by mitral regurgitation from papillary muscle infarction.

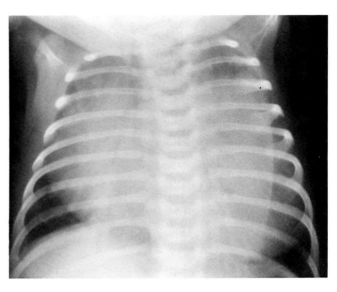

Figure 2-26. Pompey's disease (glycogen storage disease involving the myocardium). Cardiomegaly disproportionate to pulmonary vascularity is apparent.

foramen may be stretched in the setting of elevated right-sided pressures. An aneurysm may also form at the site of the thin fossa ovalis; this may occur as an isolated anomaly or may exist in association with a septal defect or patent foramen ovale. The defects are named according to their position in the atrial septum: *ostium secundum* in the region of the fossa ovalis, which is approximately the middle of the septum; *primum* in the lower part of the septum and bordering on the atrioventricular valves; *sinus venosus* in either the upper part of the septum and bordering on the ostium of the superior vena cava or in the lower septum and bordering on the ostium of the inferior vena cava. A rare type of defect occurs at a site normally occupied by the coronary sinus and coexists with absence of the wall separating the coronary sinus from the left atrium so that the associated left superior vena cava enters into the left atrium. The coexistence of large primum and secundum defects constitutes a common atrium.

Mitral valve prolapse has been detected in 20% to 30% of patients with secundum defects.[1] Atrial septal defect is the most common cardiac lesion in the Holt–Oram syndrome (radial side defect of upper limb) and common atrium is the cardiac lesion in the Ellis–van Creveld syndrome (ectodermal dysplasia with polydactyly).

The simple atrial septal defect conducts a left-to-right shunt. A stretched foramen ovale or atrial septal defect may permit predominant right-to-left shunting in complex lesions with severe right-sided obstruction, for example, tricuspid atresia. The volume of shunting across an interatrial communication usually depends upon the

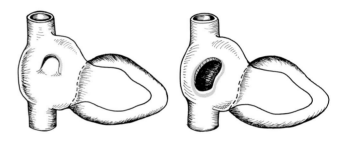
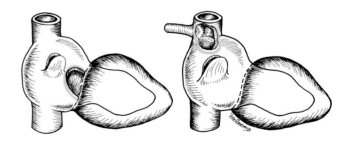

Figure 2-27. Location of the most common types of interatrial communications. Patent foramen ovale (*upper left*); primum ASD (*lower left*); secundum ASD (*upper right*); sinus venous ASD (*lower right*).

size of the defect and the relative distensibility of the two ventricles. The wall of the right ventricle is more distensible than the left ventricle during diastole, so blood preferentially flows toward the right ventricle at this time. However, obstruction of flow into or out of the right ventricle can reverse this pattern. A large atrial septal defect is defined as one that results in equalization of pressure between the atria.

Radiography. The salient radiographic features (Figs. 2-7, 2-28, 2-29) of atrial septal defect are:

1. Pulmonary arterial overcirculation. Generally a 2:1 shunt must exist before pulmonary plethora is universally present.[2] About 50% to 60% of patients with less than 2:1 shunt have only mild or no evident pulmonary plethora. Pulmonary edema rarely occurs in the simple ASD.
2. Enlargement of right atrium.
3. Enlargement of right ventricle.
4. Enlargement of main and hilar pulmonary arterial segments. In older subjects the right pulmonary artery is sometimes especially prominent (Figs. 2-28, 2-29).
5. Small ascending aorta and aortic arch.
6. Small superior vena caval shadow.

The primum defect may cause a prominent bulge along the upper right atrial border (Fig. 2-30). This may be due to the mitral regurgitant jet passing directly through the primum defect and striking the upper wall of the right atrium. The sinus venous defect may be associated with dilatation of the superior vena cava just above the connection with the atrium (superior venal caval ampulla).

Pulmonary arterial hypertension causes a further increase in the main and hilar pulmonary arterial segments. A disparity emerges between the size of the central and peripheral pulmonary vessels in this setting (Fig. 2-29). Calcification may sometimes be identified in the central pulmonary arteries (see Fig. 1-65). The Eisenmenger complex (irreversible pulmonary arterial hypertension) occurs less readily in atrial shunts than in other left-to-right and bidirectional shunts. Even in elderly patients with a lifelong shunt, it may not develop. Consequently, a marked disparity in size of central and peripheral arteries should not consign the patient to the diagnosis of Eisenmenger complex and inoperability. Persistent cardiac enlargement and prominent right-sided chambers implies persistent left-to-right shunting (see Fig. 2-28), whereas a normal cardiac size suggests little shunting due to high pulmonary vascular resistance.

Left atrial enlargement may be observed in some older adults with atrial septal defect. The left atrium is not enlarged in children with atrial septal defect.

Partial Anomalous Pulmonary Venous Connection (PAPVC).

PAPVC occurs as an isolated lesion and is also associated with additional anomalies. It can be associated with any anomaly but most frequently accompanies atrial septal defects. PAPVC exists with 10% to 15%

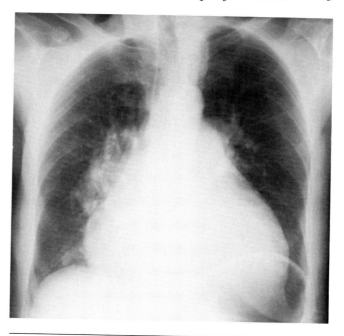

Figure 2-28. Atrial septal defect in an adult. The radiograph shows pulmonary arterial overcirculation and cardiomegaly due to right-sided chamber enlargement. Very severe dilatation of the central pulmonary arteries is a feature of this anomaly in the adult. Right pulmonary artery is very prominent.

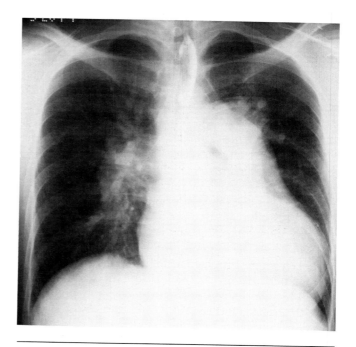

Figure 2-29. Atrial septal defect with pulmonary arterial hypertension in an adult. Aneurysmal dilatation of the main and hilar pulmonary arteries. There is disparity in the size of the hilar and segmental pulmonary arteries compared to the peripheral segments.

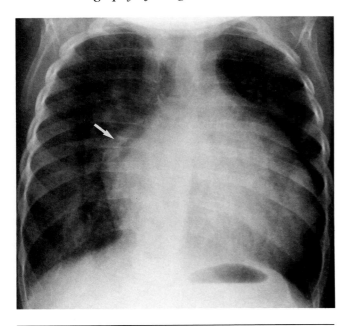

Figure 2-30. Atrioventricular septal defect–primum atrial septal defect. Radiograph shows pulmonary arterial overcirculation and cardiomegaly due to right atrial and ventricular enlargement. Vector of ventricular enlargement is lateral and superior, causing the apex to be located high above the diaphragm. Prominent bulging of upper right atrial border (*arrow*) is a feature of primum atrial septal defects.

of secundum defects and nearly 100% of sinus venosus defects. PAPVC itself is an acyanotic lesion and usually accompanies acyanotic lesions. In contradistinction, total anomalous pulmonary venous connection is a cyanotic lesion and accompanies complex cyanotic anomalies. The sites of connection to the right side of the heart are right superior vena cava (most common), azygous vein, right atrium, coronary sinus, left superior vena cava, subclavian veins, and inferior vena cava. The connection to the inferior vena cava may be above or below the diaphragm. Anomalous drainage most commonly involves the right pulmonary veins; either all veins, right upper veins (most common) or right lower veins. Anomalous drainage from the left is rare and usually the connection is to a persistent left superior vena cava. Anomalous connection of the left pulmonary veins to the left subclavian vein and coronary sinus is rare. Pulmonary venous flow is almost never obstructed, whether it exists above or below the diaphragm.

In sinus venosus ASD, the right upper pulmonary vein drains into the superior vena cava just above the junction with the right atrium. Drainage of right pulmonary veins or right lower pulmonary vein into the inferior vena cava has been named the scimitar syndrome; the connection to the inferior vena cava can be supra- or infra-diaphragmatic. This syndrome has a number of vari-

able components including hypoplasia of the right lung; hypoplasia of right pulmonary artery; dextroposition of the heart; congenital bronchostenosis and bronchiectasis; double hemidiaphragm; pulmonary sequestration; and systemic arterial supply to the sequestration.[3]

Radiography. The radiographic features of PAPVC are similar to ASD, since both are left-to-right shunts at the atrial level. As in ASD, there are right-sided cardiac enlargement and pulmonary arterial overcirculation. For an unknown reason, radiographs in some patients show greater vascular prominence in the lung for which anomalous drainage exists. Diagnosis of PAPVC from ASD depends upon recognition of abnormal course of pulmonary veins in the central portion of the lungs (see Fig. 2-9) or enlargement of a venous structure receiving the anomalous connection. The salient radiographic features are:

1. Pulmonary arterial overcirculation. This may be apparent or more severe only in the lung with anomalous drainage.
2. Enlargement of right atrium.
3. Enlargement of right ventricle.
4. Enlargement of main and hilar pulmonary arterial segments.
5. Small ascending aorta and aortic arch.
6. Enlargement of superior vena cava, azygous vein, coronary sinus or other systemic veins, depending upon site of connection.
7. Prominent left superior vena cava.
8. Abnormal course of pulmonary veins through the lung or in relation to mediastinal margins (Figs. 2-9, 2-31).

The radiographic features of the scimitar syndrome are usually pathognomonic.[3] On the frontal radiograph, the scimitar vein courses in the medial portion of the right lower lung (Fig. 2-31). The shadow of this vein mimics the shape of the Turkish sword (scimitar). The diameter of this venous shadow enlarges and it curves medially as it approaches the diaphragm. Occasionally, more than one venous shadow is evident (see Fig. 2-31). Additional features are a small right lung with an elevated right hemidiaphragm and dextroposition of the heart. Associated anomalies may be manifested, such as sequestration; pulmonary complications of the bronchial abnormalities; hypoplasia of the right pulmonary artery; and double diaphragm.

Atrioventricular Septal Defect (Endocardial Cushion Defect). The embryonic endocardial cushions contribute to the development of the medial portions of the mitral and tricuspid valves, the primum atrial septum and the inlet portion of the ventricular septum (Fig. 2-32). Defects in this region have been called endocardial

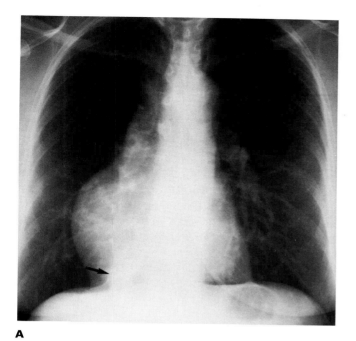

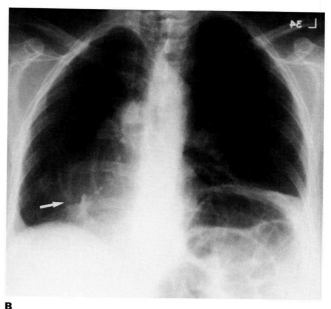

A   **B**

Figure 2-31. Two patients with scimitar syndrome. *A* shows scimitar vein near right diaphragm, dextroposed heart, and small right lung. Scimitar vein (*arrow*) enlarges in its course toward the diaphragm. *B* shows multiple anomalous veins (*arrow*) arching toward the right hemidiaphragm. The increased diameter of the veins from superior to inferior indicates that they are anomalous veins rather than pulmonary arteries. The heart is dextroposed. There is an incidental eventration of left hemidiaphragm.

cushion defects, but more recently have received the name *atrioventricular septal defects (AVSD)*. The fundamental lesion is a common atrioventricular valve and variable deficiency of the primum atrial septum and the inlet ventricular septum. The atrioventricular valve in this anomaly has five leaflets with two of the leaflets spanning the ventricular septum and the opening to both ventricles. The spanning leaflets are the anterior and posterior bridging leaflets. If there is a tongue of tissue connecting the anterior and posterior bridging leaflets and this tongue is attached to the crest of the inlet ventricular septum, then incomplete forms of the defect result. The anomaly exists in a complete form with a single atrioventricular valve, primum atrial septal defect, and inlet ventricular septal defect. In the complete form, no connecting tissue exists between the bridging leaflets. Incomplete forms are said to exist when there are two atrioventricular valves; the individual valves are formed by the connecting tongue of tissue. Portions of the valves are frequently deficient, such as underdevelopment of the septal leaflet of the tricuspid valve and a cleft in the anterior leaflet of the mitral valve. Actually, this "cleft" is the commissure between the anterior bridging leaflet and the mural leaflet of the left-sided portion of the atrioventricular valve.

The most common incomplete lesion is a primum

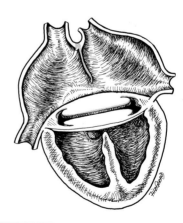

Figure 2-32. Atrioventricular septal defects. The defect consists of a primum atrial septal defect, an inlet ventricular septal defect, and a single atrioventricular valve spanning the ventricular septal defect.

atrial septal defect and a cleft in the mitral valve, causing varying degrees of mitral regurgitation. Because the primum atrial septal defect is situated immediately above the cleft, mitral regurgitation may traverse the defect and enter the right atrium. Consequently, the left atrium may not be enlarged even in patients with substantial mitral regurgitation. Direct shunting from the left ventricle to the right atrium may be caused by a defect in the atrioventricular septum, which is a small portion of the ventricular septum separating the inlet region of the left ventricle and right atrium. Even though an interventricular or atrioventricular shunt does not always exist, all patients with atrioventricular septal defect have underdevelopment of the inlet septum to some extent. This deficiency of the septum causes caudal displacement of the medial attachment of the left component of the atrioventricular valve and produces the goose-neck deformity of the left ventricle. The severity of the defect and the difficulty in surgical correction is related to the degree of underdevelopment of the inlet ventricular septum.

The physiological deficit and clinical manifestation of the AVSD depends upon the structural severity. In the complete form all four chambers communicate, causing both left-to-right and right-to-left shunts (admixture lesion). The left-to-right shunt dominates unless there is associated infundibular or valvular pulmonic stenosis or Eisenmenger's complex. Most cases are manifested as large left-to-right shunts in early infancy. Although cyanosis may not be clinically apparent, some degree of arterial desaturation is present in the complete form. The incomplete form may present in a manner similar to other ASDs but is frequently more severe. The presence of mitral regurgitation and/or left axis deviation on the electrocardiogram (ECG) are discriminatory clues.

Pulmonary arterial hypertension tends to develop in infancy or early childhood in patients with the complete form of AVSD. This is not an early complication of the primum ASD.

Mongolism is present in approximately 50% of patients with the complete form of AVSD. It is less common in the partial form. Complete AVSD is also frequently one of the cardiac anomalies in the asplenia syndrome.

Radiography. The salient radiographic features are similar to simple ASD but exaggerated. A decrease in the degree of pulmonary arterial overcirculation and extent of cardiomegaly on sequential radiographs may be a harbinger of pulmonary arterial hypertension. The salient radiographic features are:

1. Skeletal features of mongolism, such as 11 ribs, double manubrial ossification center, and tall vertebral bodies.
2. Pulmonary arterial overcirculation. This is severe in the complete forms and is frequently associated with pulmonary edema (Figs. 2-30, 2-33). Concurrent pneumonia is frequent in the complete form, especially in the child with mongolism.
3. Enlargement of right atrium. The superior margin of the right atrium is frequently very prominent (see Figs. 2-30, 2-33).

4. Enlargement of right ventricle.
5. Enlargement of main and central pulmonary arterial segments (see Fig. 2-32).
6. Left atrial enlargement may be present but is generally not severe and may be absent in spite of mitral regurgitation.
7. Small thoracic aorta (see Figs. 2-30, 2-33).
8. A cleft mitral valve without a primum defect produces the radiographic configuration of mitral regurgitation. This is rare.

Ventricular Septal Defect (VSD). Ventricular septal defects (VSDs) have been characterized by their location in the septum: perimembranous, outlet, inlet, and trabecular (Fig. 2-34). Defects in the perimembranous and outlet regions have also been described in relation to the crista supraventricularis of the right ventricle as infracristal (more frequent) and supracristal types. The defect may pass through the crista-transcristal VSD. While any perimembranous or outlet VSD can cause aortic regurgitation, the supracristal type frquently causes prolapse of the right sinus of Valsalva and aortic regurgitation. Prolapsed sinus tissue may reduce the size or obliterate the septal defect. The outlet defect may be caused by malposition of the outlet septum, resulting in

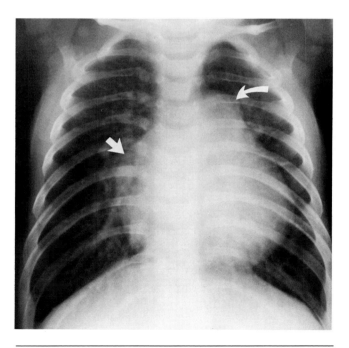

Figure 2-33. Atrioventricular septal defect (atrioventricular canal). Pulmonary arterial overcirculation and cardiomegaly due to right atrial and ventricular enlargement are present. There is marked enlargement and elongation of the main pulmonary arterial segment (*curved arrow*) and an inconspicuous ascending aorta and aortic arch. Prominent upper right atrial border (*arrow*) is characteristic of this anomaly.

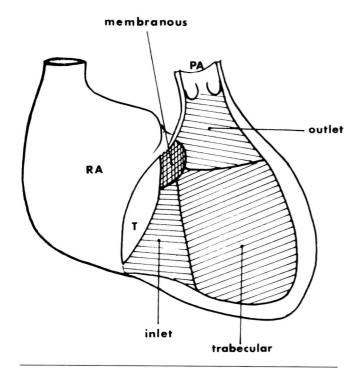

Figure 2-34. The regions of the ventricular system. The types of defect are named according to the region of the septum that is completely or partially defective. (Reproduced with permission from Higgins CB, et al. Congenital Heart Disease: Echocardiography and Magnetic Resonance Imaging. New York: Raven Press, 1990.)

a small right-ventricular outflow region and an aorta overriding the septal defect (tetralogy of Fallot). Ventricular septal defects are not uncommonly multiple. Multiple defects in the trabecular septum may produce a "Swiss cheese septum."

A small VSD is one in which the diameter or cross-sectional area is less than those of the aortic annulus. A large or nonrestrictive defect has a diameter or cross-sectional area exceeding the aortic annulus. A nonrestrictive defect permits equalization of pressures in the two ventricles.

Isolated VSD causes a left-to-right shunt of which the volume is determined by the cross-sectcional area of the defect and pulmonary vascular resistance. With large defects, shunting is not restricted by the defect but is controlled only by pulmonary vascular resistance. With low pulmonary vascular resistance the volume of the shunt is great, causing severe pulmonary overcirculation and eventually, pulmonary edema and elevated left ventricular end-diastole pressure. With higher resistance the flow is less severe and there exists pulmonary arterial hypertension. Increased pulmonary vascular resistance and pulmonary arterial hypretension may be due to pulmonary arteriolar constriction (reversible) or arteriolopathy (irreversible).

Most isolated VSDs close spontaneously. The process of closure is frequently marked by a ventricular septal aneurysm. The aneurysm usually consists of portions of the septal leaflet of the tricuspid valve adherent to the rim of the defect; a hole may develop in the adhesed leaflet. Although the supracristal defect may be obstructed by the prolapsed sinus of Valsalva, it does not actually close. The inlet VSD (part of the AVSD) rarely closes spontaneously.

In the early postpartum period, pulmonary vascular resistance has not declined completely to adult levels, and the elevated resistance limits the left-to-right shunting through large defects. Pulmonary arteriolar resistance tends to reach a nadir at 4 to 6 weeks postnatally and pulmonary overcirculation reaches a peak. Because of the process of gradual closure and a relative decrease in the defect due to cardiac growth, the defect is physiologically maximal during the first year of life. Since VSD is a volume overload lesion and the volume overload is directly related to the excess pulmonary blood flow, cardiac enlargement is proportional to the degree of overcirculation. Subsequent reduction in pulmonary arterial overcirculation and cardiomegaly may herald both good (spontaneous closure) or bad (increased pulmonary vascular resistance due to pulmonary arteriolopathy) natural history of the lesion.

Radiography. The thoracic radiograph is sometimes normal in VSDs, producing less than 2:1 shunt. The salient radiographic features of hemodynamically significant VSD are:

1. Pulmonary arterial overcirculation (see Figs. 2-2, 2-6, 2-10). With large shunts pulmonary edema is frequent during infancy.
2. Enlargement of the left atrium (see Figs. 2-6, 2-10). This may not be easy to identify during infancy.
3. Enlargement of either or both ventricles.
4. Enlargement of main and central pulmonary arterial segments. Disproportionate enlargement of central pulmonary arteries compared to peripheral vasculature suggests the Eisenmenger's complex but can also be observed with very large shunts. Pulmonary arterial calcification can occur in Eisenmenger's complex.
5. Small thoracic aorta (see Fig. 2-6). Right aortic arch is alleged to occur in about 2% of VSDs.

Cardiac size usually increases in rough proportion to the severity of pulmonary arterial overcirculation. Severe cardiomegaly in the absence of prominent overcirculation should suggest an associated lesion such as coarctation of the aorta or endocardial fibroelastosis. Left ventricular enlargement disproportionate to pulmonary overcirculation may be due to aortic regurgitation in supracristal defects. Reduction in pulmonary overcirculation and cardiac size on sequential radiographs can be a sign of spontaneous closure of the defect or pulmonary arteriolopathy (developing Eisenmenger's complex). The latter is suggested by progressive prominence of the main and central pulmonary arterial segments and right ventricle.

Patent Ductus Arteriosus (PDA). The ductus arteriosus connects the proximal descending aorta to the proximal left pulmonary artery just beyond the pulmonary arterial bifurcation. With mirror image right aortic arch the ductus usually connects the distal left innominate artery to the left pulmonary artery. With nonmirror image right arch (retroesophageal left subclavian artery) the ductus connects the proximal right descending aorta to the proximal left pulmonary artery and causes a vascular ring.

The ductus arteriosus closes within the first day of life in full-term neonates. Persistent patency of the ductus is common in the premature infant. PDA is nearly always the cause of the significant left-to-right shunting in premature infants during the early neonatal period. The shunt is predominantly left-to-right, causes pulmonary overcirculation, and if severe, pulmonary edema. However, right-to-left shunting across a PDA may be encountered in neonates with failure of the pulmonary vascular resistance to decline from levels existing during the fetal stage (persistent fetal circulation).

PDA occurs as an isolated anomaly but also frequently in association with other simple and complex anomalies. There is a propensity for the triplex of PDA, coarctation of the aorta, and VSD, to occur. PDA is also frequently present in cyanotic lesions with severe obstruction to pulmonary blood flow, such as pulmonary atresia. The PDA is life-sustaining in these instances but cannot be relied upon for maintaining pulmonary blood flow because it may severely constrict or obliterate over time.

The large-caliber PDA may conduct a large left-to-right shunt because a gradient exists between the aorta and pulmonary artery throughout the cardiac cycle. Flow through the PDA is controlled by the caliber of the ductus and pulmonary vascular resistance. The volume overload (excess pulmonary blood flow) causes enlargement of the left atrium and left ventricle. The left-to-right shunt continually recirculates to the lungs, left atrium, left ventricle, ascending aorta and aortic arch. The volume experienced by the left-sided chamber causes an elevated left ventricular diastolic pressure. With large shunts, the excess blood flow and elevated left ventricular diastolic pressure eventuates in pulmonary edema. The excess flow and elevated pulmonary venous pressure may cause considerable pulmonary arterial hypertension, which induces right ventricular hypertrophy. The eventual outcome of the process is pulmonary arteriolopathy and Eisenmenger's syndrome.

Radiography. A small-volume left-to-right shunt caused by PDA is frequently associated with a normal thoracic radiograph. The salient radiographic features of hemodynamically significant PDAs are:

1. Pulmonary arterial overcirculation (Figs. 2-11, 2-35).
2. Enlargement of left atrium (see Fig. 2-35).
3. Enlargement of left ventricle (see Figs. 2-11, 2-35).
4. Enlargement of aortic arch (Figs. 2-11, 2-35, 2-36). Although this may not be evident with infants, it is an invariable feature in the older child and adult. It may also be possible to identify prominence of the ascending aorta and lateral displacement of the descending aorta.
5. Enlargement of the main and central pulmonary arterial segments. This tends to be less prominent than in ASD.
6. Abnormal contour of the posterior aortic arch and proximal descending aorta. In many normal subjects there is a localized dilatation of the aorta at the site of attachment of the ligamentum arteriosus, the aortic spindle (also called infundibulum). This aortic spindle is enlarged in patients with PDA. The combined shadows of the

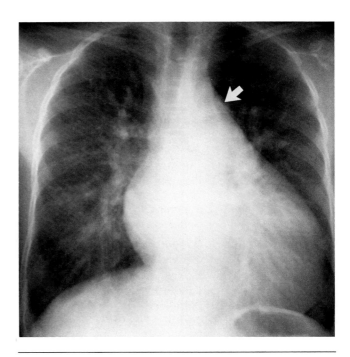

Figure 2-35. Patent ductus arteriosus. Radiographs show pulmonary arterial overcirculation, cardiomegaly, left atrial double density, and left ventricular enlargement, and posterior aortic arch enlargement (*arrow*). Vector of enlargement of the ventricle is lateral and inferior, indicating predominant left ventricular enlargement.

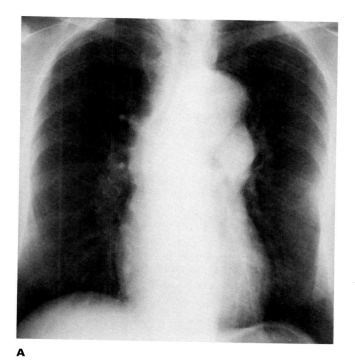

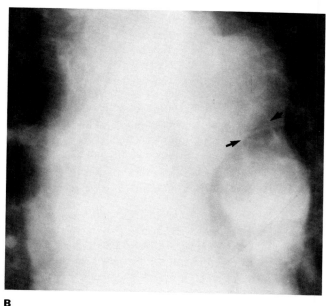

A

B

Figure 2-36. Eisenmenger's complex caused by patent ductus arteriosus. Thoracic radiograph (*A*) shows no pulmonary arterial overcirculation, but instead reveals attenuated peripheral vessels, normal heart size, and markedly enlarged main pulmonary arterial segment and aorta. Enlarged radiograph (*B*) shows parallel linear calcification (*arrows*) in the wall of the ductus arteriosus.

posterior arch and aortic spindle cause apparent elongation, prominence or atypical contour of the aortic knob. The aorticopulmonary window may be obliterated or convex due to the PDA.

7. Calcification in the aorticopulmonary window due to calcification of the walls of the ductus in older individuals (Fig. 2-36).

Although the PDA closes spontaneously during the neonatal period, especially in preterm infants, it cannot, like the VSD, be expected to close during childhood or adult life. The heart size increases in proportion to the severity of pulmonary overcirculation. Consequently, a substantial reduction in cardiomegaly on sequential radiographs must be considered an indication that pulmonary flow is being limited by increasing pulmonary vascular resistance and developing pulmonary arteriolopathy. The PDA with Eisenmenger's syndrome is characterized by normal cardiac size, right ventricular prominence, marked enlargement of central pulmonary arterial segment, and prominent aortic arch (Fig. 2-36).

Aorticopulmonary Window. This rare anomaly is a large connection between the ascending aorta and main pulmonary artery. Both semilunar valves are present, and this feature distinguishes the lesion from truncus arte-

riosus. This lesion usually causes a large left-to-right shunt and pulmonary edema in early infancy.

The physiology of this lesion is similar to PDA but is invariably severe, so nearly all cases present during early infancy. This lesion is almost never encountered in childhood or adult life. If an untreated patient is rarely encountered beyond infancy, irreversible pulmonary arterial hypertension is present.

Radiography. The radiographic features should resemble PDA if the patient survives beyond infancy. The usual radiographic appearance is severe pulmonary overcirculation and pulmonary edema. The ascending aorta and main pulmonary arterial segment are more prominent than in PDA in the infant.

Congenital Sinus of Valsalva Aneurysm and Fistula. The aneurysm begins as a funnel-shaped outpocketing at a congenital weakness at the junction of the aortic media and annulus fibrosis of the aortic valve. Congenital aneurysm arises from the right coronary sinus and noncoronary sinus. Aneurysm of the right coronary sinus ruptures into the right ventricle or right atrium, while those of the noncoronary rupture into the right atrium. This entity should be distinguished from diffuse aneurysmal dilatation of the sinuses, which occurs in Marfan's syndrome. A large acute rupture may cause intractable pulmonary edema. All fistulae to the right heart cause volume overload of the left heart, since there is volume overload of the downstream chambers. Depending upon the site of rupture, volume overload of the right ventricle and/or right atrium also occurs. These lesions may also be associated with aortic regurgitation and perimembranous or supracristal VSD.

Radiography. A large acute rupture causes pulmonary edema. Subacute or smaller communication produces pulmonary arterial overcirculation and cardiomegaly in proportion to the pulmonary arterial overcirculation. The salient radiographic findings are:

1. Pulmonary arterial overcirculation and/or edema.
2. Enlargement of left-sided cardiac chambers.
3. Enlargement of right ventricle (rupture into right ventricle or right atrium).
4. Enlargement of right atrium (rupture into right atrium).
5. Enlargement of main pulmonary and central pulmonary arterial segments.
6. Rarely, the aneurysm is sufficiently large so that there is asymmetrical dilatation at the base of the aorta.
7. Curvilinear calcification of the aneurysm occurs infrequently.

Coronary Arteriovenous Fistula. This is a fistula or angiodysplasia from a coronary artery to a coronary vein, coronary sinus, right atrium, right ventricle, or pulmonary artery. There may be multiple sites of communication. The involved coronary artery is usually dilated and tortuous. The right coronary artery is involved more frequently and most frequently enters the right atrium or ventricle. The shunt is usually small and does not produce recognizable pulmonary overcirculation or volume overload enlargement of the heart.

Radiography. Pulmonary arterial overcirculation and cardiomegaly are usually not evident. The ectatic coronary artery may infrequently be discernible on the thoracic radiograph. Ectasia of the circumflex coronary artery may cause a localized bulge in the upper left cardiac margin in the region near the site of the left atrium on the frontal radiograph. Calcification can rarely occur in the ectatic coronary artery.

Cyanotic

Tetralogy of Fallot. The major components of this anomaly are caused by a displacement of the outlet sep-

tum (conal septation) toward the right ventricle resulting in a diminutive right ventricular outflow region and failure of alignment of the outlet portion with the remainder of the ventricular septum. The latter abnormality causes a large ventricular septal defect (infracristal) and the aorta is located immediately over the defect (Fig. 2-37). Consequently, right ventricular blood is ejected directly into the aorta. There is a reciprocal relationship between the aortic and pulmonary arterial diameters; the ascending aorta is substantially enlarged in the presence of severe pulmonic stenosis and pulmonic atresia. The ventricular septal defect is nonrestrictive, so pressures are equal in the ventricles. Multiple VSDs may occur in this anomaly.

The obstruction to pulmonary blood flow is frequently diffuse and exists at multiple levels, causing subvalvular, valvular, and supravalvular stenoses. There is invariably infundibular stenosis. The annulus and proximal pulmonary artery are usually hypoplastic. The stenosis may involve the entire outflow region and include severe hypoplasia of the segmental and intraparenchymal pulmonary arteries. The extreme form of tetralogy is pulmonary atresia with a nonrestrictive VSD. Branch pulmonary arterial stenosis, especially at the origin of the left pulmonary artery, may cause asymmetric pulmonary blood flow. However, even in the absence of branch stenosis, preferential flow occurs to the right lung owing to the orientation of the right ventricular outflow tract. A right aortic arch is present in about 20% of patients with tetralogy; the incidence is about 25% with pulmonary atresia and ventricular septal defect (the extreme form of tetralogy).

The physiology of the anomaly consists of reduced pulmonary blood flow and arterial desaturation. Because

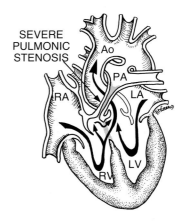

Figure 2-37. The anatomical components of tetralogy of Fallot. Stenotic pulmonary annulus and main pulmonary artery are visible. While infundibular narrowing is a constant feature, stenosis of the annulus and pulmonary artery is a variable among patients with this anomaly. The directions of blood flow through the heart are shown.

of the reduced blood flow through the lungs, the left-sided cardiac chambers are small. The right-to-left shunt is manifested by severe cyanosis.

Radiography. Tetralogy of Fallot is the most common lesion causing decreased pulmonary vascularity without substantial cardiomegaly in a cyanotic patient (Figs. 2-3, 2-38). In older patients with the anomaly, cardiomegaly may be present, especially after a systemic-to-pulmonary shunt has been constructed (Fig. 2-39). The salient radiographic features are

1. Decreased pulmonary vascularity (see Figs. 2-3, 2-38). Normal vascularity in a cyanotic individual is equated with decreased vascularity, since the distinction between normal and mildly decreased vascularity is frequently problematic.
2. Normal or nearly normal cardiac size.
3. Right ventricular enlargement or prominence. This may cause an uplifted cardiac apex (see Figs. 2-3, 2-38).
4. Concave or absent main pulmonary arterial segment (see Figs. 2-3, 2-38).
5. Small hilar pulmonary arteries. This may be most evident on the lateral view.

Table 2-4

Right Aortic Arch: Frequency in Congenital Heart Disease

Abnormality	Frequency (%)
Tetralogy of Fallot	20
Pulmonary atresia with VSD	25
Truncus arteriosus	35
Double outlet right ventricle	12
Tricuspid atresia	10–15
Transposition of great arteries	5–8
Ventricular septal defect	2

6. Prominent ascending aorta and aortic arch.
7. Right aortic arch (20%–25% of cases) (see Table 2-4).

Exceptional configuration can be observed, such as the aneurysmal main and hilar (especially the right) pulmonary arteries in patients with tetralogy and absent pulmonary valve (Fig. 2-40). Asymmetric pulmonary vascularity is frequently due to preferential flow to the right lung caused by the orientation of the elongated, narrow infundibulum of of the right ventricle (see Fig. 2-3); branch pulmonary arterial stenosis or atresia; compres-

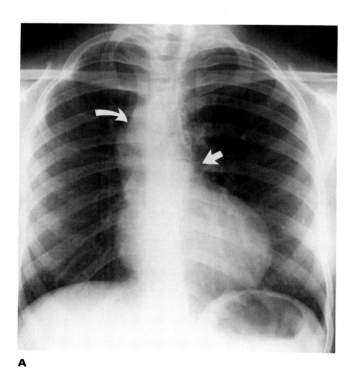

A

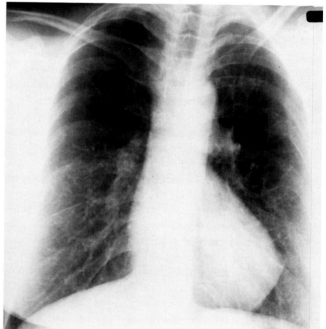

B

Figure 2-38. Two cases of tetralogy of Fallot. *A* shows reduced pulmonary vascularity, normal heart size, right ventricular prominence, and concave main pulmonary arterial segment (*arrow*) and right aortic arch (*curved arrow*). *B* shows normal vascularity, normal heart size, right ventricular prominence, and concave main pulmonary arterial segment.

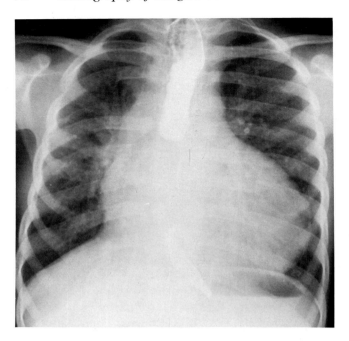

Figure 2-39. Tetralogy of Fallot after right subclavian–pulmonary arterial shunt. Asymmetric pulmonary blood flow is evident, with overcirculation on the right and cardiomegaly.

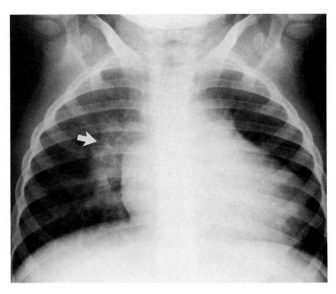

Figure 2-40. Tetralogy of Fallot with absent pulmonary valve. Aneurysmal dilatation of main and right pulmonary arterial segments (*arrow*) is diagnostic of this anomaly. Note the disparity in size of right hilar arterial region and the peripheral segments of the pulmonary arteries.

sion of the right pulmonary artery by a right aortic arch (rarely); and after a systemic-to-pulmonary artery shunt (see Fig. 2-39).

Early in life the thoracic radiograph may not be typical but becomes characteristic later (Fig. 2-41). Regression of the thymus reveals the concave main pulmonary artery segment characteristic of tetralogy of Fallot.

After surgical repair of tetralogy, a number of radiographic findings may be identified, such as aneurysm of a right ventricular outflow patch; asymmetry of pulmonary vascularity due to persistent branch pulmonary arterial stenosis; and progressive right ventricular enlargement due to pulmonary regurgitation complicating a transannular patch. Pulmonary arterial overcirculation can develop when a hemodynamically significant residual VSD exists after successful repair of outflow stenosis.

Transposition of Great Arteries (TGA). TGA is one of several abnormalities of arterioventricular connection. The others are double-outlet right ventricle, double-outlet left ventricle, and truncus arteriosus. All of these anomalies are admixture lesions. All produce cyanosis. In the absence of obstruction to blood flow, all are associated with pulmonary arterial overcirculation.

In TGA, the aorta arises from the right ventricle and the pulmonary artery arises from the left ventricle (Fig. 2-42). The base of the aorta is positioned anterior to pulmonary artery. If the aorta lies to the right of the pulmonary artery, the name d-TGA (dextro-TGA) applies, while if the aorta lies to the left of the pulmonary artery,

the name l-TGA (levo-TGA) applies. If the aorta is directly anterior to the pulmonary artery, the term a-TGA (antero-TGA) is sometimes used. Most patients with situs solitus and l-TGA also have inversion of the ventricles. With inversion of the ventricles, the right ventricle lies to the left of the left ventricle (L-ventricular loop) and is connected to the left atrium. This complex of l-TGA and inversion of the ventricles (L-ventricular loop) results in physiological correction of the flow pattern from pulmonary veins to aorta and is named corrected TGA (see Fig. 2-42*B*). The most common type of TGA is d-TGA with a normal relationship of the ventricles (D-ventricular loop), causing pulmonary venous blood to enter the pulmonary artery and desaturated systemic venous blood to enter the aorta. This anomaly is sometimes called complete TGA.

Associated lesions are frequent with TGA. All patients have an interatrial communication that must be enlarged (Rashkin balloon septostomy) after birth in order to prolong survival. The other common lesions are VSD and pulmonic stenosis. Pulmonic stenosis occurs at the subvalvular or valvular levels, or both. Pulmonic stenosis and VSD tend to occur together in about 30% of patients with TGA. Pulmonic stenosis may not be initially evident and can develop progressively during the first year. Patent ductus arteriosus is a less frequently associated lesion. About 50% of patients with tricuspid atresia have d-TGA. TGA frequently is present in patients with single ventricle.

The physiological consequence of TGA is pulmonary arterial overcirculation and cyanosis due to the combination of left-to-right and right-to-left shunts (ad-

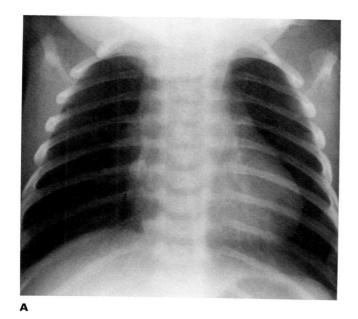
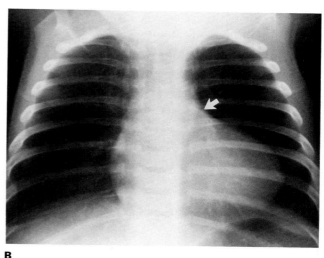

Figure 2-41. Radiographs showing tetralogy of Fallot in the first week (*A*) and at several months of age (*B*). *A* shows prominent thymus and normal cardiac configuration. *B* shows atrophy of the thymus and nearly concave main pulmonary arterial segment (*arrow*).

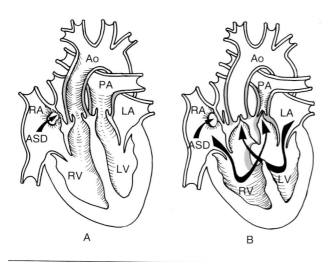

Figure 2-42. Anatomical features of transposition of the great arteries. Transposition with interatrial communication (*arrow*). Aorta originates from the right ventricle and pulmonary artery originates from the left ventricle. *B* shows pulmonary stenosis and ventricular septal defect in transposition. Direction of blood flow is shown.

mixture lesion). Because the pulmonary and systemic circulations are parallel, most of the blood ejected by the left ventricle into the pulmonary artery is recirculated. The severity of overcirculation is usually greater in the presence of VSD and reduced in the presence of pulmonic stenosis. Cardiac size increases in relation to the pulmonary overcirculation. Pulmonary arterial hypertension and arteriolopathy tend to ensue early in life in children with TGA. Pulmonary arteriolopathy and fixed hypertension not uncommonly develop at 6 to 12 months of age in TGA with VSD.

Transposition of the great arteries is the most common cyanotic heart lesion. Without surgical intervention, most of the infants would succumb in the first year of life.

Radiology. The radiographic appearance is influenced a great deal by the associated lesions. TGA is the most common anomaly causing pulmonary overcirculation in a cyanotic infant (Figs. 2-5, 2-42, 2-43, 2-44). The presence of significant pulmonic stenosis produces a radiographic appearance similar to that of tetralogy of Fallot, this is, decreased pulmonary vascularity and normal heart size in a cyanotic infant (see Fig. 2-12*B*). The radiographic appearance during the first day or first few days of life may not be characteristic, since a prominent thymus conceals the narrow great vessel region and pulmonary blood flow is still limited by high pulmonary vascular resistance persisting from intrauterine life (see Fig. 2-44). After thymic involution in the stressed newborn, the narrow base of the heart becomes evident. The salient radiographic features of d-TGA are:

1. Pulmonary arterial overcirculation. Asymmetry of pulmonary flow, greater on the right side, is sometimes apparent (Fig. 2-44).
2. Pulmonary edema is common, especially in the presence of a VSD or PDA.

3. Cardiomegaly. A cardiothoracic ratio exceeding 58% constitutes cardiomegaly in the neonatal period.
4. In the newborn, specific chamber enlargement is difficult to identify. In the older child, there is left atrial and right ventricular enlargement. Right atrium and right ventricle are enlarged.
5. Narrow vascular pedicle. The great vessels are usually but not invariably inconspicuous (Fig. 2-44). The ascending aorta occupies a more me-

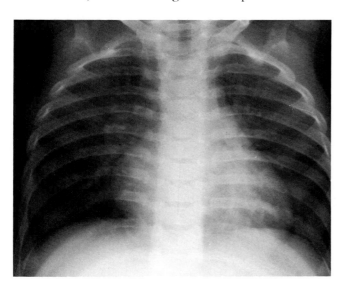

Figure 2-43. Transposition of great arteries. Pulmonary arterial overcirculation is indicated by large hilar and segmental pulmonary arteries.

dial position than normal and is hidden in the mediastinum, so a typical main pulmonary arterial segment is not present. Thus, there is the incongruity of pulmonary arterial overcirculation with a small or absent main pulmonary arterial segment. Infrequently, even in complete TGA, the aorta lies to the right or left of the pulmonary artery, causing a normal or even increased width of the pedicle.
6. Right aortic arch occurs in about 5% of patients with TGA, usually in association with pulmonic stenosis and VSD.
7. In the presence of pulmonic stenosis and VSD, there is decreased pulmonary vascular size and normal heart size, producing an appearance similar to tetralogy of Fallot (see Fig. 2-12B).

The onset of pulmonary arteriolopathy causes the radiographic appearance to alter. Peripheral pulmonary vascularity and heart size are reduced. The hilar pulmonary arteries are enlarged. The appearance may be altered after surgery. A prominent convexity may be evident along the upper right cardiac border after the Mustard (intra-atrial baffle procedure) or Senning procedures. Asymmetric or lobar pulmonary edema after a Mustard procedure (see Fig. 1-6C) should suggest obstruction to the entrance of the pulmonary veins by a redundant baffle. Right ventricular dilatation and failure is a complication occurring years after surgical correction; it is manifested radiographically by enlargement of the right ventricle and sometimes by pulmonary venous hypertension caused by associated tricuspid regurgitation.

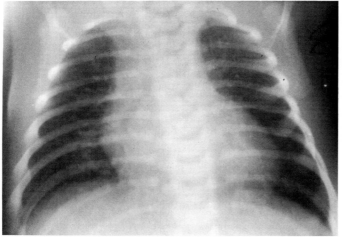

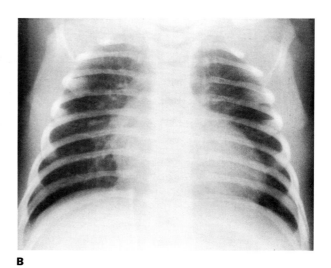

A   B

Figure 2-44. Transposition of great arteries (d-TGA). Radiograph on day one (A) and day seven (B). Initial radiograph shows prominent pulmonary vascularity but cardiac configuration is not characteristic. After involution of the thymus (B) the ovoid-shaped heart with a narrow great vessel pedicle is evident.

Corrected Transposition (I-TGA). Corrected transposition consists of arterioventricular transposition and atrioventricular discordance. The aorta originates from the right ventricle and the right ventricle is inverted with connection to the left atrium. There is an L-ventricular loop with the morphologic right ventricle to the left of the morphologic left ventricle. Thus, blood flow in the central circulation is corrected; pulmonary venous blood flows to the left atrium, to the right ventricle, and into the aorta. The majority of patients with corrected transposition have significant additional cardiac anomalies. The most frequent ones are pulmonic stenosis, VSD, Ebstein's anomaly (tricuspid regurgitation into left atrium), and complete heart block.

Radiography. The frontal radiograph is frequently diagnostic. The l-transposed aorta and inverted ventricle produce a long convexity of the upper left cardiac border (Fig. 2-45A–C).

Other features are related to the frequently associated lesions. A VSD alone may cause pulmonary arterial overcirulation, whereas VSD and pulmonic stenosis can produce reduced pulmonary vascularity. The salient radiographic features are:

1. Prominent convexity of uppr left cardiac border (see Fig. 2-45). The convexity may extend nearly to the arch (see Fig. 2-45A,B) or merely involve the base of the heart (see Fig. 2-45C).
2. Ascending aortic shadow on the right is not visible (Fig. 2-45A,C).
3. Crossing of the edge of the ascending aorta and the lateral edge of the proximal descending aorta (see Fig. 2-45C).
4. Conspicuous absence of a convex main pulmonary arterial segment, even in the presence of pulmonary arterial overcirculation. Sometimes, there is upward tilt of the right and downward tilt of the left pulmonary artery.
5. Left atrial enlargement can be caused by pulmonary overcirculation caused by the VSD, or tricuspid regurgitation caused by Ebstein's anomaly.

Double-Outlet Right Ventricle (DORV). Double-outlet right ventricle is an anomaly in which more than 50% of both great vessels originate from the right ventricle (see Fig. 2-46). The aorta is positioned further to the right of the pulmonary artery and originates completely from the right ventricle, whereas the pulmonary artery may originate entirely from the right ventricle or have a biventricular origin (Taussig–Bing malformation). A VSD is always present and other associated anomalies are common. The physiology of DORV is determined to a great degree by the position of the VSD. A VSD oriented

to the aortic valve (subaortic VSD) causes preferential flow from the left ventricle into the aorta and is often associated with significant pulmonic stenosis, resulting in physiology and radiographic appearance similar to tetralogy of Fallot. In the absence of pulmonic stenosis, preferential left ventricular to aortic flow may make cyanosis minimal. A VSD located beneath the pulmonic valve (Taussig–Bing malformation) causes preferential flow from the left ventricle into the pulmonary artery and consequently severe pulmonary arterial overcirculation. The right ventricular outflow occurs preferentially into the aorta; thus, there is also cyanosis. Coarctation or interruption of the aortic arch is sometimes associated with the subpulmonic VSD. A large VSD may be situated beneath the origin of both great vessels (doubly committed VSD) or may be displaced away from both origins (noncommitted VSD). The great arteries tend to be side by side at the base of the heart, but either vessel can be located more anteriorly.

This is an admixture lesion that causes the combination of cyanosis (right-to-left shunt) and pulmonary arterial overcirculation (left-to-right shunt). The severity of pulmonic stenosis and position of the VSD initially determine the relative severity of the two shunts. Eventually, the rise in pulmonary vascular resistance may become a prime determinant.

DORV with subaortic VSD presents in a manner similar to either a large VSD (no pulmonic stenosis) or tetralogy of Fallot (pulmonic stenosis). DORV with subpulmonic VSD presents like complete TGA.

Double-outlet left ventricle is an exceedingly rare anomaly in which both arteries originate from a morphologic left ventricle.[19] The presentation and radiologic appearance are similar to DORV.

Radiography. The radiographic appearance mimics other anomalies such as VSD, d-TGA (Fig. 2-47), and tetralogy of Fallot (Fig. 2-12C). The presentation depends upon the location of the VSD and the presence of pulmonic stenosis.

The salient features of DORV without significant pulmonic stenosis are

1. Pulmonary arterial overcirculation. It is one of the causes of cyanosis and pulmonary arterial overcirculation (Fig. 2-47).
2. Cardiomegaly.
3. Enlargement of left atrium, left ventricle and right ventricle. Distinction between left and right ventricle enlargement during infancy is usually inconclusive.
4. Widened great-artery pedicle due to side-by-side position of aorta and pulmonary artery (Fig. 2-47). This is not always evident. It can be a distinguishing feature when compared to the appearance of d-TGA.

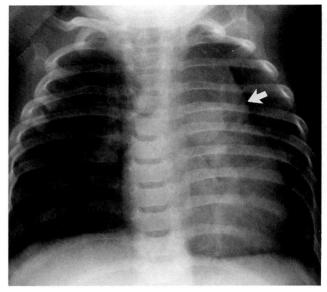

A

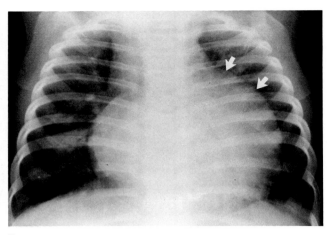

B

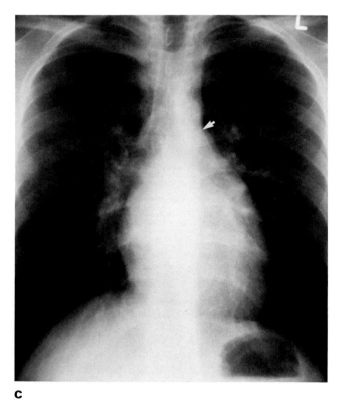

C

Figure 2-45. Three examples of the prominence of the upper left cardiac border in l-transposition of great arteries. *A:* Extreme prominence. *B:* Extreme prominence over a long segment (*arrows*). *C:* Prominence with crossing of ascending aortic line and descending aortic line (*small arrow*). The ascending aortic shadow is not observed to the right of the spine.

5. Prominent main pulmonary arterial segment. This feature can also distinguish DORV from d-TGA.
6. Signs of coarctation or interruption of the aortic arch. The salient radiographic features of DORV with pulmonic stenosis (see Fig. 2-12*C*) are:
   1. Decreased pulmonary vascularity.
   2. Normal or nearly normal cardiac size.

3. Right ventricular prominence.
4. Inconspicuous main pulmonary arterial segment.
5. Right aortic arch in about 10% to 15% of patients.

Tricuspid Atresia. Tricuspid atresia is the absence of a direct connection of the right atrium to the right ven-

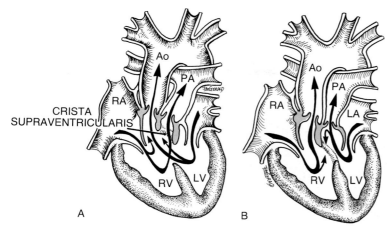

CRISTA
SUPRAVENTRICULARIS

A   B

Figure 2-46. Double-outlet right ventricle. Pulmonary artery and aorta originate from the right ventricle and ventricular septal defect. *A,* defect is located beneath the aorta so that blood from the left ventricle streams toward the aorta. *B,* defect is located beneath the pulmonary artery so that blood from the left ventricle preferentially enters the pulmonary artery. Direction of blood flow through the heart is shown.

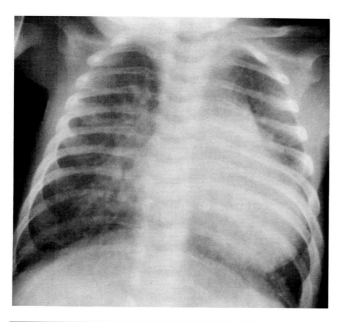

Figure 2-47. Double-outlet right ventricle. Pulmonary arterial overcirculation and cardiomegaly. Prominent great vessel region is shown rather than narrow great vessel region as seen in d-TGA.

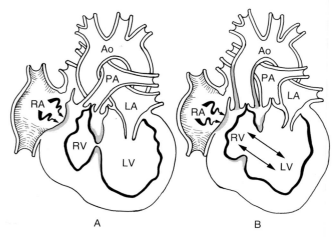

A   B

Figure 2-48. Tricuspid atresia. Patient with tricuspid atresia may have normal arterioventricular connections (*A*) or transposition of great arteries (*B*). Associated lesions are also pulmonary valvular or subvalvular stenosis, or atresia and a variable-sized ventricular septal defect.

tricle (Fig. 2-48). The atresia can be due to a membrane or a ridge of muscle between the chambers. An ASD or patent foramen ovale are always present. Other associated lesions are common and are usually important in determining the physiology and clinical presentation. The most frequently associated lesions are TGA, VSD, and pulmonic stenosis. A classification of tricuspid atresia based upon the presence or absence of these associated lesions has been proposed by Keith[20] and Edwards[21]:

I. Tricuspid atresia without TGA.
   a. With pulmonary atresia and no VSD.
   b. With pulmonary stenosis and small restrictive VSD.
   c. With no pulmonary stenosis and large nonrestrictive VSD.

II. Tricuspid atresia with TGA.
   a. With pulmonary atresia and large VSD.
   b. With pulmonary stenosis and large VSD.
   c. With no pulmonary stenosis and large VSD.

The most common form is tricuspid atresia with pulmonic stenosis and normally related great arteries and restrictive VSD. TGA is present in about 30% of patients with tricuspid atresia. It is usually associated with VSD and no pulmonic stenosis.

When the VSD is large and the pulmonary stenosis mild or nonexistent, there is pulmonary overcirculation. This is the situation both for normally related arteries and TGA. Restriction of pulmonary blood flow usually exists at pulmonic valvular and subvalvular levels or at a restrictive VSD. A small atrial septal communication also limits pulmonary flow and in addition causes the right atrium to enlarge. In spite of obstruction to the right

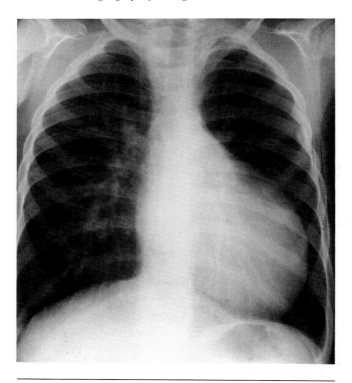

Figure 2-49. Tricuspid atresia with nonrestrictive interatrial communication, pulmonary arterial overcirculation, and cardiomegaly. The right atrial border is flat in the presence of a large ASD. Compare Figure 2-13*B,* on which the right atrium is markedly dilated in the presence of a restrictive interatrial communication.

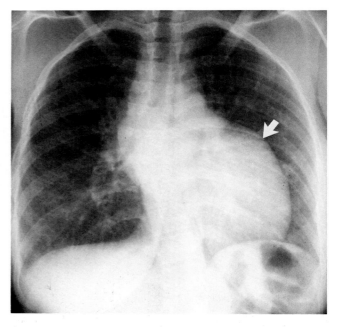

Figure 2-50. Tricuspid atresia, transposition, and juxtaposition of atrial appendages. Prominent upper left cardiac border (*arrow*) is due to the abnormal position of the right atrial appendage on the left, above the left atrial appendage. The concavity in the region of the right atrium is also characteristic of this anomaly. The appearance is accentuated by the scoliosis.

atrial outlet, the right atrium usually does not dilate, since a large interatrial communication causes the right atrium to function as a venous conduit similar to the vena cavae.

Radiography. The radiographic appearance can be variable and is determined by associated lesions (Figs. 2-13, 2-49).[22] Thus, the salient radiographic features can be:

1. With normally related great vessels, VSD, and pulmonic stenosis the appearance is similar to tetralogy of Fallot (see Fig. 2-13*A*). There is decreased pulmonary vascularity, small central pulmonary arteries, and normal or nearly normal heart size. A distinguishing feature from tetralogy, if discernible, is prominence of the left atrium and left ventricle.
2. With transposition of the great arteries, VSD and no pulmonic stenosis, the typical feature of d-TGA are present. There is pulmonary overcirculation, cardiomegaly, and a narrow vascular pedicle. A distinguishing feature may be the right atrial border. The right atrial border (right atrial enlargement) is frequently prominent in d-TGA, whereas it is not prominent or even flat

in tricuspid atresia when the interatrial communication is large (Fig. 2-49).

3. With a small (restrictive) interatrial communication, the right atrium may enlarge considerably. The right atrium enlarges to the extent of causing considerable cardiomegaly as depicted on the frontal radiograph (Fig. 2-13*B*).
4. Tricuspid atresia with TGA is sometimes associated with left juxtaposition of the atrial appendages: the right atrial appendage extends posteriorly behind the great arteries and lies above the left atrial appendage. This causes a prominent upper left cardiac border and flattening of the right cardiac border (Fig. 2-50).

Single Ventricle. Single ventricle consists of a predominant ventricle which receives both atrioventricular valves (double inlet ventricle) and a remnant portion of the other ventricle (Fig. 2-51). A more specific term for most of the anomalies grouped under this title is univentricular atrioventricular connection. The great arteries can both originate from the dominant ventricle or one may originate from the small ventricle. The ventricular loop can be D or L. The dominant ventricle can be either the left or the right. The L-loop is frequent for single ventricle of the left ventricular type, while the D-loop is usual

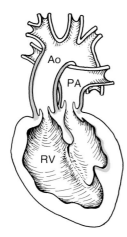

Figure 2-51. Diagram of single ventricle (univentricular atrioventricular connections). There is one complete ventricle and the outlet portion only of the second ventricle. There may be normally related great arteries, transposition, or double-outlet ventricle. The outlet chamber is frequently on the left side of the heart in single ventricle of the left ventricle type.

for single ventricle of the right ventricular type. Occasionally, the internal morphology is primitive and uncharacteristic for either ventricle; this has been called primitive single ventricle. Another entity grouped with single ventricle is more properly called common ventricle. In this anomaly, the ventricular septum is represented only by a ridge of tissue but all components of both ventricles exist and each receives an atrioventricular valve.

Single ventricle is frequently associated with an abnormality of arterioventricular connection such as TGA or DORV. Normally related great vessels are uncommon with single ventricle. The left ventricular type of single ventricle is frequently associated with an inverted right ventricular outlet chamber and l-TGA. The dominant ventricle communicates with the outlet chamber through a "bulboventricular foramen."

The physiology is determined to a substantial degree by associated obstruction of the outflow to the pulmonary artery or aorta. There is admixture of systemic and pulmonary venous blood in the dominant ventricle, so both cyanosis and pulmonary overcirculation occur. The presence and severity of the pulmonary overcirculation is regulated by pulmonary stenosis. If pulmonary stenosis is severe, the physiology and clinical presentation is similar to tetralogy of Fallot. If obstruction to pulmonary blood flow is not present, then the physiology and clinical presentation are similar to those of transposition. The physiology of the common ventricle is identical to a large VSD, which is really the proper designation of this lesion.

Radiography. The radiographic appearance is related to associated anomalies.

1. With normally related arteries and the absence of pulmonic stenosis, the appearance is like a VSD or d-TGA, depending upon the preferential streaming in the ventricle. There is pulmonary overcirculation and cardiomegaly.
2. With significant pulmonic stenosis and normally related great arteries, the appearance is reduced pulmonary vascularity and normal or nearly normal heart size. The appearance is similar to tetralogy of Fallot (see Fig. 2-12*A*).
3. With d-TGA, the appearance can be typical of d-TGA. Pulmonary blood flow may be increased or decreased.
4. With l-TGA, the appearance can be typical of l-TGA. Pulmonary blood flow may be increased or decreased (Fig. 2-52).

A notch along the upper left cardiac border may be observed owing to the intersection of the contour of an inverted right ventricular outlet chamber with the dominant ventricle (Fig. 2-53).

Truncus Arteriosus. Truncus arteriosus is a single trunk originating from the heart and supplying the pulmonary, systemic and coronary arteries. The truncus straddles a large VSD. It is an admixture lesion with both left-to-right and right-to-left shunt. Two classification sys-

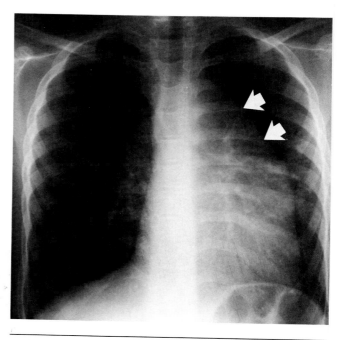

Figure 2-52. Single ventricle with inverted outlet chamber (L-loop) and l-TGA. Prominent convexity of upper left cardiac border represents the inverted RV outlet chamber and the l-transposed ascending aorta (*arrows*).

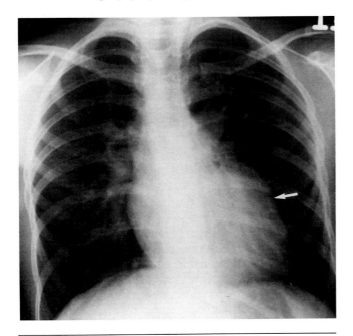

Figure 2-53. Single ventricle of the LV type with inverted RV outlet chamber. Note the notch along the left cardiac border (*arrow*) representing the transition in contour of the dominant ventricle and the outlet chamber. Note the right aortic arch.

tems for truncus arteriosus are extant currently. The older and more familiar one was proposed by Collett and Edward in 1949.[26] The four types are grouped according to the site of origin of the pulmonary arteries from the truncus (Fig. 2-54).

Type I. A main pulmonary artery originates from the proximal portion of the truncus, usually from the left posterolateral aspect.

Type II. Right and left pulmonary arteries have individual origins from the posterior aspect of the truncus.

Type III. One of both pulmonary arteries arises from the lateral aspect of the truncus.

Type IV. No pulmonary arteries arise from the ascending truncus (aorta) but rather from the descending aorta. This type is not really a truncus arteriosus but rather pulmonary atresia with VSD and major pulmonary blood flow from bronchial and other systemic arteries originating from the descending aorta.

The other classification devised by Van Pragh and Van Pragh in 1965[27] also consists of four types:

Type I. Common pulmonary artery arises from truncus.

Type II. Right and left pulmonary arteries arise separately from truncus.

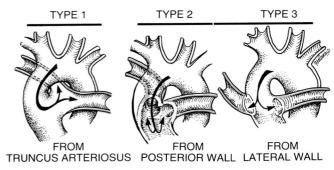

Figure 2-54. The types of truncus arteriosus. Type I—single origin of main pulmonary artery; Type II—separate origins of left and right pulmonary arteries from dorsal as part of the truncus; Type III—separate origins of left and right pulmonary arteries from the left and right side of truncus.

Type III. Absence of one pulmonary artery, other pulmonary artery arises from ductus.

Type IV. Common pulmonary artery arises from truncus with arch interruption.

The truncal valve can have two to five cusps. The valves with numbers of cusps more or fewer than three are frequently incompetent, and truncal insufficiency can be severe. Hemitruncus is not infrequent; one pulmonary artery originates from the ascending aorta and the other arises directly from the right ventricle. Stenosis at the origin of the right and/or left pulmonary arteries is common; this is especially so in types II and III of Collett and Edwards. Consequently, asymmetry of blood flow occurs with this anomaly.

The physiology is characterized by excess pulmonary blood flow and frequently by volume overload, especially of left-sided chambers. This is one of the lesions causing pulmonary arterial overcirculation in a cyanotic patient. Congestive heart failure and pulmonary edema are usually dominant.

Radiography. The radiographic features of truncus arteriosus vary among the types and to a major extent are dependent upon the presence and severity of stenosis of the pulmonary trunk stenosis and stenoses at the site of origin of individual pulmonary arteries. The level of pulmonary vascular resistance also determines the radiographic features. The appearance of type IV of Collett and Edward is not considered here.

The salient radiographic features are:

1. Pulmonary arterial overcirculation (see Fig. 2-17). Asymmetry of flow is not uncommon, even to the extent of plethora on one side and oligemia on the other.

2. Pulmonary venous hypertension or edema is frequent, especially in type I.

3. Cardiomegaly. The heart size is often, but not always, proportionate to the pulmonary overcir-

culation. Cardiomegaly may also be related to truncal insufficiency.

4. Four-chamber enlargement may be present.
5. Enlargement of left atrium and left ventricle is generally identified (see Fig. 2-17*B*).
6. Prominent main pulmonary arterial segment (type I) (Figs. 2-17*B*, 2-55) or reduced main pulmonary arterial segment (type II or III). In type I the left pulmonary artery has a higher position than usual, and a comma-shaped configuration ("hilar comma") as it curves upward and leftward (see Fig. 2-55).
7. Right aortic arch in about 35% of patients (Figs. 2-17, 2-55; see Table 2-4).
8. Dilated ascending aorta. Two cyanotic lesions are frequently associated with a large ascending aortic shadow; one causes decreased pulmonary vascularity (tetralogy of Fallot) and the other causes increased pulmonary vascularity (truncus arteriosus).

Untreated patients with truncus arteriosus frequently develop high pulmonary resistance due to arteriolopathy. This is recognized by decreasing peripheral pulmonary arterial diameter with further enlargement of central pulmonary arteries and reduction in heart size (see Fig. 2-55).

Total Anomalous Pulmonary Venous Connection.
All pulmonary veins connect to a systemic venous structure or the right atrium directly in this anomaly. This is another admixture lesion. Generally, the pulmonary veins form a central confluence before entering the systemic venous site. Infrequently, they do not all join together and may drain to different sites. This anomaly is divided into three types based upon the site of pulmonary venous drainage (Fig. 2-56):

1. Supracardiac type. Connections are to the left innominate vein, right superior vena cava, or azygous vein. A left-sided vertical vein connects the pulmonary venous confluence to the left innominate vein.
2. Cardiac type. Connections to right atrium or coronary sinus.
3. Infracardiac type. Connection is below the diaphragm to the portal vein or one of its branches, ductus venosus, or hepatic vein. In this type, a long vein courses from the pulmonary venous confluence and through the esophageal hiatus to its site of infradiaphragmatic connection. Pulmonary venous drainage is always obstructed with this type due to a variety of mechanisms, including narrowing or stenosis of the connecting vein, its site of connection with the systemic vein, or the systemic vein itself. The necessity for

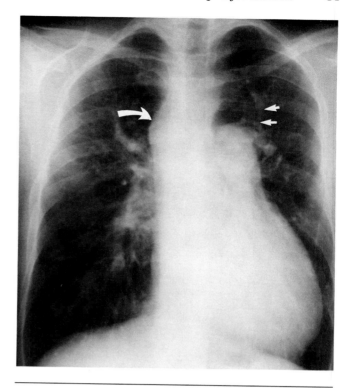

Figure 2-55. Truncus arteriosus type I with pulmonary arterial hypertension. This is a pathognomic appearance for this anomaly. There is a right aortic arch (*curved arrow*), large main pulmonary arterial segment occupying a high position, with a comma-shaped left upper lobe pulmonary artery (*arrow*). The discrepancy in diameter of the central and peripheral pulmonary arterial segments suggest Eisenmenger's complex.

passage of pulmonary venous blood through the hepatic sinusoids has also been held to be an additional site of obstruction. However, portal venous pressure is not higher than pulmonary venous pressure in normal patients. Infrequently, TAPVC above the diaphragm is associated with pulmonary venous obstruction.

The physiology of TAPVC depends upon whether or not pulmonary venous obstruction exists. Mixing systemic and pulmonary venous blood occurs in the right atrium and there is an obligatory right-to-left shunt of mixed venous blood through an interatrial connection. The size of the communication determines the volume of the flow to the left heart. Preferential flow from the right atrium is usually to the right ventricle and pulmonary artery, causing a large volume of recirculated blood. In TAPVC above the diaphragm, the volume of pulmonary blood flow is very high and is the major feature, while cyanosis may be mild. The volume overload of the lungs may be so great that pulmonary edema occurs.

In TAPVC with obstruction the major feature is pulmonary venous hypertension and edema. The flow to the

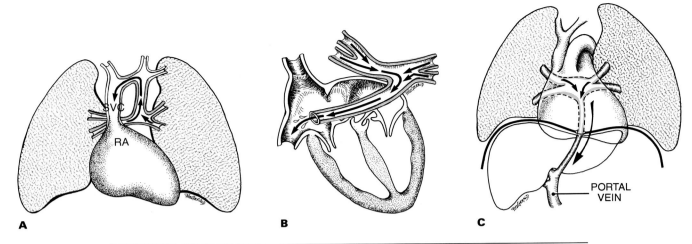

Figure 2-56. The types of total anomalous pulmonary venous connection. *A:* Supracardiac type. There is a venous confluence behind the left atrium that drains by a vertical vein to the left brachiocephalic vein. *B:* Cardiac type. There is a confluence behind the left atrium that drains to the coronary sinus or to the right atrium. *C:* Infracardiac type. There is a confluence behind the left atrium that drains by a vein connected to the portal venous system or ductus venosus.

lungs is not very great. Because there is less pulmonary venous blood to mix with the desaturated systemic venous blood, cyanosis is conspicuous. TAPVC can occur in association with a number of other cardiac anomalies. It is a common lesion in patients with the asplenia syndrome.

Radiography. The radiographic features are different in TAPVC without obstruction and TAPVC with obstruction.

The salient radiographic features of TAPVC with obstruction are:

1. Pulmonary arterial overcirculation (Figs. 2-18, 2-57). Pulmonary venous hypertension and edema may be present with extreme volume overload.
2. Cardiomegaly. This is usually proportionate to the pulmonary arterial overcirculation.
3. Enlargement of right atrium and right ventricle.
4. The enlarged systemic vein into which drainage occurs or the anomalous connecting vein may be visible as the snowman appearance (see Figs. 2-18, 2-57), dilated right superior vena cava, or dilated azygous vein or coronary sinus.

The salient radiographic features of TAPVC with obstruction are:

1. Pulmonary edema (see Fig. 2-21).
2. Normal heart size.
3. Prominence of right atrium and, less frequently, right ventricle.
4. Infrequently the connecting vein can be identified on the lateral view in a position behind the

heart. A barium swallow may show an anterior impression on the esophagus.

The appearance of the lungs in the infant with the obstructed form may mimic diffuse lung disease such as diffuse pneumonia and, especially, meconium aspiration. The hyperaeration and coarse interstitial markings may be caused by these diseases as well as TAPVC with obstruction.

Ebstein's Anomaly. Ebstein's anomaly is a deformity of the tricuspid valve in which one or more leaflets are displaced into the inflow portion of the right ventricle. The leaflet(s) have lines of attachment to the right ventricle of varying length. The displacement into the right ventricle and deformity of the valve cause tricuspid regurgitation and the mural attachments in the right ventricle may cause obstruction to pulmonary blood flow. The septal and posterior leaflet are involved while the anterior leaflet usually has a normal attachment to the atrioventricular ring. A small to substantial portion of the inflow region of the right ventricle has a thin wall and lacks ventricular myocardium (atrialization of the right ventricle). A patent foramen ovale or secundum atrial septal defect is present in about 80% of cases.

The physiological consequence of the lesion is nearly always tricuspid regurgitation and usually a small volume right-to-left shunt. Cyanosis may be absent or very mild. Occasionally the major effect is tricuspid obstruction, owing to limitation of the atrioventricular inlet to only narrow slits in the displaced leaflets of the valve. In this case the right-to-left shunt is more severe. In the

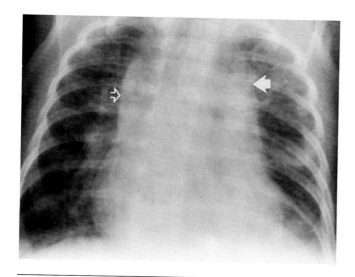

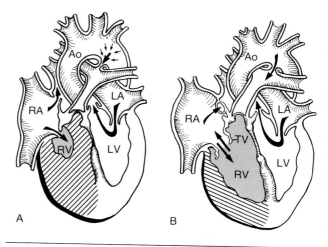

Figure 2-58. Pulmonary atresia with intact ventricular septum. Type I (*A*) is characterized by a small right ventricle and small tricuspid valve with mild or no tricuspid regurgitation. Type II (*B*) is characterized by enlarged right ventricle and right atrium caused by severe tricuspid regurgitation. An interatrial communication is present and a patent ductus arteriosus of variable diameter is frequently present. The directions of blood flow are shown.

Figure 2-57. Total anomalous pulmonary venous connection, supracardiac type (type I). Pulmonary arterial overcirculation, cardiomegaly, and enlargement of superior mediastinum ("snowman appearance"). The snowman is caused by the dilated vertical vein connecting the venous confluence to the left innominate vein (left-sided enlargement, *arrow*) and the dilated superior vena cava (right-sided enlargement, *open arrow*).

20% or so of patients without an interatrial communication, cyanosis is not present.

Radiography. This lesion is characterized by the triad of cyanosis, decreased pulmonary vascularity and cardiomegaly (see Figs. 2-4, 2-15). Because of the high pulmonary vascular resistance in the peripheral period, tricuspid regurgitation and the degree of cardiomegaly may be severe at this time (see Fig. 2-15*A*).

The salient radiographic features are:

1. Decreased pulmonary vascularity (Figs. 2-4, 2-15).
2. Cardiomegaly (Figs. 2-4, 2-15).
3. Enlarged right atrium. The right heart border is elongated, with a prominent convexity (Figs. 2-4, 2-15).
4. Enlargement of right ventricle. The right ventricle is less conspicuous than the atrium.
5. Main pulmonary arterial segment and hilar segments are small. However, the right ventricular outflow tract may produce a prominent bulge just caudal to the pulmonary arterial segment on the frontal view.
6. Small thoracic aorta.

Pulmonary Atresia with Intact Ventricular Septum. Pulmonary atresia with intact ventricular septum exists in two forms: hypoplasia of the right ventricle and tricuspid valve with little or no tricuspid regurgitation (type I); a normal or enlarged right ventricle with

significant tricuspid regurgitation (type II) (Fig. 2-58). Note that this entity is distinct from pulmonary atresia with VSD (extreme form of tetralogy of Fallot). Blood reaches the left side of the heart via a patent foramen ovale or atrial septal defect. The atresia is usually limited to the valve and the distal main and central pulmonary arteries are free of stenoses. Of patients with this anomaly, 65% to 80% have a small, very thick-walled right ventricle. Direct communication between the diminutive right ventricle and myocardial sinusoids and coronary arteries causes a right-to-left shunt into the coronaries. Desaturated blood entering the coronary arteries may be an important factor causing the substantial incidence of sudden death in patients with this anomaly.

The physiology of this lesion is reduced pulmonary blood flow, so that the volume of fully oxygenated blood entering the left atrium is small. The shunting of nearly all systemic venous blood occurs through the interatrial communication. There is admixture of desaturated and oxygenated blood in the left atrium. Because the volume of pulmonary venous blood is reduced, cyanosis is severe. Blood reaches the lung by a patent ductus arteriosus and/or bronchial arteries. Survival usually depends upon surgical construction of a systemic to pulmonary shunt in the first few days of life.

Radiography. The salient radiographic features of type I pulmonary atresia (see Fig. 2-14*A*) are:

1. Decreased pulmonary vascularity.
2. Normal cardiac size or only slight cardiomegaly.
3. Concave main pulmonary arterial segment and small hilar pulmonary arteries.

4. Uplifted apex. This appearance may be due to left ventricular enlargement in the presence of a diminutive right ventricle.
5. Thoracic aorta can be enlarged.

The salient radiographic features of type II (see Fig. 2-14*B*) are:

1. Decreased pulmonary vascularity.
2. Cardiomegaly.
3. Right atrial and right ventricular enlargement.
4. Small pulmonary arterial segment.
5. Thoracic aorta can be enlarged.

In the early neonatal period pulmonary arterial overcirculation may be present with either type because of a patent ductus arteriosus.

Pulmonic Stenosis. Pulmonary valvular stenosis exists in two distinct syndromes. The most common type presents in an innocuous manner with mild symptoms, systolic murmur and slightly abnormal thoracic radiograph. Infrequently, infants present with severe symptoms and marked cardiomegaly. The severity of the valvular stenosis is so great that the right ventricle dilates markedly and right ventricular failure ensues. Because of the elevated right-sided diastolic pressure, there is considerable right-to-left shunting across a secundum ASD or stretched foramen ovale. When the stenosis is so severe that right ventricular failure occurs, the entity is called critical pulmonary stenosis.

The physiology in the typical type is normal pulmonary blood flow, which is maintained by right ventricular hypertension and hypertrophy. Critical pulmonic stenosis does cause reduced pulmonary blood flow; the systemic venous blood is diverted to the left atrium through the interatrial connection as a right-to-left shunt.

Radiography. The radiographic appearance can be very different depending upon the two presentations.

The salient features of compensated valvular pulmonic stenosis are:

1. Normal pulmonary vascularity.
2. Normal cardiac size.
3. Right ventricular enlargement or prominence. This is usually detected initially on the lateral view as a prominent convexity of the anterior cardiac border or filling of the retrosternal space.
4. Post-stenotic dilatation of main pulmonary arterial segment (see Fig. 2-59).
5. Dilated and usually laterally displaced left pulmonary artery (Fig. 2-59*B,C*).

The salient radiographic features of critical pulmonic stenosis are:

1. Decreased pulmonary vascularity.
2. Cardiomegaly.
3. Enlargement of right atrium and ventricle.
4. Enlarged main pulmonary arterial segment. The prominent main pulmonary artery may not be identified in the neonate due to concomitantly enlarged right ventricular outflow region and overlying thymus.

Hypoplastic Left Heart. Hypoplastic left heart is a complex of lesions usually causing death in the first week of life. In recent years, palliative procedures and heart transplantation have been applied. The lesion consists of several or all of the following features: hypoplastic ascending aorta, severe aortic stenosis or atresia, hypoplastic left ventricle (thick wall and diminutive cavity), and mitral atresia (Fig. 2-60). The coronary arteries are perfused by right-to-left flow across a patent ductus arteriosus and retrograde into the ascending aorta. An atrial septal communication is present so that admixture of pulmonary and systemic venous blood occurs in the right atrium. Consequently, there is volume overload of the right-sided chambers and excess pulmonary blood flow. The usual clinical presentation is severe congestive heart failure in the first few days of life.

Radiography. This is one of the lesions which cause pulmonary overcirculation and cyanosis. The major symptomatic feature is severe congestive heart failure. However, the presenting features and the presence of pulmonary edema on the thoracic radiograph cause this anomaly to be classified as a group V lesion.

The salient radiographic features are:

1. Pulmonary arterial overcirculation. There is usually also severe pulmonary edema (Figs. 2-23, 2-61).
2. Cardiomegaly.
3. Prominent right-sided chambers, especially the right atrium (Fig. 2-23).
4. Because of the patent ductus the aortic arch may be prominent (Fig. 2-23).

Coarctation of the Aorta. Coarctation of the aorta is a narrowing of the distal aortic arch and/or proximal descending aorta due to a discrete fibromuscular ring or due to a long or short segment tunnel narrowing of the aortic isthmus. There may also be hypoplasia of the posterior portion of the aortic arch. The coarctation usually occurs near the site of attachment of the ligamentum arteriosus and distal to the left subclavian artery. The coarctation is infrequently proximal to the origin of the left suclavian artery. The coarctation can extend into the origin of the left subclavian artery, causing stenosis of this artery. Both of these situations cause a lower arterial pressure in the left compared to the right pulmonary ar-

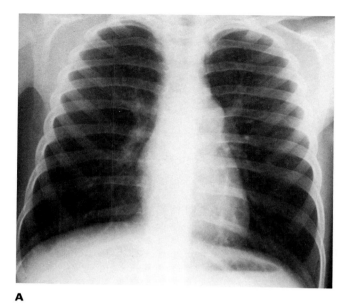

A

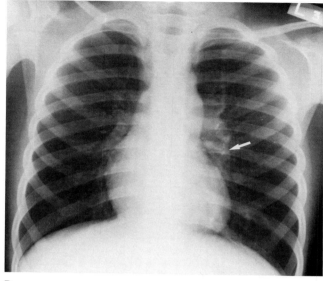

B

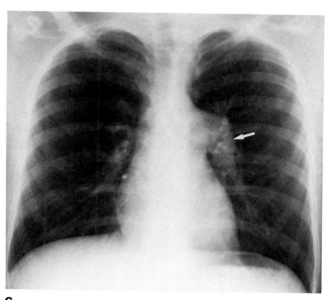

C

Figure 2-59. Valvular pulmonic stenosis in three patients. Radiographs show varying degrees of enlargement of the main and left pulmonary arterial segments. The descending branch of the left pulmonary artery is frequently very prominent (*B, C, arrows*). The left pulmonary artery sometimes projects prominently into the left lung (*C*).

tery. Anomalous origin of the right subclavian artery (retroesophageal right subclavian artery) from a site distal to the coarctation causes lower arterial pressure in the right arm.

Coarctation may be associated with a wide variety of congenital lesions but two occur with noticeable frequency; these are PDA and VSD. The triad of coarctation, VSD and PDA, has been called the coarctation syndrome and is especially common when the lesion presents in early infancy. A bicuspid aortic valve occurs in a high percentage of patients.

The physiology is hypertension in arteries originating proximal to the site of coarctation and reduced blood flow to arteries arising below the coarctation. If the coarctation occurs proximal to the site of origin of one of the subclavian arteries, then there is hypertension in only one arm and rib notching on only the side with hypertension. Hypertension causes left ventricular hypertrophy usually, but may induce left ventricular dilatation and failure if extremely severe. Left ventricular dilatation, myocardial failure, and pulmonary edema are most likely to occur in early infancy.

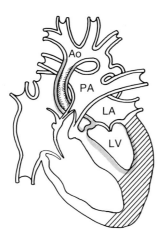

Figure 2-60. Hypoplastic left heart. Consists of hypoplasia of the left ventricular chamber, hypoplasia of the ascending aorta, severe aortic stenosis or atresia and a small or atretic mitral valve. A patent ductus arteriosus provides blood flow to the systemic circulation.

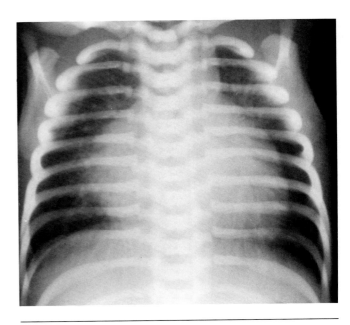

Figure 2-61. Hypoplastic left heart syndrome. Pulmonary venous congestion and marked cardiomegaly in a newborn.

Radiography. The radiographic features are dependent upon whether left ventricular decompensation has occurred. The appearance is modified by the presence of VSD and PDA. A large left-to-right shunt may be a predominant sign in this situation.

The salient radiographic features in compensated coarctation are:

1. Rib notching (Fig. 2-62). The 4th and 8th ribs are the areas usually notched. The 3rd and 9th ribs are less frequently notched. The notching consists of scalloped regions on the undersurface of the posterior portion of the ribs. The posterior upper surface may infrequently be involved. Sclerosis may outline the scalloped sites. Rib notching is unusual in patients less than 5 years of age. Rib notching depends upon the origin of the ipsilateral subclavian artery proximal to the site of the coarctation. Coarctation proximal to the left subclavian arterial origin causes right-sided rib notching only, while an anomalous origin of the right subclavian artery from a site below the coarctation produces unilateral left-sided notching.
2. Retrosternal undulating soft tissue due to dilated tortuous internal mammary arteries (site of collateral flow).
3. Abnormal appearance of the aortic arch (see Figs. 2-62, 2-74). The arch may be inconspicuous because of a more medial position than normal, along with a dilated left subclavian artery, which becomes border-forming in the region usually occupied by the posterior arch.
4. A notch on the proximal descending aorta followed by post-stenotic dilatation causes a 3 sign on the aorta (Fig. 2-62) and reverse-3 sign on the barium-filled esophagus.
5. Left ventricular prominence.
6. Prominent ascending aorta.
7. A double aortic knob may be caused by tortuosity of the posterior arch and proximal descending aorta, causing kinking of the aorta (Fig. 2-63). This is called pseudocoarctation of the aorta.

The salient radiographic features in decompensated coarctation usually presenting in early infancy are:

1. Pulmonary venous hypertension and/or edema.
2. Cardiomegaly.
3. Left ventricular enlargement.
4. Pulmonary arterial overcirculation is present with associated VSD and PDA.
5. Rib notching is not present during infancy.
6. The aortic knob is usually not characteristic. The only sign may be lateral displacement of the descending aortic stripe.

The numerous causes of rib notching are shown in Table 2-5. Rib notching confined to the upper two ribs is observed in longstanding ipsilateral Blalock–Taussig shunt. Coarctation at the lower thoracic aorta or abdominal aorta (middle aortic syndrome) is not due to the congenital anomaly called coarctation of the aorta. It can be acquired or associated with a few developmental syndromes. The causes are Takayasu's disease, Kawasaki's disease, Rubella syndrome, Williams' syndrome, and neurofibromatosis.

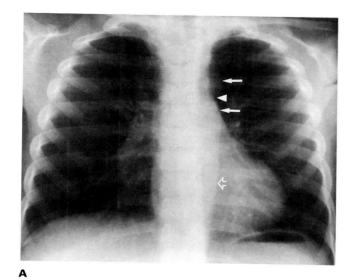

A

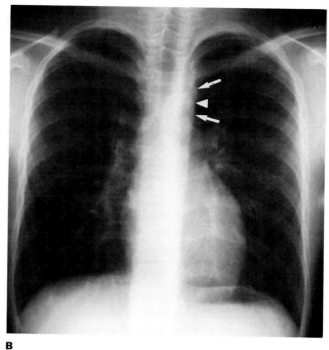

B

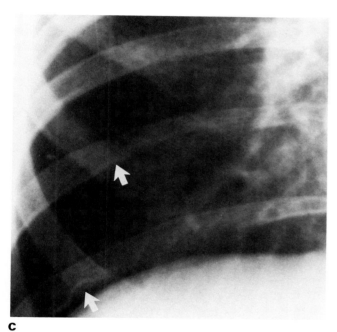

C

Figure 2-62. Three cases of coarctation of the aorta. Abnormal contour of arch and proximal descending aorta. The double aortic knob (*arrows*) is due to post-stenotic dilatation in the proximal descending aorta. There is sometimes outward displacement of the lateral margin of the descending aorta (*A, open arrow*). Note the figure 3 configuration caused by the notch (*arrowhead*) at the site of the coarctation (*A, B*). Rib notching is seen in C (*arrows*).

Interruption of Aortic Arch. The arch can be interrupted at any of three sites: beyond the left subclavian artery (type A); between the left subclavian and left common carotid arteries (type B); between the innominate artery and left carotid artery (type C). Types A and B occur with approximately equal frequency; type C is very rare. The right subclavian artery sometimes originates ectopically as a fourth aortic branch in this anomaly, which is called a type B_2 interruption. In this circumstance hypertension is confined to the carotid arteries.

This lesion can infrequently exist in an isolated form but usually is associated with VSD and PDA. There is an association with DORV with subpulmonic VSD (Taussig–Bing malformation).

The physiology is usually pulmonary arterial overcirculation and systemic hypertension which combine to produce left ventricular failure and pulmonary edema. Arterial flow to branches of the aorta below the interruption is by right-to-left shunting via the patent ductus arteriosus. Consequently, differential cyanosis of the limbs occurs, depending upon the site of origin of the arteries. Type A causes differential cyanosis of the lower limbs, while type B causes cyanosis of the left arm and lower limbs. In the isolated form of interruption the distal aortic flow is reconstituted by collaterals from branches above the interruption (branches of subclavian arteries).

The salient radiographic features are:

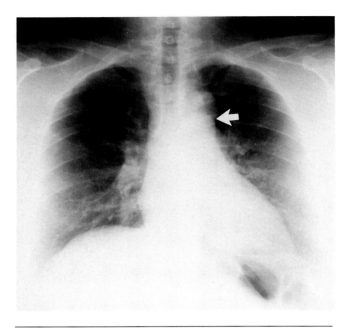

Figure 2-63. Pseudocoarctation of aorta. Tortuous distal arch and proximal ascending aorta causes an appearance similar to coarctation. Overlapping of the two contours (*arrow*) is sometimes a sign of pseudocoarctation; it is due to tortuosity of the aorta.

1. Isolated variety has the appearance as described for coarctation.
2. Interruption with VSD and PDA causes pulmonary arterial overcirculation and usually severe pulmonary edema with cardiomegaly (Fig. 2-64).
3. The trachea is sometimes identified to lie exactly in the midline and there is no indentation of the trachea.[38] This is a pathognomonic sign of this anomaly. If a PDA is present, the posterior arch may be prominent yet the trachea, not indented, lies exactly in the midline (Fig. 2-64).

Aortic Stenosis. Congenital aortic stenosis is caused by bicuspid aortic valve, unicuspid and unicommissural, or dyplastic valves.[39] It may be so severe as to induce intractable left ventricular failure in the neonate[40] (critical aortic stenosis). Stenosis also occurs at the subvalvular (discrete membranous or tunnel forms) and supravalvular sites.

Radiography. The salient radiographic features in the uncomplicated case are:

1. Normal heart size.
2. Enlargement of ascending aorta. This occurs in valvular stenosis and about half of patients with discrete membranous subvalvular stenosis.
3. Ascending aorta is small in supravalvular form (Fig. 2-65).

Table 2-5

Cause of Rib Notching

1. Aortic Obstruction
   Coarctation of the aorta
   Interruption of the aorta
   Acquired obstruction of the aorta: Takayasu's aortitis, atherosclerotic obstruction, etc.
   Unusual causes of coarctation: neurofibromatosis, Williams' syndrome, rubella syndrome
2. Subclavian arterial obstruction
   Blalock–Taussig shunt (upper two ribs)
   Takayasu's arteritis (usually unilateral)
   Atherosclerosis
3. Severely reduced pulmonary blood flow
   Tetralogy of Fallot
   Pulmonary atresia
   Tricuspid atresia
   Unilateral absence or atresia of a pulmonary artery
   Pulmonary emphysema
   Chronic pulmonary thromboembolic disease
4. Superior vena caval obstruction
5. Vascular shunts
   Pulmonary arteriovenous shunt
   Intercostal arteriovenous shunt
   Intercostal to pulmonary arterial shunt
6. Intercostal neuroma
7. Poliomyelitis (upper margin)
8. Hyperparathyroidism

Modified from Felson B. Chest roentgenology. Philadelphia: WB Saunders, 1973.

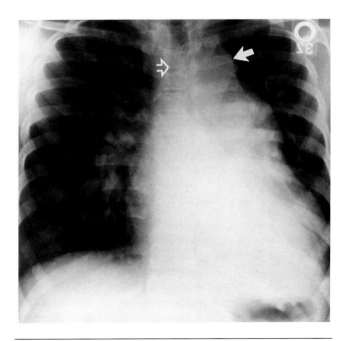

Figure 2-64. Interruption of aortic arch with VSD and PDA. Radiograph shows pulmonary arterial overcirculation, cardiomegaly due to left ventricular enlargement, enlargement of main pulmonary arterial and aortic arch segments. In spite of the enlarged aortic arch segment (*arrow*), the trachea (*open arrow*) is situated directly in the midline.

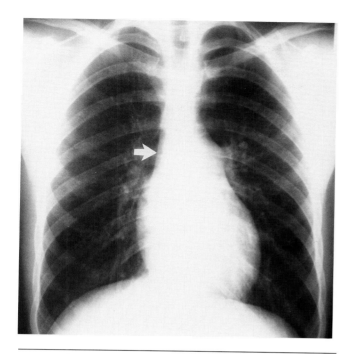

Figure 2-65. Supravalvular aortic stenosis. Concavity is seen in the region occupied by the ascending aorta (*arrow*).

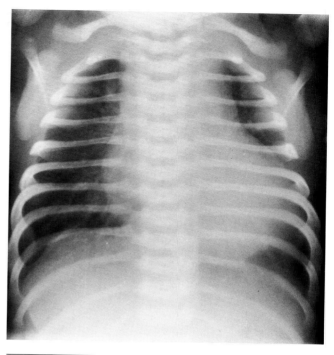

Figure 2-66. Critical aortic stenosis. Radiograph in an infant shows pulmonary edema and cardiomegaly.

In critical aortic stenosis, the radiographic features are:

1. Pulmonary venous hypertension and/or edema (Fig. 2-66).
2. Cardiomegaly.
3. Left ventricular enlargement.

Congenital Myocardial Abnormalities. The causes of congenital myocardial dysfunction include endocardial fibroelastosis; anomalous origin of left coronary artery from the pulmonary artery; and severe pressure overload of the left ventricle, such as occurs in coarctation of the aorta and critical aortic stenosis.

Radiography. The salient radiographic features are:

1. Pulmonary venous hypertension and edema (see Figs. 2-24, 2-25).
2. Cardiomegaly.
3. Enlargement of left ventricle and sometimes the left atrium. Certitude regarding which ventricle is enlarged may not be possible in neonates. The left atrium is enlarged in endocardial fibroelastosis and origin of the left coronary artery from the pulmonary as a consequence of mitral regurgitation (see Fig. 2-25).

Pulmonary Arteriovenous Malformation. Pulmonary arteriovenous malformation occurs as a single discrete lesion; multiple discrete lesions; and diffuse telangiectasias throughout the lungs. This lesion causes a right-to-left shunt and, consequently, cyanosis.

The radiographic appearance is one or more lung nodules. Discrete vascular shadows can sometimes be traced into the nodules. Multiple malformations and enlarged vessels can cause the appearance of pulmonary plethora in a cyanotic patient. Cardiac size is usually normal except in the presence of a very large malformation or the rare talangiectatic form in an infant.

References

1. Bertria A, Wible ED, Felderholf CH, McLaughlin MJ. Prolapse of the posterior leaflet of the mitral valve associated with secondum atrial septal defect. Am J Cardiol 1975;35:363.
2. Jefferson K, Rees S. Clincal cardiac radiology. London: Butterworths, 1973:77.
3. Svellen HA, van Ingren HC, Hoetsmit EC. Patterns of anomalous pulmonary venous drainage. Circulation 1968;38:45.
4. Kiely B, Filler J, Stone S, Doyle EF. Syndrome of anomalous venous drainage of the right lung to the inferior vena cava. Am J Cardiol 1967;20:102.
5. Baron MG. Endocardial cushion defect. Radiol Clin North Am 1968;6(3):343.
6. Rastelli GC, Kirklin JW, Titus JC. Anatomic observations of complete form of persistent atrioventricular canal with special reference to atrioventricular valves. Mayo Clin Proc 1966;41:296.

14. Lakier JB, Stanger P, Heymann MA, et al. Tetralogy of Fallot with absent pulmonary valve: natural history and hemodynamic consideration. Circulation 1974;50:167.

15. Van Praagh R. Transposition of the great arteries. Am J Cardiol 1971;23:409.

16. Tonkin IL, Kelley MJ, Bream PR, et al. The frontal chest film as a method of suspecting transposition complexes. Circulation 1976;53:1016.

17. Allwork SP, Bentall HH, Backer AE, et al. Congenitally corrected transposition of the great arteries: morphologic study of 32 cases. Am J Cardiol 1976;38:910.

18. Sondheimer HM, Freedom RM, Olley PM. Double outlet right ventricle: clinical spectrum and prognosis. Am J Cardiol 1977;39:709.

19. Brandt PWT, Calder AL, Barratt–Boyes BG, Neutze JM. Double outlet left ventricle: morphology, cineangiographic diagnosis and surgical treatment. Am J Cardiol 1976;38:897.

20. Keith JD, Rowe RD, Vlad P. Heart disease in infancy and childhood. 2nd ed. New York: Macmillan, 1967:647.

21. Edwards JE, Burchell HB. Congenital tricuspid atresia: a classification. Med Clin North Am 1949;33:1177.

22. Dick M, Fyler DC, Nadar AS. Tricuspid atresia: clinical course in 101 patients. Am J Cardiol 1975;36:327.

23. Van Praagh R, Ongley PA, Swan HJC. Anatomic types of single or common ventricle in man. Am J Cardiol 1964;13:367.

24. McCartney FJ, Partridge JB, Scott O, Deverall PB. Common or single ventricle: an angiographic and hemodynamic study of 42 patients. Circulation 1976;53:543.

25. Soto B, Pacifico AD, DiSciascio G. Univentricular heart: an angiographic study. Am J Cardiol 1982;49:787.

26. Collett RW, Edward JE. Persistent truncus arteriosus: classification according to anatomic types. Surg Clin North Am 1949;29:1245.

27. Calder L, Van Praagh R, Van Praagh S, et al. Truncus arteriosus communis: clinical, angiographic, and pathologic findings in 100 patients. Am Heart J 1976;92:23.

28. Weaver MD, Chen JTT, Anderson PAW, Lester RG. Total anomalous pulmonary venous return to left vertical vein. Radiology 1976;18:679.

29. Bonham–Carter RE, Capriles M, Noe Y. Total anomalous pulmonary venous drainage: a clinical and anatomical study of 75 children. Br Heart J 1969;31:45.

30. Anderson KR, Zuberbuhler JR, Anderson RH, et al. Morphologic spectrum of Ebstein's anomaly of the heart. Mayo Clin Proc 1979;54:174.

31. Ellis K, Griffith SP, Burris JO, et al. Ebstein's anomaly of the tricuspid valve: angiographic considerations. Am J Roentgenol 1964;92:1338.

32. Elliott LB, Adams P, Edward JE. Pulmonary atresia with intact ventricular septum. Br Heart J 1963;25:489.

33. Freedom KM, Harrington DP. Contribution of intramyocardial sinusoids in pulmonary atresia and intact ventricular septum to a right-sided circular shunt. Br Heart J 1974;36:1061.

34. Roberts WC, Perry LW, Chandler RS, et al. Aortic valve atresia: a new classification based on necropsy study of 73 cases. Am J Cardiol 1976;37:753.

35. Figley MM. Accessory roentgen signs of coarctation of the aorta. Radiology 1954;62:671.

36. Baron MG. Obscuration of the aortic knob in coarctation of the aorta. Circulation 1971;43:311.

37. Higgins CB, French JW, Silverman JF, Wexler L. Interruption of the aortic arch: preoperative and postoperative clinical hemodynamics, and angiographic features. Am J Cardiol 1977;39:563.

38. Jaffe RB. Complete interruption of the aortic arch: characteristic radiographic findings in 21 patients. Circulation 1975;52:714.

39. Lakier JB, Lewis AB, Heymann MA, et al. Isolated aortic stenosis in the neonate. Circulation 1974;50:801.

40. Broderick TW, Higgins CB, Guthaner DF, et al. Critical aortic stenosis in the neonate. Radiology 1978;129:393.

41. Moller JH, Lucas RV, Adams P, et al. Endocardial fibroelastosis: a clinical and anatomic study of 47 patients with emphasis on its relationship to mitral insufficiency. Circulation 1964;30:759.

42. Talner NS, Halloran KH, Mabday M, et al. Anomalous origin of left coronary artery from the pulmonary artery: a clinical spectrum. Am J Cardiol 1965;15:689.

43. Higgins CB, Wexler L. Clinical and angiographic features of pulmonary arteriovenous fistulas in children. Radiology 1976;119:171.

Chapter 3

Intensive and Coronary Care Radiology

Jeffrey S. Klein

Technical Considerations

The vast majority of chest radiographs obtained in the critical care setting are portable anteroposterior (AP) radiographs, obtained with the patient in a semierect position. For most patients, a daily, morning chest radiograph is obtained to evaluate deterioration or improvement in cardiopulmonary status, and to check the position of monitoring and support devices. In addition, a film is obtained routinely immediately after the placement of catheters and tubes in order to assess position and to detect complications related to placement.

There are both specific technical and patient-related limitations of portable bedside radiography in critically ill patients. The limited maximal kvp of portable units often requires longer exposures to obtain adequate radiographic penetration of cardiomediastinal structures. This can result in greater motion artifact, especially in ventilated patients and patients who cannot sustain a brief apneic period. The short focus-to-film distance (typically 40″) causes a 5% increase in apparent cardiac size.[1] Anteroposterior radiographs increase the apparent cardiac diameter by 15% to 20% compared to posteroanterior (PA) chest radiographs. This is due to magnification of the anteriorly situated heart combined with a reduction in the projected transverse diameter of the thorax on AP films. This reduction occurs because the maximum transverse diameter of the thorax lies posterior to the midcoronal plane. When assessing AP radiographs for cardiomegaly, the upper limit of normal for the cardiothoracic ratio should be 57%.[2]

The critically ill patient is often supine when a portable radiograph is obtained. The supine position makes it more difficult for the patient to inspire deeply because of the restraining effect of intra-abdominal organs on diaphragmatic movement. Thus, these films tend to show smaller lung volumes and are difficult to interpret. The recognition of mild pulmonary venous hypertension is difficult in the supine patient, where a 30% increase in pulmonary blood flow and the absence of gravitational effects lead to an even distribution of pulmonary blood flow.[2] The 30% increase in systemic venous return to the heart in the supine position leads to distention of the azygous vein and superior vena cava, causing a widening of the upper mediastinum or "vascular pedicle" on frontal radiographs. The detection of small or moderate pleural effusions may be difficult on a supine radiograph, owing to the tendency of free flowing pleural fluid to layer posteriorly with the patient supine. The only clue to the presence of an effusion may be a subtle veil of increased opacity over the affected hemithorax, a small "cap" of fluid over the lung apex, or obscuration of the hemidiaphragm.[3] The presence of an effusion can be confirmed by obtaining upright or decubitus films, or by portable bedside sonography. Similarly, a pneumothorax may be difficult to detect when the patient is supine. Since free intrapleural air rises to a nondependent position, the only radiographic finding may be anteromedial or inferolateral radiolucency, including an abnormally deep and radiolucent lateral costophrenic sulcus ("deep sulcus sign").[4] As with suspected effusions, upright or decubitus films (with the affected side up) should be obtained when a pneumothorax is suspected and the visceral pleural reflection is not visible (Fig. 3-1). A hydropneumothorax in a supine patient is recognized when air outlines the visceral pleura, and the increased density of pleural fluid is seen lateral to this reflection.[5]

Because of difficulty in properly positioning criti-

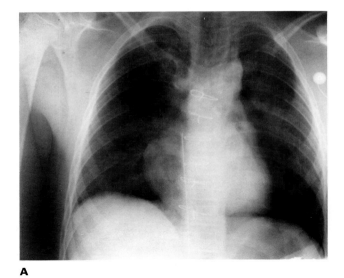

A

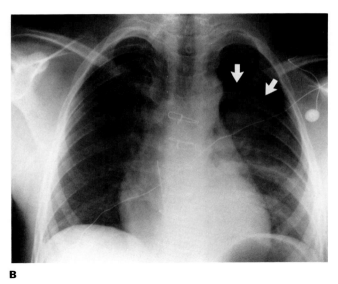

B

Figure 3-1. Pneumothorax in a supine patient. *A:* Supine film immediately following midline sternotomy. A deep, lucent left lateral costophrenic sulcus is noted. *B:* Upright film obtained one hour later. As the left pneumothorax rises to a nondependent portion of the pleural space, the visceral pleural reflection (*arrows*) is evident.

cally ill patients for portable radiographs, the patient is often rotated from the midline. On an AP radiograph, the side rotated anteriorly (i.e., away from the film-screen cassette) will appear more radiolucent than the side adjacent to the film. This is mostly due to diminished absorption of the x-ray beam by the pectoral muscles on the side rotated away from the film. A similar phenomenon occurs as a result of lateral decentering of the x-ray beam in relation to the patient.[6] This artifact must be distinguished from unilateral decreased density due to a pneumothorax or a hyperlucent lung, or, conversely, from unilateral increased opacity due to chest wall, pleural, or parenchymal lung disease. Inaccuracies in directing the x-ray beam perpendicular to the patient can result in kyphotic or lordotic films. The effect of lordosis is to foreshorten the visible height of the lung, increase cardiac magnification, and cause apparent obscuration of the left hemidiaphragm. The latter effect can be caused by the limited interface between the left lower lobe and the left hemidiaphragm with the patient projected lordotically.[7] Kyphotic films are rarely seen in the critical care setting, since technicians are more likely to overestimate the erectness of the patient, and thus angle the x-ray tube more horizontally than is necessary.

Portable radiographs performed in many coronary or intensive care units have a label attached that indicates the kVp, mAs, focal-film distance, and an estimate of the patient's angle from the supine (Fig. 3-2). This helps the radiologist compare different films on the same patient, and guide the technician as to the appropriate technique to use on a given patient. An additional device that accu-

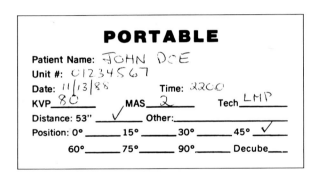

Figure 3-2. Label for portable chest radiographs. The technician records patient information and technical data on a self-adhesive label attached to each portable chest radiograph.

rately determines patient recumbency is the inclinometer.[8] This device, which contains ten holes, each with a small lead ball and each angled 10° relative to its neighbor, can be clipped to the film cassette and aids in the interpretation of portable radiographs (Fig. 3-3).

Tubes, Lines, and Catheters

Endotracheal Tubes

The position of the tip of the endotracheal tube in relation to the carina should be checked routinely on each film obtained in a patient on mechanical ventilation. Most endotracheal tubes have a radio-opaque line that extends

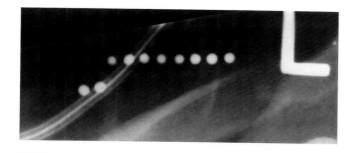

Figure 3-3. Inclinometer. Close up of inclinometer as seen on portable radiograph. This device contains ten lead balls, each within a self-contained cylinder angled 10° toward the vertical from the ball immediately to its left. The most leftward cylinder is angled 10° past horizontal (Trendelenburg), with the last ball in a cylinder 90° vertical. This film was obtained with the patient 10° upright. Note two balls in the dependent part of the inclinometer, indicating the cassette was 10°–20° upright at the time of exposure.

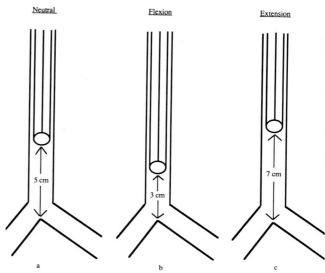

Figure 3-4. Movement of endotracheal tube with changes in head position. *A:* With the head in a neutral position (mandible over C5–C6), the endotracheal tube is ideally positioned with its tip 5 cm above the carina. *B:* Full flexion (mandible over T1–T2) will push the tip of the endotracheal tube 2 cm inferior from its position with the head neutral. *C:* Full extension (mandible over C2–C3) will draw the tube 2 cm cephalad from the neutral position.

vertically to its tip. The ideal location for the tip is 5 to 7 cm above the carina with the head in a neutral position (i.e., the inferior mandible overlying the lower cervical spine).[9] This allows for the maximal cephalocaudad tube excursion of 4 cm that occurs as the head moves from full extenstion to full flexion (Fig. 3-4). In addition, this tube position avoids traumatizing the vocal cords or tracheal carina. In addition to carinal irritation and ulceration from the tube and suction catheters, a tube placed too low may lead to right main stem intubation with head flexion, resulting in left lung collapse and right lung overinflation (Fig. 3-5). Too high a position may cause hypopharyngeal intubation with extension, resulting in ineffective ventilation and gastric overdistention.

The carina is located by following the lower margin of the left main bronchus proximally to its junction with the right main stem bronchus. If the carina cannot be identified (usually owing to an underpenetrated film), its position can be estimated to be between the T5 and T7 level.[10] Inadvertent right main bronchus or esophageal intubation is usually clinically evident, but on occasion the radiologist will be the first to detect these complications. Although right main bronchus intubation is readily evident radiographically, esophageal placement may be difficult to recognize. Projection of the tube to the left of the tracheal air column on a slight right posterior oblique view with esophageal and gastric air distention are the radiographic findings of esophageal intubation.[11]

The diameter of the endotracheal tube should be two-thirds of the tracheal cross-sectional diameter. The tube should lie parallel to the tracheal walls, with the cuff filling but not distending the tracheal lumen (Fig. 3-6). After the position, appearance, and alignment of the endotracheal tube have been checked, the radiologist should search for complications of the intubation itself, or of the positive pressure ventilation instituted following intubation.

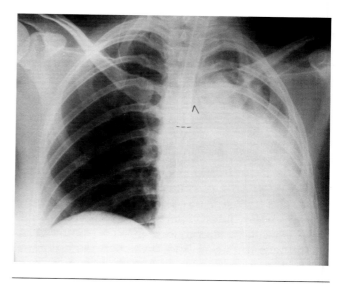

Figure 3-5. Endotracheal tube in right main stem bronchus. Postintubation film demonstrating the endotracheal tube in the right main stem bronchus, resulting in occlusion of the left main stem bronchus and left lung collapse.

Perforation of the hypopharynx may occur after a difficult intubation and is suggested when subcutaneous emphysema is noted shortly after intubation. This may progress to pneumomediastinum, pneumothorax, or mediastinitis if unrecognized. Pharyngography should be performed as soon as the diagnosis is suspected.

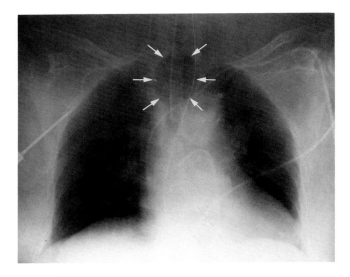

Figure 3-6. Overdistended endotracheal tube balloon. The cuff on the endotracheal tube (*arrows*) has overdistended the trachea; if not corrected, tracheomalacia or rupture could result. Also note the right subclavian central venous catheter ascending in the right internal jugular vein.

The most common complication of positive pressure ventilation is alveolar rupture resulting in interstitial emphysema, pneumomediastinum, and pneumothorax (Fig. 3-7). Since the development of pneumothorax in these patients (usually under tension) is almost always preceded by pneumomediastinum, early recognition of mediastinal air is critical.

Chest Tubes

Pleural tubes are often placed intraoperatively to evacuate air and fluid that accumulate in the mediastinum and left pleural space following cardiac surgery. Most often two mediastinal tubes are placed prior to sternal closure; a straight tube placed anteriorly and an angled tube placed over the diaphragm to lie in a more posterior position (Fig. 3-8). These tubes exit the chest just below the xiphoid process and are removed in the early postoperative period unless excessive drainage is encountered. Pleural drainage catheters similarly can be placed through the lower end of the sternotomy wound, or via a left intercostal approach. Although the optimal tube position for pleural drainage in the supine patient is posteroinferior for fluid and anterosuperior for air, these tubes tend to function well in any position within the pleural space.

On the postoperative radiograph, the chest tube should project over the pleural space. A radio-opaque stripe along the length of the tube marks the tip and outlines the most proximal side hole. If this hole projects

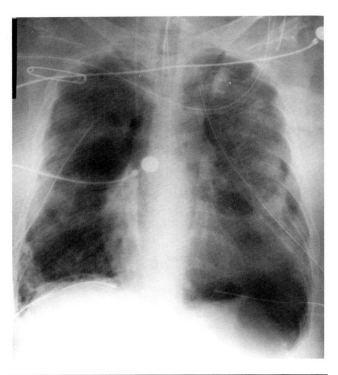

Figure 3-7. Ventilator-induced pneumomediastinum and pneumothorax. In this patient with the adult respiratory distress syndrome, high ventilatory pressures and noncompliant lungs have led to pneumomediastinum and pneumothorax despite multiple chest tubes.

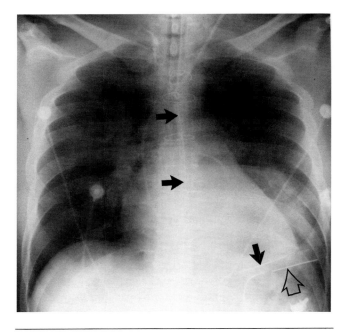

Figure 3-8. In this post-coronary bypass patient, one straight and one angled mediastinal drain (*solid arrows*), left pleural tube (*open arrow*), endotracheal tube, and Swan–Ganz catheter are positioned ideally.

beyond the lung, pleural air or fluid may accumulate in the subcutaneous tissues of the chest wall. An intrathoracic location can be confirmed by noting the wall of the tube outlined by air within the lumen of the tube and the lung. Inability to visualize the tube wall where it overlies the lung suggests an extrathoracic position, since the soft tissues of the chest wall are of similar radio-opacity as the polyvinylchloride tube and silhouette its wall.[12] Kinked tubes and tubes placed intraparenchymally or intrafissurally function poorly. An intrafissural location is recognized by noting an oblique upward course of the tube on frontal radiograph.[13] A lateral film, fluoroscopy, or computed tomography (CT) scan can be used to confirm an intrafissural position. An intraparenchymal tube is usually not recognized on plain radiographs but rather is first noted on CT. Lung laceration or herniation into the tube lumen with infarction may result.

Central Venous Catheterization

Central venous catheters (CVCs) are used commonly in the critical care setting. They allow monitoring of right atrial filling pressures, providing an estimate of circulating blood volume. The high flow rates within the subclavian and brachiocephalic veins and superior vena cava, where these catheters are placed, allow for the administration of hyperalimentation, antibiotics, and chemotherapeutic agents that cannot be safely infused into small peripheral veins. In addition, a central venous catheter may be placed for venous access in a patient lacking a peripheral access.

Virtually all CVCs are placed percutaneously into the internal jugular, subclavian, or external jugular veins. Occasionally, a catheter may be threaded into a central location by way of the arm or groin, particularly when catheterization from the neck is unsuccessful or impossible for anatomic reasons.

The optimal location for a CVC inserted for central venous pressure monitoring is with its tip beyond any valves that might preclude accurate measurement of right atrial pressure. Since the most proximal valves within the internal jugular and subclavian veins lie 2.5 cm proximal to their junction to form the brachiocephalic vein,[14] the catheter tip should lie in the superior vena cava, brachiocephalic vein, or proximal internal jugular or subclavian vein (Fig. 3-9). Although placement of the catheter tip in the right atrium might seem desirable, the risk of atrial arrhythmias and atrial perforation from catheter migration make this position less than optimal. Additionally, certain compounds administered directly to the heart and lungs as an undiluted bolus can cause life-threatening cardiac arrhythmias.[15]

A postcatheterization chest radiograph is necessary to confirm adequate CVC position and detect catheter

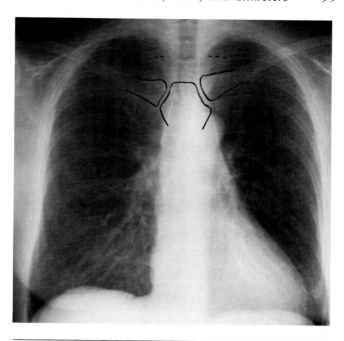

Figure 3-9. Position of catheters for central venous pressure monitoring. The tip of the central venous catheter should be positioned within at least 2.5 cm of either brachiocephalic vein (broken lines), in order to avoid inaccurate readings of right atrial pressure due to intervening valves.

misplacement. An atypical catheter course or tip position may signify catheterization of a mediastinal venous tributary, inadvertent arterial catheterization, or extravascular (e.g., pleural or mediastinal) placement. Complications that can be detected on chest radiographs include pneumothorax; hydrothorax from blood, chyle or infusate; extrapleural, cervical, or mediastinal hemorrhage (Fig. 3-10); superior vena caval thrombosis; brachial plexus or phrenic nerve injury; pericardial tamponade; and catheter kinking, knotting, breakage, or embolization.

A detailed knowledge of normal thoracic venous anatomy is necessary to recognize aberrant catheter positioning. In cases where an atypical position is suspected, review of prior radiographs may resolve the issue. On occasion, lateral radiographs, contrast injection under fluoroscopy, or CT may be necessary to accurately localize the catheter.

Normal Central Venous Anatomy. The normal thoracic venous anatomy is shown in Figure 3-11. Each subclavian vein begins at the lateral border of the first rib, and joins the ipsilateral jugular vein to form the brachiocephalic vein behind the sternoclavicular joint. From its point of origin, the right brachiocephalic vein courses inferiorly and slightly posteriorly to join the left brachiocephalic vein behind the right first costochondral junction. The left brachiocephalic vein runs toward the right

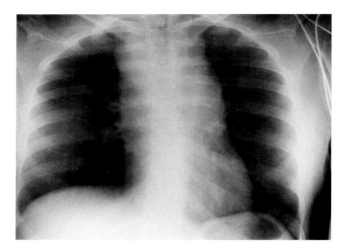

Figure 3-10. Mediastinal hematoma complicating attempted central venous catheterization. Smooth, symmetric mediastinal widening represents hemorrhage from laceration of the right carotid artery during an unsuccessful attempt at internal jugular catheterization.

and inferiorly behind the manubrium before arching posteriorly to join the right brachiocephalic vein and form the superior vena cava.

Aberrant Catheter Placement. Commonly recognized atypical catheter tip positions include a subclavian catheter ascending in the ipsilateral internal jugular vein (see Fig. 3-7), or retrograde catheterization of the subclavian vein from the ipsilateral internal jugular vein. Both are more likely to occur when the angle at their junction is obtuse. Similarly, a catheter placed in the subclavian vein may traverse the junction of the brachiocephalic veins and lie within the contralateral brachiocephalic or subclavian vein.

Catheterization of small venous tributaries of the great veins is undesirable since it may lead to venous thrombosis or catheter occlusion. Additionally, such placement will not accurately reflect central venous pressure. On the right side, a catheter that appears looped within the superior vena cava at the level of the right tracheobronchial angle may actually lie within the arch of the azygous vein. This is easily confirmed by a lateral radiograph showing the catheter coursing posteriorly along the arch of the azygous vein at a level just below the aortic arch. Another anomalous right-sided catheter position is in the right internal mammary vein; this vein drains into the right brachiocephalic vein behind the right first costochondral junction. Catheterization of this vein is recognized by noting a vertically oriented, parasternal catheter that lies lateral to the outer margin of the superior vena cava. A lateral radiograph will confirm the typical anterior and parasternal course.

On the left side, the catheter may enter one of several mediastinal veins that drain into the left brachiocephalic vein, or may enter a left-sided superior vena cava. If the catheter arches superiorly from the brachiocephalic vein in the midline, it may have entered one of the inferior thyroid veins. A catheter coursing around the aortic arch may lie in the left superior intercostal vein; this is uncommon unless this vein acts as collateral venous drainage due to obstruction of the superior vena cava. As on the right, internal mammary catheterization is recognized when a left-sided catheter follows a vertical course inferiorly, just behind and lateral to the sternum. Pericardiophrenic vein catheterization has an appearance similar to catheterization of the left internal mammary vein; these can be distinguished by noting that the pericardiophrenic vein courses around the left heart margin and appears to bisect the heart on a lateral film.

A left-sided superior vena cava (SVC) is the most common congenital vascular anomaly of the thorax. A catheter placed through the left jugular or subclavian vein in a patient with a persistent left SVC will be seen to have the CVC coursing in a vertical fashion from above inferiorly along the left side of the mediastinum[16] (Fig. 3-12). On frontal radiograph this may be indistinguishable from internal mammary or pericardiophrenic catheterization. On lateral radiograph, a left SVC will course along the posterior aspect of the heart to empty into the coronary sinus.

Extravenous Catheter Placement. When the postcatheter placement films show the catheter to course in a direction separate from the great veins and their tributaries, the catheter must be presumed to lie in an extravascular location (Fig. 3-13). Inadvertent arterial catheterization is usually evident clinically, but on occasion, the radiologist will be the first to suspect arterial placement by noting the catheter positioned within the aorta. An extravenous placement is often difficult to detect clinically, since catheters that have perforated the vein may lie within a communicating pseudoaneurysm and thus provide blood return on aspiration. The administration of intravenous contrast material under fluoroscopy can confirm an extravascular position. Occasionally, an extravascular location is not suspected until extravascular infusion of intravenous solution leads to mediastinal widening or, if the catheter tip is intrapleural, a "glucothorax" (Fig. 3-13).

Complications of Central Venous Catheters. Complications of central venous catheterization may be secondary to CVC placement or may occur while the catheter is indwelling. Pneumothorax from pleural laceration during venipuncture accounts for 30% of all CVC-related complications.[17] This is usually detected on an immediate postcatheterization chest film, which is optimally

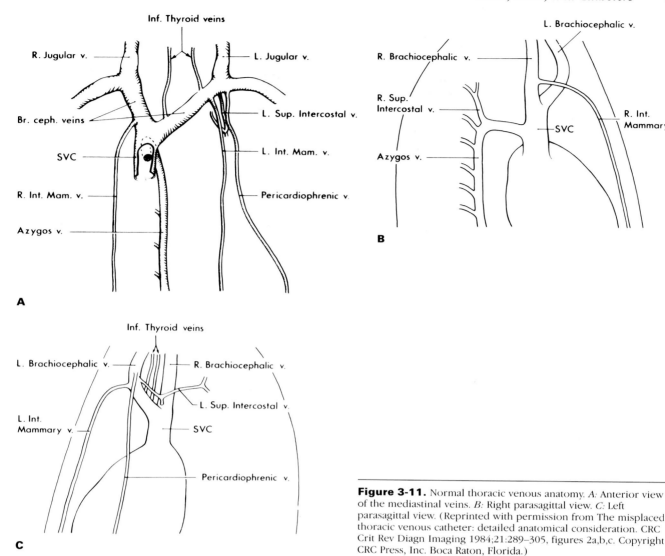

Figure 3-11. Normal thoracic venous anatomy. *A:* Anterior view of the mediastinal veins. *B:* Right parasagittal view. *C:* Left parasagittal view. (Reprinted with permission from The misplaced thoracic venous catheter: detailed anatomical consideration. CRC Crit Rev Diagn Imaging 1984;21:289–305, figures 2a,b,c. Copyright CRC Press, Inc. Boca Raton, Florida.)

performed as a frontal, expiratory film with the patient upright. If the patient cannot be placed upright, a decubitus film with the noncatheterized side down should be obtained so that a small pneumothorax, which accumulates anteromedially or inferiorly with the supine patient, is not missed. Recognition of a pneumothorax is especially important when initial catheterization has been unsuccessful, and an attempt at catheterization on the contralateral side follows immediately.

Vascular laceration usually occurs after multiple unsuccessful attempts at catheterization, and may present as neck swelling, an apical extrapleural cap, hemothorax, or mediastinal widening. Any of these findings may be immediate or delayed. The bleeding is usually self-limited, but occasionally surgical repair is necessary.

If a CVC is withdrawn through the beveled introducing needle, the catheter may sheer off in the vein and

embolize to the heart or lungs. Immediate transvenous retrieval should be performed.

A catheter that is advanced too far, or is repeatedly advanced and withdrawn may end up looped or knotted within the great veins or heart. A knotted catheter can give falsely high central venous pressure readings. It is also more likely to traumatize the vein and lead to venous thrombosis or perforation. Once recognized, the knot usually can be undone transvenously.

Other, rare complications of CVC placement include injury of the phrenic, vagus, or recurrent laryngeal nerve or brachial plexus, thoracic duct laceration with chylothorax, and venous air embolism.[17]

Venous thrombosis occurs in up to 20% of patients with long-term indwelling CVCs. Thrombosis of subclavian vein or superior vena cava is usually first suspected clinically. Radiographic clues to the development of SVC

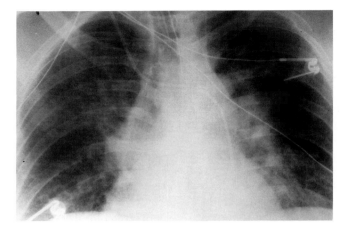

Figure 3-12. Catheter in persistent left superior vena cava. A right internal jugular Swan–Ganz catheter and a left internal jugular LeVeen (peritoneojugular) shunt catheter course along the left side of the mediastinum within a persistent left SVC.

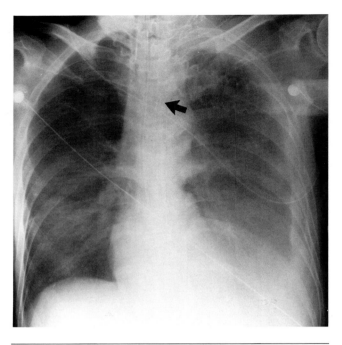

Figure 3-13. Extravascular central venous catheter placement. The tip of a left internal jugular catheter lies in an atypical location (*arrow*). Mediastinal widening and left pleural effusion are secondary to extravasation of infusate ("glucothorax").

thrombosis include dilatation of the SVC and enlargement of collateral venous channels such as the azygous vein and left superior intercostal vein. Contrast-enhanced CT, MRI, or venography can provide the diagnosis. Streptokinase or urokinase applied locally to the thrombus can successfully lyse clots in a majority of cases.

Catheter-associated infection occurs in approximately 10% of cases, either from catheter contamination at the time of insertion or from breaks in the infusion system.[17] Septicemia, endocarditis, septic emboli, or pneumonia may develop. Catheter removal and antibiotic therapy should be instituted as soon as the diagnosis is suspected.

Recognition of a gentle curve at the tip of a CVC in the SVC on frontal or lateral chest films should prompt catheter repositioning or removal; this sign was noted in six of nine cases of catheter perforation of the SVC reviewed retrospectively.[18]

As mentioned previously, recognition of the catheter tip in the right atrium should prompt catheter withdrawal, since the catheter or the infused solutions may cause arrhythmias, and rigid catheters may perforate the atrium and lead to fatal pericardial tamponade.

Swan-Ganz Catheters

Flow-directed pulmonary artery catheters are common in the cardiac care unit. Their use has revolutionized the fluid and pharmacologic management of critically ill patients. The radiologist interfacing with his or her critical care colleagues should be knowledgeable about the normal appearance of the catheter, the proper positioning within the pulmonary arterial circulation, and complica-

tions related to catheter placement or due to the indwelling catheter itself.

Complications from Introduction. As balloon-tipped flow-directed pulmonary artery catheters are introduced from the internal jugular or subclavian veins, the complications from introduction of these catheters are essentially the same as discussed for the placement of CVCs. Since the catheter traverses the right ventricle on its path toward the pulmonary artery, other possible complications encountered during placement include irritation of the right-sided conducting system, resulting in ventricular ectopy and, in patients with preexisting left bundle branch block, catheter-induced complete heart block.

Normal Appearance and Position. In a majority of patients with catheters placed from the neck, the natural curve of the catheter leads the tip from the right ventricle into the right pulmonary artery. Catheters placed via the femoral vein tend to follow the relatively straight course from the right ventricular outflow tract to the left pulmonary artery. The resting position of the catheter tip is ideally in a central right or left pulmonary artery.[19] Radiographically, this position is no farther distal than the proximal interlobar pulmonary artery (Fig. 3-14). Such a position allows brisk flow around the catheter

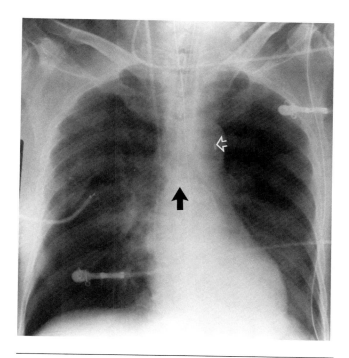

Figure 3-14. Normal position of Swan–Ganz catheter. In a patient requiring intra-aortic balloon counterpulsation (*solid arrow*) for cardiogenic shock, a Swan–Ganz catheter is ideally positioned with its tip (*open arrow*) in the proximal right main pulmonary artery.

tip, preventing thrombus formation, and allows for safe inflation of the balloon for pulmonary capillary wedge pressure (PCWP) measurement. Also, a position within the main or interlobar pulmonary artery assures that when wedged, the catheter will be in a zone III vessel and therefore give accurate measurements of pulmonary venous and left atrial pressures. If the catheter wedges in an upper lobe, lingular, or middle lobe vessel (zones I and II), inaccurate left atrial and left ventricular pressure readings will be obtained. This is because in nondependent regions of the lung, intra-alveolar pressure exceeds pulmonary venous pressure and compression of the pulmonary veins occurs when arterial inflow is occluded by the balloon. A continuous column of blood will not exist, and the resultant PCWP will reflect intra-alveolar rather than intravascular pressure. A catheter tip which is too proximal (in the right atrium, right ventricle, or SVC) is undesirable and should be advanced into the pulmonary artery.[20] The catheter should follow a smooth course without kinks, loops, or redundancies. The inflated, radiolucent balloon just proximal to the catheter tip should never be seen radiographically, as this may lead to vascular occlusion or arterial wall trauma.

Clinical Uses. Swan–Ganz catheters currently used contain five lumens, each of which is dedicated to providing specific hemodynamic measurements. When attached to a transducer and oscilloscope, the distal lu-

men provides continuous pulmonary arterial pressure tracings and, when wedged in a distal vessel, PCWP tracings. When wedged in a vessel that is dependent in relation to the left atrium (a lower lobe vessel in a supine or upright patient), the PCWP accurately reflects pulmonary venous, left atrial, and left ventricular diastolic pressures. Cardiac output may be measured by a thermodilution technique, in which a known amount of fluid at a given temperature is injected into a proximal lumen, and the resultant temperature change is measured by a distal thermister. Systemic vascular resistance is simply calculated once cardiac output and systemic blood pressure are known. Another proximal lumen with a port in the SVC or right atrium measures right atrial filling pressures and is used for intravenous infusions. Finally, most current catheters contain a separate lumen that may be used for the introduction of a temporary pacemaker.

Complications. The major complication rate from Swan–Ganz catheters ranges from 3% to 17%.[21,22] In addition to complications related to venipuncture and introduction of the catheter, a number of serious complications have been ascribed to indwelling pulmonary artery catheters. A catheter coiled or looped in the right atrium or ventricle can irritate the chamber wall and induce arrhythmias, and predisposes to knot formation. A redundant catheter loop may also lead to distal migration, with persistent catheter wedging and vascular occlusion. The tip of the catheter can traumatize the tricuspid or pulmonic valve, especially if the catheter is advanced without the balloon inflated. Similarly, the papillary muscles or chordae tendineae can be damaged by the catheter.

A relatively common serious complication of Swan–Ganz catheters is catheter-induced vascular thrombosis, resulting in ischemia and infarction (Fig. 3-15). Foote et al. retrospectively analyzed 125 patients with Swan–Ganz catheters and found 9 cases (7.2%) of documented catheter-related pulmonary ischemia or infarction.[23] A catheter tip placed too far distally, or migrating from a more central position to wedge peripherally, may obstruct flow. This usually occurs within 24 to 48 hours after placement because of the tendency of the catheter loop to tighten, particularly if a big intracardiac loop or coil in the catheter exists. If the balloon just at the tip of the catheter is incompletely deflated after use, vascular occlusion can result (Fig. 3-16). Clinically, this may be recognized by noting a persistent PCWP tracing, inability to aspirate the same volume of air used for balloon inflation, or increased resistance to the injection of air. Radiographically, the radiolucent balloon should never be seen; if recognized, immediate deflation or catheter withdrawal should follow. Finally, thrombus can form in or about the catheter, leading to vascular occlusion. To reduce thrombus formation, a heparinized intravenous solution should be infused through all unused lumina.

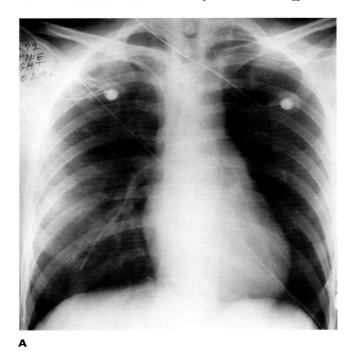

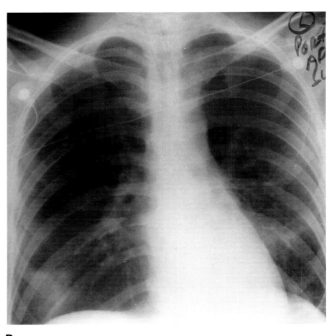

A

B

Figure 3-15. Pulmonary infarct secondary to Swan–Ganz catheter placement. *A:* Initial film after catheter introduction shows the tip of the catheter distally in a segmental right lower lobe pulmonary artery. *B:* Three days later, after catheter removal, a wedge-shaped opacity representing an infarct is seen in the lower lobe segment distal to the previous catheter position.

A rare but reported complication of Swan–Ganz catheters is laceration of a pulmonary artery with hemorrhage and pseudoaneurysm formation. Dieden et al. described ten cases of pulmonary artery pseudoaneurysms secondary to use of Swan–Ganz catheters.[24] In six of the ten, the radiographic findings were the presenting features; typically this was a focal dense air-space consolidation that evolved into a focal nodule or mass immediately adjacent to the catheter tip.

As with any percutaneously placed intravascular catheter, a line infection can develop. Frequent changing of indwelling catheters reduces the incidence of catheter-related sepsis. Radiographically, the development of cavitating lung nodules consistent with septic emboli should suggest the diagnosis. The catheter should be withdrawn, its tip cultured, and intravenous antibiotics started.

Cardiac Pacemakers

Many patients in cardiac care units have permanent pacemakers, or require temporary pacing for ischemia-induced arrhythmias. The radiologist should be familiar with the normal position and appearance of cardiac pacemakers, and plays an important role in the evaluation of pacemaker failure and complications.

Types of Pacemakers. Previously, permanent pacemakers were directly sutured or screwed into the myocardium by an open thoracotomy. Currently, the vast majority of pacemakers are placed transvenously via the subclavian or, less commonly, the jugular or cephalic veins. The generator is placed in a subcutaneous pocket. The pacing system is comprised of a pulse generator with a lithium iodide power source, the lead wire (or wires, as with an atrioventricular sequential pacemaker), and the tip electrode.

Temporary pacemakers are placed by means of an indwelling central venous sheath or through a lumen of a Swan–Ganz catheter. In many patients undergoing cardiac surgery at most institutions, temporary epicardial leads are placed over the anteroinferior heart and tunneled subcutaneously to the upper abdominal wall. These leads are removed percutaneously prior to discharge from the hospital.

Normal Appearance and Positioning. Transvenous pacemaker leads should follow a gentle, smooth course through the superior vena cava, right atrium, and right ventricle to its apex.[25] A number of abnormal positions have been recognized (Fig. 3-17). A pacemaker placed on the left may enter a persistent left superior vena cava, which is present in 0.5% of the population. In

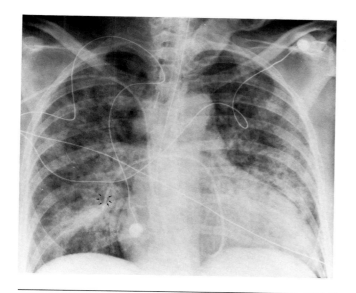

Figure 3-16. Inflated Swan–Ganz catheter balloon. The inflated balloon, located just proximal to the tip of the catheter, is seen as a round radiolucency (*arrows*) within the right lower lobe pulmonary artery. Its visibility is enhanced in this patient by surrounding air-space opacification.

this situation, the wire traverses the left side of the mediastinum and coronary sinus before entering the right atrium. Inadvertent arterial placement is recognized on ECG by noting a right bundle branch block pattern, and on radiograph by noting an oblique course to the wire lead across the mediastinum from right to left as it traverses the ascending aorta and aortic valve to enter the left ventricle.

Proper tip position in the right ventricular apex is recognized by noting an inferior and lateral position of the tip on the frontal view, with a slight inferior and anterior course of the distal portion of the wire on the lateral film. If only a frontal view is available, wires in the middle cardiac vein or coronary sinus may be indistin-

guishable from apical placement (Figs. 3-17, 3-18). When an ectopic tip location is suspected, a lateral radiograph usually clarifies its location. A pacemaker wire in the middle cardiac vein runs along the undersurface of the heart in a slightly posterior direction on the lateral view.[25] A coronary sinus position is recognized by a wire looped cephalad toward the right ventricular outflow tract on the frontal view, which loops posteriorly to run in the atrioventricular groove of the heart on the lateral view (see Figs. 3-17, 3-18). It is important that the radiologist interpreting the film be aware of the desired location of the tip; coronary sinus placement may be intended for patients with sick sinus syndrome. If the wire is too short (i.e., lacks a smooth curve), the tip may become dislodged. Too long a wire or a looped wire is also undesirable (see below).

Detection of Complications. The complications of pacemaker implantation include those of central venous puncture and catheterization; those related to the lead wire, including dislodgement, fracture, and myocardial perforation; and inflammation and infection within the generator pouch. Electrode tip dislodgement occurs in 3% to 14% of patients, usually before a fibrous sheath has formed over the electrode tip to secure it to the endocardium within 2 weeks of placement. Predisposing factors include too short a wire, leading to dislodgement during ventricular systole, or retraction of the wire into the subcutaneous tissues.

Lead fracture has an incidence of 2% to 3% and in transvenous pacemakers tends to occur at the point of lead connection to the generator, within a loop, or at the point of venous entry.[25] Epicardial lead fractures tend to occur at the point of lead fixation to the myocardium. Myocardial perforation is first suspected when diaphragmatic pacing or pacing failure occurs. It occurs within several days of implantation and is usually asymptomatic, although pericarditis or pericardial hemorrhage with

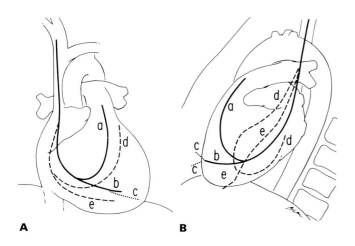

A   B

Figure 3-17. Diagramatic representation of the normal and abnormal positions of pacemaker leads as shown on frontal (*A*) and lateral (*B*) views. (a, pulmonary outflow tract; b, normal position (right ventricular apex); c, cardiac perforation; d, coronary sinus; e, middle cardiac vein.) (Reproduced with permission from M. J. Hewitt. Coronary sinus atrial pacing: radiographic considerations. Am J Radiol 1981;136:323–328. Copyright 1981 by the American Roentgen Ray Society.)

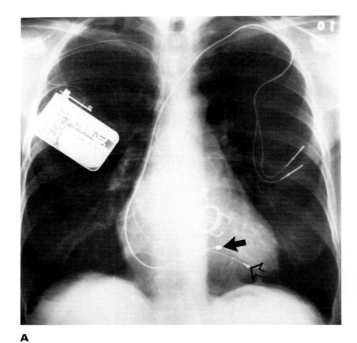

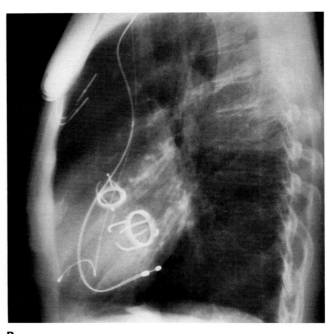

A

B

Figure 3-18. Pacemaker position in coronary sinus. A frontal chest film (*A*) demonstrates two pacemaker wires: the tip of the old wire (*solid arrow*) arches cephalad to the new wire (*open arrow*), which is attached to a subcutaneous pacemaker (*arrowhead*). The lateral film (*B*) shows the old wire (*solid arrow*) in the typical posterior course of the coronary sinus.

tamponade can result. Radiographically, an extracardiac lead position may be obvious, but most often the electrode tip appears to be in a normal position. Lateral radiographs or fluoroscopic spot films may be able to demonstrate that the tip lies within or beyond the subepicardial layer of fat, thereby confirming myocardial perforation.[26] Two-dimensional echocardiography and CT can confirm the extracardiac tip position. Infection within the subcutaneous pouch housing the generator causes pain, swelling, and erythema over the site. Radiographically, air or an air-fluid level may be present about the generator.

Automatic Implantable Cardioverter Defibrillators

Automatic implantable cardioverter defibrillators (AICD) devices are increasingly being placed for the treatment of life-threatening ventricular tachyarrhythmias. Earlier devices comprised transvenous right ventricular sensing and SVC defibrillating electrodes and an epicardial patch defibrillating electrode, all attached to a pulse generator placed in an abdominal subcutaneous pouch. Current devices are completely epicardial, with screw-tipped sensing electrodes and anterior (right ventricular) and posterior (left ventricular) defibrillating electrodes (Fig. 3-19). The defibrillating electrodes are radiolucent mesh

wire patches that contain an embedded rectangular radio-opaque wire that marks its position. The apparent "gap" between the lead wire from the AICD and the radio-opaque marker is factitious and should not be confused with lead fracture[27] (see Fig. 3-19). These devices are placed by way of a subxiphoid approach, median sternotomy, or left anterolateral thoracotomy.

Lurie et al. reported atelectasis, infiltrates, or effusions on radiographs in 17 of 22 patients (77%) with AICD devices.[27] Four (18%) developed pneumothoraces from thoracotomy or median sternotomy. In the postoperative evaluation of these devices, the detection of crumpling of the rectangular marker is usually of clinical significance. This finding associated with fever, leukocytosis, or signs of infection around the generator pouch strongly suggests intrapericardial infection.[28] In the absence of signs or symptoms of infection, a crumpled pad may be the first indicator of pericardial fibrosis, which may cause an increased energy requirement for defibrillation, or lead to constrictive pericarditis. CT may be valuable in the diagnosis of late postoperative AICD infection, since most pericardial fluid collections in asymptomatic patients resolve within 4 weeks postoperatively. CT can also be used to demonstrate the position of the pads in relation to the myocardium and to demonstrate thickened pericardium in patients with the complication of constrictive pericarditis.

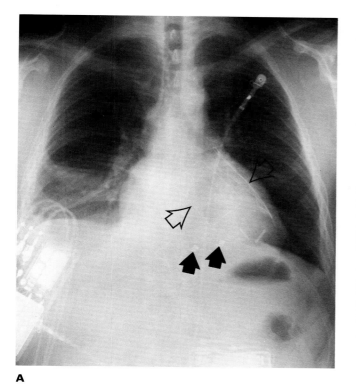
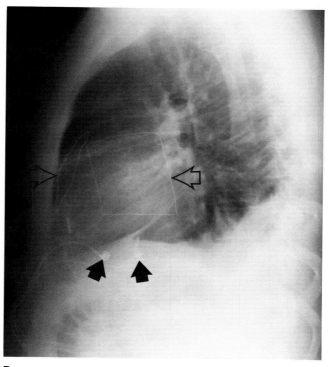

Figure 3-19. PA (*A*) and lateral (*B*) radiographs of a patient with an automatic implantable cardioverter defibrillator (AICD) device. Note sensing (*solid arrows*) and defibrillating (*open arrows*) electrodes.

Intraaortic Counterpulsation Balloon Pump

The intra-aortic balloon pump (IABP) has been used since 1962 for the management of cardiogenic shock and in high-risk patients undergoing cardiac surgery.[29] The balloons are introduced percutaneously through femoral artery and positioned in the descending thoracic aorta. A 26-cm balloon inflates with carbon dioxide during diastole. If a radiograph is exposed during diastole, the gas-filled balloon is seen as a sausage-shaped radiolucency within the descending thoracic aorta (Fig. 3-20). Diastolic inflation increases coronary artery flow and myocardial perfusion, and improves systemic perfusion by increasing diastolic runoff. Active deflation during systole decreases ventricular afterload, thereby decreasing myocardial work and oxygen demand.[30]

The tip of the catheter, which can be identified on chest film by its radio-opaque marker, is ideally positioned just distal to the origin of the left subclavian artery (see Fig. 3-20). This position provides maximal perfusion to the coronary circulation while avoiding occlusion of the left subclavian and renal arteries. A catheter with its tip at or within the left subclavian orifice may occlude or thrombose the vessel.

Aortic dissection from the catheter has been reported and should be suspected when the outer margin of the aorta becomes ill-defined, especially after a difficult placement. An aortogram should be performed if aortic dissection or perforation is suspected. Additional complications include renal and mesenteric ischemia, atherosclerotic emboli to the kidneys or lower extremities, femoral artery thrombosis and bleeding, and balloon rupture.

The Chest Radiograph in Acute Myocardial Infarction

The radiographic changes associated with elevated pulmonary venous pressures due to left ventricular decompensation from ischemia occur in a predictable sequence. Correlative studies in patients with acute myocardial infarction have shown that when PCWP, as measured by flow-directed balloon catheters, is normal (< 12 mm Hg), the chest radiograph is normal.[31] Patients with mild elevation of PCWP (12–18 mm Hg) demonstrate constriction of lower lobe vessels, either due to

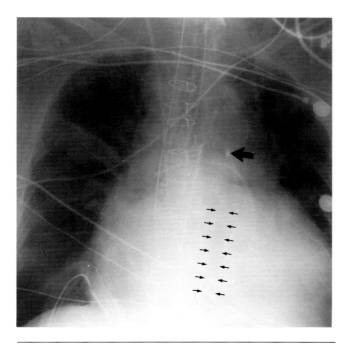

Figure 3-20. Intra-aortic counterpulsation balloon pump. In a postoperative patient with a porcine mitral valve prosthesis, an inflated intra-aortic balloon (*small arrows*) is seen in position. The tip of the catheter, denoted by a radio-opaque marker (*solid arrow*), is well positioned below the origin of the left subclavian artery.

mild perivenous edema, eliminating the normal tethering effect of the lung on the pulmonary veins, or from reflex vasoconstriction. This in turn leads to redistribution of blood flow to lower resistance upper lobe vessels in the upright patient. Moderate elevation of PCWP (19–25 mm Hg) leads to loss of vascular definition in the perihilar and lower zones, peribronchial cuffing, and the development of Kerley's A and B lines (Fig. 3-21). Severe pulmonary venous hypertension (PCWP > 25 mm Hg) results in perihilar or generalized alveolar edema.[2]

Although the sequence of radiographic changes are fairly predictable, the chest radiograph may over- or underestimate the severity of pulmonary venous hypertension in certain situations. In one study, the radiograph accurately predicted the PCWP in only 43% of patients with acute myocardial infarction.[32] Normal radiographs in postinfarction patients with elevated PCWP may be due to a "diagnostic lag" of up to 12 hours following acute myocardial infarction.[31] In their study correlating PCWP with radiographic assessment of pulmonary vascular congestion, Kostuk et al. found that of 23 postinfarction patients with PCWP of 13 to 18 mm Hg had normal radiographs.[32]

Radiographic overestimation of PCWP has been attributed to a "post-therapeutic phase lag" in which there is persistent clinical and radiographic evidence of pulmonary edema after PCWP has returned to normal following treatment.[31] This time interval may range from 21

hours to 4 days after correction of PCWP. Additionally, persistent edema due to increased capillary permeability from cardiogenic shock and hypoxemia may complicate the picture and give pulmonary edema in the presence of normal PCWP. Finally, patients with underlying chronic interstitial fibrosis from any etiology may be thought to demonstrate persistent elevation of PCWP and interstitial edema, even though PCWP is normal.

Although a normal chest radiograph may be encountered early after myocardial infarction in the presence of an elevated PCWP, the chest radiograph is clearly the most sensitive noninvasive indicator of early left ventricular dysfunction following myocardial infarction. In a study by Harrison et al., of 37 patients with acute myocardial infarction and radiographic evidence of pulmonary edema, the radiographic findings preceded clinical signs of left ventricular failure in 14 (38%).[33] In none of the patients was failure evident clinically without concomitant radiographic findings of left ventricular failure (i.e., pulmonary venous hypertension, interstitial and airspace pulmonary edema). This provides the rationale for routine chest radiographs in asymptomatic postinfarction patients for the early detection and treatment of pulmonary edema.

The development of congestive heart failure is associated with a poor prognosis for early and late survival following myocardial infarction. Assessment of films obtained within 24 hours of an acute myocardial infarction for cardiac enlargement and evidence of pulmonary venous hypertension or pulmonary edema are useful in identifying groups with increased short- (30 days) and long-term (1 yr) mortality. Patients with interstitial or air-space edema have a significantly higher short- and long-term mortality; when generalized alveolar edema develops within 24 hours of acute myocardial infarction, patients do not survive beyond 1 year.[34] Cardiac enlargement after acute myocardial infarction, defined as a cardiothoracic ratio of greater than 50%, appears to be a predictor of early and late mortality independent of pulmonary venous hypertension and pulmonary edema. The fact that the radiographic findings of pulmonary venous congestion and cardiomegaly portend a poor outcome after acute myocardial infarction makes inherent sense; these findings reflect the extent of myocardial damage, which is the predominant prognostic factor following myocardial infarction.

The radiographic changes associated with pulmonary venous hypertension and pulmonary edema require an intact pulmonary vascular bed and normal pulmonary architecture. Subsequently, the pattern of disease may be atypical in patients with underlying pulmonary vascular, parenchymal, or pleural disease. Additionally, normal gravitational forces govern the distribution of interstitial and air-space edema. Absence of portions of the pulmonary arterial bed, as in pulmonary arterial hypoplasia (e.g., Swyer–James syndrome), emphysema, or throm-

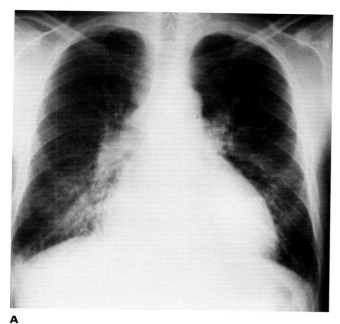

A

Figure 3-21. Radiographic findings in mild pulmonary venous hypertension. Following an acute myocardial infarction, distention of upper lobe vessels, indistinct vascular markings, subpleural edema, and the presence of Kerley B lines reflect elevated pulmonary capillary wedge pressure due to a noncompliant left ventricle.

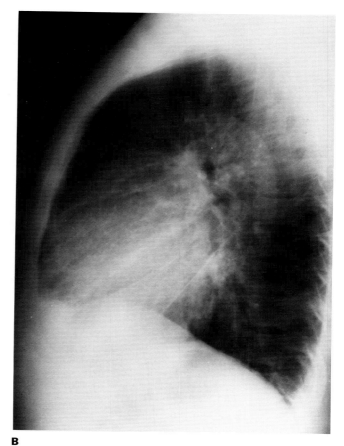

B

boembolic disease, will protect those areas from developing vascular engorgement and subsequently the transudation of fluid. In these patients, air-space pulmonary edema may be misdiagnosed as multilobar pneumonia (Fig. 3-22). Chronic parenchymal lung disease may result in a reticular or even miliary pattern of disease.[35] Extensive fibrothorax, as from previous tuberculous pleural disease, may lead to restricted ventilation and secondary underperfusion, resulting in unilateral pulmonary edema.

Unilateral pulmonary edema may also be due to prolonged positioning in the decubitus position, and it is difficult to distinguish this from pneumonia radiographically. A similar, predominantly unilateral pattern may be seen after the rapid evacuation of large, subacute or chronic (> 48 hr) pleural air or fluid collections. Prolonged collapse of the underlying lung with secondary surfactant depletion and the requirement for applying large negative intrapleural pressure for reexpansion are the proposed mechanisms.

Localized air-space edema of the right upper lobe in patients following acute myocardial infarction has been demonstrated when acute mitral valvular dysfunction occurs secondary to ischemia or infarction and rupture of the posterior papillary muscle (Fig. 3-23). The

regurgitant flow of blood across the incompetent anterolateral leaflet of the mitral valve leads to selective right superior pulmonary venous hypertension. The diagnosis should be considered when focal right upper lobe airspace opacification develops on a background of interstitial pulmonary edema following acute myocardial infarction, in the absence of signs of infection.[36] A mitral regurgitation murmur may be noted, and two-dimensional echocardiography confirms the diagnosis.

Complications Following Myocardial Infarction

Cardiac Rupture. Cardiac rupture following transmural myocardial infarction occurs in approximately 5% of patients.[37] Rupture most commonly occurs at the free wall of the left ventricle, but the interventricular septum and papillary muscle may be affected. Rupture of the left ventricular wall typically occurs within 2 to 4 days of infarction, and may involve the anterior, lateral, or posterior wall. Most patients develop fatal hemopericardium; however, in one autopsy study, 32% of patients developed a false ventricular aneurysm.[38] It is in this latter group of patients that radiographic detection of a focal evagination emanating from the left ventricle in the post-

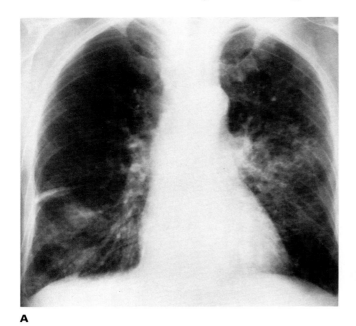
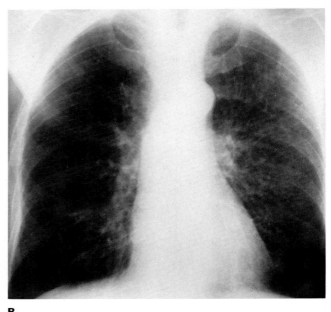

A   **B**

Figure 3-22. Pulmonary edema in patient with underlying emphysema. *A:* Initial radiograph demonstrates patchy air-space opacification in the right lower lobe and left perihilar region. Note small bilateral pleural effusions. *B:* Followup film obtained three days later shows resolution of air-space process and pleural effusions. Note supernormal lung volumes and attenuated right upper lobe vessels evident after diuresis. The patient had suffered an acute myocardial infarction resulting in atypical pulmonary edema that spared emphysematous regions.

infarction period can lead to life-saving surgical intervention.

Rupture of the interventricular septum occurs within 1 week of onset of AMI.[38] Sudden clinical deterioration with biventricular failure, associated with a pansystolic murmur and thrill, are characteristic findings. Half of the patients die within 1 week of onset. Chest radiographs may demonstrate pulmonary arterial and venous engorgement from a combination of shunt vascularity and left ventricular failure. The presence of alveolar pulmonary edema precludes recognition of these vascular changes, and the radiographs are likely to be interpreted solely as worsening left ventricular function. The diagnosis is confirmed by noting an increase in oxygen saturation between the SVC and right atrium as compared to the right ventricle and pulmonary artery.[38] Echocardiography demonstrates the septal defect and the left-to-right shunt.

Rupture of a papillary muscle usually occurs within 5 days of acute myocardial infarction, although in 2 of 7 cases in one series, rupture occurred months after infarction. It is as common as septal rupture.[37] The posteromedial papillary muscle is almost always involved, and it is always associated with infarction of the adjacent posterior wall of the left ventricle. Clinically, distinction from ventricular septal rupture may be difficult. Radiographically, worsening pulmonary edema, particularly affecting

the right upper lobe out of proportion to the remainder of the lung, is usually seen, with little change in the size of the left atrium or left ventricle.

Aneurysms. True and false ventricular aneurysms result from transmural myocardial infarction. True aneurysms consist of fibrous replacement of the infarcted myocardium, which contains some elements of the original wall. They are wide mouthed and appear radiographically as focal bulges along the left ventricular contour. Calcification may be detected within the wall of the aneurysm, although calcification may be seen within infarcted myocardium without aneurysm formation.[39] True aneurysms rarely rupture. However, stasis of blood within the asystolic aneurysm sac may lead to the formation of mural thrombi. Congestive heart failure may develop because of paradoxical filling of the aneurysm during systole. Reentrant tachyarrhythmias may emanate from the aneurysm wall. When aneurysms are associated with congestive failure, systemic emboli from intraaneurysmal mural thrombi, or medically resistant tachyarrhythmias, aneurysmectomy should be considered.

False aneurysms or pseudoaneurysms represent contained rupture of the left ventricular wall in which the parietal pericardium and mediastinal connective tissue form the wall of the aneurysm. They may occur over any portion of the left ventricular wall, although they tend to

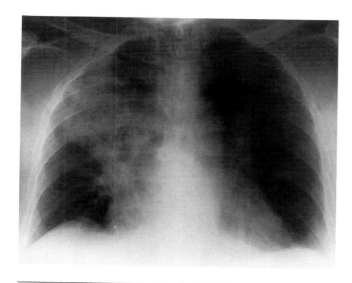

Figure 3-23. Right upper lobe pulmonary edema secondary to mitral regurgitation. Three days following inferior/posterior myocardial infarction, a mitral regurgitation murmur was noted on physical exam. Chest radiograph demonstrates pulmonary venous hypertension with focal right upper lobe air-space opacification. Echocardiogram documented a regurgitant flow across the mitral valve.

involve the diaphragmatic or posterolateral wall following right coronary artery infarcts. The mouth of a false aneurysm more narrow than its fundus, which is typically quite large in diameter (on the order of 10 cm).[40] The importance of the correct diagnosis of a false aneurysm lies in its propensity to rupture, early surgical intervention being the key to improved survival.[41] Noninvasive imaging by echocardiography, CT, and magnetic resonance imaging are key to the diagnosis.[42] Contrast ventriculography demonstrates filling of the false aneurysm through one or more narrow channels, and shows the avascular nature of the wall of the pesudoaneurysm. This latter finding helps distinguish false aneurysm from true aneurysm, in which the coronary arteries are seen to drape over the aneurysm.[40]

References

1. Milne ENC. A physiological approach to reading critical care unit films. J Thorac Imag 1986;1(3):60.
2. Higgins CB, Battler A. The chest radiograph in acute myocardial infarction. In: Karlinski JS, Gregoratus G, eds. Coronary Care. 1st ed. New York: Churchill Livingstone, 1981.
3. Ruskin JA, Gurney JW, Thornsen MK, Goodman LR. Detection of pleural effusion on supine chest radiographs. Am J Radiol 1987;148:681.
4. Tocino IM, Miller MH, Fairfax WR. Distribution of pneumothorax in the supine and semirecumbent critically ill adult. Am J Radiol 1985;144:901.
5. Onik G, Goodman PC, Webb WR, Brasch RC. Hydropneumothorax: detection on supine radiographs. Radiology 1984;152:31.
6. Joseph AEA, Lacey BJ, Bryant THE, et al. The hypertransradiant hemithorax: the importance of lateral decentering, and the explanation for its appearance due to rotation. Clin Radiol 1978;29:125.
7. Zylak CJ, Littleton JT, Durizch ML. Illusory consolidation of the left lower lobe: a pitfall of portable radiography. Radiology 1988;167:653.
8. Gallant TE, Dietrich PA, Shinozaki T, Deane RSD. Simple device to measure patient position on portable radiography. Am J Radiol 1978;131:169.
9. Goodman LR. Pulmonary support and monitoring apparatus. In: Goodman LR, Putman CE, eds. Intensive care radiology: imaging of the critically ill. 2nd ed. Philadelphia: WB Saunders, 1983:19.
10. Goodman LR, Conrardy PA, Laing F, Singer MM. Radiographic evaluation of endotracheal tube position. Am J Radiol 1976;127:433.
11. Smith GM, Reed JC, Choplin RH. Radiographic detection of esophageal malpositioning of endotracheal tubes. Am J Radiol 1990;154:23.
12. Webb WR, LaBerge J. Radiographic recognition of chest tube malposition in the major fissure. Chest 1984;85(1):81.
13. Webb WR, Godwin JD. The obscured outer edge: a sign of improperly placed pleural drainage tubes. Am J Radiol 1980;134:1062.
14. Goss CM. In: Clemente S, ed. Gray's anatomy. 29th ed. Philadelphia: Lea and Febiger, 1976:697,704.
15. Marx GF. Clinical Anesth Conf: Hazards associated with venous pressure monitoring. New York J Med 1969;69:955.
16. Wechsler RJ, Steiner RM, Kinori I. Monitoring the monitors: the radiology of thoracic catheters, wires, and tubes. Semin Roentgenol 1988;23(1):61.
17. Mitchell SE, Clark RA. Complications of central venous catheterization. Am J Radiol 1979;133:467.
18. Tocino IM, Watanabe A. Impending catheter perforation of superior vena cava: radiographic recognition. Am J Radiol 1986;146:487.
19. McLoud TC, Putman CE. Radiology of the Swan–Ganz catheter and associated pulmonary complications. Radiology 1975;116:19.
20. Henry DA, LeBolt S. Invasive hemodynamic monitoring: radiologist's perspective. Radiographics 1986;6(4):535.
21. Sise MJ, Hollingsworth P, Brimm JE, Peters RM, Virgilio RW, Sheckford SR. Complications of the flow-directed pulmonary artery catheter: a prospective analysis in 219 patients. Crit Care Med 1981;9:315.
22. Boyd KD, Thomas SJ, Gold J, Boyd AD. A prospective study of complications of pulmonary artery catheterizations in 500 consecutive patients. Chest 1983;84:245.
23. Foote GA, Schabel SI, Hodges M. Pulmonary complications of the flow directed balloon-tipped catheter. N Engl J Med 1974;290:927.
24. Dieden JD, Friloux LA, Remer JW. Pulmonary artery false aneurysms secondary to Swan–Ganz pulmonary artery catheters. Am J Radiol 1987;149:901.
25. Steiner RM, Tegtmeyer CJ, Morse D, et al. The radiology of cardiac pacemakers. Radiographics 1986;6(3):373.
26. Ormond RS, Rubenfire M, Anbe DT, Drake EH. Radiographic demonstration of myocardial penetration by permanent endocardial pacemakers. Radiology 1971;98:35.
27. Lurie AL, Udoff EJ, Reid PJ. Automatic implantable cardioverter–defibrillator: appearance and complications. Am J Radiol 1985;145:723.
28. Goodman LR, Almassi GH, Troup PJ, et al. Complications of automatic implantable cardioverter–defibrillators: radiographic, CT, and echocardiographic evaluation. Radiology 1989;170:447.

29. Hyson EA, Ravin CE, Kelley MJ, McB Curis A. Intraaortic counterpulsation balloon: radiographic considerations. Am J Radiol 1977;128:915.

30. Weber KT, Janicki JS. Intraaortic balloon counterpulsation: a review of physiological principles, clinical results, and device safety. Ann Thorac Surg 1974;17(6):602.

31. McHugh TJ, Forrester JS, Adler L, Zion D, Swan HJC. Pulmonary vascular congestion in acute myocardial infarction: hemodynamic and radiologic correlations. Ann Intern Med 1972;76:29.

32. Kostuk W, Barr JW, Simon AL, Ross J. Correlations between the chest film and hemodynamics in acute myocardial infarction. Circulation 1973;48:624.

33. Harrison MO, Conte PJ, Heitzman ER. Radiological detection of clinically occult cardiac failure following myocardial infarction. Br J Radiol 1971;44:265.

34. Battler A, Karliner JS, Higgins CB, et al. The initial chest x-ray in acute myocardial infarction: prediction of early and late mortality and survival. Circulation 1980;61(5):1004.

35. Hublitz UF, Shapiro JH. Atypical pulmonary patterns of congestive failure in chronic lung disease: influence of pre-existing disease on the appearance and distribution of pulmonary disease. Radiology 1969;93:995.

36. Gurney JW, Goodman LR. Pulmonary edema localized in the right upper lobe accompanying mitral regurgitation. Radiology 1989;171:397.

37. VanTassel RA, Edwards JE. Rupture of heart complicating myocardial infarction: analysis of 40 cases including nine examples of left ventricular false aneurysm. Chest 1972;61(2):104.

38. Heikkila J, Karesoja M, Luomanmaki K. Ruptured interventricular septum complicating acute myocardial infarction: clinical spectrum and hemodynamic evaluation with bedside cardiac catheterization. Chest 1974;66(6):675.

39. Baron MG. Postinfarction aneurysm of the left ventricle. Circulation 1971;43:762.

40. Spindola–Franco H, Kronacher N. Pseudoaneurysm of the left ventricle: radiographic and angiocardiographic diagnosis. Radiology 1978;127:29.

41. Vlodaver Z, Coe JI, Edwards JE. True and false left ventricular aneurysms: propensity for the latter to rupture. Circulation 1975;51:567.

42. Higgins CB, Lipton MJ, Johnson AD, Peterson KL, Vieweg WVR. False aneurysm of the left ventricle: identification of distinctive clinical, radiographic, and angiographic features. Radiology 1978;127:21.

Chapter 4

Angiography of Acquired Heart Disease

Charles B. Higgins

Cardiac catheterization, for the past four decades, has been the cornerstone upon which cardiac diagnosis has been based. The three major components of catheterization are measurement of pressures with fluid-filled or solid-state catheters; estimation of blood flow by oximetry (Fick method) and indicator dilution techniques; and examination of cardiac morphology and contractile function by angiography. The importance of the angiographic data acquired at cardiac catheterization has assumed increasing significance in the last decade. However, the role of ventricular angiography in the medical and surgical management of acquired cardiac disease has had its peak and will decline in the future because of the recognition of the capabilities of noninvasive imaging studies. Although cardiac angiography is still held to be the gold standard against which noninvasive techniques are validated, some of the newer tomographic techniques provide a three-dimensional rather than two-dimensional representation of the heart and thereby are quantitatively more precise and reproducible.

The methodology of cardiac angiography has had three notable phases: nonselective angiography (intravenous injection of contrast media); selective angiography (intrachamber injection); and selective angiography with digital enhancement. Digital enhancement has permitted reduction in the volumes of contrast media needed for optimal chamber opacification. Registration of angiographic image has passed through two phases—serial radiography ("cut films") and cine films and is now moving toward digital display and archiving.

Contrast angiography provides high resolution, two-dimensional images of the cardiac chambers and coronary arteries from which morphologic, dimensional, and functional data can be derived. Subjective assessment of the cardiac angiogram is usually employed on a daily basis in order to secure a diagnosis and to review decisions about management. Quantitative methods have been developed and extensively verified for the measurement of volumes of atria and ventricles, stroke volume, ejection fraction and regional wall motion of the ventricles. Although estimation of the severity of valvular stenosis is not reliable from the angiographic appearance, estimation of the severity of regurgitation can be provided by angiography. Sophisticated measurements of cardiac dimensions and function can be derived from angiography, such as ventricular mass, wall thickness and thickening, ventricular wall tension and stress, pressure-volume work and power curves, and compliance.

Technique

Selective angiography is done by placing the injecting catheter into the ventricle to be evaluated. Selective catheterization is now done preferably by the femoral route, using a percutaneous approach (Seldinger technique). The right ventricle is entered by a catheter passed antegrade through the femoral vein, and the left ventricle is entered by a catheter passed retrograde through the femoral artery. Retrograde arterial catheterization may be impeded or inadvisable owing to a heightened chance of complications in patients with obstructive ileofemoral arterial disease or abdominal aortic aneurysm. Under such circumstances, catheterization is done by way of the brachial artery (arteriotomy) or axillary artery (percutaneous Seldinger technique). Catheterization of the left ventricle may also be difficult because of aortic stenosis, a prosthetic aortic valve, or aortic ectasia. Selective catheterization of the left-sided cardiac chambers can also be accomplished by puncture of the atrial septum with a catheter introduced through the femoral vein, or as a last option, transthoracic needle puncture of the left ventricular apex.

Left atrial angiography is performed infrequently for the evaluation of acquired heart disease; it is used for the identification of myxoma and thrombus. For this purpose contrast media are injected into the main pulmonary artery and the left atrium is opacified on the transit of the contrast media through the left side of the heart (levo phase). Selective left atrial opacification can be performed either by catheter passage across a patent foramen ovale or by transseptal puncture or retrograde passage of a catheter across the mitral valve.

Catheters

For delivery of contrast media a catheter with multiple side holes and adequate internal caliber is employed in order to deliver a sufficient injection rate. Although a single end-hole catheter is essential for pressure measurements, this kind of catheter is avoided for injection of contrast media in order to minimize the possibility of intramural injection of the media. A coiled tipped (pigtail) catheter is used to reduce movement and contact of the catheter with the ventricular wall during injection in order to minimize arrhythmias and intramyocardial penetration of contrast media during angiography. Intramural injection of contrast media and instability of the catheter position are especially troublesome during right ventriculography; balloon-tipped catheters have been employed to reduce these problems. Catheters used for pressure measurements and ventriculography are shown in Figure 4-1. Single end-hole catheters are designed for acquiring pressure measurements and multiple-hole catheters are employed for angiography. Balloon-tip catheters were designed for flotation of the catheter downstream with blood flow and, in the case of the Berman angiographic catheter, for decreasing the problem of intramyocardial injection of contrast media.

Radiographic Factors

Contrast angiography is performed using either single-plane or biplane views with registration of images on

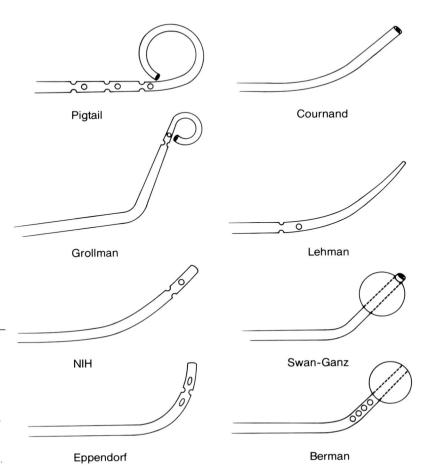

Pigtail

Cournand

Grollman

Lehman

NIH

Swan-Ganz

Eppendorf

Berman

Figure 4-1. Catheters used for left and right ventricular catheterization and angiography. Cournand and Swan–Ganz catheters have end holes only and are used for measuring pressures. Other catheters are designed for angiography with multiple end and/or side holes. Grollman and Pigtail catheters are designed to prevent myocardial penetration during manipulation and intramyocardial injection of contrast medium for right and left ventriculography, respectively. The balloon of the Berman catheter also minimizes the possibility of intramyocardial injection.

cine film. The filming rate for ventriculography is 30 to 60 frames per second. In order to enhance contrast between the opacified blood pool and surrounding structures, the kVp should be maintained as low as possible. This provides contrast based upon K edge effect of iodine in the contrast media. To maximize the K edge effect, the kVp should ideally be less than 70, but this is usually impractical in large adults. In order to maintain adequate film exposure, the mAS must be high. This can be done by using high milliamperage (mA) and long exposure time (S). However, the time must be kept very short (5–10 μsec) in order to diminish motion unsharpness of the beating heart. Consequently, x-ray generators capable of delivering very high mA and with excellent heat loading capability are needed to maintain and deliver mA repeatedly during the relatively long period of cine recording.

Digital registration, enhancement, and analysis of ventriculograms has been used in recent years. Because of digital image enhancement and subtraction processes, excellent contrast can be achieved with a reduction in the volume and concentration of the contrast medium. Digital contrast ventriculography has been effective by injection of contrast media intravenously or into the ventricle. However, the selective injection of the contrast media into the cardiac chambers is preferred even when using digital enhancement processes, and the intravenous route has been nearly abandoned except under unusual circumstances.

Timing of the film exposures can be recorded in relation to the precise phases within the cardiac cycle. This provides precise selection of the end-diastolic and end-systolic frames. A record of timing of exposures is seldom needed except for experimental protocols that require construction of pressure-volume curves.

Views

Biplane filming is generally the most frequently employed protocol. The advantage of the biplane mode is the more accurate measurement of volumes and examination of a more extensive area of the ventricle. The need for biplane angiography is becoming less critical because of the now-recognized high level of accuracy of noninvasive techniques for imaging the left ventricle. Biplane contrast ventriculography is important for the full evaluation of valvular disease, cardiomyopathy, and ischemic heart disease with a prior myocardial infarction. Single-plane left ventriculography has been considered adequate for the evaluation of patients with suspected coronary arterial disease without a history of prior myocardial infarction.

The left anterior oblique (LAO) and right anterior oblique (RAO) are preferred in most circumstances. The 30° RAO view is used to improve the visualization of the various segments of the left ventricle (Fig. 4-2). In this view segmental contraction can be evaluated in the region of distribution of the three major coronary arteries (right coronary, left anterior descending, and circumflex coronary arteries). The left ventricle is moved away from the spine and separately displays five segments of the left ventricle. This view is also effective for displaying motion of the mitral valve and for assessing severity of mitral regurgitation. The 60° LAO view separates the right and left

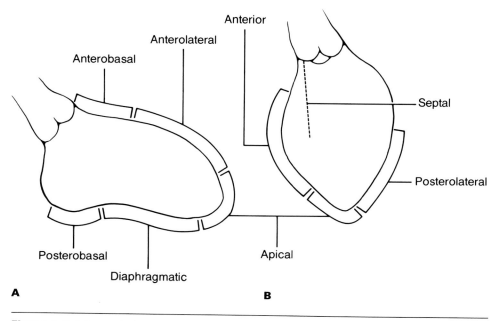

Figure 4-2. Left ventricular segments in the RAO (*A*) and LAO (*B*) views.

ventricles and is used to assess shunts between these chambers. It is the optimal view for assessing function of the aortic valve. It also provides direct visualization of the anterior, posterolateral, and part of the septal segment of the left ventricle (see Fig. 4-2).

Axial ventriculography is not often needed for the assessment of acquired heart disease, but may be useful in some instances. Axial or double oblique angiography employs double angulation (obliquity) of the x-ray beam relative to the sagittal plane of the body. The obliquity is designated by the relationship of the image registration device (image intensifier) to the subject. Angulation of the mechanically linked x-ray tube and intensifier is effected in both the transverse and sagittal planes of the subject (Fig. 4-3). If the image intensifier has been rotated to the left anterior side of the subject and in a cranial direction, the view is called cranial LAO view. If the image intensifier is rotated to the right anterior side of the subject and in a caudal direction, the view is called caudal RAO view. Cranial and caudal angulation minimize overlap of ventricular regions. The cranial LAO view improves visualization of the septal region of the left ventricle and the mitral valve. The RAO caudal view provides slight improvement in visualization of left ventricular segments and the mitral valve.

Contrast Media

Iodinated contrast media with a concentration of 320 to 370 mg/ml iodine (approximately 64%–76% contrast media solution) is generally employed. A lower concentration may be effective with the use of digital enhancement techniques. Ionic contrast media are still used with great frequency in the United States, but nonionic media are used preferentially in many European countries. Because of the reduced frequency of adverse effects and lesser hemodynamic action of the nonionic media, it is advisable to use them in patients at increased risk for complications, such as those with severe aortic stenosis, severe myocardial dysfunction, recent acute myocardial infarction, history of prior contrast media reaction, diabetes, or renal insufficiency. The hemodynamic effects of ionic and nonionic contrast media are beyond the scope of this chapter and can be found in publications on this topic.[1,2]

Contrast media are injected in the lowest volume and at the lowest rate necessary to provide optimal opacification of the left ventricle. For left ventriculography in adults of average size, the volume is 40 to 50 ml and the injection rate is 12 to 15 ml/sec. The injection rate is maintained as low as possible in order to minimize catheter recoil and thereby avoid or reduce premature ven-

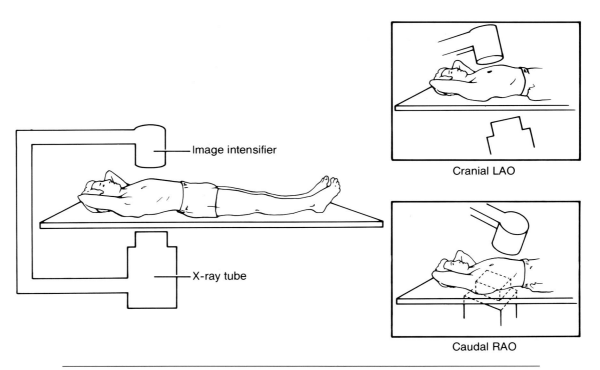

Image intensifier

X-ray tube

Cranial LAO

Caudal RAO

Figure 4-3. Positions of the image intensifier and x-ray tube for the cranial LAO and caudal RAO views. The views are named according to the position of the image intensifier in relation to the body of the patient. For the cranial LAO view the intensifier is rotated toward the patient's head and left anterior side. For the caudal RAO view the intensifier is rotated toward the patient's feet and right anterior side.

tricular contractions (PVCs) during ventricular opacification. Although such PVCs are usually unsustained, they complicate analysis of the ventriculogram by inducing artifactual mitral regurgitation and an abnormal segmental contraction pattern.

The volume and injection rate of the contrast media must be increased in larger patients and in the presence of dilated ventricles, severe valvular regurgitation, or shunt lesions. Attempts to reduce the total volume of contrast media are important for patients with hyperviscosity states (macroglobulinemia), multiple myeloma, and renal insufficiency, especially patients with diabetes and renal insufficiency. The volume of contrast media can be reduced substantially by using digital contrast enhancement and subtraction techniques.

The Left Ventriculogram

The salient features of the left ventriculogram are:

1. Biplane in AP and lateral views or 30° RAO and 60° LAO views.
2. Pigtail catheter.
3. Contrast volume = 45 to 50 ml.
4. Injection rate = 12 to 15 ml/sec.
5. Filming rate = 30 to 60 frames/sec. It is now usually done at 30 frames/sec.

The subjective assessment of the left ventriculogram must be done in a stepwise systematic fashion. The analysis consists of the following five sequential steps:

1. Identification of calcification. This is done on images acquired prior to contrast injection.
2. Evaluation of motion, thickness, and competency of the mitral valve.
3. Evaluation of thickness and motion of the aortic valve.
4. Evaluation of left ventricular size. Size of left atrium may also be defined by mitral regurgitation.
5. Evaluation of global and regional wall motion. This includes the extent and pattern of diastolic expansion as well as systolic contraction.

Calcification

Prior to opacification of the left ventricle, calcification can be identified moving within the cardiac silhouette. Cardiac calcification must be differentiated from noncardiac calcification such as calcified hilar lymph nodes or pleural calcification; the former move with cardiac pulsation while the latter are immobile or move slightly with respiration. Some calcifications of the heart are important

either for diagnosis or to provide a sign of the likely severity of a lesion.

Identification of the site of calcification is done by recognition of the position and the nature of motion of the calcification (Fig. 4-4). Valvular calcification moves rapidly as expected for valvular motion. However, the motion of the valve may be very slight in the presence of severe stenosis. The aortic valve is located in the LAO view; it is located at the base of the aorta, which is readily recognized in this view. Dense calcification of the aortic valve in patients younger than 60 years indicates hemodynamically significant stenosis. Aortic annular calcification is discerned by a circular configuration. A caudal extension from the circular calcification is sometimes seen when the calcification has penetrated into the base of the ventricular septum, where it may cause heart block. Mitral valvular calcification is identified most readily in the RAO view at the junction of the left atrium and left ventricle. Again, the motion is rapid and occurs toward the apex during diastole. Mitral annular calcification is frequently very dense, extensive, and conforms to a C shape. This calcification shows a slower swaying motion toward the apex during systole. When mitral annular and valvular calcification coexist, differentiation may be difficult, but may be possible by viewing the valve in the RAO view. In this view the rapid motion of calcification within the C-shaped calcification of the annulus can be discerned.

Curvilinear calcification in the region of the left atrium is observed in some patients with rheumatic mitral stenosis. This calcification of the left atrial wall or appendage is frequently associated with left atrial thrombus. Amorphous and highly mobile calcification in the left atrium is seen in a minority of patients with left atrial myxoma.

Coronary arterial calcification is observed most frequently. The location and configuration (double parallel lines of calcium) may be characteristic. The site of the calcium in the RAO and LAO views can be used to localize it to one of the major coronary arteries (Fig. 4-4). The extent and density of the calcification has a relationship to the likelihood of hemodynamically significant coronary arterial disease.[3,4] Coronary arterial calcification detected in men and women under 50 years of age has been associated with a 6 to 50 times increased likelihood of coronary arterial disease. After 60, it has limited predictive value. Calcification of the left main coronary artery and calcification in the sinuses of Valsalva are indicators of increased likelihood of stenosis of the left main coronary artery.

Calcification at the margin of the heart indicates pericardial or ventricular mural calcification. To confirm a marginal location, an oblique view in which the incident x-ray beam is tangent to the heart must be used. Pericardial calcification in specific locations is nearly diagnostic of constrictive pericardial disease. It is observed

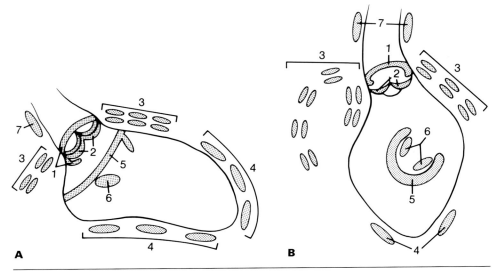

Figure 4-4. Location of cardiac calcifications in the RAO (*A*) and LAO (*B*) views. (1, aortic annulus; 2, aortic valve; 3, coronary arteries; 4, pericardium; 5, mitral annulus; 6, mitral valve; 7, aortic wall.)

in about 50% of patients with constrictive pericarditis.[5] Calcification in this disease occurs most frequently in the atrioventricular and interventricular grooves. However, the calcification is occasionally focal and uncharacteristic. Focal calcification in the pericardium may occur within pericardial plaques for no apparent reason or at the site of a prior hematoma incurred with cardiac surgery.

Curvilinear calcification at the left ventricular margin is characteristic for calcification of a transmural myocardial infarction or left ventricular aneurysm. Calcification may also occur in an organized ventricular mural thrombus.

Rare causes of calcification include mass lesions of the pericardium, such as teratoma and echinococcal cysts; myocardial masses such as fibroma and tuberculoma; and Loeffer's eosinophilic fibroplasia of the left ventricle.

Valvular Function

Thickening and reduced motion of the aortic cusps or the mitral leaflets indicates disease of the valves. However, motion of the valves is difficult to estimate or quantify from the angiographic appearance. The severity of aortic and mitral stenosis is assessed by measuring the pressure gradient and estimating blood flow across the valve in relation to the pressure gradient. On the other hand, the angiogram is used to estimate the severity of valvular regurgitation.

Valvular motion and insufficiency can be evaluated most effectively by injecting the contrast media immediately downstream of the valve. For the evaluation of the aortic valve, the contrast media are injected through a

multi-holed coiled catheter placed near the sinotubular junction of the ascending aorta. Since there is no problem with induction of PVCs, the contrast media should be injected at a high rate through the aortic catheter. An injection rate of 25 to 30 ml/sec for a total volume of 50 to 60 ml is effective. For evaluation of the mitral valve, the contrast media are injected through a coiled (pigtail) catheter placed in the inflow region of the left ventricle. An injection rate of 12 to 15 ml/sec for a total volume of 40 to 50 ml provides effective ventricular opacification, and such a low flow rate minimizes provocation of PVCs.

Estimation of the Severity of Valvular Stenosis

The severity of valvular stenosis is determined by the measurement of a pressure gradient across the valve and an estimation of the orifice size of the valve. Calculation of the orifice area is based upon measurement of the pressure gradient and flow across the valve. Measuring a pressure gradient alone means risking underestimating the severity by finding a small gradient in the presence of a low flow rate across the valve.

The Gorlin equations for calculating orifice area are:

$$\text{Aortic valve area} = \frac{F}{44.5\sqrt{\Delta P}}$$

$$\text{Mitral valve area} = \frac{F}{38.0\sqrt{\Delta P}}$$

where F = flow across the orifice in ml/sec and ΔP = mean pressure gradient in mm Hg across the orifice. For this measurement, F is derived from the cardiac output and estimation of the time of opening of the specific valve in the following way:

$$Flow\ (F)\ (ml/sec) = \frac{cardiac\ output\ (ml/min)}{DFP\ (sec/min)\ or\ SEP\ (sec/min)}$$

The DFP (diastolic filling period) or SEP (systolic ejection period) is measured in sec/beat from the pressure tracings. The DFP is used for the calculation of F across the mitral valve and SEP is used for calculation of F across the aortic valve.

Valve areas are corrected for body surface area (m^2). This results in a valve area index (area/m^2).

Estimation of the Severity of Valvular Regurgitation

Subjective (visual) estimation of severity is done by comparing the degree of opacification of the chamber or vessel into which contrast media are injected with the chamber receiving regurgitant flow.

Aortic Regurgitation

Injection into proximal ascending aorta:

Grade I   Regurgitant contrast media does not opacify the apical portion of the LV. No accumulation among beats.

Grade II   Contrast media accumulate in the LV among beats. Density of the contrast media in the LV is less than that of the ascending aorta at the end of the injection period (2–3 beats).

Grade III   Contrast media accumulate to the extent that the density of the LV is equal to that of the aorta.

Grade IV   At the end of the injection, the density of the LV is greater than that of the ascending aorta.

Mitral Regurgitation

Injection into the left ventricle:

Grade I   Regurgitant contrast media do not fill the entire left atrium. No accumulation of contrast media among beats.

Grade II   Contrast media accumulate and fill most of the left atrium. Density of contrast media in the left atrium is less than that of the left ventricle at the end of the injection.

Grade III   Contrast media accumulate to the extent that density of opacification of the left atrium equals that of the left ventricle at the end of the injection period (2–3 beats).

Grade IV   At the end of the injection period, density of left atrial opacification is greater than that of left ventricular opacification. An additional sign of grade IV mitral regurgitation is the entrance of contrast media into the pulmonary veins. The reliability of this sign is questionable because entrance of contrast media into the pulmonary veins is influenced by the size of the left atrium and the direction of the regurgitant jet.

The qualitative (visual) grading of the severity of regurgitation is used routinely in most laboratories and is the most frequently employed practical guide in management decisions. However, comparisons between quantitative measurements of regurgitant flow and the visual grading have revealed only fair correlations.[6,7] Lack of agreement and potential inaccuracies of visual interpretation seem to be related to the influence of chamber size because of rapid dilution of contrast media as they enter a very dilated recipient chamber and the depressed contractile state of the left ventricle, causing inordinately long retention. Heart rate and arterial pressure are other variables that influence the extent of regurgitation as assessed by both qualitative and quantitative techniques.

Quantitative methods for defining the severity of regurgitation are based upon the differences in left ventricular stroke volume as calculated by angiographic measurement of left ventricular stroke volume (total stroke volume) and stroke volume derived from the Fick or indicator dilution methods (effective forward stroke volume).[8] The regurgitant volume per heart beat is calculated by subtracting the forward (effective) stroke volume determined by the Fick, or indicator dilution, method from the stroke volume of the left ventricle as measured by angiographic volumes. The angiographic stroke volume measures the entire output of the ventricle and includes both the forward volume and the regurgitant volume. When both mitral and aortic regurgitation coexist, a combined regurgitant volume can be calculated, but the individual regurgitant volume cannot be measured.

Evaluation of Ventricular Size

A qualitative (visual) estimation of ventricular size is done in the interpretation of the ventriculogram and provides an impression that has some value for those with considerable experience. However, measurement of ventricular volume is required to establish reliability and provide comparisons among sequential studies. The measurements that are done are:

End diastolic volume (EDV)
End systolic volume (ESV)

from which are calculated stroke volume (SV) and ejection fraction (EF):

$$SV = EDV - ESV$$

$$EF = \frac{SV}{EDV}$$

The area length method for calculating left ventricular volume was derived and validated by Dodge and his colleagues.[9] The basic formulae are:

$$volume = \frac{\pi}{6}(L \times D_a \times D_b)$$

where L = length of the major axis of the LV (aortic-mitral valve junction to apex), and D_a and D_b are the transverse diameters in the orthogonal planes when the measurements are done using biplane filming. D is derived from the planimetered area of the ventricle using the formula

$$D = \frac{4A}{\pi L}$$

The area is measured by outlining the interface between the opacified left ventricular chamber and the endocardium on end-diastolic and end-systolic frames. Papillary muscle and trabeculae are included within the outline of the chamber.

Calculations have been accurate using biplane filming in the anteroposterior and lateral views[9]; single plane in the anteroposterior view[10]; and biplane right and left anterior oblique views.[11]

Comparison of measurements derived from these equations with the measured volume of cast models indicates the need to use regression equations to adjust for systematic overestimation of volume by the angiographic calculation. The angiographic measurements overestimate volume before correction, owing in part to the in-clusion of papillary muscle and trabeculae. The regression equations used for the various views are:

biplane AP	$V^1 = 0.928V - 3.8$
single-plane AP	$V^1 = 0.951V - 3.0$
single-plane RAO	$V^1 = 0.81V + 1.9$

where V^1 is the true volume and V is the calculated volume in the various planes.

Calibration of the radiographic projection system is required to obtain accurate measurements. This is done by projecting an opaque measurement grid at a position related to the x-ray tube and image intensifier that is equivalent to the position of the left ventricle during filming. Filming of the grid provides calibration for the measurements and can also be used to correct image distortion resulting from nonparallel x-ray beams and the image intensifier.

The normal values for left ventricular volumes in adults are given in Table 4-1.

Evaluation of Wall Motion

Wall motion is usually assessed qualitatively (visually) in clinical practice. Management decisions are usually based upon the quantification of ejection fraction derived by angiographic volumetrics and visual interpretation of the extent of wall motion. However, visual assessment of wall motion has shown a substantial variability rate among observers.[12] Quantitative methods to measure wall motion exist and have been facilitated using image processing computers, but are actually employed by few laboratories except for research purposes.[13,14]

Abnormalities of wall motion are classified as global and segmental (regional). The former is expected to be the consequence of the failing ventricle caused by cardiomyopathies, valvular heart disease, hypertension,

Table 4-1

Normal Volumes and Dimensions of the Left Ventricle Defined by Cineangiography

	Adults	Children (<2 yrs)	Children (>2 yrs)
End diastolic vol.	70 ± 20	42 ± 10	73 ± 11
End systolic vol.	45 ± 13	28 ± 6	44 ± 5
Ejection fraction (%)	0.67 ± 0.08	0.68 ± 0.05	0.63 ± 0.05
Wall thickness (mm)	10.9 ± 2.0		
Mass (g)	92 ± 16	96 ± 11	86 ± 11

From Dodge HT, Sheehan FH. Quantitative angiographic techniques. In: Fozzard HA, et al, eds. The Heart and Cardiovascular System. New York: Raven Press, 1986.

and other diseases affecting the entire left ventricle. The latter is usually caused by ischemic heart disease.

The terminology for wall motion abnormalities (Fig. 4-5) is:

Hypokinesis: reduced extent of inward wall motion during systole.
Akinesis: no wall motion during systole.
Dyskinesis: outward (paradoxical) wall motion during systole.
Asynchrony: motion of segments slightly out of phase with each other during systole.

The various segments of the left ventricle are displayed in the 30° RAO and 60° LAO views. These are shown diagrammatically in Figure 4-2. Fixed anatomic boundaries between segments have not been uniformly employed owing to variable internal morphology of the left ventricle, but a practical convention in approximating the location of segments exists.

Numerous objective measurements of wall motion have been introduced. These methods attempt to mea-

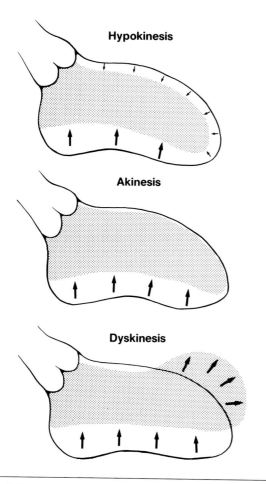

Figure 4-5. Contraction abnormalities of the left ventricle in the RAO view. (Hypokinesis, decreased inward motion; akinesis, no inward motion; dyskinesis, outward motion during systole.)

sure the motion of the same segment of myocardium throughout the cardiac cycle, but because of the complicated motion of the myocardium, none of these methods succeed in doing so. Moreover, all methods measure the two-dimensional display of motion, which actually occurs in three dimensions. Validation of the various methods has been based upon the demonstration of inter- and intra-observer reproducibility rather than a strict comparison with a truth standard and the ability of a method to identify wall motion abnormalities of patients with coronary artery stenoses or previous myocardial infarctions.

Methods are used to realign the end-diastolic and end-systolic images to each other in order to correct for translational motion. Images are also realigned and measured in relation to an external reference system.

Orthogonal and radial motion vectors have been employed to measure wall motion. Regional area changes or regional ejection fraction have also been used to quantitate regional contraction. The orthogonal methods measure the change in length of hemiaxes constructed perpendicular to the long axis of the ventricle. The radial method measures motion toward a single point within the left ventricle; from this single point radii are drawn to the endocardial surface at predetermined fixed radial angles. The changes in length of the hemiaxes or radii are expressed as a shortening fraction. Methods have also been developed that do not assume that motion occurs along predetermined axes or radii.

Regional wall motion in normal subjects has been found to be variable in absolute value from the different regions of the ventricle. Consequently, abnormalities of wall motion are defined as values deviating from the mean value ± 1 or 2 standard deviations for a hemiaxis (chord) or radius in a particular region of the ventricle in order to establish reduced motion (hypokinesis). The normal mean value is determined from the values calculated in a group of normal subjects.

Objective measurement of asynchrony of segmental wall motion necessitate measurements of segmental motion on multiple images during systole rather than just comparison of end-diastolic and end-systolic images, as is done to identify hypokinesis. Normal subjects demonstrate some asynchrony of contraction but marked asynchrony is observed with bundle branch blocks, abnormal conduction pathways, and sometimes ischemic heart disease.

Angiographic Features of Specific Diseases

Ischemic Heart Disease

The left ventriculogram is obtained in most patients who undergo coronary arteriography. It is used to define dimensions and function of the left ventricle and to identify the morphologic consequences and complications of previous myocardial infarctions. The frequency of its application has waned in recent years because of increasing confidence in noninvasive techniques, two-dimensional echocardiography, and gated blood pool radionuclide images for the evaluation of global and, to a more limited degree, regional ventricular function. The importance of evaluation of left ventricular function in ischemic heart disease is indicated by the findings in repeated studies that two of the major prognostic indices in patients treated with coronary artery bypass surgery are ejection fraction and end-systolic volume.[15,16] Although these parameters can be derived with reasonable accuracy from the gated radionuclide blood pool study, precise evaluation of regional wall motion is accomplished most reliably from the biplane left ventriculogram. Left ventricular catheterization also provides sampling of the left ventricular end-diastolic pressure in the baseline state and after the stress induced by the injection of contrast media into the left ventricle.

Left ventriculography is optimally acquired in the 30° RAO and 60° LAO biplane mode. Single-plane (30° RAO) filming is done in many laboratories and is usually adequate. The 30° RAO view is most useful because it demonstrates most of the representative left ventricular segments (see Fig. 4-2). The biplane mode is preferable in patients with a history of previous infarction and especially in patients with multiple infarctions, episodes of congestive heart failure, or low ejection fraction. Under some circumstances, left ventriculography is not done because of concern about increased morbidity associated with the procedure. Left ventriculography is frequently deferred in chronic renal failure, especially the combination of diabetes and renal failure; congestive heart failure; and severe aortic stenosis. In these situations the results of noninvasive tests usually suffice.

Left ventriculography is usually done in a resting state. Several provocative maneuvers have been used to elicit regional contraction abnormalities in patients with coronary artery disease. These are usually maneuvers to augment myocardial oxygen requirements in order to evoke temporary ischemia in regions served by stenotic coronary arteries. The provocative maneuvers have included atrial pacing, exercise, and the use of pressor or sympathomimetic drugs to increase myocardial oxygen requirements and ergonovine to provoke coronary spasm in predisposed patients.[17–19]

The salient angiographic features of ischemic heart disease are:

1. Volumes of the left ventricle are frequently normal even in patients with severe multiple vessel coronary disease. The volumes are increased in some patients with prior myocardial infarctions and ischemic cardiomyopathy. The increase of end-systolic volume is related to long-term prognosis and short- and long-term survival after myocardial revascularization.[15,16]

2. Left ventricular shape is frequently altered in patients with prior infarction (Fig. 4-6). Remodeling of the left ventricle is related to wall thinning and stretching (bulging) of the infarcted segment and compensatory hypertrophy of the remaining normal segments of the ventricle.

3. Regional contraction abnormalities (asynergy) occur in most but not all patients after acute myocardial

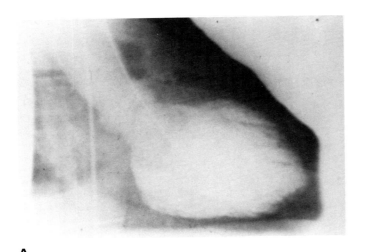
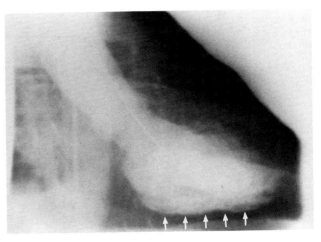

A   **B**

Figure 4-6. Left ventriculogram in the RAO view in diastole (*A*) and systole (*B*). There is no motion of the diaphragmatic segment (*arrows*) comparing the two phases of the cardiac cycle, indicating akinesis.

infarction and in some patients with coronary arterial stenoses that reduce luminal diameter by greater than 85%.

As indicated above, the contraction abnormalities consist of hypokinesis, akinesis, and dyskinesis. At the sites of hypokinesis viable myocardium is presumed to exist, but portions of the wall frequently contain fibrosis. Dyskinetic segments (systolic expansion) are nearly always composed of scar and can be presumed to represent nonviable, nonsalvageable myocardium. Akinetic segments usually represent scar but may contain some viable and salvageable myocardium. The "stunned" myocardium (decreased or absent segmental contraction after a recent episode of ischemia) and "hibernating" myocardium (decreased or absent segmental contraction due to depressed contractile state associated with chronic ischemia) are abnormalities of regional function that are considered reversible. Differentiation of asynergic, ischemic but viable myocardium from myocardial scar has been attempted using maneuvers to induce contraction of the region. These maneuvers include post-extrasystolic potentiation (the beat following a premature ventricular contraction shows greater extent of contraction) and administration of nitroglycerin (reduction in afterload) and epinephrine (catecholamine stimulation of contractile state).[20,21] If the akinetic region displays contraction on the second ventriculogram (or the first ventriculogram after a premature ventricular contraction), then the region is presumed to contain some viable myocardium and is alleged to be predictive of recovery of function after myocardial revascularization.

Asynchrony is another, more subtle, indicator of hemodynamically significant coronary obstruction. This is dependent upon delayed onset of contraction (tardokinesis) during mid- to late-systole in ischemic regions in comparison to normal myocardial regions. The interpretation of the significance of regions of tardokinesis is usually inconclusive.

4. Identification of the complications of recent or remote myocardial infarction is reliably provided by the left ventriculogram. These complications are mural thrombus; true aneurysm; false aneurysm; mitral regurgitation from papillary muscle ischemia; and ventricular septal rupture.

Mural Thrombus. The angiographic identification of left ventricular thrombus is unreliable in sensitivity and specificity. More than 70% of thrombi observed at surgery were not detected by angiography, and about 10% of those diagnosed by angiography were not confirmed at operation.[21a] Mural thrombus is recognized as a filling defect projecting into the opacified left ventricular chamber (Fig. 4-7). Such filling defects must be differentiated from papillary muscles and trabeculations. The thrombus should be attached to a region of abnormal contraction, whereas trabeculations and papillary muscle may be related to regions with normal contraction. Papillary muscles and trabeculations increase in size from diastole to systole, whereas the thrombus should not. Flattening of the apical curvature (squaring) of the left ventricle is a sign of mural thrombus (see Fig. 4-8). This finding usually indicates chronic thrombus that has been firmly incorporated into the ventricular wall. A polypoid filling defect is a more ominous finding in terms of potential peripheral embolization.[22] Thrombus most frequently occurs at the ventricular apex and occurs in about 50% of patients with ventricular aneurysm.

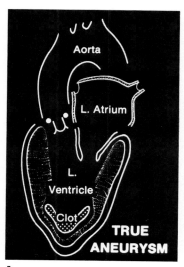

A

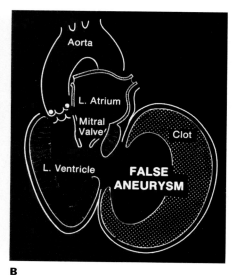

B

Figure 4-7. Diagram of the features of the true (*A*) and false (*B*) aneurysms of the left ventricle. The true aneurysm usually involves the apical or anterior segment and has a wide ostium. The false aneurysm usually involves the posterior or diaphragmatic segment and has a narrow ostium. Thrombus is usually present in both types. (L, left.)

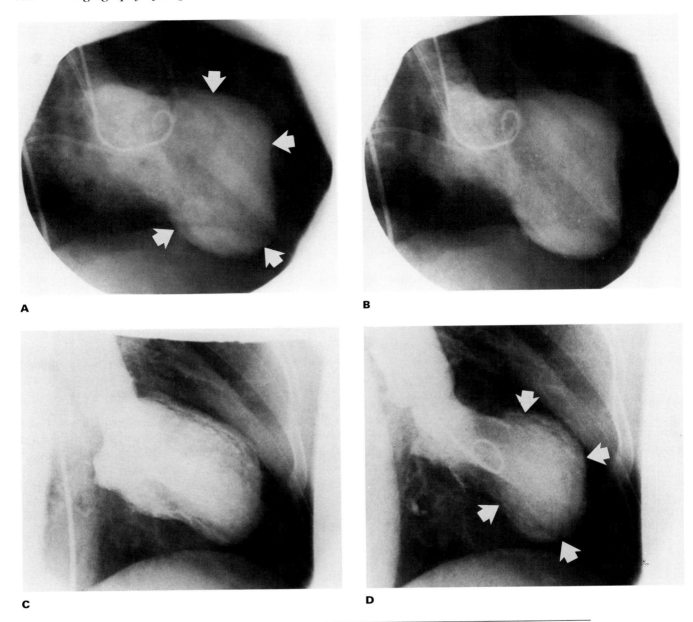

Figure 4-8. True aneurysm of the left ventricle. Left ventriculograms in the RAO view in two patients with true aneurysms of the left ventricle. The true aneurysm (*arrows*) involves the anterolateral and apical segments of the left ventricle. Systolic frames are *B* and *D*. The huge aneurysm (*A, B*) involves most of the ventricle, including the anterior, lateral, apical, and part of the diaphragmatic segments. The moderate-size aneurysm (*C, D*) involves the anterior, lateral, and apical segments. It causes only a slight diastolic deformity but is obvious in systole. (Courtesy of Eleanor Paquet, M.D., Montreal Heart Institute.)

True Aneurysm. Left ventricular aneurysm is defined as a bulge of the left ventricle contour in diastole (see Figs. 4-7, 4-8). The true aneurysm is composed of fibrous tissue, but the myocardial wall is intact. Aneurysms display dyskinesis (paradoxical bulging in systole).

The true aneurysm has a wide ostium and is usually located in the apical or anterolateral segments of the left ventricle (see Fig. 4-8). The true aneurysm not frequently

results from occlusion of the left anterior descending artery. Because of stasis of unopacified blood in a large aneurysm, the aneurysm may be poorly opacified. The aneurysm usually contains thrombus, but distinction of thrombus from poorly opacified blood in the aneurysm may be problematic. A true aneurysm of the ventricular septum bulges into the right ventricular cavity.

The left ventriculogram defines the location and ex-

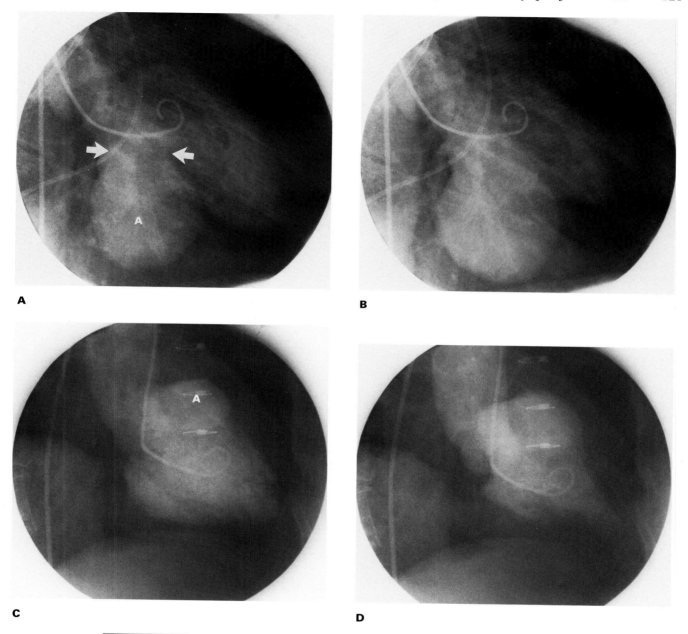

Figure 4-9. False aneurysms of the left ventricle. Left ventriculograms in the RAO view in diastole (*A, C*) and systole (*B, D*). The false aneurysm (*A*) has a small ostial connection (*arrows*) with the ventricular chamber. In one case the false aneurysm originates from the diaphragmatic segment (*A, B*) and in the other from the lateral segment (*C, D*). (Courtesy of Eleanor Paquet, M.D., Montreal Heart Institute.)

tent of the aneurysm (Figs. 4-8, 4-9). Some aneurysms have sharp margins with a clear interface between normal and dyskinetic myocardium, whereas others have poorly defined margins. In the latter, the aneurysm is frequently large and the left ventricular contraction abnormality is diffuse. Prognosis after resection of the aneurysm has been related to the contractility of the remainder of the ventricle.[22a] The ejection fraction of the nonaneurysmal portion of the ventricle is measured for this purpose.

Left ventricular aneurysm in the United States is nearly always due to myocardial infarction. Infrequent or rare causes are congenital apical aneurysm (Ravitch syndrome); congenital annular atrioventricular subvalvular aneurysm; apical aneurysm in Chagas' disease; apical aneurysm in midventricular type of hypertrophic cardiomyopathy; trauma; myocarditis; and residua of myocardial abscess.

False Aneurysm (Pseudoaneurysm). The false aneurysm is a focal rupture of the myocardial wall with localization of the blood by the fused visceral and parietal pericardial layers (see Figs. 4-7, 4-9).[23] The fused pericardial layers are markedly expanded, causing large aneurysms. False aneurysms are usually larger than true aneurysms and may reach astounding dimensions (see Fig. 4-9). The angiographic characteristics are relatively narrow ostium between the left ventricular chamber and the aneurysm, enormous size of the aneurysm, and location in the diaphragmatic or posterior region of the ventricle. When the diameter of the fundus of the aneurysm is greater than twice the diameter of the ostium, a pseudoaneurysm should be considered. A false aneurysm can originate from any region of the ventricle, but posterior or diaphragmatic sites are most common. The occlusion involves the right or left circumflex coronary arteries with disporportionate frequency. Coronary arteriography demonstrates that coronary arterial branches are displaced by the false aneurysm, but usually stretched over the true aneurysm.

False aneurysms are usually caused by myocardial infarction. They can also be caused by penetrating trauma.

Papillary Muscle Dysfsunction or Rupture. This complication causes mitral regurgitation. Papillary muscle ischemia causes chronic regurgitation of variable severity. Rupture causes severe regurgitation and usually intractable pulmonary edema. The posterolateral papillary muscle is responsible for ischemic regurgitation in about 70% of cases and the anteromedial papillary muscle in about 30% of cases. The left ventriculogram reveals the presence and severity of regurgitation. Sometimes the jet is directed superiorly in dysfunction of the posterior papillary muscle. The site of the associated wall motion abnormality incriminates one of the papillary muscles; diaphragmatic wall motion abnormalities implicate the posterior papillary muscle. Papillary muscle dysfunction can cause mitral valve prolapse, which is recognized as leaflet tissue ballooning behind the plane of the atrioventricular annulus during systole (Figs. 4-10, 4-11). Papillary muscle rupture causes "flail" of the mitral leaflet, which is recognized as movement of the tip of a leaflet into the left atrium in systole.

Ventricular Septal Defect (Rupture). Ventricular septal defect involves the muscular (trabecular) septum and is frequently located near the ventricular apex. The defect involves more frequently the anterior (left an-

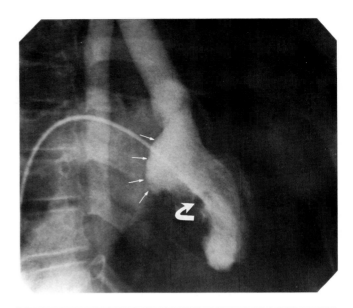

Figure 4-10. Mitral valve prolapse. Left ventriculogram in the RAO view shows the prominent, prolapsing scallops (*small arrows*) of the posterior leaflet of the mitral valve. The ventricle assumes a "ballerina foot" deformity during systole, which is a feature of the ventriculogram in some patients with mitral valve prolapse. This contraction abnormality is caused by exaggerated contraction of the diaphragmatic surface (*curved arrow*) and bulging of the opposite anterolateral wall.

terior descending coronary arterial occlusion) than the posterior (right coronary arterial occlusion) portion of the septum. Most septal defects are associated with an aneurysm. Ventriculography in the cranial (30°)–LAO (60°) view is usually optimal for demonstrating the site and size of the defect. Left-to-right shunting of contrast media is demonstrated in the muscular (trabecular) portion of the septum.

Valvular Heart Disease

The severity of stenotic valvular lesions is not assessed effectively by angiography, whereas that of regurgitant lesions can be evaluated by angiography. The criterion for assigning severity of regurgitant lesions is described above. For the evaluation of the left ventricle in valvular disease, biplane angiography in the 30° RAO and 60° LAO views is usually done. Cranial angulation in the LAO and caudal angulation in the RAO views may improve visualization of valves.

Aortic Stenosis. Isolated aortic stenosis is usually caused by early degeneration of an abnormally structured aortic valve, whereas combined aortic and mitral stenosis are usually caused by rheumatic fever. The aortic valve itself is evaluated better by the ascending aortogram than by the left ventriculogram.

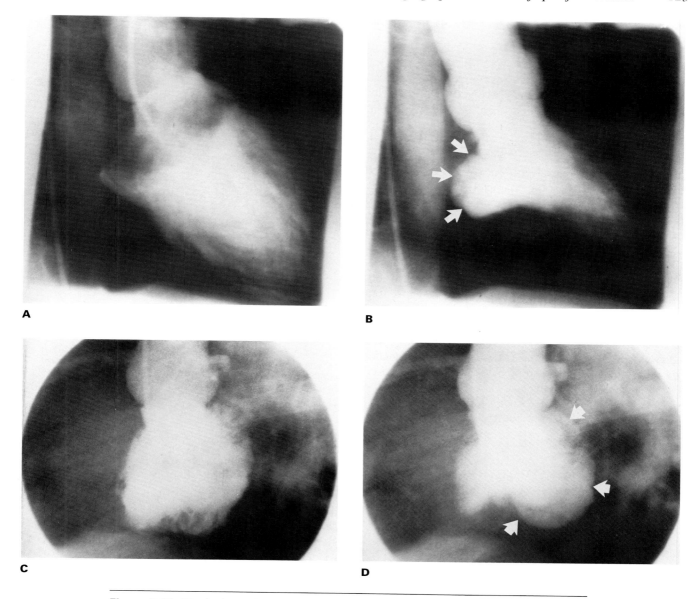

Figure 4-11. Mitral valve prolapse. Left ventriculogram in two patients in the RAO (*A, B*) and lateral (*C, D*) views. The prolapsed leaflets (*arrows*) are evident in systole (*B, D*). Prolapse is moderate (*A, B*) in one patient and severe (*C, D*) in the other. The latter case also has mitral regurgitation (*D*). (Courtesy of Eleanor Paquet, M.D., Montreal Heart Institute.)

The salient angiographic features of the aortic stenosis are:

1. Thickened and restricted motion of the aortic valve (Fig. 4-12).
2. Left ventricular hypertrophy as indicated by enlarged papillary muscle and distal cavity obliteration during systole (Fig. 4-12).
3. Hyperdynamic left ventricular contraction (Fig. 4-12*B,C*).
4. Relatively small left ventricular EDV and ESV.
5. The left ventriculogram defines the site of left ventricular outflow obstruction as supravalvular, valvular, or subvalvular. The cranial LAO view is particularly effective in demonstrating a subvalvular membrane or subvalvular septal hypertrophy, which may coexist with valvular stenosis.

6. Increased left ventricular volumes, reduced ejection fraction, and generalized hypokinesis may be recognized in decompensated aortic valve disease or could indicate associated idiopathic or ischemic cardiomyopathy. Rarely, left ventricular contraction is depressed by imbalance in left ventricular oxygen demand compared to myocardial blood supply.

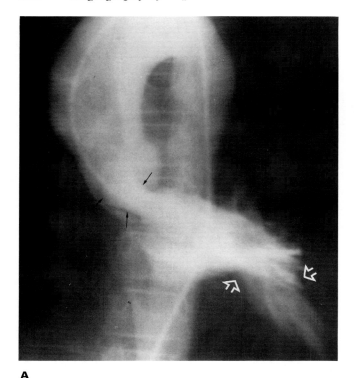

A

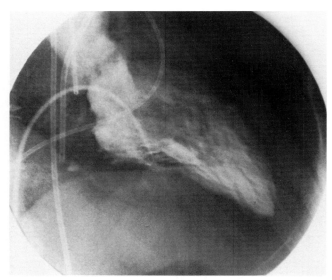

B

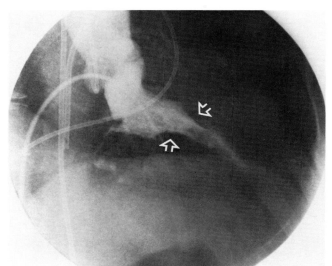

C

Figure 4-12. *A:* Aortic stenosis. Left ventriculogram in the AP view shows thickened, domed aortic valve cusps (*arrows*) in systole and dilatation of the ascending aorta. Left ventricular hypertrophy is indicated by the thickened papillary muscle (*open arrows*). Diastolic (*B*) and systolic (*C*) frames in another patient with aortic stenosis. The distal cavity obliteration during systole and enlarged papillary muscles (*open arrows*) indicate severe left ventricular hypertrophy.

7. Segmental contraction abnormalities usually indicate underlying ischemic heart disease.

8. Aortography demonstrates thickening and doming of the valve; an eccentric jet (of nonopacified blood) across the valve; and poststenotic dilatation of the ascending aorta (see Fig. 4-12).

The aortogram in the LAO view demonstrates the features of the bicuspid aortic valve. Normally, there are three well-formed sinuses of Valsalva. The posterior (noncoronary) sinus is normally larger than the other two. However, the disparity in size is exaggerated with the bicuspid aortic valve. Upon opening of the bicuspid valve, one of the cusps spans the full distance from the anterior to the posterior wall (see Fig. 5-32). The opened valve has a "fish mouth" appearance.

Aortic Insufficiency. Evaluation of this lesion requires ascending aortography in order to assess the severity of regurgitation. It is also used to identify aortic or aortoannular abnormalities, which are frequently the cause of aortic regurgitation. Aortography may demonstrate signs indicating its etiology, such as uniform dilatation of the aortic annulus and proximal ascending aorta in aortoannular ectasia, aneurysmal dilatation of the ascending aorta but a normal aortic annulus in syphilitic aortitis, intimal flap and false channel in aortic dissection,

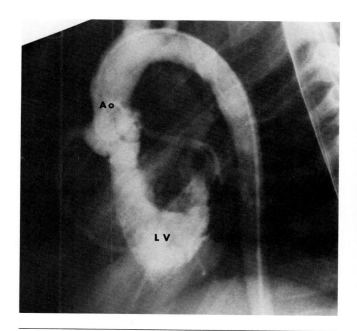

Figure 4-13. Aortic regurgitation. Aortogram in moderately severe, grade 3 +, aortic regurgitation. Grade 3 + is indicated by equal density of the left ventricle and ascending aorta. (Ao, ascending aorta; LV, left ventricle.)

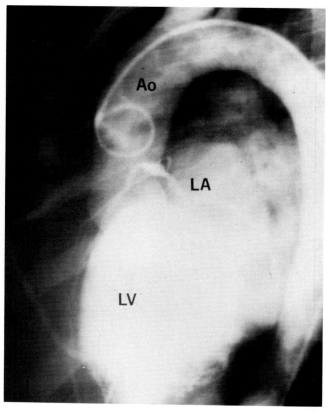

Figure 4-14. Severe aortic regurgitation. Grade 4 + is indicated by greater density of the left ventricle than of the ascending aorta. There is also mitral regurgitation. (Ao, ascending aorta; LA, left atrium; LV, left ventricle.)

and perivalvular abscess or vegetations in bacterial endocarditis.

The salient angiographic features of aortic regurgitation are:

1. Increased left ventricular EDV, ESV, and stroke volume.

2. Normal ejection fraction and wall motion in compensated disease. The decompensated left ventricle is indicated by reduced ejection fraction and diffuse hypokinesis.

3. Structural abnormalities of the left ventricle may indicate the etiology, such as ventricular septal defect (especially supracristal type), myocardial abscess in bacterial endocarditis, and subvalvular membrane.

4. Aortic valve may or may not be thickened and usually displays normal excursion. Thickening and doming of the valve are characteristic for a rheumatic etiology. Etiologic characteristics are gleaned also from the aortogram (described above).

5. Regurgitation of blood from the aorta into the left ventricle. This is usually displayed best in the 60° LAO view (Figs. 4-13, 4-14). The qualitative grading scheme for regurgitation is described above.

Mitral Stenosis. The mitral valve is visualized well in the 30° RAO view. The usual etiology of mitral stenosis is rheumatic heart disease, which frequently causes some regurgitation as well as stenosis.

The salient angiographic features are:

1. Prior to opacification of the left ventricle, the valve region is inspected for either valvular or periannular calcification.

2. Thickened leaflet with doming during diastole (Fig. 4-15). The normal mitral leaflets are virtually invisible in diastole as they open and abut the ventricular walls. A narrowed stream of nonopacified blood flow into the left ventricle during diastole ("wash in" jet) signifies stenosis.

3. Normal or reduced EDV and ESV in isolated stenosis.

4. Normal wall motion. Reduced wall motion has been described in a minority of patients with rheumatic mitral stenosis and attributed to direct rheumatic affliction of the myocardium. This mechanism has been invoked in patients demonstrating hypokinesis of the posterobasal region of the left ventricle.

5. Thickened and fused chords of the mitral valve may be shown as lucent extension of the papillary muscles up to the level of the leaflets.[24] This finding indicates

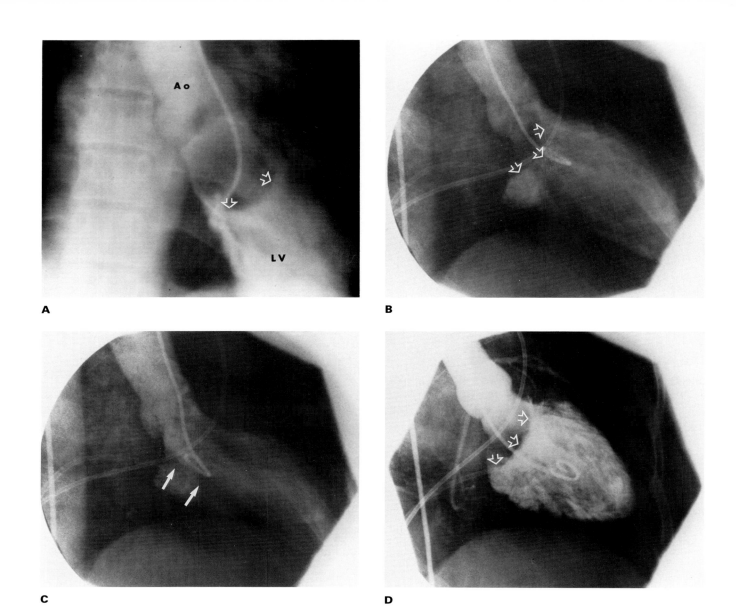

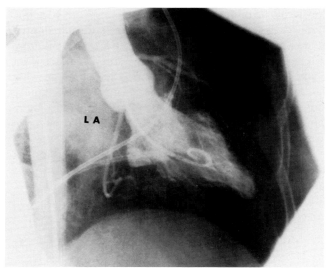

Figure 4-15. Mitral stenosis, three cases. Left ventriculogram in the RAO view (*A*) in mitral stenosis shows doming of the mitral valve (*open arrows*) in diastole. (Ao, aorta; LV, left ventricle.) RAO views show, in diastole (*B*), doming mitral valve (*open arrows*) and, in systole (*C*), a lucent band (*closed arrows*) extending from papillary muscle to the valve region, indicating subvalvular chordal fusion. RAO views in diastole (*D*) and systole (*E*) show restricted diastolic motion and doming of the mitral valve (*open arrows*) and regurgitation. (LA, left atrium.)

the likelihood of significant subvalvular obstruction in addition to valvular stenosis.

6. Abnormal motion pattern of the anterior leaflet of the mitral valve. This observation is made on the cine-angiogram in the LAO view. The normal valve displays biphasic motion in diastole with opening toward the mitral valve in early diastole, followed by a drift back toward the annulus and then a second presystolic reopening motion with atrial systole. In mitral stenosis, the motion is continuous and persistently occurs toward the left ventricle in diastole because the gradient between the left atrium and left ventricle is maintained during the entire diastolic phase.

Mitral Regurgitation. Evaluation of the presence and severity of this lesion requires left ventricular angiography. The most common cause of mitral regurgitation during opacification of the left ventricle is malposition of the catheter across or in the path of motion of the mitral valve or premature ventricular contractions induced by whipping of the catheter during injection. For assessment of motion and insufficiency of the mitral valve, biplane ventriculography in the 30° RAO and 60° LAO views is optimal.

The salient angiographic features of mitral regurgitation are:

1. Enlarged left atrium.

2. Increased left ventricular EDV, ESV, and stroke volume.

3. Normal ejection fraction and wall motion in the compensated disease.

4. Reduced ejection fraction and generalized hypokinesis in the decompensated phase.

5. Regurgitation of contrast media into the left atrium (Figs. 4-11, 4-16). Grading of the severity is described above.

6. The mitral valve is usually thickened. Excursion is frequently reduced when rheumatic valve disease is the etiology.

7. Structural abnormalities of the valve or left ventricle may indicate the etiology, such as mitral valve prolapse (see Figs. 4-10, 4-11), flail leaflet of the mitral valve, vegetation of the valve in bacterial endocarditis, regional wall motion abnormality adjacent to a papillary muscle in ischemic heart disease, calcification of the mitral annulus, and signs of hypertrophic cardiomyopathy, such as asymmetrical septal hypertrophy.

Mitral annular calcification is occasionally the sole cause of regurgitation. The cause of the calcification is usually unknown, but such calcification occurs with increased frequency in hypertension, aortic stenosis, hypertrophic cardiomyopathy, hyperlipidemia, and hypercalcemia. Mitral valve prolapse and flail can be distinguished from each other. Prolapse is ballooning of the

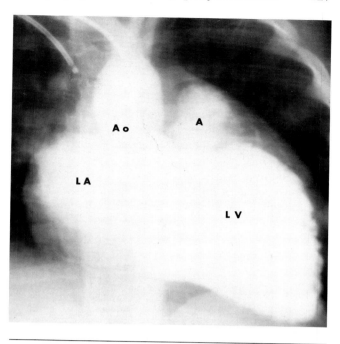

Figure 4-16. Left ventriculogram in the AP view shows dense opacification of the left atrium. Moderately severe regurgitation is indicated by equal density of the left ventricle and left atrium. (A, left atrial appendage; Ao, aorta; LA, left atrium; LV, left ventricle.)

middle of the valve beyond the annulus during systole; the tips of the leaflets to which the chordae attach do not pass beyond the annulus (see Figs. 4-10, 4-11). Flail is indicated by passage of the tips of the mitral leaflets beyond the annulus and into the left atrium during systole.

Mitral Valve Prolapse. This abnormality of the mitral valve is observed on approximately 5% of left ventriculograms.[25] Pathologically, it is caused by myxomatous degeneration of the mitral valve leaflets and chordae tendinae. A minority of patients with prolapse have mitral regurgitation, which is frequently mild. However, rupture of a chordae tendinae is a complication that can induce severe regurgitation. Aside from chordal rupture causing severe regurgitation, other complications include supraventricular and ventricular arrhythmias, bacterial endocarditis, and cerebral emboli. Abnormal contraction of segments of the left ventricle and abnormal shape of the left ventricle have been observed in some patients with mitral valve prolapse (see Figs. 4-10, 4-11).[26]

Salient radiographic features are:

1. Displacement of portions of the mitral leaflet into the left atrium during systole (see Figs. 4-10, 4-11). The posterior leaflet is usually involved, but in a minority of cases both leaflets prolapse. The posterior leaflet is divided into three portions (scallops), and one or more of these prolapse during systole. The scallops are desig-

nated as anterolateral, middle, and posteromedial. Prolapse is identified on the RAO view, on which the posteromedial leaflet is visualized optimally. The posteromedial scallop most frequently demonstrates prolapse.

2. Thickening of the leaflet of the mitral valve with normal excursion.

3. Mitral regurgitation. Regurgitation commences in mid- or late systole (see Fig. 4-10).

4. Infrequently there are regional contraction abnormalities of the left ventricle. A variety of patterns exist. The most common are a hypercontractile ring beneath the mitral valve and a prominent contractile region in the midportion of the diaphragmatic surface with diminished contraction at an opposing site on the anterolateral wall of the left ventricle ("ballerina foot deformity") (see Fig. 4-10).

Artificial Valves

The various types of artificial valves are displayed in Figures 4-17 through 4-33.

The complications of the prosthetic valves are:

1. Insufficiency
   Valve leak
   Perivalvular leak

(*Text continues on page 134*)

Figures 4-17 through 4-33. Prosthetic heart valves. For each valve the panels show the PA radiograph (*A*), lateral radiograph (*B*), and photograph (*C*). (Reproduced by permission of the American Heart Association from Mehlman DJ, Resnekov L. A guide to the radiographic recognition of prosthetic heart valves. Circulation 1978;57:613.)

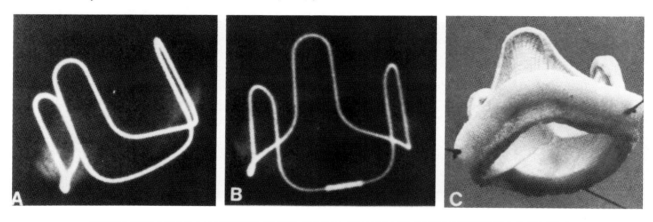

Figure 4-17. Edwards xenograft.

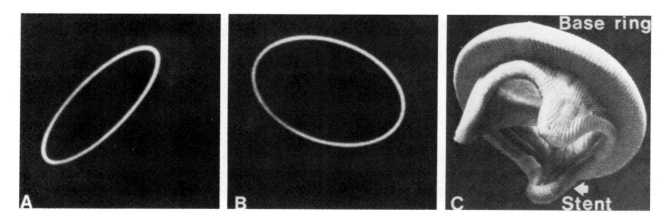

Figure 4-18. Hancock xenograft.

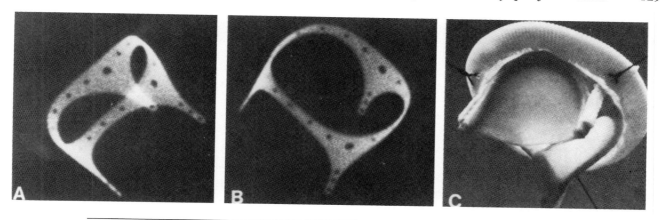

Figure 4-19. Ionescu–Shiley xenograft.

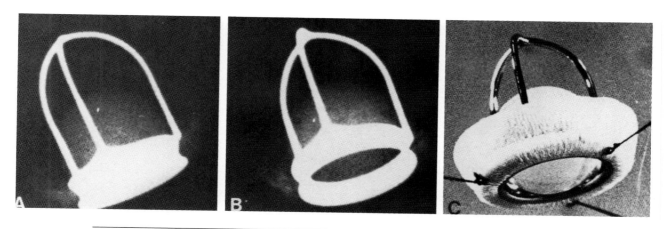

Figure 4-20. Starr–Edwards model 1200.

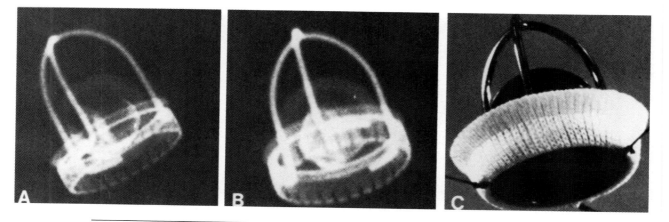

Figure 4-21. DeBakey–Surgitool.

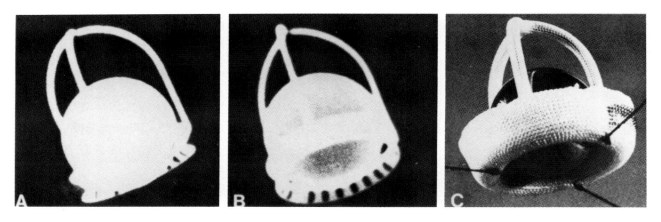

Figure 4-22. Starr–Edwards model 2300.

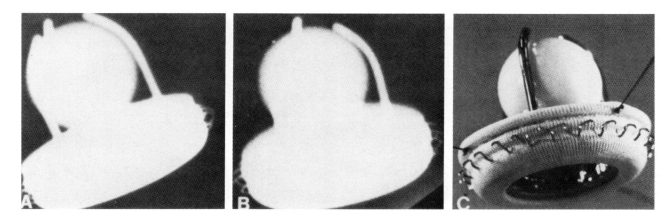

Figure 4-23. McGovern–Cromie.

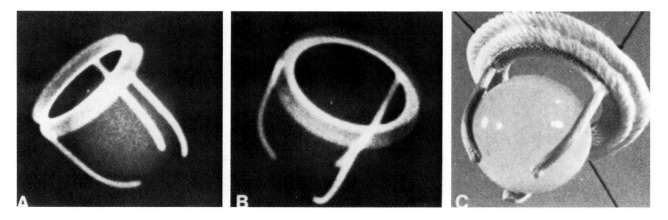

Figure 4-24. Braunwald–Cutter.

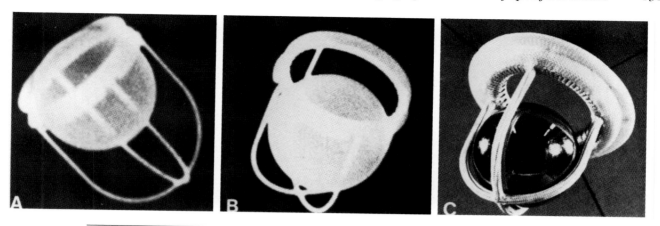

Figure 4-25. Starr–Edwards model 6310.

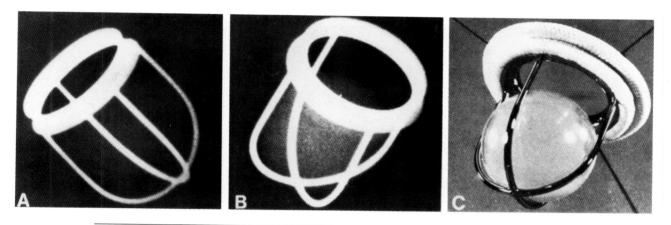

Figure 4-26. Starr–Edwards model 6000.

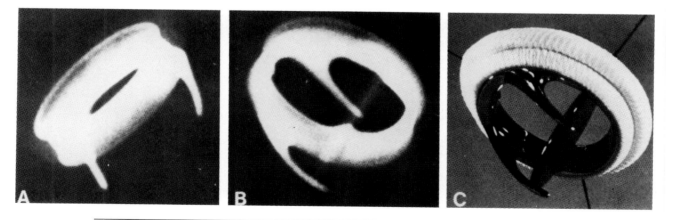

Figure 4-27. Lillehei–Kaster

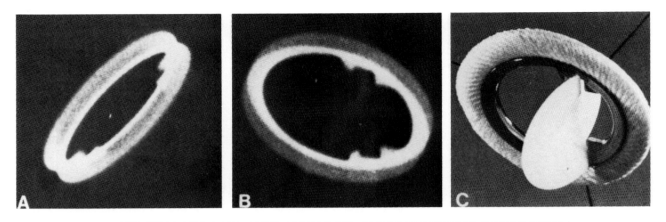

Figure 4-28. Wada–Cutter.

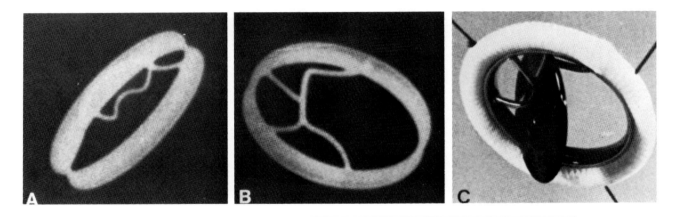

Figure 4-29. Björk–Shiley.

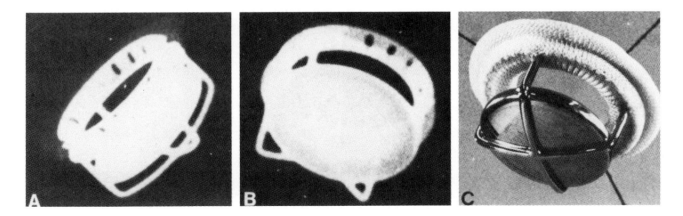

Figure 4-30. Starr–Edwards model 6500.

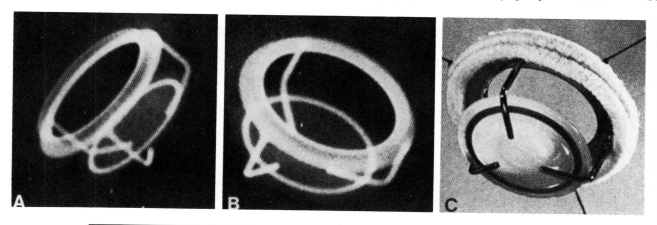

Figure 4-31. Cross–Jones.

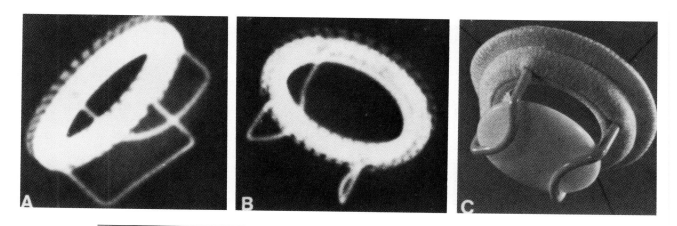

Figure 4-32. Beall model 103.

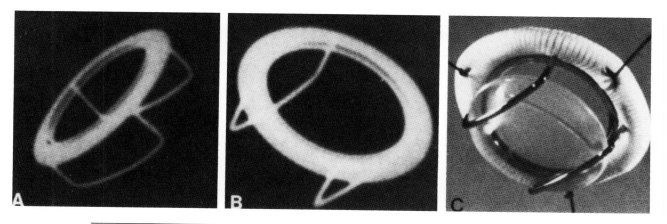

Figure 4-33. Kay–Shiley T series.

2. Stenosis

   Poppet or ball enlargement

   Thrombus or tissue closure or narrowing of valves

3. Thrombus–embolism

4. Fatigue and disintegration of components of prosthetic valves. This may cause embolization of struts, poppet, or ball.

5. Degeneration of bioprosthesis

6. Bacterial endocarditis

The valve is usually assessed optimally by opacification of the chamber or great artery immediately downstream from the valve. For an artificial mitral valve, the contrast media are injected into the left ventricle. For an aortic valve, they are injected into the supravalvular portion of the ascending aorta.

Salient angiographic features of complications of prosthetic valves are:

1. A wide stream of regurgitation across the valve is usually caused by insufficiency of the valve itself (Fig. 4-34). However, a large perivalvular leak may not always be clearly discernible from a valvular leak. A narrow jet of regurgitation at the periphery of the valve indicates a perivalvular leak.

2. Disruption of the suture ring is shown by displacement of the valve above a hinge point. This "trap door" movement of the valve indicates disruption of greater than 180° of the suture ring at the base of the valve.

3. Failure of complete seating of the poppet or ball of the valve is a cause of regurgitation that can be identified on the angiogram.

4. Restricted motion of the radio-opaque moving component of the valve can be recognized as causes of both regurgitation and stenosis. A poppet, or any other moving component held in a fixed or partially open position can cause both stenosis and regurgitation.

5. Stenosis is recognized by a narrowed stream or jet of contrast media passing through the artificial valve. It may also be recognized by a narrow jet of unopacified blood entering an opacified region. Restricted motion of components of the valve and filling defects attached to the valve may indicate the cause of stenosis.

6. Filling defects attached to the valve can also be recognized as the cause of embolization.

7. Rarely, components of the valve, such as struts, discs, or poppets can be observed at remote intravascular sites. Such major disruption of prosthetic valves is usually a catastrophic event, causing cardiovascular collapse and precluding catheterization and angiography.

8. Bacterial endocarditis may be associated with vegetations on the valve, perivalvular abscess(es), or fistula(e). Delayed emptying of contrast media from the perivalvular abscess usually makes them readily visible on the angiogram. The abscesses are usually located in the myocardium or the posterior or diaphragmatic wall of the left ventricle for infected mitral valves and in the ventricular septum or between the aorta and left atrium for infected aortic valves.

Cardiomyopathies

A diverse group of diseases are included under the title cardiomyopathies. These are chronic diseases of cardiac muscle; the etiology of the myocardial abnormalities is sometimes known, but frequently the cause is not known. Nearly all diseases afflicting the heart, if present for a prolonged period and if sufficiently severe, cause myocardial dysfunction. Certaintly, valvular, ischemic, hypertensive, and congenital heart disease at the end stage are associated with myocardial disease and failure. Primary cardiomyopathies are those in which the myocardium is afflicted directly rather than as a consequence of a long-term hemodynamic stress such as valvular regurgitation. The heart is the only organ afflicted in primary cardiomyopathies, while secondary cardiomyopathies are the result of myocardial involvement in systemic diseases such as rheumatoid arthritis, sarcoidosis, and amyloidosis. A cardiomyopathic process restricted to the right ventricle—right ventricular dysplasia—has been recognized.[26a] This is usually associated with arrhythmias originating in the right ventricle.

A clinicopathologic classification of cardiomyopathies exists[27]:

1. Hypertrophic cardiomyopathy.

2. Congestive cardiomyopathy. This form is also called idiopathic dilated cardiomyopathy.

3. Restrictive cardiomyopathy. Some of the secondary types involve infiltration of the myocardium by various substances (amyloidosis) or cells (sarcoidosis) and cause a restrictive physiology.

4. Obliterative cardiomyopathy. This is a very rare form which has been observed for the most part in Africa.

A list of the various etiologies of secondary cardiomyopathies is given in Table 4-2.

The salient features of hypertrophic cardiomyopathy are:

1. The left ventriculogram demonstrates abnormalities of structure and function in both systole and diastole.[28] During diastole there is evidence of restricted or prolonged filling of a left ventricular chamber with a diastolic volume frequently less than normal and less than in concentric hypertrophy due to valvular aortic stenosis. The normal or reduced end-diastolic volume contrasts with the increased volume of congestive cardiomyopa-

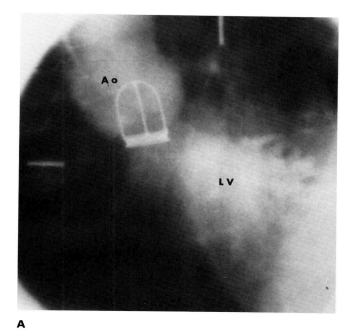

A

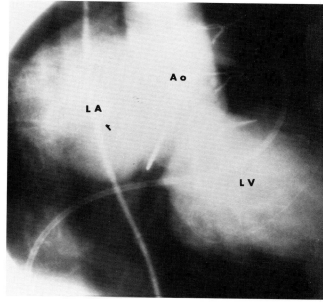

B

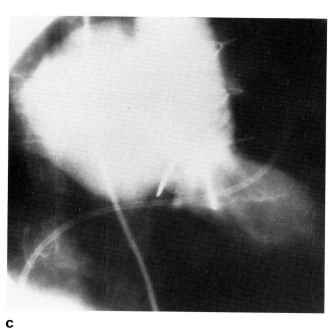

C

Figure 4-34. Regurgitation across prosthetic aortic (*A*) and mitral (*B, C*) valves. Aortogram in LAO view shows aortic regurgitation (grade 3) across a Starr–Edwards valve. Left ventriculogram in diastole (*B*) and systole (*C*) shows mitral regurgitation (grade 3) across a Hancock porcine valve. (Ao, aorta; LA, left atrium; LV, left ventricle.) (Courtesy of Eleanor Paquet, M.D., Montreal Heart Institute.)

thies. Pressure-volume studies confirm the visible reduction in diastolic compliance.[29]

2. Increased wall thickness of the left ventricle, usually to a greater degree than in valvular stenosis. The ratio of cavity diameter to wall thickness is substantially below the normal range and also lower than in most patients with aortic stenosis. There is no clear relationship between the gradient across the outflow tract and the diastolic thickness of the left ventricular myocardium.

3. The diastolic contour of the left ventricle in the frontal projection is usually abnormal, with a prominent filling defect on the inferior margin and a convexity or an additional filling defect along the left superior margin (Fig. 4-35). This abnormality of contour is the result of the asymmetrical hypertrophied septum bulging into the left ventricular chamber.

4. The markedly hypertrophied papillary muscles displaced by the asymmetrically hypertrophied septum

Table 4-2

Specific (Secondary) Cardiomyopathies

I. Infections (?)*
   1. Viral (especially Coxsackie B virus)
   2. Bacterial (diphtheric; associated with endocarditis)
   3. Parasitic (Chagasic, trichinosis, echinococcosis, schistosomiasis)
   4. Mycotic (histoplasmosis, actinomycosis, aspergillosis, blastomycosis)
II. Metabolic
   1. Hyperthyroidism or hypothyroidism
   2. Glycogen storage diseases
   3. Mucopolysaccharidosis (Hurler's disease)
   4. Nutritional deficiencies (thiamine deficiency, tryptophan deficiency, kwashiorkor)
   5. Acromegaly
   6. Pheochromocytoma
III. Collagen diseases
   1. Disseminated lupus erythematosis
   2. Periarteritis nodosa
   3. Dermatomyositis
   4. Scleroderma
   5. Ankylosing spondylitis
   6. Rheumatoid arthritis
IV. Neuromuscular disease
   1. Muscular dystrophies
   2. Mytonia dystrophica
   3. Friedreich's ataxia
V. Toxic
   1. Alcohol
   2. Cobalt, aresenic
   3. Drugs (catecholamines, others)
VI. Infiltrative
   1. Amyloidosis
   2. Sarcoidosis
   3. Hemochromatosis
   4. Whipple's disease

Infectious etiology of cardiomyopathies is unproven at the current time.

often have an abnormal orientation; instead of pointing normally toward the mitral annulus they are displaced leftward and point to the left of the mitral annulus in the frontal projection.

5. The lateral view during diastole characteristically demonstrates an inverted cone in the outflow tract, formed by contrast between the hypertrophied septum anteriorly and the open anterior leaflet of the mitral valve posteriorly. The site of obstruction may be demonstrated very well in the cranial LAO view.[30]

6. The end-systolic volume is nearly always less than normal, and obliteration of all but the proximal part of the inflow tract is frequently observed. The ejection fraction is typically increased. During systole there is exaggerated circumferential contraction and essentially no apex-to-base shortening, producing a cylindrical or bananalike appearance of the chamber at end systole. A variety of other bizarre configurations, including septation of the left ventricle into two chambers (hourglass ap-

pearance) or a spade-shaped left ventricle due to apical hypertrophy during systole, have been described.[30a,30b]

7. Systolic frames in the frontal projection display a scalloped, V-shaped or W-shaped radiolucent band across the left ventricular outflow tract (see Fig. 4-35) produced by contact of the thickened leading edge of the anterior mitral valve leaflet against the hypertrophied septum. The lateral view during systole again shows the hypertrophied septum bulging into the outflow tract and posteriorly, a shelflike deformity caused by the forward tethering of the anterior leaflet of the mitral valve. The mitral valve leaflets, exposed to turbulent flow in the left ventricular outflow tract, may be thickened. Infusions of inotropic agents in this disorder exaggerate or actually induce the obstructive deformity of the outflow tract. Moreover, during the infusion of epinephrine and with a post-premature ventricular contraction, the ejection time of the left ventricle is increased rather than decreased as in normal patients and patients with valvular aortic stenosis.

8. Right ventriculography demonstrates compression and anterior displacement of the right ventricle by the asymmetrically hypertrophied septum. The entire right ventricle or its infundibular portion may be narrowed by the bulging septum. In advanced cases, the right ventricle exhibits marked generalized hypertrophy.

The salient features of congestive cardiomyopathy are:

1. Increased end-diastolic and end-systolic volumes and reduced ejection fraction (Fig. 4-36). Because of the large increase in the left ventricular diameter, calculated end-diastolic circumferential wall tension and stress are considerably increased.[31] The increased wall tension is not compensated by appropriate left ventricular hypertrophy; the left ventricle wall is considerably thinner than expected for the size of the chamber. The lack of appropriate hypertrophy contrasts strikingly with other diseases (aortic regurgitation), in which left ventricular hypertrophy matches dilatation until a late stage of the disease. Patients with thin ventricular walls have had a poor prognosis, while some degree of hypertrophy has been associated with a more favorable prognosis.[32]

2. Generalized hypokinesis is evident in most symptomatic patients (see Fig. 4-36). The hypokinesis usually includes the basal segments in congestive cardiomyopathies; the contraction of the basal segments is characteristically preserved in the severe left ventricular dysfunction of advanced coronary artery disease. Although considered unique to coronary artery disease, localized areas of hypokinesis, akinesis, and even aneurysm formation (chronic chagasic cardiomyopathy) have been rarely encountered with cardiomyopathies.

3. The left ventricle has a spherical contour and not

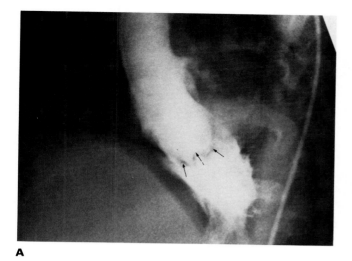

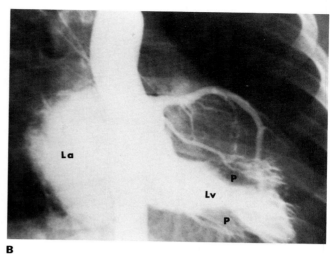

Figure 4-35. Left ventriculogram in the LAO (*A*) and RAO (*B*) views in hypertrophic cardiomyopathy. The W-shaped lucency (*arrows*) in the LV outflow region in systole shown in the LAO view is due to apposition of the anterior leaflet of the mitral valve with the hypertrophied septum. The papillary muscles (P) and upper portion of ventricular septum are prominent, and there is moderate mitral regurgitation. (La, left atrium; Lv, left ventricle.)

infrequently contains mural or apical filling defects representing thrombus.

4. Mitral regurgitation due to dilatation of the annulus and loss of subvalvular muscle support is rarely severe and characteristically less than expected for the degree of left ventricular dilatation.

5. Right ventricular dilatation and hypokinesis are also observed in advanced disease. In contradistinction to the left ventricle, the right ventricular wall is sometimes thicker than normal, which is likely a response to pulmonary hypertension.

Poor prognosis has been directly related to the extent of elevation of end-diastolic left ventricular volume and the presence of significant mitral regurgitation. It has been inversely related to left ventricular wall thickness and ejection fraction.

Coronary arteriography, essential to establishing the diagnosis of congestive cardiomyopathy, has revealed large-caliber coronary arteries (Fig. 4-36C,D). This finding correlates with the high myocardial oxygen requirements in this disease as a consequence of excessive myocardial wall tension. Typical angina and pathologic Q waves on ECG are occasionally encountered in cardiomyopathic patients with normal coronary arteries.

The salient features of restrictive cardiomyopathy are:

1. The end-diastolic volume of the ventricles may be normal, decreased, or increased.

2. The distinctive feature is apparent rigidity of the myocardium as reflected by diminished diastolic expansion. The abrupt cessation of diastolic filling ("diastolic snap") has been observed with restrictive cardiomyopathies as well as with constrictive pericarditis.

3. The distinction between restrictive cardiomyopathy and constrictive pericarditis without pericardial calcification is difficult, but may be facilitated by demonstrating a thick pericardial shadow extending more than 1 cm beyond the opacified right atrium or a cardiac border. In restrictive cardiomyopathy the thickness of the soft-tissue shadow adjacent to the opacified right atrium is less than 4 to 5 mm.

The salient features of obliterative cardiomyopathy are:

1. Angiocardiography in obliterative cardiomyopathies has revealed an enlarged right atrium that frequently contains thrombi in the appendage.

2. Contrast clears very slowly from the right side of the heart, and the high venous pressure may be reflected by reflux of contrast down the inferior vena cava.

3. The right ventricular chamber is small and deformed, with obliteration of the apex in advanced cases. Segmental dysfunction has been an unexpected feature in some patients.

4. Pericardial effusion is a frequently associated finding in right-sided and biventricular disease.

5. In left-sided disease the left ventricular end-diastolic volume is reduced.

6. The chamber is usually smooth-walled and/or contains filling defects due to mural thrombi.

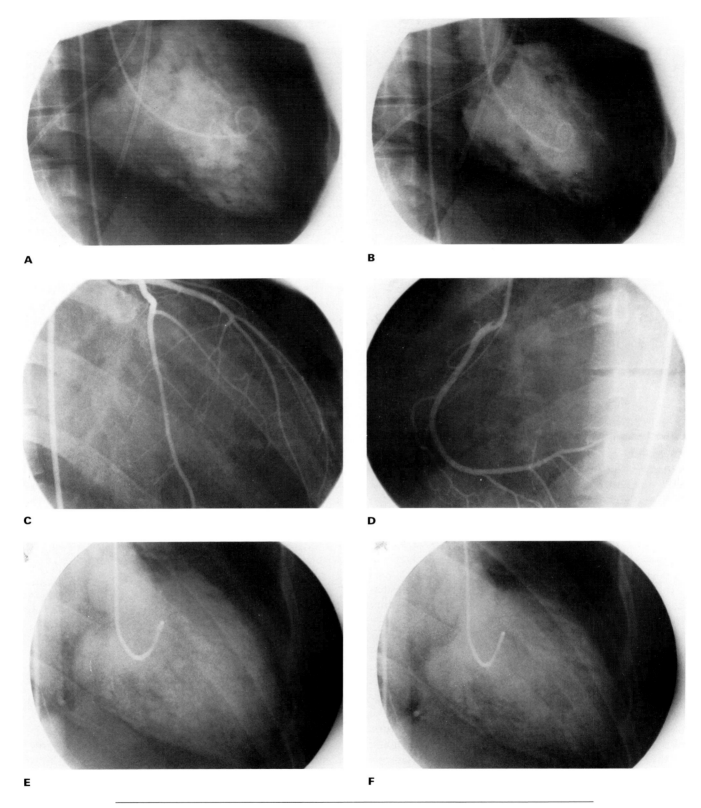

Figure 4-36. Congestive cardiomyopathy in two patients. Moderately severe cardiomyopathy. Left ventriculogram on RAO view in diastole (*A*) and systole (*B*) in a patient with congestive (dilated) cardiomyopathy shows diffuse hypokinesis and reduced ejection fraction. Left coronary arteriogram in RAO view and right coronary arteriogram in LAO view display normal coronary arteries. Left ventriculogram (*E, F*) in RAO view in diastole (*E*) and systole (*F*) in a patient with severe cardiomyopathy shows little change in volume during the cardiac cycle, indicating a very low ejection fraction. (Courtesy of Eleanor Pacquet, M.D., Montreal Heart Institute.)

7. The posterior papillary muscle and leaflet may be deformed and mitral regurgitation is common.

Cardiac Masses

Angiography is sometimes performed in order to confirm the presence of a cardiac mass initially detected by echocardiography or magnetic resonance imaging, or to exclude a cardiac origin of a thrombus in patients after one or more episodes of peripheral embolization. Angiography may also be performed to define the extent of a paracardiac or intracardiac mass. It is very questionable whether angiography should be done for cardiac masses, considering the several accurate noninvasive studies now available. The masses usually are of three varieties: tumor, thrombus, or infective vegetation. The most common primary tumor is the myxoma. The second most common is the rhabdomyoma; it is the one most frequently encountered in children. Eighty percent of primary tumors are benign. Fibroma is a rare benign primary tumor. Cardiac tumors are more frequently secondary (40 times more frequent) than primary in origin. Secondary tumors involve the heart by direct extension to the heart or pericardium from the lungs or mediastinum; growth along the inferior vena cava and into the right atrium, usually from a primary tumor of the liver, adrenal gland, or kidney; or hematogenous metastasis to the myocardium or cardiac chambers. The most common tumors causing secondary cardiac involvement are breast carcinoma, lung carcinoma, renal cell carcinoma, melanoma, and lymphoma. Sarcomas sometimes metastasize to cardiac chambers, especially the right-sided chambers.

The most common sites of origin of peripheral emboli are the left atrium in patients with mitral valve disease or atrial fibrillation, and the left ventricle in patients with recent myocardial infarction or congestive cardiomyopathy. Nearly all left ventricular aneurysms contain thrombi. A less common cause is paradoxical arterial embolization of emboli from a venous origin through a patent foramen ovale. Unexpected right-to-left embolization is caused by transient rise in the right atrial pressure during such events as a Valsalva maneuver.

For the evaluation of intracardiac masses, contrast media are usually injected upstream from the chamber with the suspected mass or, in the case of ventricles, directly into the ventricular chamber. Caution is necessary when injecting into the involved chamber to prevent embolization of parts of the mass. For left atrial masses, visualization is usually achieved by injecting into the pulmonary artery. With left atrial myxoma, the left atrium may be visualized after injection into the left ventricle due to mitral regurgitation, which is frequently caused by the tumor.

The angiographic features of intracardiac masses are:

1. Filling defect projecting into the opacified chamber (Fig. 4-37). A spherical filling defect in the left atrium with a stalk attached to the atrial septum is characteristic of a left atrial myxoma (see Fig. 4-37). The shape may infrequently be filiform with a broad-based attachment to the middle of the septum or at the junction of the septum and the anterior mitral valve leaflet. The tumor moves into the cone of the mitral valve in diastole or may even move across the valve into the left ventricle (see Fig. 4-37). The position of the tumor in the mitral valve apparatus during diastole causes obstruction of the valve. Large tumors fall to the back of the left atrium in systole, where they may partially obstruct the entrance of the pulmonary veins and accentuate pulmonary venous hypertension. A broad-based attachment to the atrial septum may be observed with the malignant variety (myxosarcoma). Invasion of such myxosarcomas beyond the left atrium may be difficult to define by angiography and is more readily evident on computed tomography or magnetic resonance imaging.

2. Focal thickening of the ventricular wall with distortion of the shape of a cardiac chamber is observed with intramural tumors. The rhabdomyoma is frequently small and located in the wall of the ventricle. The angiogram is often normal. If this tumor is large, focal thickening of the myocardial wall may cause a distortion in the shape of the left or right ventricular chambers. Sarcoma of the right atrium can cause bizarre distortion of the right atrium and varying degrees of obliteration of the chamber.

3. Hypervascularity and/or venous lakes on coronary angiography can be caused by any tumor, but are most frequently observed with myxoma.[32a] A similar appearance can be caused by chronic left atrial thrombus.[32b]

4. Increase in the distance between an opacified chamber and the soft-tissue shadow of the heart. This is most frequently caused by pericardial effusion or thickening but can also be caused by a mural tumor.

Thrombus

1. Filling defect in a cardiac chamber, usually the left atrium or left ventricle.

2. Thrombus in the left atrial appendage may prevent opacification of this structure during the levo-phase of an injection into the pulmonary artery.

3. Focal thickening of the left ventricular wall at the site of a regional contraction abnormality. This is caused by a chronic thrombus engrafted upon a transmural myocardial infarction. Mural thrombus in the left ventricle can cause a flat endocardial contour (see Fig. 4-8A,B).

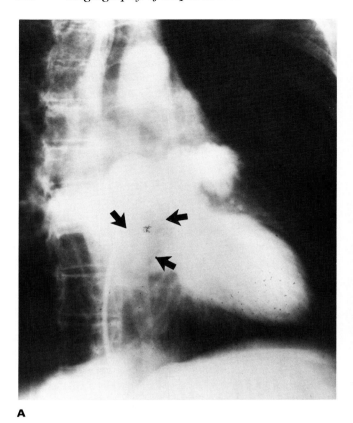

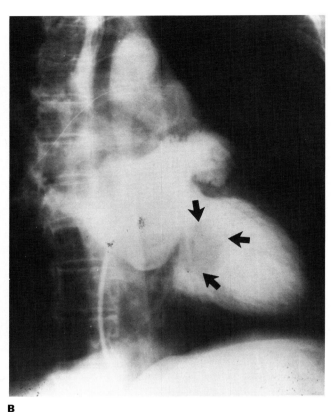

A

B

Figure 4-37. Left atrial myxoma. Levo-phase opacification of the left atrium and left ventricle in a patient with left atrial myxoma. In systole (*A*) a large filling defect (*arrows*) is recognized in the left atrium. In diastole (*B*) the filling defect (*arrows*) moves across the mitral valve into the left ventricle.

Pericardial Abnormalities

Angiography is used infrequently for the diagnosis of pericardial abnormalities because of the greater effectiveness of noninvasive imaging modalities such as echocardiography, computed tomography, and magnetic resonance imaging. The pericardial abnormalities detectable by angiography are constrictive pericardial disease, pericardial effusion, pericardial cysts and tumors, and partial absence of the left pericardium.

Right atrial opacification can be used to identify pericardial abnormalities. Angiography of any cardiac chamber can be used to determine that an abnormal cardiac contour is not caused by a cardiac chamber.

The angiographic features of constrictive pericarditis are:

1. Pericardial calcification (Fig. 4-38). This is most frequently observed in the atrioventricular or interventricular grooves of the heart.

2. Distance of greater than 4 mm from the opacified right atrial cavity to the adjacent soft-tissue shadow of the edge of the heart.[33] The observation can be made in the frontal or left anterior oblique projections. A soft-tissue shadow with a thickness greater than 10 mm is usually caused by a pericardial effusion rather than purely pericardial thickening.

3. Soft-tissue shadow external to the opacified coronary arteries. The wall must be placed tangential to the x-ray beam in order to accurately estimate the coronary artery–soft tissue interface.

4. Failure of normal coiling (systole bending) of some or all of coronary arterial segments during systole.[34]

5. Enlarged right atrium with normal or small ventricular volumes. The ventricle may display a tubular shape.

6. Ventricular diastolic filling pattern is abnormal. There is abrupt expansion of the left ventricle in early diastole with little or no filling in the remainder of diastole and no presystolic expansion. In the normal ventricle, presystolic expansion of the diastolic volume occurs coincident with atrial systole.

7. Right and left ventricles are normal or small in size. The ventricles, especially the right ventricle, may be narrow.

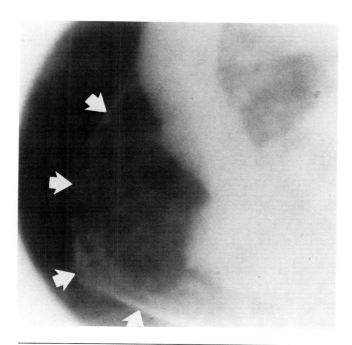

Figure 4-38. Left ventriculogram in the LAO (A) view in a patient with constrictive pericarditis. The left ventricle is reduced in volume and dense calcification (*arrows*) surrounds the heart.

8. Differentiation between constrictive pericarditis and restrictive cardiomyopathy is frequently difficult by angiography. Both may cause diminished motion of the right ventricular wall. However, the contraction of the region of crista supraventricularis is preserved in constrictive pericarditis but diminished in restrictive cardiomyopathy.[35] Another potential differentiating feature is the diastolic filling pattern. Early diastolic filling is considered abnormally rapid in constrictive disease, whereas it is reduced below the normal range in restrictive cardiomyopathy.[36]

References

1. Higgins CB. Overview and methods used for the study of the cardiovascular actions of contrast materials. Invest Radiol (Suppl) 1980;15(6):S188.
2. Higgins CB. Contrast media in the cardiovascular system. In: Sovak M, ed. Radiocontrast agents: Handbook of experimental pharmacology. Berlin: Springer-Verlag, 1984.
3. Hamby RI, Tabrah F, Wiskoff BG, et al. Coronary artery calcification: clinical implications and angiographic correlates. Am J Heart J 1974;87:565.
4. Green CE, Kelley MJ. A renewed role for fluoroscopy in the evaluation of cardiac disease. Radiol Clin N Amer 1980;18(3):345.
5. Cornell SH, Rossi NP. Roentgenographic findings in constrictive pericarditis: analysis of 21 cases. Am J Roentgenol 1968;102:301.
6. Hunt D, Boxley WA, Kennedy JW, et al. Quantitative evaluation of cineaortography in the assessment of aortic regurgitation. Am J Cardiol 1973;31:696.
7. Craft CH, Lipscomb K, Mathis K, et al. Limitations of qualitative angiographic grading in aortic or mitral regurgitations. Am J Cardiol 1984;53:1593.
8. Hay RE, Rackley CE. Quantitation of valvular insufficiency in man by angiocardiography. Am Heart J 1963;65:501.
9. Dodge HT, Sandler H, Ballew DW, Lord JD Jr. The use of biplane angiocardiography for the measurement of left ventricular volume in man. Am Heart J 1960;60:762.
10. Kasser IS, Kennedy JW. Measurements of left ventricular volumes in man by single plane angiocardiography. Invest Radiol 1969;4:83.
11. Wynne J, Green LH, Mann J, et al. Estimation of left ventricular volumes in man from biplane cineangiograms filmed in oblique projections. Am J Cardiol 1978;41:726.
12. Chaitman BR, DeMota H, Bristow JD, Rosch J, Rahimtoola SH. Objective and subjective analysis of left ventricular angiograms. Circulation 1975;52:420.
13. Leighton RF, Wilts SM, Lewis RP. Detection of hypokinesis by a quantitative analysis of left ventricular cineangiograms. Circulation 1974;50:121.
14. Gelberg HJ, Brundage BH, Glantz S, Parmley WW. Quantitative left ventricular wall motion analysis: a comparison of area, cord, and radial methods. Circulation 1979;59:991.
15. Kennedy JW, Kaiser CG, Fisher CD, et al. Clinical and angiographic predictors of operative mortality from the Collaborative Study in Coronary Artery Stenosis (CASS). Circulation 1981; 63:793.
16. White HD, Norris RM, Brown MA, et al. Left ventricular end systolic volume as the major determinant of survival after recovery from myocardial infarction. Circulation 1987;76:44.
17. Sharma B, Goodwin JF, Raphail MJ, et al. Left ventricular angiography on exercise: a new method for assessing left ventricular function in ischemic heart disease. Br Heart J 1976;38:59.
18. Helfant RH, Pine R, Meister SG, et al. Nitroglycerin to unmask reversible asynergy: correlation with post bypass ventriculography. Circulation 1974;50:108.
19. Higgins CB, Wexler L, Silverman JF, Hayden W, Anderson WL, Schroeder JS. Spontaneously and pharmacologically provoked coronary arterial spasm in Prinzmetal variant angina. Radiology 1976;199:521.
20. Hamby RI, Aintablian A, Wisoff BG, Hartstein ML. Response of the left ventricle in coronary artery disease to post extra systolic potentiation. Circulation 1975;51:428.
21. Horn HR, Teichholz LE, Cohn PF, et al. Augmentation of left ventricular contraction pattern in coronary artery disease by an inotropic catecholamine. Circulation 1974;49:1063.
21a. Simpson MT, Oberman A, Kouchoukos NT, et al. Prevalence of mural thrombi and left ventricular aneurysms: effects of anticoagulation therapy. Chest 1980;77:463.
22. Cabin HS, Roberts WC. Left ventricular aneurysm, extra-aneurysmal thrombus and systemic embolus in coronary heart disease. Chest 1980;77:586.
22a. Baratt–Boyes BG, White HD, Agnew TM, et al. The results of surgical treatment of left ventricular aneurysms: an assessment of risk factors affecting early and late mortality. J Thorac Cardiovasc Surg 1984;87:87.
23. Higgins CB, Lipton MJ, Johnson AD, Peterson KL, Vieweg WVR. False aneurysms of the left ventricle: identification of distinctive clinical radiographic and angiographic features. Radiology 1978;127:21.
24. Akins CW, Korklin JW, Block PC, et al. Preoperative evaluation of subvalvular fibrosis in mitral stenosis: a predictive factor in conservative vs replacement surgical therapy. Circulation 1978; 60:71.

142 *Angiography of Acquired Heart Disease*

25. Spindola–Franco H, Bjork L, Adam DF, Abrams HL. Classification of the radiological morphology of the mitral valve: differentiation between true and pseudo prolapse. Br Heart J 1980;44:30.

26. Scampardoni G, Yang SS, Moranhao V, et al. Left ventricular abnormalities in prolapsed mitral leaflet syndrome. Circulation 1973;48:287.

26a. Marcus FI, Fontaine GH, Guiraudon G, et al. Right ventricular dysplasia: a report of 24 adult cases. Circulation 1982;65:384.

27. Goodwin JF. Prospects and predictions for the cardiomyopathies. Circulation 1974;50:210.

28. Simon AL, Ross J Jr, Goult JH. Angiographic anatomy of the left ventricle and mitral valve in idiopathic hypertrophic subaortic stenosis. Circulation 1967;36:852.

29. Sanderson JF, Gibson DG, Brown DJ, Goodwin JF. Left ventricular filling in hypertrophic cardiomyopathy: an angiographic study. Br Heart J 1977;39:661.

30. Green CE, Elliott LP, Coughlan HC. Improved cineangiographic evaluation of hypertrophic cardiomyopathy by caudo-cranial left anterior oblique view. Am Heart J 1981;102:1015.

30a. Falecov R, Resnekov L, Bharati S, Lev M. Mid zone ventricular obstruction: a variant of obstructive cardiomyopathy. Am J Cardiol 1976;37:432.

30b. Yamaguchi H, Ishimura T, Nishiyama S, et al. Hypertrophic non-obstructive cardiomyopathy with giant negative T waves (apical hypertrophy). Am J Cardiol 1979;44:401.

31. Gould KL, Lipscomb K, Hamilton GW, Kennedy JW. Relation of left ventricular shape, function, and wall stress in man. Am J Cardiol 1974;34:627.

32. Kreulen TH, Gorlin R, Herman MV. Ventriculographic patterns and hemodynamics in primary myocardial disease. Circulation 1973;47:299.

32a. Marshall WH, Steiner RM, Wexler L. Tumor vascularity in left atrial myxoma demonstrated by selective coronary arteriography. Radiology 1969;93:815.

32b. Cipriano PR, Guthaner DF. Organized left atrial mural thrombus demonstrated by coronary arteriography. Am Heart J 1978;96:166.

33. Figley MM, Bagshaw MA. Angiographic aspects of constrictive pericarditis. Radiology 1957;69:46.

34. Alexander J, Kelley MJ, Cohen LS, Langon RA. The angiographic appearance of the coronary arteries in constrictive pericarditis. Radiology 1979;131:609.

35. Chang LW, Grollman JH Jr. Angiographic differentiation of constrictive pericarditis and restrictive cardiomyopathy due to amyloidosis. Am J Radiol 1978;130:451.

36. Tyberg TI, Goodyer AVN, Hurst VW, et al. Left ventricular filling in differentiating restrictive amyloid cardiomyopathy and constrictive pericarditis. Am J Cardiol 1981;47:791.

Chapter 5

Angiography of Congenital Heart Disease

Charles B. Higgins

For more than three decades, angiography has been the technique relied upon for the definitive diagnosis of congenital heart disease. For much of this time it has been the only technique that provides adequate depiction of cardiovascular morphology, and consequently it has served as the diagnostic guide upon which cardiovascular surgery has depended. The enormous advances in cardiovascular surgical techniques during the past decade have demanded ever more precise definition of abnormal morphology, stimulating improvements in cardiovascular angiographic techniques for congenital heart disease. A major technical advance for the evaluation of congenital heart disease was the introduction of doubly angulated (axial) angiography by Bergeron.[1,2] Because of the widespread use of two-dimensional echocardiography, the type of congenital heart disease is generally already known prior to catheterization; catheterization is frequently done in order to define more precisely the abnormal morphology of the lesion(s).

Technique

Angiography in congenital heart disease requires the biplane mode. For many years angiography was performed in the anteroposterior and lateral views. These views are now supplemented or substituted with doubly angulated views.

Cineangiography is now the standard technique for recording images. Cineangiography is recorded on 35 mm film at a rate of approximately 30 frames per second.

In order to maximize the contrast between the blood pool and cardiac structures, the radiographic technique uses a low kilovolt peak (kvp) and high milliam-perage-second (mas). The kilovolt peak is set in the range of 60 to 70 in order to provide an average kev near the K edge of iodine. This approach causes the maximum absorption of x-rays by the contrast medium in the blood pool and thereby maximizes contrast between the blood pool and surrounding tissues.

Contrast Medium

A contrast medium containing 300 to 370 mg/ml iodine is required. Usually a concentration of 370 mg/ml is used. Nonionic iodinated contrast media are being used with increasing frequency in infants and children. Nonionioc media are advisable for all infants and for children with ventricular failure. Some laboratories use nonionic media for all cardioangiography.

Contrast medium is administered at a total volume of 1 to 1.5 ml/kg for each angiogram. The injection should be sufficiently high in order to deliver the contrast medium in a single heartbeat in order to minimize dilution of the contrast effect by the inflow of unopacified blood into the target chamber.

Views

The anteroposterior and lateral views have limited utility because of substantial overlap of cardiac structures and foreshortening of most cardiac chambers, especially the left ventricle. Most structures can be evaluated better using the doubly angulated views. The limitation of the axial view is that a greater mass of tissue must be penetrated by the obliquely oriented x-ray beam. This inevitably increases the radiation dose. It can also decrease image quality and contrast because of a need to increase the kvp when limited x-ray generators are used. In general, x-ray exposure should be increased by raising mas rather than kvp in order to maintain the kev in the optimal range for x-ray absorption by contrast medium.

Doubly angulated angiography involves angulation in two planes in order to align the x-ray beam perpendicular to a specific cardiovascular structure or region. The angulations accomplish two goals: alignment of the long axis of the heart with the x-ray beam; and rotation of the patient or the image intensifier so that the area of interest is perpendicular or nearly perpendicular to the x-ray beam.

Three doubly angulated views are used frequently:

1. Four chamber view.
2. Long-axial oblique view.
3. Cranial anteroposterior (sit-up) view.

These views can be accomplished by rotating the patient in relation to a fixed x-ray tube–image intensifier system (Fig. 5-1) or by rotating the image intensifier in both the craniocaudal and transverse planes (Fig. 5-2) or by a combination of the two. The nomenclature for these views based on double angulation is described by the position of the image intensifier in relation to the patient's body. The positions of the patient in relation to fixed x-ray tube and image intensifier for the various views is shown in Figure 5-1. At present, most laboratories are equipped with x-ray equipment capable of rotating in multiple planes, so this technique is described below in some detail.

Four-Chamber View. The image intensifier is rotated approximately 40° cranially and approximately 45° leftward (in relation to the patient) in the transverse plane (see Fig. 5-2). Alternatively, the patient is rotated 20° into a left anterior oblique (LAO) position, and the image intensifier is rotated only 25° leftward. This view aligns the atrial septum and the posterior (inlet) portion of the ventricular septum perpendicular to the x-ray beam. The view displays the attachments of the atrioventricular valves to the ventricular septum and the relationship of each atrioventricular valve or, if present, a single atrioventricular valve, to the inlet portion of the ventricles.

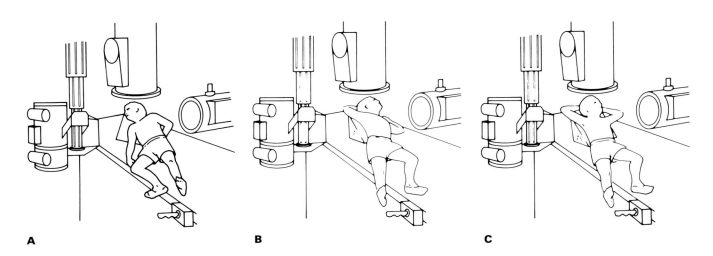

A　　　　　　　　　　**B**　　　　　　　　　　**C**

Figure 5-1. Diagrams display the positioning of the patient for the angled angiographic views using a fixed x-ray tube-image intensifier system. *A:* Four-chamber view. The long axis of the body is angled across the x-ray table such that the head is toward the left margin of the table and the feet toward the right margin. This causes the body to be skewed at a 20° angle in relation to the x-ray table. Using a cushion, the patient is elevated approximately 40° to 45° and rotated approximately 40° to 45° to the right. This causes the heart to have a double angulation in relationship to the overhead image intensifier. The double angulation is 40° to 45° cranial and 40° to 45° left anterior oblique (LAO). *B:* Long-axial oblique view produced by double angulation of the patient in relationship to a fixed x-ray tube-image intensifier system. For this view the patient is rotated in relation to the lateral image intensifier. The long axis of the body is angulated in relation to the x-ray table with the head toward the left side of the table and the foot toward the right side of the table. This causes the body to be skewed about 25° to 30° in relation to the x-ray table. A cushion is used to elevate the patient about 40° to 45° and to rotate the patient toward the left side by about 20°. This results in a doubly angulated cranial LAO view of the body in relation to the image intensifier, which lies to the left side of the patient. This is a 40° cranial 70° left right anterior oblique (RAO) view. *C:* Cranial anteroposterior (sit-up) view. A cushion is used to raise the upper portion of the body approximately 40° to 45° in relation to the x-ray table. This produces a 45° cranial anteroposterior view in relation to the overhead image intensifier.

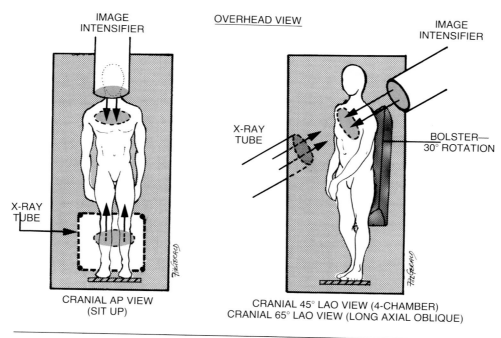

Figure 5-2. Diagram showing the techniques for obtaining the angulated angiographic views using rotation of the image intensifier and x-ray tube in two planes. For these views the image intensifier and x-ray tube are linked to each other through a C or U arm, which permits angulation in both the craniocaudal and transverse directions. *Left,* cranial arteroposterior view; *right,* cranial LAO view. The angulation can be done using a bolster to partially rotate the patient and further angulation by rotation of the image intensifies.

When this view is used, the contrast medium is usually injected into the left ventricle in order to display inlet types of ventricular septal defects or to demonstrate the morphology and relationship of the atrioventricular valve to the left ventricle. Contrast medium is also injected into the left upper pulmonary vein by means of a catheter placed across an interatrial communication (septal defect or patent foramen ovale) to demonstrate the site and relative size of atrial septal defects. Alternatively, contrast medium can be injected into the left atrial chamber.

The use of the four-chamber view is indicated for the following cardiac lesions:

1. Ventricular septal defect, especially if a posterior defect is suspected.
2. Atrioventricular septal (endocardial cushion) defect.
3. Atrial septal defect.
4. Overriding or straddling atrioventricular valve.
5. Pulmonary arterial and proximal left pulmonary arterial stenosis.

Long Axial Oblique View. The frontal image intensifier is rotated cranial 20° to 30° and 60° to 65° leftward (see Fig. 5-2). Because of the extreme angulation of the image intensifier required for this view, it may be necessary or even advisable to rotate the patient into about a 30° LAO position and then rotate the intensifier 30° cranially and 30° to 35° leftward, thus accomplishing a 30° cranial, 65° LAO view. The exact degree of LAO positioning and cranial angulation depends upon the orientation of the heart in the thorax. Horizontal hearts require greater cranial angulation. This view is intended to render the long axis of the left ventricle (a line coursing from the junction of the aortic and mitral valves to the apex) perpendicular to the x-ray beam and the anterior ventricular septum in profile.

The perimembranous and outlet portions of the ventricular septum are optimally visualized in this view. Likewise, the left ventricular outflow tract is optimally visualized. It shows the relationship of the anterior leaflet of the mitral valve to the aortic valve and the ventricualr septum. This view also displays the aortic arch, the region of the ductus arteriosus, and the left coronary artery. When this view is used, contrast medium is injected into the left ventricle.

The long axial oblique view is indicated for the following:

1. Perimembranous and outlet ventricular septal defects.
2. Abnormalities of arterioventricular connections.
3. Subvalvular aortic stenosis.
4. Hypertrophic cardiomyopathy.

5. Patent ductus arteriosus. For this diagnosis other views are also adequate.
6. Definition of coronary arterial anatomy. This is needed for the preoperative assessment of tetralogy of Fallot and transposition of the great arteries when the arterial switch (Jatene) procedure is contemplated.

Cranial Anteroposterior (Sit Up) View. The frontal image intensifier is rotated 40° to 45° cranially (see Fig. 5-2). Alternatively, the patient is raised 15° to 20° on a bolster and the intensifier is rotated 25° to 30°. This view obviates the foreshortening and overlapping of the right ventricular outflow tract and pulmonary artery, which is present in the standard anteroposterior view. This view is optimal for demonstrating the full length of the main pulmonary artery and its bifurcation, since it eliminates the superimposition of the proximal and distal segments of the pulmonary artery. It also spatially separates the sites of aortopulmonary collateral arteries and the central pulmonary arteries in patients with pulmonary atresia.

The use of the cranial anteroposterior view is indicated for the following:

1. Right ventricular outflow obstruction, especially tetralogy of Fallot.
2. Pulmonary stenosis. The standard lateral view can suffice for this diagnosis.
3. Pulmonary atresia.
4. Branch pulmonary arterial stenosis.

Caudal Right Anterior Oblique View. The frontal image intensifier is rotated 30° caudally and 40° rightward. If the patient is rotated for the long axial oblique view, the lateral image intensifier can be used. The caudal right anterior oblique view displays most of the segments of the left ventricle, parts of the mitral valve, the crista supraventricularis and other parts of the right ventricular infundibulum.

This view may be indicated in the following:

1. Differentiation of supracristal and infracristal ventricular septal defect.
2. Evaluation of regional left ventricular contraction.
3. Evaluation of the mitral valve.

Angiographic Features of Specific Lesions

The anatomy and the clinical features of specific cardiac lesions are discussed in Chapter 2. This section deals only with the angiographic features of each lesion.

Atrial Septal Defect

There are four types of possible atrial septal defects (ASDs): secundum, primum, sinus venosus, and coronary sinus. The sinus venosus type may be either superior or, rarely, inferior vena caval in location. Partial anomalous pulmonary venous connection is associated with nearly 100% of sinus venous defects and about 10% of secundum defects. Elliott et al.[3] have described the appearance of ASDs using the four-chamber view.

The goals of angiographic imaging are:

1. Identification of the ASD or ASDs.
2. Determination of the site (type of ASD).
3. Determination of the size of the defect.
4. Identification of the entrance of all pulmonary veins.
5. Identification of associated defects.

Optimal views and sites of injection are:

1. Four-chamber view with injection into the right upper pulmonary vein. This is done to depict the site of the defect.

2. Anteroposterior and lateral views with injection into the right ventricle or main pulmonary artery. This is done to demonstrate the entrance of the pulmonary veins.

3. Four-chamber view with injection into the left ventricle. This view is used with suspected primum ASD in order to demonstrate the characteristic contour ("gooseneck deformity") of the left ventricle in the defect.

Salient angiographic features are:

Secundum ASD

1. Contrast medium shunts across the middle of the atrial septum, which is outlined in profile on the four-chamber view (Fig. 5-3).

2. If the pulmonary veins are not identified entering the left atrium on the frontal view of the injection into the main pulmonary artery, anomalous connection must be considered. This diagnosis is indicated when the right upper lobe vein is shown to be draining into the superior vena cava or azygous vein (Fig. 5-4). Right pulmonary veins draining directly into the right atrium may not be obvious in the presence of an ASD. If anomalous connection of the right pulmonary veins is recognized on injection into the main pulmonary artery, an injection into the left pulmonary veins may be required to verify that an ASD is also present. During the levo-phase of this injection, appearance of contrast medium in the right atrium confirms an atrial level shunt in addition to the anomalous pulmonary venous connection of the right pulmonary veins.

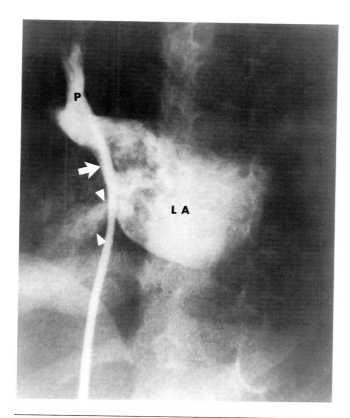

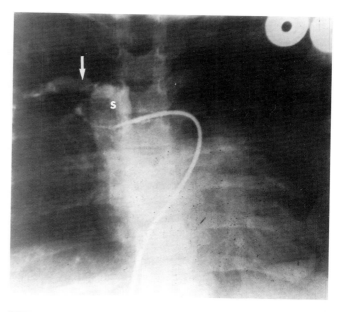

Figure 5-4. Partial anomalous pulmonary venous connection from the right upper-lobe pulmonary vein to the superior vena cava. The levo-phase after the injection of contrast medium into the right pulmonary artery demonstrates the right upper-lobe pulmonary vein (*arrow*) connecting to the superior vena cava (S).

Figure 5-3. Atrial septal defect, secundum type. Cranial LAO (four-chamber) view with injection into the right upper lobe pulmonary vein. The catheter has passed across the interatrial communication and lies in the right upper lobe pulmonary vein, where the contrast medium is injected. The contrast medium outlines the ventricular septum (*arrows*) and displays left-to-right shunting of the medium (*arrowheads*) through a secundum atrial septal defect. (LA, left atrium; P, pulmonary vein.)

Primum ASD

1. Contrast medium shunts across the most caudal portion of the atrial septum after injection into the right upper pulmonary vein in the four-chamber view.

2. Caudal displacement of the medial attachment of the mitral valve is shown in the four-chamber view after injection into the left ventricle (Figs. 5-5, 5-6). This caudal displacement causes an orientation of the left component of the atrioventricular valve, which is diagnostic of some form of the atrioventricular septal (endocardial cushion) defect. In the four-chamber view a line drawn through the middle of the mitral valve (the left-sided component of the atrioventricular valve) is directed toward the right shoulder in the atrioventricular septal defect. A line through the middle of the mitral valve in the normal ventricle points to the head or toward the left shoulder in this view.

3. A right anterior oblique (RAO) or anteroposterior view of the left ventricle depicts the goose-neck deformity caused by the large anterosuperior portion of the left atrioventricular valve as it unfurls during diastole (see Fig. 5-6), causing a narrowed and elongated appearance of the left ventricular outflow region. A cleft or prominent serration of the mitral valve leaflet is recognized in systole (see Fig. 5-6).

4. Mitral regurgitation. Mitral regurgitation along with the primum ASD may cause a jet of contrast medium to pass from the left ventricle into the right atrium.

5. Direct atrial shunting from the left ventricle to the right atrium indicates a defect in the atrioventricular septum.

Sinus Venous Defect[4]

1. Contrast medium shunts across the most cranial portion of the atrial septum as observed in the four-chamber view. Because of the anomalous connection of the right upper pulmonary vein, the injection is made into the left atrium.

2. Superior vena cava straddles the atrial septal defect because the defect removes the separation between the superior vena cava and the top of the left atrium.

3. Anomalous connection of the right upper pulmonary vein to the superior vena cava at its junction with the atria.

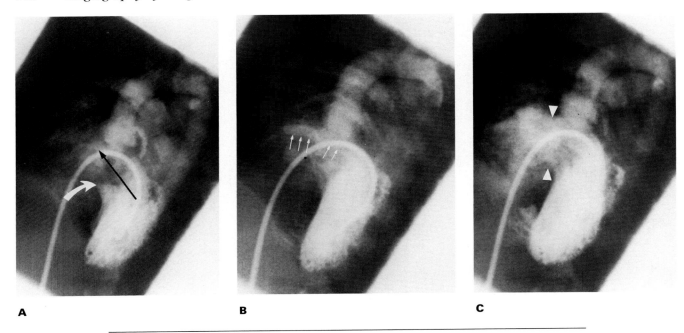

A   **B**   **C**

Figure 5-5. Atrioventricular septal defect (endocardial cushion defect). *A:* Cranial LAO view with injection of contrast medium into the left ventricle. Catheter has passed from the right-sided cardiac chambers across a primum atrial septal defect and into the left ventricle through the left component of the atrioventricular valve. Contrast medium trapped beneath the atrioventricular valve outlines the large anterior leaflet of the common atrioventricular valve. A vector (*long black arrow*) drawn through the middle of the left component of the atrioventricular valve points toward the right shoulder of the patient. This is due to the caudal displacement of the attachments of the atrioventricular valve to the foreshortened inlet ventricular septum (*curved arrow*). Normally, such a vector drawn through the middle of the mitral valve will point directly toward the head or slightly toward the left shoulder. Frames of a cineangiogram obtained early (*B*) and later (*C*) after the injection of contrast medium into the left ventricle in the cranial LAO view. Contrast medium outlines the anterior large leaflet of the common atrioventricular valve (*small arrows*), spanning both ventricles. Substantial left-to-right shunting (*arrowheads*) across the large defect in the inlet portion of the ventricular septum is evident during systole. Note the position of the crest of the inlet ventricular septum, indicating considerable deficiency of this portion of the septum.

Partial Anomalous Pulmonary Venous Connection

The most common site of partial anomalous pulmonary venous connection (PAPVC) is the right upper lobe vein to the superior vena cava.[5,6] Other sites of anomalous drainage from the right lung are the azygous arch, the right atrium, the coronary sinus, and the inferior vena cava (scimitar syndrome). Anomalous drainage from the left lung is rare, and drainage is usually into a persistent left superior vena cava. Anomalous connection of left veins to the left subclavian artery and coronary sinus can rarely occur.

Goals of angiographic imaging are:

1. Identification of the site of anomalous connection.

2. Identification of associated atrial septal defect.

Optimal view and injection sites are:

1. Anteroposterior view with injection into the main pulmonary artery or ipsilateral pulmonary artery (Fig. 5-4).

2. Direct cannulation and injection of the anomalous pulmonary vein with filming in the anteroposterior or four-chamber views.

3. In the presence of anomalous right pulmonary venous connection, injection into the left pulmonary artery is done for identification of an associated ASD.

Salient angiographic features are:

1. Connection of all four pulmonary veins to the left atrium should be recognized during the levo-phase after injection into the pulmonary artery in order to exclude partial anomalous connection.

2. Early appearance of contrast medium in the superior vena cava or azygous vein indicates anomalous pulmonary venous connection. The site of connection of the anomalous right pulmonary vein may be visualized (Fig. 5-4).

3. Direct cannulation and injection of the anomalous vein identifies precisely the site of connection.

4. Appearance of contrast medium in the right

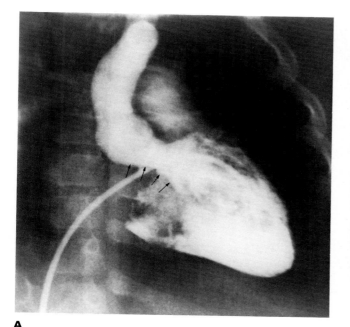

A

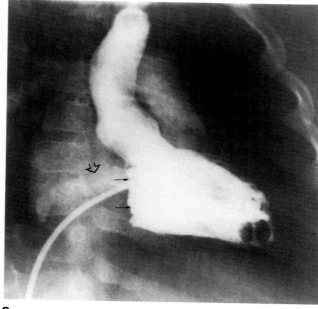

B

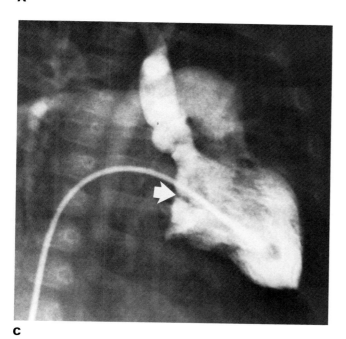

C

Figure 5-6. Atrioventricular septal defect. RAO views with injection of contrast medium into the left ventricle. The catheter has passed into the right-sided cardiac chambers across a primum atrial septal defect and into the left ventricle through the left component of the atrioventricular valve. Diastolic frame (*A*) demonstrates the goose-neck deformity caused by the superior portion of the large anterior leaflet (*arrows*) of the atrioventricular valve as it unfurls into the left ventricle. This produces elongation and narrowing of the left ventricular outflow region. The outflow region also has a more horizontal orientation compared to the normal situation in this view. Contrast medium opacifies the right ventricular outlet region and the pulmonary artery because of the ventricular septal defect. Note the shorter length of the medial wall of the left ventricle in comparison to the lateral wall. This indicates deficiency or foreshortening of the inlet portion of the ventricular septum. Systolic (*B*) frame demonstrates prominent serrations (*small arrows*) of the left component of the atrioventricular valve with a cleft due to thickened tissue at this site. A jet of regurgitant flow (*open arrow*) from left ventricle to left atrium is evident. Systolic frame in RAO view of another patient (*C*) shows a lucent cleft (*arrow*) at the site of coarctation of two components of the left part of the atrioventricular valve.

atrium during the levo-phase after pulmonary arterial injection can be caused by PAPVC to the right atrium or ASD, or both. Absence of right atrial opacification after selective injection of contrast medium into the left pulmonary artery excludes an ASD. Usually, partial anomalous pulmonary venous connection involves the right pulmonary veins. Consequently, in the presence of PAPVC of right-sided veins, injection into the left pulmonary artery is done to demonstrate or exclude an associated atrial septal defect.

Ventricular Septal Defect

The sites of the ventricular septal defects (VSDs) form the basis of their classification.[7,8] For this discussion, the defects are considered according to their position in the septum: perimembranous, outlet, supracristal, inlet, and trabecular ("muscular"). Outlet defects have been divided into supracristal and malignant types. Because of the high incidence of progressive aortic regurgitation in supracristal VSD, it is important to determine whether the defect is located cranial (supracristal) or caudal (infracristal) to the crista supraventricularis of the right ventricle. Infracristal VSDs include any defect located below the crista and consequently can include malignant, perimembranous, and inlet types.

Goals of imaging studies are:

1. Identification of the VSD.
2. Exclusion of multiple sites of VSDs.
3. Demonstration of the site(s) of the VSD(s).
4. Definition of the size of the VSD.
5. Identification of associated anomalies.

Optimal views and sites of injection are:

1. Long axial oblique view with injection into the left ventricle.

2. Four-chamber view when an inlet ventricular septal defect is suspected or a small right ventricular size suggests a straddling tricuspid valve.

3. Caudal RAO view with injection into the left ventricle in order to depict a supracristal VSD.

4. Anteroposterior view or LAO view with injection into the ascending aorta in order to exclude an associated patent ductus arteriosus and aortic regurgitation caused by prolapse of a sinus of Valsalva. There may be loss of support for the right or posterior sinus of Valsalva in the presence of a VSD. This occurs with substantial frequency in supracristal VSD and less frequently in infracristal perimembranous VSD.

Salient angiographic features are:

1. In the long axial oblique view the outlet and perimembranous VSDs cause disruption of the line representing the anterior portion of the septum (Figs. 5-7, 5-8).

2. In the long axial oblique view a defect in the center of the outflow region indicates a perimembranous VSD (see Fig. 5-7).

3. The supracristal defect is located high in the outlet region; it appears just beneath the aortic valve. The shunted blood is directed primarily into the pulmonary artery; little or none is directed into the body of the right ventricle (Fig. 5-9).

4. In the four-chamber view a defect in the portion of the septum brought into profile (posterior or inlet septum) in this view indicates an inlet VSD (Fig. 5-10).

5. A defect in the midportion or lower in the septum toward the apex indicates a trabecular (muscular) VSD. If the defect is seen on the long axial oblique view it involves the anterior portion of the muscular septum. If it is visualized on the four-chamber view, it is located in the posterior portion of the muscular septum.

6. In the caudal RAO view the body of the crista is seen separating the pulmonary and aortic valves (Fig.

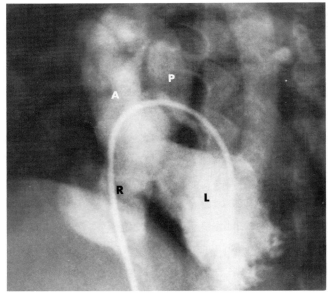

A

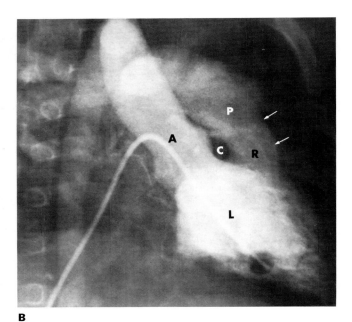

B

Figure 5-7. Perimembranous ventricular septal defect. Cranial LAO view (*A*) and RAO view (*B*) with injection of contrast media into the left ventricle. Contrast medium flows from the left ventricle to the right ventricle across a perimembranous ventricular septal defect. Note in the RAO view that the shunted opacified blood (*arrows*) flows below the crista supraventricularis (*C*). (A, aorta; L, left ventricle; P, pulmonary artery; R, right ventricle.)

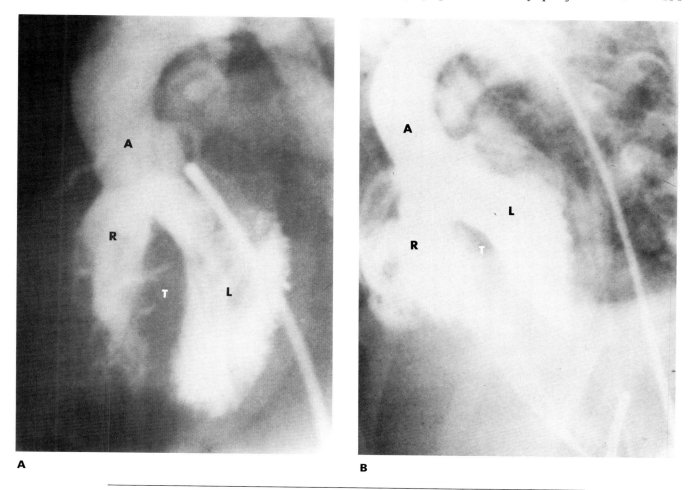

A   B

Figure 5-8. *A:* Malalignment type of outlet defect of the ventricular septum in a patient with tetralogy of Fallot. Cranial LAO view with injection of contrast medium into the left ventricle. There is a large defect in the outlet (anterior) portion of the ventricular septum that conducts a large bidirectional shunt. In this frame, considerable shunting from the left ventricle to the right ventricle is evident. Note that the enlarged aorta overrides the ventricular septal defect. *B:* Large perimembranous ventricular septal defect with some extension into the outlet septum. Cranial LAO view with injection of contrast medium into the left ventricle. A large defect is evident in the portion of the ventricular septum outlined in this view. This indicates a perimembranous location with extension primarily into the outlet septum. There is a large-volume left-to-right shunt that produces considerable opacification of the right ventricle. The trabecular portion (T) of the ventricular septum is intact. (A, ascending aorta; L, left ventricle; R, right ventricle; T, trabecular septum.)

5-9). A shunt through the expected region of the crista indicates a supracristal defect. Predominant opacification of the main pulmonary artery and no or little opacification of the right ventricular body by flow through the defect suggest a supracristal VSD. In the long axial oblique view, the shunt is located high in the outlet septum and the shunt opacifies the distal right ventricular outlet region and the pulmonary artery (Fig. 5-9).

Patent Ductus Arteriosus

The location of the patent ductus arteriosus may be variable, depending upon the presence of associated anom-

alies. Patent ductus in the presence of severe pulmonary stenosis or pulmonary atresia is located at the undersurface of the aortic arch.[9] As an isolated anomaly, the ductus is located just distal to the origin of the left subclavian artery.

Goals of angiographic imaging are:

1. Demonstration of the presence and location of the ductus.

2. Exclusion of associated anomalies, especially VSD and coarctation of the aorta.

Optimal view and injection site are:

1. Long axial oblique view with injection into the ascending or descending aorta.

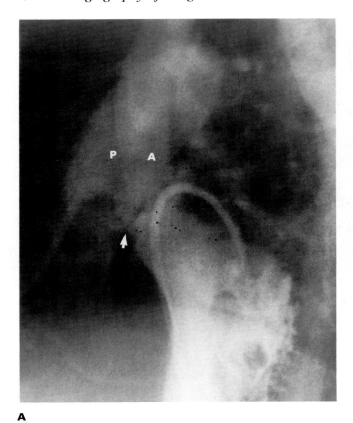

A

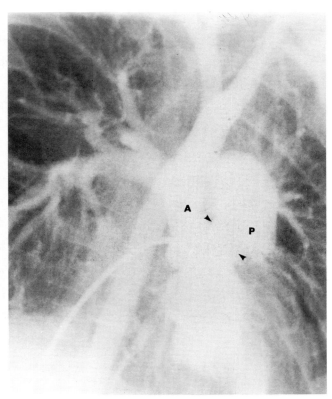

B

Figure 5-9. Supracristal ventricular septal defect. Cranial LAO view (*A*) and caudal RAO (*B*) views with injection into the left ventricle. In the LAO view the jet of shunted blood (arrow) is evident passing from high in the outlet portion of the ventricular septum into the pulmonary artery (P) with little opacification of the right ventricle. This flow pattern of shunted blood is characteristic of the supracristal ventricular septal defect. The defect is located just beneath the right sinus of Valsalva of the aorta. The caudal RAO view demonstrates that the shunted contrast (*arrowheads*) passes through the region of the body of the crista supraventricularis. The muscle of the crista, which is generally recognized separating the aorta from the pulmonary valve (see Fig. 5-7), in this view is obliterated owing to the passage of contrast media across this region. (A, aorta.)

2. Anteroposterior and lateral view with injection into the ascending aorta.

Salient angiographic features are:

1. Shunt from proximal descending to the proximal portion of the left pulmonary artery (Fig. 5-11).

2. Ductus is attached to the undersurface of the aorta when associated with severe pulmonary stenosis and pulmonary atresia. The site of attachment to the aorta is depicted as the long axial oblique and lateral views.

3. In the long axial oblique view the length of the ductus is visualized and focal constrictions at either end can be discerned.

Atrioventricular Septal Defect (Endocardial Cushion Defect)

This defect involves varying degrees of malformation of the center of the heart.[10–12] It consists of a primum septal defect, a single atrioventricular valve annulus, and deficiency of the inlet ventricular septum. The anterior and posterior leaflets of the valve of the single atrioventricular orifice are usually attached to the crest of the inlet ventricular septum. Bridging tissue between the anterior and posterior leaflet may be present, and this tissue attaches to the ventricular septum and effectively divides the valve into left and right components. Absence of this bridging tissue and an interrupted line of attachment of the valve leaflet to the inlet septum results in an interventricular communication (inlet VSD). The division of the atrioventricular orifice may be disproportionate in regard to the two ventricles, resulting in a small right ventricle (left ventricular dominant type), or a small left ventricle (right ventricular dominant type). The type of attachment of the atrioventricular valve to the septum has formed the basis of the Rastelli classification of the complete forms of atrioventricular septal defect.[12] Rastelli type A is characterized by attachment of the anterior common leaflet to the crest of the inlet septum. Type B con-

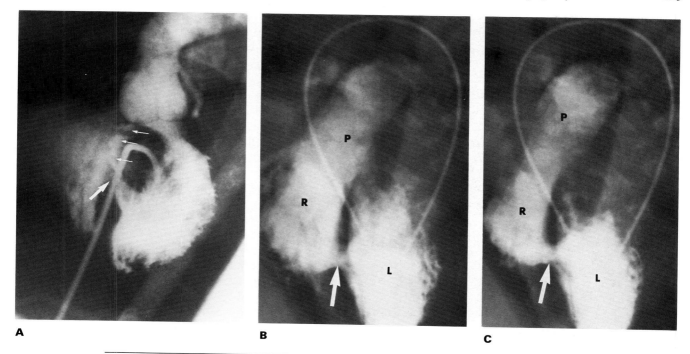

Figure 5-10. Inlet ventricular septal defect in a patient with the complete form of atrioventricular septal defect (*A*). Cranial LAO view with injection of contrast medium into the left ventricle. The catheter has passed from the right-sided cardiac chambers across the primum atrial septal defect and into the left ventricle. Injection of contrast medium into the left ventricle outlines the bridging tissue (*large arrow*) attached to the crest of the ventricular septum. This tissue separates the left component of the atrioventricular valve from the right ventricular portion. Although this bridging tissue is present, there is an interventricular connection through the inlet portion (*arrow*) of the ventricular septum, producing a left-ventricular-to-right-ventricular shunt. Isolated inlet ventricular septal defect in another patient is shown in the cranial 45° LAO (four-chamber) views in early (*B*) and later (*C*) frames. The inlet (posterior) defect (*arrow*) between the right (R) and left (L) ventricle is evident. (P, pulmonary artery.)

sists of attachment of the anterior leaflet to papillary muscles on the right side of the septum. In type C, the anterior leaflet is not attached to the septum and is considered to be free floating.

Other anomalies may coexist with this defect. The most common are an additional VSD and right ventricular outflow obstruction.

Goals of angiographic imaging are:

1. Identification of the several components of the defect, such as the primum ASD, inlet VSD, and atrioventricular valve deformity.
2. Demonstration of the severity of mitral regurgitation (left-sided atrioventricular valve regurgitation).
3. Definition of the size of the right and left ventricles.
4. Determination of the type of atrioventricular valve deformity.
5. Identification of associated anomalies, such as an additional VSD or obstruction to the right ventricular outflow tract.

Optimal views and injection sites are:

1. Four-chamber view with injection into the right upper pulmonary vein.
2. Four-chamber view with injection into the left ventricle.
3. Long axial oblique view with injection into the left ventricle may be required to exclude a second VSD.
4. Sit-up view with injection into the right ventricle may be used to define obstruction to the right ventricular outlet if this is suspected by hemodynamic measurements.

Salient angiographic features are:

1. Left-to-right shunting at the caudal portions of the atrial septum is shown in the four-chamber view and indicates a primum ASD.
2. Left-to-right shunting is shown in the inlet portion of the ventricular septum (see Figs. 5-5, 5-6, 5-10). The defect may be seen just inferior to the point of attachment of the atrioventricular valve leaflet to the septum in some cases. The size of the inlet defect is variable, and its size is generally proportional to the severity of the atrioventricular septal anomaly.
3. Mitral regurgitation. Regurgitant flow may opac-

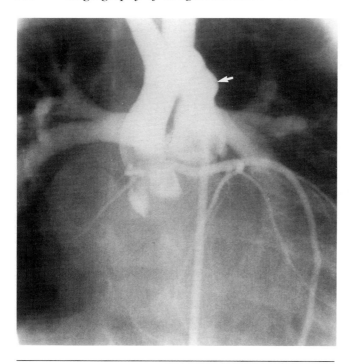

Figure 5-11. Patent ductus arteriosus. Anteroposterior view after injection of contrast media into the distal ascending aorta. Contrast medium appears almost simultaneously within the ascending aorta and the pulmonary artery. A localized dilatation (*arrow*) of the proximal portion of the descending thoracic aorta indicates the site of the patent ductus arteriosus.

ify the left atrial body, but frequently immediately traverses the primum ASD and opacifies the right atrium (see Fig. 5-6).

4. Direct left ventricular to right atrial shunting may occur through a defect in the atrioventricular septum.

5. Gooseneck deformity of the left ventricle is evident during diastole in the anteroposterior or the RAO view. This is caused by movement of the large untethered superior component of the clefted anterior leaflet into the left ventricular outflow region (see Fig. 5-6).

6. Cleft or prominent serrations of the anterior leaflet of the left (mitral) component of the atrioventricular valve is observed during systole (see Fig. 5-6).

7. A large anterior leaflet spanning both ventricles observed on the four-chamber view is a sign of a single atrioventricular defect and indicates a complete form of the defect (see Figs. 5-5, 5-6).

8. Rastelli type A causes the gooseneck deformity. Types B and C do not usually cause this characteristic deformity of the left ventricular contour.

9. In the four-chamber view, the common atrioventricular annulus is indicated by a continuous line formed by the posterior annulus across the crest of the ventricular septum (see Fig. 5-5). This view also shows the relative commitment of the common valve to the two ventricles.

Tetralogy of Fallot

This anomaly consists of obstruction to the right ventricular outflow tract; ventricular septal defect; dextraposed aorta overriding the VSD; and right ventricular hypertrophy. The VSD is a malalignment defect caused by anterosuperior displacement of the infundibular septum; the anterior displacement of the septum causes reduction in the width of the right ventricular outflow region and causes the aorta to override the defect and the remainder of the septum.[13]

The obstruction to the pulmonary blood flow may exist at multiple levels, including the infundibulum, pulmonic annulus, pulmonic valve, and pulmonary arteries. Stenoses at the origin of the right and left pulmonary arteries (the most common site) and segmental arteries, occur frequently. Diffuse hypoplasia of the pulmonary circulation may be present and, rarely, the pulmonary artery contralateral to the aortic arch is absent. Important anomalies of the origin of the coronary arteries occur in 2% to 5% of patients with this anomaly.[14] A prominent right-ventricular branch of the right coronary artery has been reported in 30% to 40% of cases.[15]

Goals of angiographic imaging are:

1. Demonstration of the site of VSD. Exclusion of multiple VSDs.

2. Demonstration of the sites of obstruction to pulmonary blood flow.

3. Determination of the size of the pulmonary annulus and the pulmonary arteries. Identification of branch or peripheral pulmonary arterial stenosis(es).

4. Exclusion of coronary arterial anomalies.

5. Exclusion of aortic arch anomalies. Determination of the origin of arch branches may be important for construction of systemic–pulmonary arterial shunts.

6. Status of palliative shunts.

7. Identification of acquired pulmonary arterial stenoses situated at shunt anastomoses or caused by twisting or tethering of pulmonary arteries by the shunts.

Optimal views and injection sites are:

1. Long axial oblique view (cranial 60° LAO view) with injection into the left ventricle.

2. Anteroposterior or sit-up anteroposterior view and lateral view with injection into the right ventricle.

3. Left anterior oblique and anteroposterior view with injection into the proximal ascending aorta. This is used to display the coronary arterial anatomy.

Salient angiographic features are:

1. The presence, site and severity of the right ventricular outflow region are demonstrated in the anteroposterior and lateral views of the right ventriculogram (Figs. 5-12, 5-13). This view is also used to assess the size

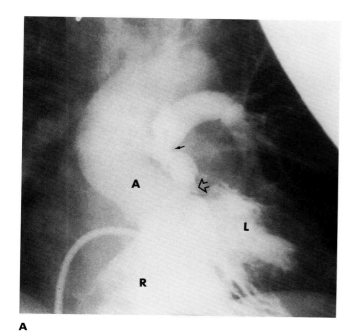

A

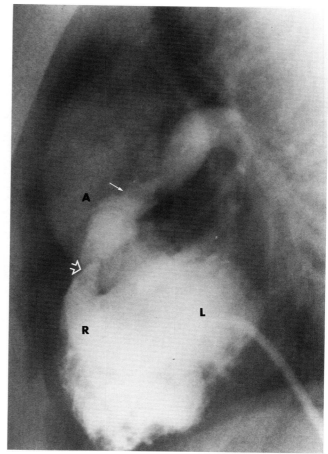

B

Figure 5-12. Tetralogy of Fallot. Cranial anteroposterior (*A*) and lateral (*B*) views demonstrate narrowing of the right ventricular outflow tract at multiple levels. There is severe stenosis in the infundibulum (*open arrow*) of the right ventricle and in the proximal portion (*small arrow*) of the main pulmonary artery. The annulus of the pulmonic valve is small. The injection into the right ventricle produces direct filling of the ascending aorta due to the aortic overriding. Contrast medium also outlines the left ventricle as a consequence of right-to-left shunting. On the cranial anterior posterior (sit-up) view the entire right ventricular outflow tract and the main pulmonary artery, along with the origin of the left pulmonary artery, are visualized. (A, aorta; L, left ventricle; R, right ventricle.)

of the pulmonic annulus. It may also disclose pulmonic valvular stenosis and, occasionally, an abnormally positioned hypertrophied muscle bundle, producing obstruction in the body of the right ventricle.

2. The cranial anteroposterior (sit-up) view demonstrates the pulmonary artery and the bifurcation region (see Figs. 5-12, 5-13), which is a common site of the pulmonary arterial stenosis. Small caliber of the intraparenchymal pulmonary arteries may indicate hypoplasia or may be due to severe underperfusion as a consequence of proximal obstruction.

3. The long axial oblique (cranial LAO) view demonstrates malalignment outlet VSD and shows the enlarged aorta overriding the remainder of the septum and the defect (see Fig. 5-8). Additional VSDs (usually trabecular) can be demonstrated with this view.

4. The LAO view of the aortic injection demonstrates an enlarged aorta. The diameter of the ascending aorta is enlarged reciprocally in relation to the severity of the right ventricular obstruction and size of the main pulmonary artery. An aortic injection is essential for excluding coronary arterial anomalies. A variety of anomalies

can be encountered, but the one that is critical is the origin of the left anterior descending coronary artery from the right sinus or right coronary artery. The anomalous course of the left anterior descending (LAD) artery across the right ventricular infundibulum is evident in the LAO view. It is essential to identify the normal bifurcation of the left coronary artery into the LAD and circumflex coronary arteries in order to exclude this anomaly. The LAD artery courses vertically from the root of the aorta to the apex. A prominent muscular branch arises from the proximal right coronary artery and courses across the right ventricle in 30% to 40% of patients with tetralogy of Fallot.[15] This can easily be confused with the LAD artery.

5. A small right ventricle is unusual in tetralogy of Fallot. It should suggest an associated tricuspid valve abnormality such as straddling or overriding tricuspid valve, tricuspid stenosis, or Ebstein's anomaly.

6. A right aortic arch is present in 20% to 25% of patients. It is usually mirror-image, but right arch with retroesophageal left subclavian artery also occurs.

7. The aortogram indicates the types of palliative systemic to pulmonary shunts and demonstrates the pres-

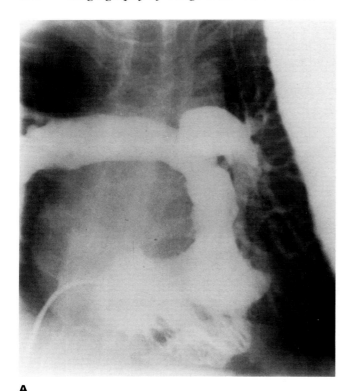

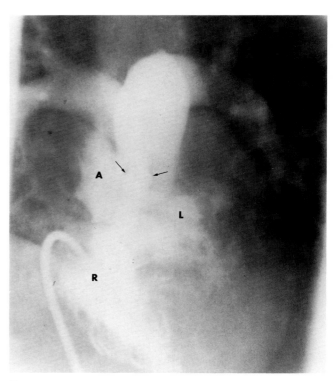

A   **B**

Figure 5-13. Cranial anteroposterior (sit-up) views in two patients with tetralogy of Fallot. Contrast medium is injected into the right ventricle. *A* demonstrates relatively normal caliber of the right ventricular outflow tract and the pulmonary artery after repair of tetralogy of Fallot. *B* demonstrates narrowing of the right ventricular outflow tract and doming of the pulmonic valve (*arrows*). Contrast medium faintly outlines the left ventricle as a consequence of right-to-left shunting through the ventricular septal defect. There is also faint opacification of the ascending aorta as a consequence of direct shunting from the right ventricle to the aorta. (A, aorta; R, right ventricle; L, left ventricle.)

ence and size of bronchial collateral arteries to the lungs. The course and distal connections of bronchial arteries are disclosed by injections into the descending aorta or selectively into the enlarged bronchial or intercostal arteries. Differentiation of bronchial and pulmonary arteries may not always be possible. In general, at the level of the hila the pulmonary arteries are situated ventral to the bronchi, whereas the bronchial arteries are situated dorsal to the bronchi.

When a Blalock–Taussig anastomosis is contemplated, it is essential to exclude an aortic arch anomaly such as a retroesophageal subclavian artery.

Complications Associated with Palliative Shunts

The types of palliative shunts used to augment pulmonary blood flow are:

1. Blalock–Taussig anastomosis, which is an anastomosis between the subclavian and the ipsilateral pulmonary artery. It is performed on the site opposite the aortic arch. An alternative method is the interposition of

a graft between the underside of the proximal subclavian artery and the pulmonary artery (Fig. 5-14).

2. Waterston shunt, which is a side-to-side anastomosis of the ascending aorta to the right pulmonary artery.

3. Potts shunt is a side-to-side anastomosis between the descending aorta and the left pulmonary artery.

4. Central shunt is an interposed graft connecting the ascending aorta to the main, right, or left pulmonary artery (see Fig. 5-14).

5. Glenn shunt, which is an end-to-side anastomosis between the superior vena cava and ipsilateral pulmonary artery (Fig. 5-15).

Angiographic Features

1. Stenosis of the anastomosis.
2. Stenosis of the subclavian or the pulmonary artery near the site of the anastomosis.
3. Distortion, occlusion, stenosis, tethering of the pulmonary artery at the anastomosis. Distortion and/or

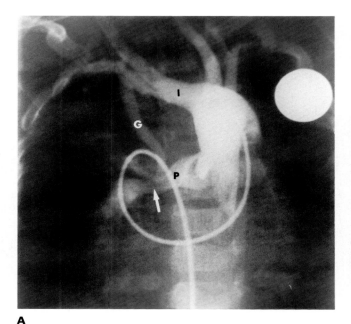

A

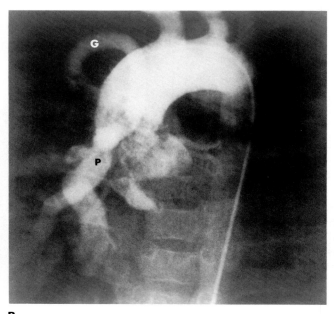

B

Figure 5-14. Anteroposterior view of injection into the ascending aorta. *A:* A graft connecting the right subclavian to the right pulmonary artery is demonstrated. Note the stenosis (*arrow*) of the right pulmonary artery at the site of the anastomosis. *B:* Anteroposterior view after injection into the ascending aorta. There is a redundant graft connecting the ascending aorta to the right pulmonary artery. (I, innominate artery; G, graft; P, right pulmonary artery.)

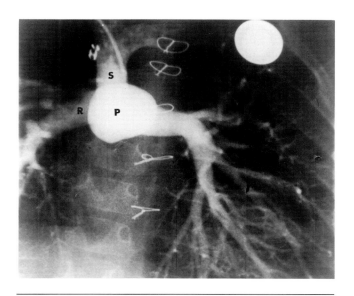

Figure 5-15. Anteroposterior view after injection of contrast medium into the superior vena cava. Anastomosis from the superior vena cava to the right pulmonary artery (Glenn procedure) is demonstrated. (P, pulmonary artery; R, right pulmonary artery; S, superior vena cava.)

stenosis of the proximal right pulmonary artery is common after the Waterston shunt.

4. Enlargement with or without reduced function of the left ventricle due to volume overload caused by a large shunt.

5. Hypoplasia of one lung, which receives little of the shunt flow owing to a stenosis between the shunt and the contralateral pulmonary circulation.

6. Pulmonary arteriolopathy of the ipsilateral lung due to excessive pulmonary blood flow caused by a large shunt. This is infrequent with the Blalock–Taussig shunt, but not uncommon with the Waterston and Potts shunts.

Variants of Tetralogy of Fallot

There are two important variant forms of tetralogy: absent pulmonary valve, and pulmonary atresia with ventricular septal defect. Absent pulmonary valve is usually associated with a ventricular septal defect and dextroposed aorta.[16] In this anomaly, the annulus is small and contains no formed valve tissue; consequently, pulmonary stenosis and regurgitation are present. It is accompanied by aneurysmal dilatation of the main and one or more of the central pulmonary arteries, usually at least the right pulmonary artery (Fig. 5-16). There is usually abrupt narrowing of the pulmonary arteries beyond the hila. Although there is malalignment of the infundibular septum, the right ventricular outlet region may be larger than typically encountered in tetralogy owing to the pulmonic regurgitation. The features of tetralogy exist in about 75% of patients with an absent pulmonary valve. It rarely (< 5%) exists as an isolated anomaly and may co-

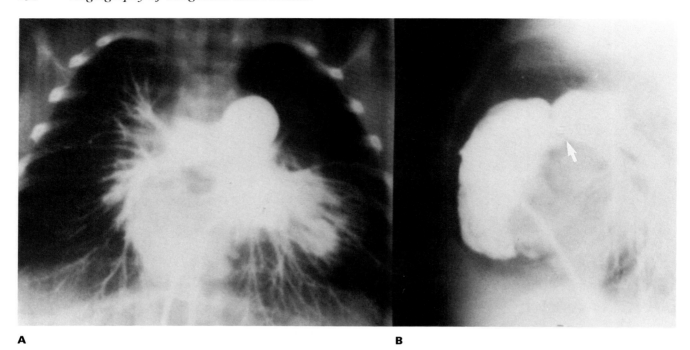

A   **B**

Figure 5-16. Anteroposterior (*A*) and lateral (*B*) views after injection into the right ventricle in a patient with absence of the pulmonary valve and ventricular septal defect. There is aneurysmal dilatation of the main pulmonary artery and very narrow caliber interparenchymal pulmonary arteries. No valve tissue is recognized at the level of the pulmonary annulus (*arrow*).

exist with other congenital defects. The ductus arteriosus may be absent.

The aneurysmal pulmonary arteries cause bronchial compression and respiratory distress, severe atelectasis, and recurrent or persistent pneumonia. Compression of the distal trachea and right bronchus is the most common situation. During the neonatal period the respiratory complications are preeminent and frequently cause death in early infancy.

Salient angiographic features of tetralogy of Fallot with absent pulmonary valve are:

1. Small pulmonary valve annulus (see Fig. 5-16). Valve tissue is not observed in the annulus.

2. Jet of contrast across the annulus, indicating stenosis.

3. Severe pulmonary regurgitation.

4. Aneurysmal dilatation of the main, left and/or right pulmonary artery (see Fig. 5-16). The status of the pulmonary arteries is displayed optimally in the cranially (sitting up) anteroposterior view. The compression of the distal trachea and bronchi (most frequently the right bronchus) is shown on the lateral view.

5. Other features of tetralogy of Fallot.

Pulmonary Atresia with Ventricular Septal Defect

The atresia may exist only at the valve level as a membranous obstruction or may involve a part or the entire length of the main pulmonary artery, including the bifurcation.[17] The infundibular portion of the right ventricle is present, although it is usually hypoplastic. The malalignment of the infundibular septum is severe.

There is generally an inverse relationship between the various potential sources of blood to the intraparenchymal pulmonary arteries (embryonic pulmonary plexus). If the aortopulmonary connections are prominent, then the central pulmonary arteries are usually very small or nonexistent, and a ductus arteriosus is absent.

Goals of angiographic imaging are:

1. Demonstrate atresia of the pulmonary valve.

2. Demonstrate the length of the atresia.

3. Identify the main pulmonary artery or a central confluence of the right and left branches if it exists.

4. Demonstrate the size of the central and distal pulmonary arterial circulation.

5. Demonstrate the systemic collaterals to the lungs.

6. Identify the hypoplastic right ventricular infundibulum, ventricular septal defect(s), and the other features of tetralogy of Fallot.

Optimal views and injection sites are:

1. Those described for tetralogy of Fallot.

2. Cranial (sit-up) anteroposterior view with injection into the descending aorta or with injection into large aortopulmonary collateral arteries is essential to dem-

onstrate the right and left pulmonary arteries and disclose a central confluence. Injection of a ductus arteriosus, if present, also demonstrates the central pulmonary arteries.

3. Wedge injection into a pulmonary vein may be needed to demonstrate the central pulmonary artery(ies).

Salient angiographic features are:

1. Those described for tetralogy of Fallot.

2. Severely hypoplastic infundibulum. Since it is so small, it may not be readily recognized but can usually be identified at the base of the right ventricle on the lateral and anteroposterior or RAO view of a right ventriculogram.

3. A ductus arteriosus, if present, connects the undersurface of the aorta to the proximal left pulmonary artery in the presence of a left aortic arch. The ductus arises from the undersurface of the arch, courses vertically, and is longer and sometimes tortuous in the presence of pulmonary atresia and severe pulmonary stenosis (tetralogy). In the presence of a right arch, the ductus arises from the proximal portion of the left innominate artery. Bilateral ducts can be present, with both providing origins for an ipsilateral pulmonary artery.

4. The aortopulmonary collateral usually arises from the proximal or mid-descending aorta at the level of or just below the carina (Figs. 5-17, 5-18). There is generally a reciprocal relationship between the size of the aortopulmonary collateral arteries and the central pulmonary arteries. These collaterals are large in the absence of a patent ductus arteriosus.

5. The distribution of aortopulmonary collaterals to the pulmonary segments is usually quite unequal. Some pulmonary segments may have dual arterial supply from both central pulmonary arteries and aortopulmonary collateral arteries.

6. Confluence of the central pulmonary arteries causes a "seagull" configuration on the sit-up anteroposterior view (see Fig. 5-17). The sit-up view displaces this central confluence cranial to the aortopulmonary collaterals. This view eliminates the overlap of the two vascular segments generally present in the standard anteroposterior view.

Pulmonary Atresia with Intact Ventricular Septum

Pulmonary atresia with intact ventricular septum is associated with a variably sized right ventricle and tricuspid valve annulus.[18,19] At one extreme is a severely hypoplastic right ventricle with a small annulus and tricuspid stenosis, and at the other end is a substantially enlarged right ventricle and enormous right atrium with profound tricuspid regurgitation. The overall heart size and right atrial size is related to the severity of tricuspid regurgitation. The atresia can be isolated to the valve level or involve the infundibulum as well. There are nearly always normal (concordant) atrioventricular and arterioventricular connections. An interatrial communication is nearly always present.

The right ventricle is small in about 70% of patients. The small chamber and large myocardial sinusoid indicates the inadequate cavitation of the right ventricle. The hypoplastic right ventricles contain a stenotic tricuspid valve and annulus. Persistent communications between the chamber and myocardial sinusoids of the right ventricular wall conduct blood retrograde into the coronary arteries.

In the neonate, pulmonary blood flow depends on a patent ductus arteriosus and is augmented by aortopulmonary collaterals. The pulmonary arterial circulation above the level of the pulmonary valve is generally free of atretic or stenotic segments.

Functional pulmonary atresia is a condition of the neonate in which blood does not flow across the pulmonic valve because of severe tricuspid regurgitation (Ebstein's anomaly, dysplasia of the tricuspid valve, transient tricuspid regurgitation of the neonate), or maldevelopment of the right ventricle (Uhl's anomaly).[20] This condition can be misdiagnosed as pulmonary atresia from a right ventriculogram that shows no opacification of the pulmonary artery.

Goals of angiographic imaging are:

1. Identify the presence and length of the pulmonary atresia.

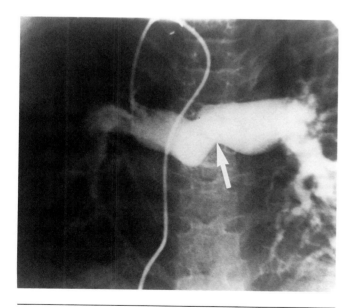

Figure 5-17. Injection into the right pulmonary artery through a catheter that has been placed across a right subclavian to right pulmonary artery shunt. The injection demonstrates right and left pulmonary arteries of adequate caliber in a patient with pulmonary atresia. Note that there is confluence between the right and left pulmonary arteries with a mild stenosis at the point of confluence (*arrow*). There is no filling of the proximal portion of the main pulmonary artery.

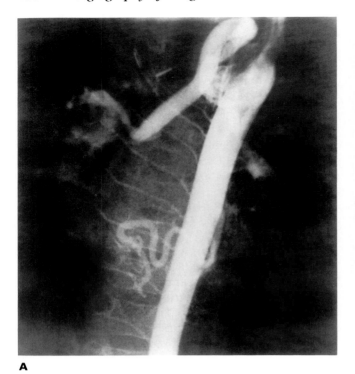

A

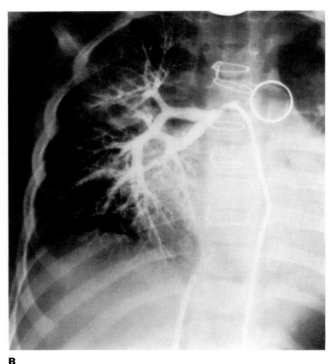

B

Figure 5-18. Injection into the descending aorta in a patient with pulmonary atresia. *A:* Contrast medium opacifies a large, tortuous bronchial artery. The bronchial artery courses toward the right hilum. *B:* Selective injection of a large right bronchial artery arising from the descending aorta. This bronchial artery provides considerable blood to the right lung. Note the multiple branches supplying both the upper and lower portions of the right lung.

2. Demonstrate the sources of blood supply to the lungs and the size of the pulmonary arteries.

3. Demonstrate the size of the right ventricle.

4. Identify the size of the tricuspid valve and annulus.

5. Define the presence and extent of right ventricular–sinusoidal fistulous communications with the coronary arteries.

Optimal views and injection sites are:

1. Anteroposterior and lateral views with injection into the right ventricle. A small volume of contrast media must be used for the hypoplastic ventricle; injection of excess volumes of contrast media into a hypoplastic ventricle has caused death ("suicide right ventricle").

2. Anteroposterior or sitting-up anteroposterior and lateral views with injection into the ascending or descending aorta.

3. Injection into the left brachiocephalic vein is indicated to exclude a left superior vena cava in patients in whom a Fontan procedure is being considered.

Salient angiographic features are:

1. Atresia isolated to the valve level is indicated by opacification of the infundibulum and doming of atretic valve tissue (Fig. 5-19).

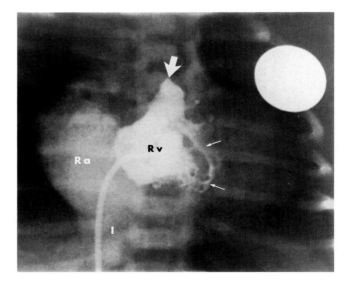

Figure 5-19. Anteroposterior view of injection into a hypoplastic right ventricle in a patient with pulmonary atresia. The injection demonstrates the blindly ending right ventricular outflow region (*arrow*) and severe tricuspid regurgitation, which outlines a substantially dilated right atrium and inferior vena cava. There is also flow of contrast from the right ventricle into the myocardial sinusoids (*small arrows*). (Ra, right atrium; Rv, right ventricle; I, inferior vena cava.)

2. Lack of opacification of the infundibulum or opacification of an attenuated infundibulum suggests a long segment of atresia.

3. Hypoplastic right ventricle with small tricuspid annulus and stenotic tricuspid valve is observed in the majority of cases (see Fig. 5-20). A restricted jet and doming of the valve are shown in diastole. Usually, there is only mild regurgitation, or none, in this type of ventricle.

4. Enlarged right ventricle with tricuspid regurgitation is found in the minority of cases. Tricuspid regurgitation may be profound, causing a gigantic right atrium (Fig. 5-20).

5. Right-to-left shunting across an interatrial communication.

6. Injection into the thoracic aorta usually demonstrates a patent ductus arteriosus in the neonate. The ductus is kept patent by the infusion of prostaglandin E. Aortopulmonary collateral or a surgically created shunt may be visible.

7. A plexus of myocardial sinusoids is evident in association with hypoplastic right ventricle. Contrast medium passes from the sinusoids and fills the coronary arteries (see Fig. 5-20). The major branches of the coronary arteries opacify retrograde from the right ventricular injection; contrast media may even flow retrograde as far as the sinuses of Valsalva. Dense retrograde opacification of the coronary arteries in this fashion without flow continuing into the aorta raises the question of absence of a proximal connection to the aorta, which occurs in some patients with pulmonary atresia.

8. The exclusion of functional pulmonary atresia (lack of antegrade flow across a patent valve due to severe tricuspid regurgitation) may be accomplished by demonstrating pulmonic regurgitation, which is usually present in this condition. The pulmonary artery can be opacified by aortography if a patent ductus arteriosus exists.

Tricuspid Atresia

Tricuspid atresia exists as a muscular or membranous barrier between the right atrium and right ventricle.[21,22] An imperforate but formed tricuspid valve is one type of membranous atresia. Tricuspid atresia exists in both situs solitus and inversus, as well as with D- or L-ventricular loops. There is almost invariably an interatrial communication, either a patent foramen ovale or an atrial septal defect. About 70% of patients with tricuspid atresia have normal arterioventricular connections; most of the re-

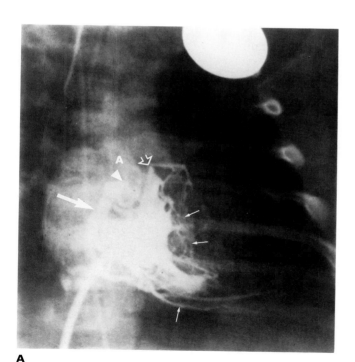
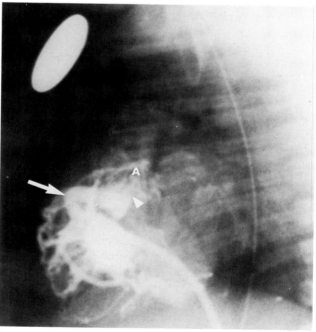

A   **B**

Figure 5-20. Anteroposterior (*A*) and lateral (*B*) views after injection into the right ventricle in a patient with pulmonary atresia with an intact ventricular septum. Contrast medium outlines the severely hypoplastic right ventricle. Contrast medium has flowed retrograde through myocardial sinusoids and coronary arterial branches (*small arrow*), and outlines the right coronary artery (*arrow*). Retrograde flow in the right coronary artery produces faint opacification of the ascending aorta (A). Note the connection of the dilated right coronary artery with the ascending aorta (*arrowhead*). The blindly ending right ventricular outflow region is demonstrated (*open arrow*).

mainder have transposition of the great arteries. Pulmonary stenosis or atresia is frequently associated with tricuspid atresia.

The majority of patients with normal arterioventricular connections have some degree of pulmonary stenosis or atresia. Obstruction to pulmonary blood flow can exist at the site of the ventricular septal defect (bulboventricular foramen), infundibular, or pulmonary valvular levels. A minority of patients with normal arterioventricular connections have excess pulmonary blood flow due to a nonrestrictive VSD. In patients with abnormal arterioventricular connections (usually transposition), there may also be pulmonary stenosis. In transposition with tricuspid atresia, blood flows to the aorta through the bulboventricular foramen. If the foramen has a diameter less than the diameter of the aortic annulus, then the foramen is flow restrictive and in effect produces subaortic stenosis. Progressive narrowing of this foramen can occur, and acquired narrowing may be accelerated by left ventricular hypertrophy induced by pulmonary arterial banding.

Goals of angiographic imaging are:

1. Identification of tricuspid atresia.
2. Determination of arterioventricular connections.
3. Determination of the relative size of the bulboventricular foramen.
4. Identification of pulmonic stenosis or atresia.
5. Determination of sources of blood flow to the lungs.
6. Determination of the size of the interatrial communications.
7. Identification of associated anomalies.
8. Exclusion of a left superior vena cava (this is essential when a Fontan procedure is being considered).

Optimal views and injection sites are:

1. Four-chamber view or anteroposterior view with injection into right atrium or superior vena cava.
2. Long axial oblique view with injection into the left ventricle.
3. Anteroposterior or sit-up anteroposterior view and lateral view with injection into the right ventricular outlet chamber.
4. Anteroposterior view with injection into the left brachiocephalic vein. This is done to exclude a left superior vena cava when a Fontan procedure is being considered.

Salient angiographic features are:

1. Injection into the right atrium produces prominent reflux into the inferior vena cava and hepatic vein but no flow of contrast across the tricuspid valve. The flow of contrast is right atrium → left atrium → left ventricle → right ventricular outlet region.

2. In the anteroposterior view, the opacification of the right atrium, left atrium, and left ventricle produces a nonopacified triangular bare area.

3. Injection into the left ventricle in the long axial oblique or four-chamber view demonstrates the ventricular septal defect. The size of the defect can be compared with the annulus of the artery arising from the right ventricle in order to determine whether the defect is obstructive.

4. In the presence of normal arterioventricular connections, obstruction of pulmonary blood flow is frequently recognized at the subvalvular or valvular levels (pulmonary valve).

5. Right ventricular size is small due to inadequate development of the inlet portion of the right ventricle. No "wash in" of unopacified blood is observed in the region of the tricuspid valve when the right ventricle is opacified by flow across the ventricular septal defect.

6. The atrial septal defect is visualized in the four-chamber view. As the right atrium opacifies the left atrium through a high defect, a "waterfall" appearance may be produced.

7. Abnormal arterioventricular connection is evident in 30% of cases. This is usually transposition of the great arteries, but double-outlet left or right ventricle or truncus arteriosus is present rarely.

Ebstein's Anomaly

This anomaly involves displacement of the attachment of the tricuspid leaflet from the annulus into the inlet region of the right ventricle.[23,24] The normal right ventricle is tripartite, consisting of inlet, trabecular (apical), and outlet regions. In this anomaly the tricuspid leaflets are attached at the junction of the inlet and trabecular portions and the inlet myocardium is thinned so that it resembles the musculature of the right atrium (atrialization of the right ventricle). The abnormal attachments of the leaflets cause tricuspid stenosis and/or regurgitation. The anomaly can occur on the left side of the heart in corrected transposition (l-transposition) and causes functional mitral regurgitation (regurgitation into the left atrium).

A secundum atrial septal defect or stretched foramen ovale is usually, but not invariably, present. Other anomalies can be associated with this lesion, including pulmonary stenosis, pulmonary atresia, and tetralogy of Fallot.

The degree of displacement of the leaflets into the right ventricle is highly variable. The septal and posterior leaflets are involved in the anomaly and are attached to the right ventricular wall to a varying degree. The anterior leaflet most often is attached normally, but is malformed. The attachment of this leaflet by abnormal chordae or through a continuous attachment to a papillary muscle can severely restrict flow or produce an imperforate atrioventricular orifice.

Goals of angiographic imaging are:

1. Identify the displacement of the attachment of the tricuspid valve leaflets.

2. Determine the severity of tricuspid regurgitation and stenosis.

3. Define the extent of atrialization of the right ventricle.

4. Identify an interatrial communication.

5. Exclude associated anomalies.

Optimal views and injection sites are:

1. Anteroposterior and lateral views with injection into the right ventricle.

2. Anteroposterior and lateral views with injection into the right atrium.

Salient angiographic features are:

1. The tricuspid valve annulus can be recognized as an indentation on the inferior surface of the heart located between the right atrium and right ventricle (Fig. 5-21). The tricuspid leaflets are displaced away from the annu-

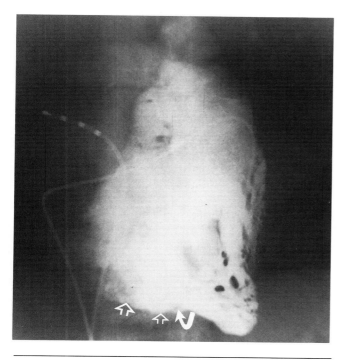

Figure 5-21. Anteroposterior view of a right ventriculogram in a patient with Ebstein's anomaly. Contrast medium outlines the markedly dilated right ventricle. Note the normal trabecular pattern of the apical portion and outlet portion of the right ventricle, but complete absence of trabeculation in the inlet portion (*open arrows*). This is the atrialized portion of the right ventricle (*open arrows*). The site of insertion of one of the leaflets of the tricuspid valve is visualized (*curved arrow*). The outlet portion of the right ventricle is dilated.

lus and lie within the right ventricle. The anterior leaflet usually appears as a curvilinear lucency within the right ventricle. A tricuspid leaflet may produce a second notch on the inferior surface.

2. The tricuspid valve may be difficult to identify fully owing to adherence of the posterior and septal leaflets to the right ventricular wall.

3. The inlet portion of the right ventricle lacks normal trabeculation (see Fig. 5-21) and displays akinesis or dyskinesis during systole. The systolic motion of the segment is disparate to the remainder of the right ventricle.

4. Tricuspid regurgitation, usually severe, is demonstrated on the right ventriculogram.

5. Dilatation and prominent diastolic expansion of the outlet portion of the right ventricle are frequently observed.

6. The tricuspid orifice may be restricted or consist of several fenestrations, indicating tricuspid stenosis.

7. Marked right atrial enlargement.

8. Right-to-left shunting at the atrial level.

9. In the infant with elevated pulmonary vascular resistance and severe tricuspid regurgitation caused by Ebstein's anomaly, there may be no antegrade flow across the tricuspid valve. This can cause pulmonary atresia to be erroneously diagnosed (pseudopulmonary atresia or functional pulmonary atresia).

Tricuspid Valve Dysplasia

This anomaly involves stunted development of the tricuspid leaflet. The leaflets are thickened and nodular and do not close the tricuspid orifice in diastole. There is frequently severe tricuspid regurgitation in the newborn, causing an enormously enlarged right atrium and cardiac contour. Ischemia of the right ventricular papillary muscle caused by severe pulmonary hypertension, such as occurs with persistent fetal circulation, can cause severe tricuspid regurgitation in the newborn and mimic this lesion (transient tricuspid regurgitation of the newborn).

Optimal views and injection sites are the same as those used for Ebstein's anomaly.

Salient angiographic features are:

1. Severe tricuspid regurgitation with normal attachments of the tricuspid valve.

2. Dilated right ventricle but normal trabeculation of the inlet portion.

Straddling Tricuspid Valve

Straddling tricuspid valve is characterized by the attachment of chordae of the tricuspid valve to both ventricles.[25] This entity is subtly distinguished from the overriding tricuspid valve, in which the annulus overrides the inlet septum but the chordae are attached only within the right ventricle. In both conditions, right atrial blood flows into both ventricles. Straddling tricuspid valve usually causes a relatively small right ventricle. It is always associated with an inlet ventricular septal defect. It can occur with an inlet VSD alone but is usually associated with abnormal atrioventricular connections. This anomaly occurs with atrioventricular discordance, criss-cross atrioventricular relations, and univentricular hearts.

Optimal views and injection sites are:

1. Four-chamber view with injection into the right atrium.

2. Four-chamber view with injection into the left ventricle.

Salient angiographic features are:

1. The lesion should be suspected in any case in which an inlet ventricular septal defect is associated with a small right ventricle.

2. Right atrial injection in the four-chamber view shows two streams of contrast medium flowing into the right and left ventricles.

3. Left ventriculography in the four-chamber view or long axial oblique view displays the tricuspid orifice straddling the ventricular septum, and unopacified blood enters the left ventricle through this orifice during diastole.

Complete Transposition of the Great Arteries

The aorta originates from the right ventricle, and the pulmonary artery arises posteriorly from the left ventricle.[26,27] In complete transposition of the great arteries (TGA), the aortic valve is usually anterior and rightward in relation to the pulmonary valve but can infrequently be directly anterior or even anterior and leftward. About 60% to 70% of cases of TGA have no VSD and no obstruction to pulmonary blood flow. Aside from an obligatory interatrial communication, the most frequently associated lesions are VSD and valvular or subvalvular pulmonic stenosis. Less frequently, there is a patent ductus arteriosus.

Left ventricular outflow tract stenosis (obstruction of pulmonary blood flow) can occur at valvular and subvalvular levels.[27] It can be discrete or variable in length in the left ventricular outlet region. It may be caused by fibrous rings or tunnels, excess tissue from either atrioventricular valves bulging into the region, or displacement or hypertrophy of various portions of the ventricular septum.

Goals of angiographic imaging are:

1. Identification of atrioventricular connections.
2. Identification of arterioventricular connections.

3. Identification of atrioventricular valves and their attachment to one or both ventricles.

4. Evaluation of left ventricular outlet obstruction.

5. Identification of the presence and site of ventricular septal defect(s).

6. Determination of whether two fully developed ventricles are present.

7. Definition of coronary arterial anatomy.

8. Identification of associated anomalies.

Optimal views and injection sites are:

1. Anteroposterior and lateral view with injection into the right ventricle.

2. Anteroposterior and lateral view with injection into the ascending aorta.

3. Long axial oblique view with injection into the left ventricle.

Salient angiographic features are:

1. Arterioventricular discordance (complete transposition) is evident by right ventricular origin of the aorta and left ventricular origin of the pulmonary artery (Fig. 5-22A). The right ventriculogram displays an infundibulum beneath the aortic valve, separating it from the tricuspid valve (Figs. 5-22B, 5-23). The left ventriculogram depicts the pulmonary–mitral valve continuity.

2. The aorta is located anterior and to the right of the pulmonary artery in most cases (d-transposition). It is located directly anterior (a-transposition) or anterior and to the left of the pulmonary artery (l-transposition) in the minority.

3. In situs solitus the ventricular loop is D (right ventricle is located rightward in relation to the left ventricle). The left ventricle is identified by a posterior position and no infundibulum, whereas the right ventricle is located anteriorly and has an infundibulum. Rarely, the relationship is severely distorted, with ventricles positioned superior–inferior in relationship to one another; this occurs usually in criss-cross atrioventricular relationships.

4. Left ventriculogram in the long axial oblique view shows the obstruction to the left ventricular outlet region (see Fig. 5-22B). This may consist of valvular or subvalvular stenosis. There may be diffuse narrowing of the outlet region or a discrete subpulmonic membrane, causing a thin transverse lucency in the outlet or a fibromuscular ring, causing a discrete thick (hourglass) narrowing. Irregular lobulated filling defects in the outlet region can be caused by extravalvular tissue extending either from the atrioventricular valve or from an aneurysm of the membranous septum. The anterior septum may be asymmetrically hypertrophied and bulge into the outlet region, where further narrowing occurs in systole because of systolic anterior motion of the anterior leaflet of the mitral valve.

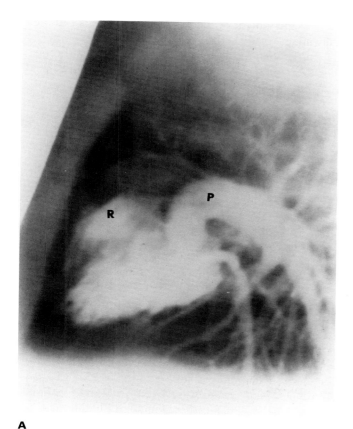

A

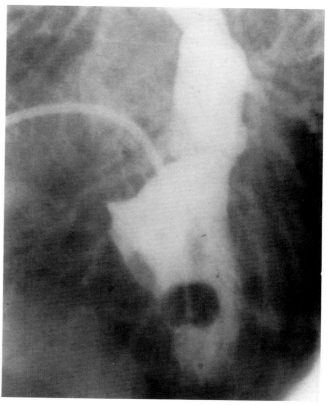

B

Figure 5-22. Transposition of the great arteries. *A:* Lateral view of an injection into the left ventricle in a patient with transposition of the great arteries. Note the opacification of the right ventricle (R) through a ventricular septal defect. The pulmonary artery (P) arises posteriorly from the left ventricle. *B:* Caudal RAO view of an injection into the left ventricle in another patient with transposition of the great arteries. Note the direct continuity between the mitral valve and the pulmonic valve. The pulmonic artery arising from the left ventricle indicates transposition of the great arteries.

5. The presence and location(s) of VSDs is shown by selective right and left ventriculograms (see Fig. 5-22A). Because of reversal in pressure relationships, the defect may be displayed better, or only, during right ventriculography. Most VSDs in TGA involve the perimembranous septum or outlet (infundibular) septum.

6. Aortography demonstrates the origin of the coronary arteries from the posterolateral aspects of the base of the aorta; the two orifices are situated nearly across from each other. The anterior sinus is the noncoronary sinus in TGA. This is a reversal of the normal relationship, in which the posterior sinus is the noncoronary one.

7. In corrected transposition,[28] the aorta is positioned anterior and to the left of the pulmonary artery. The right ventricle is situated to the left of the left ventricle (L-ventricular loop). Pulmonary stenosis and VSD and Ebstein's anomaly of the left-sided atrioventricular valve are associated lesions that can be demonstrated by ventriculography.

Double-Outlet Right Ventricle

Double-outlet right ventricle (DORV) includes a spectrum of lesions in which both great arteries arise from the right ventricle.[29,30] The angiographic criterion for this diagnosis has been variable among investigators. The most frequently applied criterion is the presence of infundibula beneath both great arteries, causing absence of semilunar–atrioventricular valve continuity. An alternate angiographic criterion is the origin of one great artery completely from the right ventricle and predominant (> 50%) origin of the other great artery from the right ventricle, with no concern for semilunar–atrioventricular continuity. This latter definition has been slightly differently stated as the origin of more than half of each great artery from the right ventricle.

VSDs exist with DORV. The type of DORV is defined by the position of the VSD in relation to the great arteries.[30] The locations of the VSD are (1) subaortic—beneath

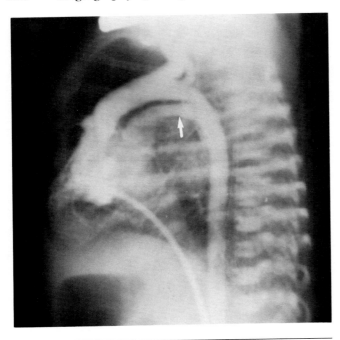

Figure 5-23. Lateral view of right ventricular injection in a patient with transposition of the great arteries. The aorta originates from the right ventricle. Note that the aorta is located anteriorly and occupies an abnormally cranial position. This indicates transposition of the great arteries. A patent ductus arteriosus is evident (*arrow*).

the aortic valve; (2) subpulmonic—beneath the pulmonic valve; (3) doubly committed—beneath both great arteries; and (4) noncommitted or remote from both great arteries. The great arteries can be oriented to each other in any of four ways: aorta to the right and posterior to the pulmonary artery; aorta and pulmonary artery side by side with the aorta to the right; aorta to the right and anteriorly; aorta to the left and anteriorly.

Pulmonary stenosis, usually both infundibular and valvular, occurs in DORV, especially the form with subaortic VSD. Coarctation or interruption of the aortic arch is also associated with DORV, especially the type with subpulmonic VSD (Taussig–Bing malformation).

A right aortic arch has been reported in 12% to 20% of patients with DORV. It usually occurs in DORV with subaortic VSD and pulmonic stenosis. Abnormalities of the mitral valve occur in DORV; these include overriding or straddling mitral valve, mitral atresia, and double-inlet ventricle.

Goals of angiographic imaging are:

1. Identification of the presence of DORV.
2. Determination of the site of VSD in relation to the origin of each great artery.
3. Identification and assessment of severity of pulmonic stenosis.
4. Identification of anomalies of the aorta, especially right aortic arch, coarctation, or interruption of the aorta.

5. Assessment of the location and status of the mitral valve.
6. Definition of the size and function of the ventricles.

Optimal views and injection sites are:

1. Long axial oblique view with injection into the left ventricle.
2. Anteroposterior and lateral views with injection into the right ventricle.
3. Long axial oblique view or anteroposterior and lateral views with injection into the ascending aorta.

Salient angiographic features are:

1. Demonstration of the origin of more than half of each great artery from the right ventricle. Imaging of the ventricular septum in profile provides spatial separation of the two ventricles, which enables the determination of the site of origin of the great arteries from the right ventricle (Fig. 5-24). Usually, one great artery arises entirely from the right ventricle while more than 50% of the annulus of the other artery lies to the right of the ventricular septum. Alignment of the septum in profile can usually be achieved optimally with the long axial oblique view. It may be difficult to angiographically differentiate between DORV with subaortic VSD and pulmonic stenosis from tetralogy of Fallot.

2. On right ventriculography in the anteroposterior and lateral views, the two semilunar valves lie at the same caudocranial level and infundibula exist beneath both valves (Fig. 5-25). However, in some cases the length of the infundibula are not equal, so one great artery is situated at a higher level than the others.

3. Infundibular septum separates the origin of the two great arteries. This is shown on the right ventriculogram (see Fig. 5-25).

4. The relationship of the great arteries is characteristically side by side, with the aorta to the right. However, either artery may be more anterior and either may lie to the right or left.

5. The relationship of the VSD to the origin of the great arteries is shown on the long axial oblique view (Fig. 5-24). Side by side relationship of the great arteries is usually associated with subaortic VSD. This occurs in about 50% of patients with DORV. Anterior orientation of the aorta is associated with subpulmonic or subaortic VSD. This type occurs in 35% of cases.

6. Valvular or infundibular pulmonic stenosis is demonstrated using the anteroposterior and lateral right ventriculogram. In patients with pulmonary atresia, the site of the infundibulum in relationship to the ventricular septum must be determined to establish the diagnosis of DORV.

7. Hypoplasia of the left ventricle in the presence of DORV should suggest the possibility of associated mi-

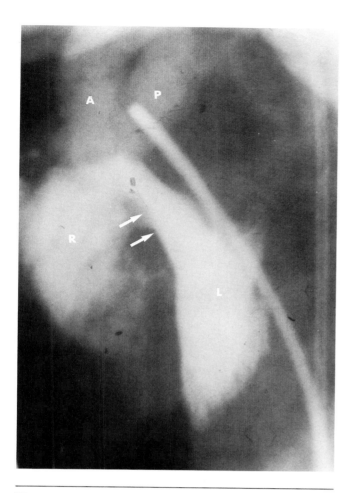

Figure 5-24. Cranial LAO view of an injection into the left ventricle in a patient with double-outlet right ventricle. Both the aorta (A) and the pulmonary artery (P) are connected to the right ventricle (R). A ventricular septal defect (*arrows*) connects the left ventricle to the right ventricle (L) and the great vessels.

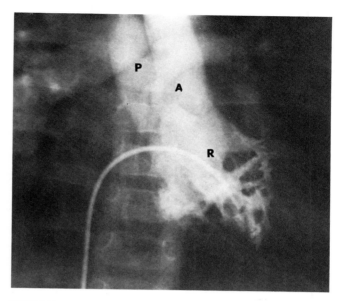

Figure 5-25. Anteroposterior view of an injection into the right ventricle in a patient with double outlet right ventricle. The injection into the right ventricle (R) demonstrates that the aorta (A) and pulmonary artery (P) are at approximately the same craniocaudal level and both are immediately and almost equally opacified during the right ventricular injection. The catheter has passed from the inferior vena cava to the right atrium across the tricuspid valve and into the right ventricle.

tral stenosis, mitral atresia, or straddling of the mitral valve.

8. Coarctation or interruption of the aorta. These occur usually with DORV with subpulmonic VSD and reflect the decreased aortic blood flow during embryonic life. Blood from the left ventricle preferentially flows into the pulmonary artery because of the subpulmonic location of the VSD.

9. Equivalent oxygen saturation of blood from the aorta and pulmonary artery is a feature of some cases of DORV.

10. The origin of the coronary arteries can be characteristic for DORV. The noncoronary sinus is generally the one farthest from the pulmonary artery. So in DORV with side-by-side orientation of the great arteries (the most common type), the noncoronary sinus is the right sinus of Valsalva when the aorta is rightward from the pulmonary artery.

Double-Outlet Left Ventricle

Double-outlet left ventricle (DOLV) is defined as origin of more than 50% of both great arteries from the left ventricle.[31] A VSD is nearly always present. This anomaly can exist with absence of an infundibulum, subaortic infundibulum, subpulmonic infundibulum, or bilateral infundibula. The aorta can lie anterior, rightward, or leftward to the pulmonary artery. The VSD is most frequently subaortic in DOLV. This type is frequently associated with pulmonic stenosis, and this form of DOLV mimics tetralogy of Fallot.

Optimal view and injection sites are the long axial oblique view with injection into the left ventricle. This view provides a profile view of the septum so that there is spatial separation of the two ventricles.

Salient angiographic features are:

1. Demonstration of more than 50% origin of each great artery from the left side of the ventricular septum in the long axial oblique view.

2. Demonstration of the presence and site of the VSD in relationship to the two semilunar valves.

Truncus Arteriosus

Truncus arteriosus is a single arterial trunk originating from the heart and providing origin for the coronary, pulmonary, and systemic arterial vessels.[32,33] Truncus arteriosus has only a single semilunar valve, whereas aortic and pulmonic atresia differ by the presence of a second atretic semilunar valve. An outlet ventricular septal defect is nearly always present owing to absence or severe underdevelopment of the infundibular septum. Two classifications of truncus arteriosus have been proposed. These are described in Chapter 2.

The truncal valve can exhibit a variable number of cusps: tricuspid in 50%, quadricuspid in 30%, bicuspid in 10%, others or indeterminate in 10%. The truncal valve is frequently insufficient but rarely stenotic. Stenoses of the main and/or branches of the pulmonary artery are common. Absence of one of the pulmonary arteries, usually the left, sometimes occurs.

A mirror-image right aortic arch is present in 35% to 40% of cases. Coarctation and arch interruption infrequently occur.

Goals of angiographic imaging are:

1. Demonstration of truncus ateriosus.

2. Definition of the presence of a main pulmonary artery or the site of origin of the right and left pulmonary arteries.

3. Identification of stenosis(es) of the origin of main or branch pulmonary arteries. Demonstration of the presence of both pulmonary arteries.

4. Demonstration of the presence, site, and size of the VSD.

5. Exclusion of multiple VSDs.

6. Identification and assessment of severity of truncal regurgitation.

Optimal views and injection sites are:

1. Anteroposterior and lateral views with injection into the truncus. This angiogram is critical for establishing the diagnosis of truncus arteriosus.

2. Long-axial oblique view with injection into the left ventricle.

Salient angiographic features are:

1. Single large arterial trunk arising above both ventricles (Fig. 5-26). The trunk supplies the pulmonary arteries, aorta, and coronary arteries.

2. Large VSD located immediately beneath the truncus.

3. Truncal regurgitation of variable severity. Regurgitation occurs into both ventricles.

4. Left ventricular enlargement due to volume overload of the left ventricle caused by left-to-right shunt and, in some cases, truncal regurgitation.

5. Stenoses at the site of origin of either or both pulmonary arteries may be demonstrated. This may be recognized by asymmetric opacification of the arteries of the two lungs.

6. Right aortic arch in some cases.

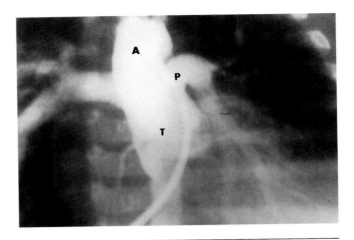

Figure 5-26. Anteroposterior view of an injection into the truncus in a patient with truncus arteriosus. Note the origin of the pulmonary arteries from the truncus arteriosus. Only a single semilunar valve (truncal valve) is demonstrated. (A, aorta; P, pulmonary artery; T, truncus.)

Aorticopulmonary Window

An aorticopulmonary window is a communication between the ascending aorta and the main pulmonary artery.[34] It differs from truncus arteriosus in that two separate semilunar valves are present. Associated lesions include ventricular septal defect, patent ductus arteriosus, and coarctation or interruption of the aorta.

Goals of angiographic imaging are:

1. Demonstration of two semilunar valves, which differentiates aorticopulmonary window from truncus arteriosus.

2. Exclusion of associated anomalies, such as patent ductus arteriosus.

Optimal views and site of injection are:

1. Anterorosterior and lateral view with injection into ascending aorta.

2. Long axial oblique view with injection into the left ventricle.

3. Anteroposterior or lateral view with injection into the proximal descending aorta.

Salient angiographic features are:

1. Connection between the ascending aorta and the main pulmonary artery. The connection is usually on the left side of the proximal ascending aorta. Opacification of the pulmonary arteries occurs before contrast appears in the proximal descending aorta. This finding differentiates the lesion from patent ductus arteriosus.

2. Demonstration of two semilunar valves. This finding is crucial for distinguishing this lesion from truncus arteriosus.

Total Anomalous Pulmonary Venous Connection

Total anomalous pulmonary venous connection (TAPVC) consists of all pulmonary veins connecting to some structure other than the left atrium.[35,36] Almost always there is an interarterial communication. The anomalous connection is divided among (1) supracardiac, (2) cardiac, (3) infracardiac, and (4) mixed sites of connection. Supracardiac connection is to the left innominate vein, right superior vena cava, or azygous vein. The left innominate vein is connected by a left vertical vein or left superior vena cava. Cardiac connection is to the coronary sinus or right atrium. Infracardiac connection is to the portal vein or one of its branches, ductus venosus, or inferior vena cava. In the mixed type, pulmonary veins drain to more than one site. TAPVC occurs as an isolated anomaly in two-thirds of cases and in association with other anomalies in one third. In TAPVC of any type, there is frequently a horizontal vein that connects the right- and left-sided veins and lies directly behind the left atrium.

TAPVC may be associated with obstruction to pulmonary venous drainage. This is nearly always true of the infracardiac type and sometimes occurs with the supracardiac type. Obstruction may be due to intrinsic stenosis or extrinsic compression of the anomalously connecting venous structure.

Goals of angiographic imaging are:

1. Identification of the site of drainage of all four pulmonary veins.

2. Evaluation of the caliber of the connection(s) to systemic venous site and the caliber of anomalous connecting veins.

3. Determination of left atrial dimensions.

4. Exclusion of additional anomalies.

Optimal views and injection sites are:

1. Anteroposterior and lateral views with injection into the main pulmonary artery. Occlusive injection through a balloon catheter may facilitate visualization of pulmonary venous drainage. Selective injection of the right and left pulmonary arteries may improve visualization of the anomalous venous connections.

2. Anteroposterior and lateral views with injection into the anomalously connecting vein. Direct injection into the anomalous vein is usually the best way to demonstrate sites of obstruction along the anomalous pathway.

Salient angiographic features are:

1. Supracardiac type is characterized by a horizontal vein that connects the right and left pulmonary veins. This is situated behind or above the left atrium. It is opacified during the levo-phase after injection into the pulmonary artery. This vein connects to a vertical vein or left superior vena cava, which is attached to the left innomi-

nate view. The sequence of opacification is confluence of pulmonary vein (horizontal vein) to the vertical vein to the right superior vena cava to the right atrium (Fig. 5-27).

Stenosis occurs usually at the connection of the vertical vein to the left innominate vein. Extrinsic compression can also occur when the vertical vein courses between the left bronchus and the left pulmonary vein, resulting in a viselike compression by the two structures. When the vein courses anterior to the left bronchus, this mechanism of obstruction does not occur. Supracardiac connection may less frequently be shown as a common vein connecting to the right superior vena cava or azygous vein.

2. Cardiac type is characterized by a confluence of pulmonary veins behind the right atrium with direct connection usually to the posterior or superior wall of the right atrium. The other site of drainage by a common connecting vein is the coronary sinus. In the latter case, the levo-phase shows early and dense opacification of a dilated coronary sinus. The coronary sinus is recognized as a circular structure located to the left of the spine and just above the diaphragm on the frontal view. Drainage into the right atrium is suggested by early opacification of that atrium.

3. Infracardiac type is characterized by confluence of pulmonary veins behind the atria with connection to a descending vertical vein that courses through the diaphragm and connects to the portal venous, ductus venosus, or inferior vena cava. Because obstruction is nearly always present with this type, the opacification of these structures may be delayed and not very dense. The site of obstruction may be at the junction of the connecting vein to the abdominal systemic vein. The obstruction has

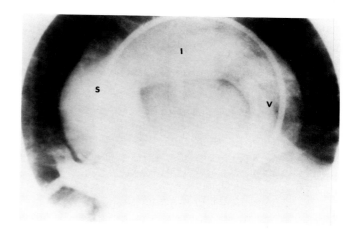

Figure 5-27. Anteroposterior view after injection into the vertical vein in a patient with the supracardiac type of total anomalous pulmonary venous connection. This injection demonstrates the vertical vein connecting with a markedly dilated left innominate vein, which connects to the markedly dilated superior vena cava. (I, left innominate vein; S, left superior vena cava; V, vertical vein.)

also been alleged to be due to drainage of blood through the portal venous bed. Closure of the ductus venosus during early postnatal life can also obstruct drainage when drainage is into this structure.

Single Ventricle (Univentricular Heart)

Controversy surrounds the nomenclature of this entity, but this controversy will not be addressed here. This section will consider one system of nomenclature, which is useful in understanding the angiographic features. The angiographic features have been described in detail.[37,38] Single ventricle is the anomaly in which only a single complete ventricle is present and the other ventricle, or a major portion of it, is absent. The completely formed dominant ventricle receives both atrioventricular valves or a single valve if one is atretic or a common atrioventricular valve exists. Therefore, the incomplete ventricle does not have an atrioventricular valve, nor does it contain the vestige of an atretic atrioventricular valve.

Ventriculography displays three components in a ventricle (this structure is referred to as tripartite).[39] These are the inlet portion containing the atrioventricular valve, the apical portion, and the outlet portion. In single ventricle, the inlet portion of one of the ventricles is absent.

The types of single ventricle are:

1. Left ventricular type (about 70%). The dominant left ventricle is connected to a right ventricular outlet chamber through a VSD (bulboventricular foramen) of variable diameter. The outlet chamber is usually located directly anterior or anterior leftward (situs solitus) or anterior rightward (situs inversus).

2. Right ventricular type (about 20%). The dominant right ventricle is connected by a VSD to a dimunitive left ventricular chamber located posteriorly.

3. Primitive single ventricle (about 10%). The ventricle has indeterminate features and a second dimunitive chamber is not evident.

A single ventricular chamber due to nearly complete absence of the ventricular septum is called a common ventricle rather than a single ventricle. In this anomaly, all components of both ventricles are present and each receives an atrioventricular valve.

Although normally related great arteries occur in single ventricle, anomalies of arterioventricular connection are common. The usual associated anomaly is transposition of the great arteries.

Single ventricle is frequently an anomaly of a considerably malformed central cardiovascular system. Single ventricle (univentricular heart) is common in patients with asplenia and right atrial isomerism. Consequently, the description of the cardiac anatomy must be assidu-ously based upon a consideration of segmental connections and organ situs.

This requires a segmental approach to determine:

1. Types of situs: solitus, inversus, and ambiguous.
2. Atrioventricular connection: concordant or discordant.
3. Arterioventricular connection: concordant or discordant or double outlet. Concordant = origin of aorta from left ventricle. Discordant = origin of aorta from infundibular chamber (left ventricular type of single ventricle) or right ventricle (right ventricular type of single ventricle).
4. Position of the heart in the chest: mirror-image dextrocardia, isolated dextrocardia, mesocardia, levocardia.

These patients frequently have additional cardiac anomalies, most often:

1. Valvular or subvalvular pulmonic stenoses.
2. Atrial septal defects.
3. Anomalies of systemic veins (bilateral superior vena cava and interrupted inferior vena cava) and pulmonary venous connections.
4. Coarctation of the aorta. This occurs in single ventricle of the left ventricular type with transposition and a restrictive bulboventricular foramen.

The diameter of connection between the dominant and dimunitive ventricle is an important determinant of the hemodynamic impairment. The bulboventricular foramen connecting the dominant left ventricle and the infundibular chamber is sometimes restrictive initially or may progressively decrease in size relative to the orifice of the great artery arising from the infundibular chamber.[40] Since transposition is frequently present in this type of single ventricle, a restrictive foramen causes subaortic stenosis. The foramen is restrictive if its diameter is less than that of the aortic valve.

Goals of angiographic imaging are:

1. Identification of the type of single ventricle. This requires the recognition of ventricular morphology, which depends primarily upon the identification of an infundibulum (right ventricle).
2. Identification of the other dimunitive partial ventricle.
3. Determination of situs, atrioventricular connection, and arterioventricular connection.
4. Demonstration of the presence and connection of the atrioventricular valves.
5. Determination of the size of the ventricular septal defect (or bulboventricular foramen).
6. Definition of systemic and pulmonary venous connections.
7. Exclusion of valvular or subpulmonic or subaortic obstruction.

Optimal views and injection sites are:

1. Anteroposterior and lateral views with injection into dominant chamber.

2. Anteroposterior and lateral views with injection into the infundibular chamber in the left ventricular type of single ventricle.

3. Long axial oblique view with injection into the dominant ventricle.

4. A view perpendicular to the orientation of the bulboventricular foramen is needed to define its size.

Salient angiographic features are:

1. Single ventricle of the left ventricular type is characterized by a dominant ventricle with the morphology of a left ventricle (Fig. 5-28). This ventricle has semilunar–mitral valve continuity (lacks a conus) and usually a posterior location. The rudimentary right ventricular infundibulum is located directly anterior, anterior and leftward, or anterior and rightward in relation to the left ventricle. In this type of single ventricle, a discrete bulboventricular foramen is usually visualized. Transposition of the great arteries frequently occurs in this type of single ventricle; the aorta originates from the infundibular chamber (Fig. 5-28). Depending upon the position of the infundibular chamber, there is d-transposition (infundibular chamber anterior and rightward) or l-transposition (infundibular chamber anterior and leftward).

2. Single ventricle of the right ventricular type is characterized by a dominant ventricle with morphology of a right ventricle, containing an infundibulum. This ventricle is usually located anteriorly and a diminutive left ventricle is located posteriorly. In this type of single ventricle, both great vessels frequently originate from the right ventricle.

3. The primitive type of single ventricle has a very disordered internal morphology and shape. It shows morphologic features of both the right and left ventricles.

4. Both atrioventricular valves can be seen to enter the dominant ventricle. In other instances there may be a single atrioventricular valve, or one of the valves may be atretic.

5. The left ventricular outflow is narrowed over a variable length in the left ventricular type with transposition causing subvalvular pulmonic stenosis. In this type of single ventricle, a diameter of the bulboventricular foramen less than that of the aortic annulus (valve) indicates limitation of systemic flow at the bulboventricular foramen. This causes the equivalent of subaortic stenosis.

6. The presence of atrioventricular valve atresia in single ventricle may be visualized by selective injection into the atrium connected to the atretic valve. This may be depicted best in the four-chamber (hepatoclavicular) view, which minimizes overlap of the cardiac chambers. Demonstration of atrioventricular valve atresia may be difficult in the presence of a large atrial septal defect.

7. Injection into the pulmonary artery demonstrates the connection of the pulmonary vein on the levo-

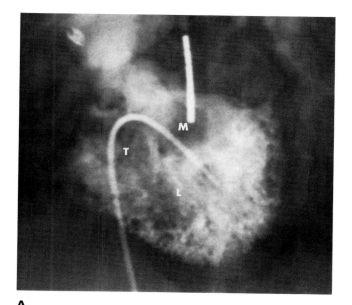

A

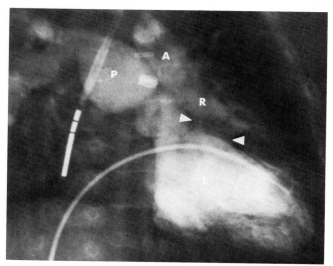

B

Figure 5-28. Single ventricle of the left ventricular type (double-inlet left ventricle) and transposition of the great arteries. LAO (*A*) and RAO (*B*) views. The LAO views demonstrate both the tricuspid (T) and mitral (M) valves entering the left ventricle (L). The RAO view shows the bulboventricular foramen (*arrowheads*) connecting the dominant left ventricle to the right ventricle outlet chamber (R). (A, aorta; P, pulmonary artery.)

phase, which is important, since anomalous venous connection is not uncommon in single ventricles.

8. In patients with single ventricle of the left ventricular type, transposition, and restrictive bulboventricular foramen, an aortogram may be indicated in order to exclude coarctation of the aorta.

Asplenia and Polysplenia

Splenic syndromes consist of asplenia, polysplenia, and other abnormalities of splenic size and shape.[41–43] These syndromes are usually associated with visceral heterotaxy or visceral isomerism.[44] These splenic syndromes are nearly always associated with severe congenital heart disease. Asplenia is usually accompanied by complex cyanotic heart disease. Polysplenia may also be associated with complex cyanotic disease, but the structural anomalies are on average less severe and sometimes consist of a single acyanotic lesion.

Atrial situs abnormalities such as situs ambiguous or atrial isomerism are characteristic. While normal situs and situs solitus can occur, right atrial isomerism tends to occur with asplenia and left atrial isomerism with polysplenia. However, asplenia and polysplenia can be associated with any atrial situs. Left isomerism is associated with bilateral hypoarterial bronchi (bilateral left-pulmonary arterial morphology) and right isomerism with bilateral epiarterial bronchi (bilateral right-pulmonary arterial morphology).

The diagnosis of splenic abnormalities can be established definitively by nuclear scintigraphy, computed tomography, and magnetic resonance imaging. Angiography is not indicated for this purpose.

Asplenia is characterized by:

1. Right-sided atrial isomerism and bilateral epiarterial bronchi. However, asplenia can occur with any atrial situs.
2. Midline transverse liver.
3. Midline gallbladder.
4. Midline stomach, usually small.
5. Malrotation of the intestine.
6. Bilateral superior vena cavae. The coronary sinus is usually not present (unroofed coronary sinus) so neither cava enters the coronary sinus. The superior cavae enter directly into the top of both sides of the atrium or atria.
7. Inferior vena cava ipsilateral to the abdominal aorta.
8. Anomalous pulmonary venous connection occurs in over 70% of patients with right atrial isomerism. It is usually total anomalous connection. Obstructive pulmonary venous connection is frequent.
9. Complex cardiac anomalies are common in patients with asplenia. These are common atrium, complete atrioventricular septal (endocardial cushion) defect (single atrioventricular valve), single ventricle, transposition of the great arteries, and severe pulmonary outflow obstruction or atresia. Of patients with asplenia and/or right atrial isomerism, 70% to 80% have severe obstruction of pulmonary blood flow.
10. Most patients with right atrial isomerism have arterioventricular abnormalities: transposition or double outlet ventricle.

Polysplenia is characterized by:

1. Left-side atrial isomerism and bilateral hyparterial bronchi. However, polysplenia may be associated with any atrial situs.
2. Absence of the gallbladder or biliary atresia.
3. Malrotation of the intestine.
4. Infrahepatic interruption of the inferior vena cava with azygous continuation. This does not occur with asplenia.
5. Anomalous pulmonary venous connection. Partial anomalous connection is more common than total anomalous connection.
6. Cardiac anomalies are less severe than those of asplenia. Any of the anomalies discussed in regard to asplenia can occur. However, atrial and ventricular septal defects may be expected rather than common atrium and single ventricle. Arterioventricular connections are normal in the majority of patients. Obstruction to pulmonary blood flow is less common and subaortic stenosis more common in polysplenia than in asplenia.

Right Ventricular Outflow Obstruction

Obstruction to pulmonary blood flow occurs as an isolated anomaly and is also frequently a component of complex congenital heart disease. This section focuses upon the isolated form and forms associated with simple intracardiac shunts.

The obstruction usually falls into three major types:

1. Valvular stenosis.
2. Infundibular stenosis.
3. Anomalous right ventricular muscle bundles.

Valvular stenosis occurs with a wide spectrum of severity from critical stenosis causing severe right ventricular failure in the neonate, to mild stenosis remaining asymptomatic in the adult.[45,46] Valvular stenosis secondarily causes hypertrophy of the right ventricle, especially the infundibular portion. Such compensatory infundibular hypertrophy can act as a second site of stenosis and can persist or even become intensified after removal of the valvular obstruction. There is an increased incidence of branch pulmonary arterial stenosis in patients with valvular stenosis.

Anomalous right ventricular muscle bundles are

also called double-chambered right ventricle. The anomalous muscle bundles course diagonally or horizontally across the right ventricular chamber from the septum to the free wall. It is essentially a hypertrophied, malpositioned moderator band. It is located at the junction between the inlet and outlet portions of the right ventricle. This lesion is frequently associated with a VSD that can occur either proximal or distal to the muscle bundle. It also occurs in association with valvular pulmonic stenosis. A fibrous membrane is a rare cause of subvalvular pulmonic stenosis.

Goals of angiographic imaging are:

1. Demonstration of the presence, location, morphology, and severity of the right ventricular outlet obstruction.

2. Identification of additional sites of stenosis, fixed or dynamic.

3. Assessment of severity of right ventricular hypertrophy and function.

4. Exclusion of branch pulmonary arterial stenosis(es).

5. Exclusion of intracardiac shunts or other associated anomalies.

Optimal views and injection sites are:

1. Anteroposterior or cranial anteroposterior (sit-up) view.

2. Cranial anteroposterior (sit up) and cranial LAO views with injection into the main pulmonary artery or right ventricle are useful for excluding branch pulmonary arterial stenosis(es).

Salient angiographic features are:

Valvular Stenosis

1. Thickened pulmonic valve leaflets with dome-shaped appearance in systole (Fig. 5-29).

2. Narrow jet of opacified blood passing across the stenotic valve into the pulmonary artery is seen upon injection into the right ventricle. Upon injection into the pulmonary artery, a negative jet is recognized in the proximal part of the pulmonary artery.

3. Dilated main and left pulmonary atery (see Fig. 5-29). Sometimes the right pulmonary artery is also dilated but less so than the left pulmonary artery.

4. Dynamic narrowing of the infundibulum during systole. Due to hypertrophy, there may also be mild to moderate narrowing even in diastole (see Fig. 5-29). After valvuloplasty, the infundibular narrowing may initially become more severe owing to decrease in distending pressure after reduction in the valvular stenosis.

5. In critical pulmonic stenosis, which occurs during infancy, the right ventricle is dilated and diffusely hypokinetic.[46] In this circumstance, there is generally also tricuspid regurgitation and right-to-left shunting across

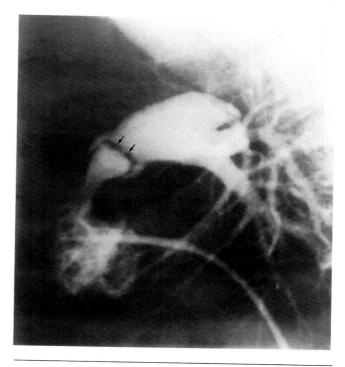

Figure 5-29. Lateral view of right ventricular injection in a patient with valvular pulmonic stenosis. Note the marked thickening and doming of the pulmonic valve (*small arrows*). There is poststenotic dilatation of the main pulmonary artery. During systole there is dynamic narrowing of the infundibulum.

an interatrial communication (defect or stretched foramen ovale).

6. Dysplastic pulmonic valve is severely thickened and shows very little movement during systole.[47] It has the appearance of a washer.

Infundibular Stenosis

1. Fixed narrowing of the infundibulum is unusual in the presence of associated lesions such as tetralogy of Fallot. However, it can occur as an isolated anomaly.

2. Discrete membranous or fibromuscular rings located a few centimeters beneath the pulmonic valve are rare causes of right ventricular outlet obstruction.

3. The lateral view may demonstrate the maximal narrowing at the ostium leading into the infundibulum in some patients.

Anomalous Right Ventricular Muscle Bundles[48]

1. Aberrant hypertrophied muscle bundles divide the right ventricle into proximal (inlet region) and distal (outlet region) chambers (Fig. 5-30). The site of obstruction is variable.

2. On the frontal view, large circular myocardial structures are visible, narrowing the proximal portion of the outlet region (see Fig. 5-30). This appearance is due to end-face visualization of hypertrophied muscle bundles coursing through the right ventricle in an antero-posterior orientation.

3. In the lateral view, the muscle bundles may be displayed coursing diagonally just below the infundibulum. It may also demonstrate circumferential narrowing below the infundibulum.

4. Most patients (70%–80%) with this anomaly also have a ventricular septal defect. Subaortic stenosis also occurs in some patients. Consequently, left ventriculography in the long axial oblique view is useful for excluding both ventricular septal defect and subaortic stenosis.

Left Ventricular Outlet Obstruction

The obstruction occurs at three sites:

1. Valvular aortic stenosis.
2. Subvalvular aortic stenosis.[49,50]
3. Supravalvular aortic stenosis.[51]

Valvular aortic stenosis is usually caused by a bicuspid aortic valve. However, aortic stenosis presenting in the first few years of life may be caused by more primitive deformities of the valve, such as a dysplastic or unicuspid valve, as well as a bicuspid valve. Aortic stenosis usually causes left ventricular hypertrophy with a hyperdynamic contractile pattern causing systolic cavity oblit-

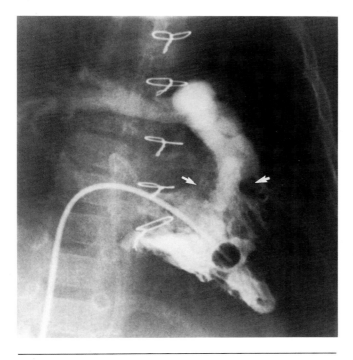

Figure 5-30. Anteroposterior view of an injection into the right ventricle in a patient with a double-chambered right ventricle. Note the severe stenosis produced by hypertrophied muscle bands (*arrows*) separating the inflow portion of the right ventricle from the outflow portion.

eration. However, the several stenoses presenting during the neonatal period sometimes cause left ventricular dilation and diffuse or regional hypokinesis and may be associated with endocardial fibroelastosis. This syndrome has been called critical aortic stenosis and is caused by an imbalance in myocardial oxygen supply:demand ratio, with consequent subendocardial ischemia. Valvular aortic stenosis may be associated with a variety of other left-sided obstructive lesions, including mitral valve obstruction such as parachute mitral valve, subaortic stenosis, coarctation, and interruption of the aorta.

Subaortic stenosis exists in several forms: discrete membranous stenosis, discrete fibromuscular ring, long fibromuscular tunnel, asymmetric septal hypertrophy, or a combination of these. Subaortic stenosis causes a jet across or against the aortic valve that thickens and damages the aortic valve. Consequently, a variable degree of aortic regurgitation is common. Subaortic stenosis becomes progressively more severe with time.

Supravalvular aortic stenosis occurs in three configurations: hourglass constriction of the proximal ascending aorta (the most common type), diffuse narrowing of nearly the entire ascending aorta, and discrete membranous narrowing of the proximal ascending aorta. The stenosis starts at the top of the sinuses of Valsalva. Stenosis may be present at the origin of aortic arch branches, coronary arteries, pulmonary arteries, and abdominal aortic branches.

Goals of angiographic imaging are:

1. Identify the presence and site of outlet obstruction.

2. Exclude multiple sites of obstruction and aortic arch obstruction and mitral valve abnormalities.

3. Exclude stenosis at origin of aortic branches in patients with supravalvular aortic stenosis.

4. Evaluate left ventricular dimensions and function.

Optimal views and injection sites are:

1. LAO view with injection into the ascending aorta is used to evaluate the aortic valve and thoracic aorta.

2. Long axial oblique view provides visualization of the left ventricular outlet region with minimal foreshortening and overlap by the mitral apparatus, and is indicated for the demonstration of subvalvular aortic stenosis.

Salient angiographic features are:

Valvular Stenosis

1. Thickened and domed contour of the aortic valve in systole (Fig. 5-31).

2. Narrow jet of opacified or unopacified blood traversing the aortic valve during systole upon injection of contrast media into the left ventricular or ascending aorta, respectively.

3. Poststenotic dilatation of the ascending aorta.

4. Left ventricular hypertrophy is indicated by thickened papillary muscle and apical cavity obliteration during systole.

5. A typical appearance of a bicuspid aortic valve is indicated by a leaflet that spans the entire chamber or 180° of the circumference of the aortic annulus. This causes a fish-mouth opening of the valve (Fig. 5-32). Another feature is disproportionately large sinus of Valsalva. The posterior sinus is normally larger than the other two. This is disproportionately so with the bicuspid valve. It may not always be possible to distinguish between a bicuspid and tricuspid valve.

Subaortic Stenosis

1. Membranous stenosis is indicated by a narrow lucency positioned across the outflow region of the left ventricle at approximately 1 to 3 cm below the valve. It is visualized best on the long axial oblique view[52] (Fig. 5-33). The aortic valve cusps are usually thickened.

2. Aortic regurgitation is present in most patients with membranous subaortic stenosis. The membrane may be outlined by the regurgitant jet of contrast media after injection into the proximal ascending aorta.

3. An elongated, smoothly or irregularly narrowed outflow region of the left ventricle indicates the tunnel type of subaortic stenosis (Fig. 5-34).

4. Hypertrophic muscular subaortic stenosis is indicated by asymmetric bulging and hypertrophy of the

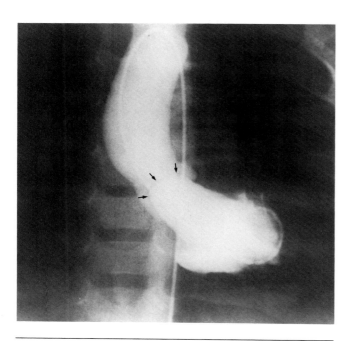

Figure 5-31. Anteroposterior view of an injection into the left ventricle in a patient with valvular aortic stenosis. Note the doming and thickening of an aortic valve (*small arrows*) and poststenotic dilatation of the ascending aorta.

septum with apposition of the mitral tricuspid valve anterior leaflet against the septum in systole. This apposition causes a W- or V-shaped lucent line in the lower portion of the outflow region. There is anterior motion of the anterior leaflet of the mitral valve in systole. This is demonstrated in the lateral view of the left ventriculogram.

5. A ventricular septal defect and subpulmonic stenosis are occasionally observed in association with subaortic stenosis.

Supravalvular Stenosis

1. An hourglass narrowing of the ascending aorta located at the top of the sinus of Valsalva is the most frequent appearance (Fig. 5-35).

2. Less common types are characterized by a membranous focal lucent defect in the proximal ascending aorta or long-segment narrowing of the ascending aorta.

3. The thoracic aortogram may indicate narrowing of the origin of a coronary artery or the arch arteries. An abdominal aortogram may indicate narrowing of the renal or visceral arteries. Coarctation in the distal thoracic aorta or midabdominal aorta can occur in association with supravalvular aortic stenosis.

Hypoplastic Left Heart Syndrome

The anatomic severity of hypoplastic left heart syndrome (HLHS) is variable.[53] It usually consists of a severely hypoplastic ascending aorta and aortic annulus; severe aortic stenosis or atresia; mitral stenosis or atresia; hypoplasia of the left ventricle. Coarctation or interruption of the aortic arch is present sometimes. The left ventricle consists of a very small cavity and disproportionately great myocardial mass. The systemic circulation is supported by a patent ductus arteriosus in the early neonatal period. Endocardial fibroelastosis is a common associated abnormality. The right-sided cardiac chambers are usually dilated.

The diagnosis of this syndrome precipitates three possible paths of management: no treatment; initial cardiac transplantation; palliative procedure (Norwood stage I procedure) followed by cardiac transplantation, or the stage II Norwood procedure. The Norwood procedure consists of creation of a large atrial septal defect; pulmonary artery to ascending aorta (end-to-side) anastomosis; graft from aorta to pulmonary arteries.

Goals of angiographic imaging are:

1. Demonstration of the severely hypoplastic ascending aorta, which establishes the diagnosis.

2. If a palliative procedure is being considered, exclusion of coarctation or aortic arch interruption is essential in planning the operative procedure (Norwood procedure).

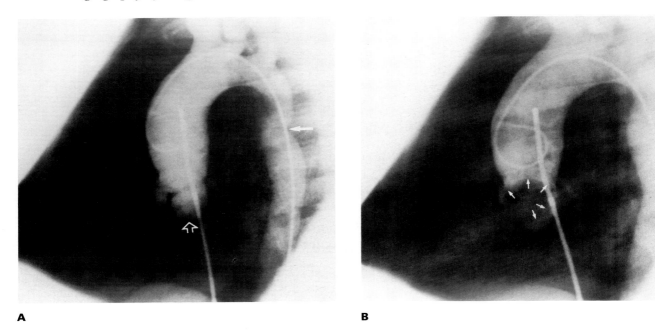

A

B

Figure 5-32. Diastolic (*A*) and systolic (*B*) frames of a thoracic aortogram in a patient with bicuspid aortic valve and mild aortic coarctation. There is buckling and mild stenosis in the proximal of the descending aorta (*arrow*). Note the disproportionately large posterior sinus of Valsalva (*open arrow*). There is doming of the aortic valve, producing a "fish mouth" (*small arrows*), demonstrated during systole.

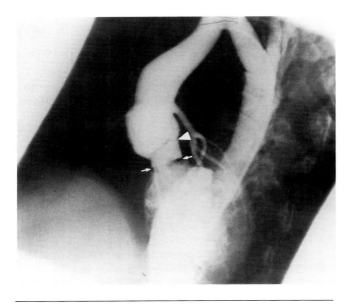

Figure 5-33. Cranial LAO view in a patient with subaortic stenosis. There is a discrete membrane (*small arrows*) located a few centimeters below the aortic valve (*arrowhead*).

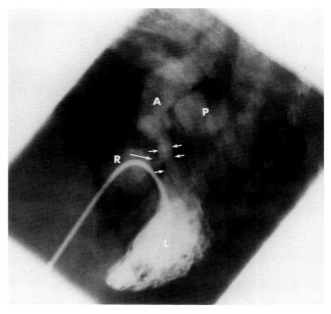

Figure 5-34. Cranial LAO view after injection into the left ventricle in a patient with ventricular septal defect and the tunnel type of subaortic stenosis. Because of posterior malalignment of the ventricular septum there is a narrowing in the long segment (*small arrows*) of the left ventricular outflow tract. Shunting across a ventricular septal defect is also evident (*long arrow*). (A, aorta; L, left ventricle; P, pulmonary artery; R, right ventricle.)

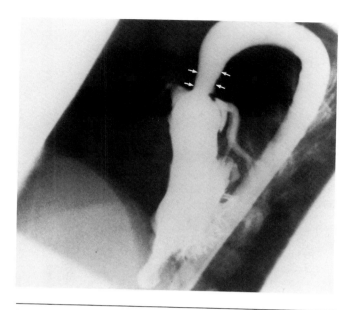

Figure 5-35. LAO view after injection into the left ventricle in a patient with supravalvular aortic stenosis. There is narrowing in the long segment in the proximal portion of the ascending aorta. The narrowing begins at the sinotubular junction and extends through the proximal third of the ascending aorta (*arrows*).

3. If a palliative procedure is being considered, exclusion of right-sided lesions such as tricuspid abnormalities or pulmonary arterial stenosis, is essential.

Optimal views and injection sites are:

1. Anteroposterior and lateral views after injection into the aortic arch or proximal descending aorta. The catheter is advanced from the right side through a patent ductus and into the proximal descending aorta. After balloon occlusion of the proximal descending aorta (using a Berman catheter), injected contrast medium flows retrograde into the hypoplastic aorta.

Salient angiographic features are:

1. Hypoplastic ascending aorta is outlined after injection into the ductus arteriosus or the proximal ascending aorta (through a catheter placed across the ductus [Fig. 5-36]).
2. Coarctation or interruption of the aortic arch.
3. If contrast medium flows retrograde to the level of the aortic valve and no wash-in defect is noted, this indicates aortic atresia.
4. Atrial septal defect with left-to-right shunting is shown after injection into the pulmonary artery.
5. Enlarged right-sided cardiac chamber.

References

1. Bargeron LM Jr, Elliott LP, Soto B, et al. Axial cineangiography in congenital heart disease. I. Concept, technical and anatomic consideration. Circulation 1977;56:1075.

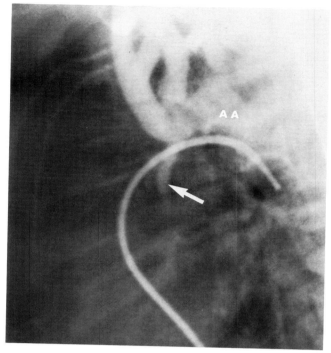

Figure 5-36. Hypoplastic left heart. Lateral view of aorta after injection into the aortic arch (AA) with balloon occlusion of the descending aorta. With occlusion of the descending aorta contrast medium is forced retrograde into the hypoplastic ascending aorta (*arrow*).

2. Elliott LP, Bargeron LM, Green CE. Angled angiography: general approach and findings. In: Friedman WF, Higgins CB, eds. Pediatric cardiac imaging. Philadelphia: WB Saunders, 1984.
3. Elliott LP, Bargeron LM Jr, Bream PR, et al. Axial cineangiography in congenital heart disease. II. Specific lesions. Circulation 1977;56:1084.
4. Davia JE, Cheitlin MD, Bedynek JL. Sinus venosus atrial septal defect: analysis of fifty cases. Am Heart J 1973;85:177.
5. Nakib A, Moller JH, Kanjuh VI, Edwards JE. Anomalies of pulmonary veins. Am J Cardiol 1967;20:77.
6. Neill CA. Development of pulmonary veins, with reference to the embryology of anomalies of pulmonary venous return. Pediatrics 1956;18:880.
7. Soto B, Becker AE, Moulaert AJ, et al. Classification of ventricular septal defects. Br Heart J 1980;43:332.
8. Santamaria H, Soto B, Ceballos R, Bargeron LM Jr, Coghlan HC, Kirklin JW. Angiographic differentiation of types of ventricular septal defects. Am J Radiol 1983;141:273.
9. Rudolph AM. In: Congenital diseases of the heart. Chicago: Year Book Medical Publishers, 1974:405.
10. Soto B, Bargeron LM Jr, Pacifico AD, et al. Angiography of atrioventricular defects. Am J Cardiol 1981;48:492.
11. Baron MG, Wolf BS, Steinfeld L, Van Mierop LHS. Endocardial cushion defects. Specific diagnosis by angiocardiography. Am J Cardiol 1964;13:162.
12. Rastelli GC, Kincaid OW, Ritter DG. Angiocardiography of persistent common atrioventricular canal. In: Feldt RH, ed. Atrioventricular canal defects. Philadelphia: WB Saunders, 1976:110.
13. Soto B, Pacifico AD, Ceballos R, et al. Tetralogy of Fallot: an angiographic pathologic correlative study. Circulation 1981; 64:558.
14. Fellows KE, Freed MD, Keane JF, Van Praag R, Bernhard WF, Cas-

tenada AC. Results of routine preoperative coronary angiography in tetralogy of Fallot. Circulation 1975;51:561.

15. Dabizzi RP, Caprioli G, Aizzi L, Castelli C, Baldrighi G, Parenzan C, et al. Distribution and anomalies of coronary arteries in tetralogy of Fallot. Circulation 1980;60:95.

16. Ruttenberg HD, Carey LS, Adams P Jr, Edwards JE. Absence of the pulmonary valve in the tetralogy of Fallot. Am J Roentgenol 1964;91:500.

17. Soto B, Pacifico AD, Luna RF, Bargeron LM Jr. A radiographic study of congenital pulmonary atresia with ventricular septal defect. Am J Roentgenol 1977;129:1027.

18. Ellis K, Casarella WJ, Hayes CJ, Gersony WM, Bowman FO Jr, Malm JR. Pulmonary atresia with intact ventricular septum: new development in diagnosis and treatment. Am J Roentgenol 1972;116:501.

19. Lauer RM, Fink HP, Petry EL, Dunn MI, Diehl AM. Angiographic demonstration of intramyocardial sinusoids in pulmonary-valve atresia with intact ventricular septum and hypoplastic right ventricle. N Engl J Med 1964;271:69.

20. Haworth SG, Shinebourne EA, Miller GA: Right-to-left interatrial shunting with normal right ventricular pressure: a puzzling haemodynamic picture associated with some rare congenital malformation of the right ventricle and tricuspid valve. Br Heart J 1975;37:386.

21. Anderson RH, Wilkinson JL, Gerlis IM, Smith A, Becker AE. Atresia of the right atrioventricular orifice. Br Heart J 1977;39:414.

22. Guller B, Kincaid OW, Ritter DG. Angiocardiographic findings in tricuspid atresia: correlation with hemodynamic and morphologic features. Radiology 1969;93:531.

23. Deutsch V, Wexler L, Blieden LE, Yahmi JH, Neufeld HN. Ebstein's anomaly of tricuspid valve: critical review of roentgenological features and additional angiographic signs. Am J Radiol 1975;125:395.

24. Hippona FA, Arthachinta S. Ebstein's anomaly of the tricuspid valve: a report of 16 cases and review of the literature. Prog Cardiovasc Dis 1965;7:434.

25. La Corte MA, Fellows KE, Williams RG. Overriding tricuspid valve: echocardiographic and angiocardiographic features. Am J Cardiol 1976;37:911.

26. Theine G, Razzolin R, Dalla–Volta S. Aorto-pulmonary relationship, arterioventricular alignment, and ventricular septal defects in complete transposition of the great arteries. Eur J Cardiol 1976;4:13.

27. Sansa M, Tonkin IL, Bargeron LM Jr, et al. Left ventricular outflow tract obstruction in transposition of the great arteries: an angiographic study of 74 cases. Am J Cardiol 1979;44:88.

28. Soto B, Bargeron LM Jr, Bream PR, Elliott LP. Conditions with atrioventricular discordance: angiographic study. In: Anderson RH, Shinebourne EA, eds. Paediatric cardiology, 1977. Edinburgh: Churchill Livingstone, 1978:207.

29. Sridaromont S, Ritter DG, Feldt RH, Davis GD, Edwards JE. Double outlet right ventricle: anatomic and angiocardiographic correlations. Mayo Clin Proc 1978;53:555.

30. Sondheimer HM, Freedom RM, Olley PM. Double outlet right ventricle: clinical spectrum and prognosis. Am J Cardiol 1977;39:709.

31. Bargeron LM Jr, Soto B: A double outlet ventricle. Pediatr Cardiol 1979/80;1:161.

32. Calder L, Van Praagh R, Van Praagh S, Sears WP, Corwin R, Levy A, et al. Truncus arteriosus communis. Clinical, angiocardiographic and pathologic findings in 100 patients. Am Heart J 1976;92:23.

33. Ceballos R, Soto B, Kirklin JW, Bargeron LM Jr. Truncus arteriosus. An anatomical–angiographic study. Br Heart J 1983;49:589.

34. Bleiden LC, Moller JH: Aorticopulmonary septal defect: an experience with 17 patients. Br Heart J 1974;36:630.

35. Bonham–Carter RE, Capriles M, Noe Y. Total anomalous pulmonary venous drainage: a clinical and anatomical study of 75 children. Br Heart J 1969;31:45.

36. Delisle G, Ando M, Calder AL, Zuberbuhler JR, Rochenmacher S, Alday LE, et al. Total anomalous pulmonary venous connection. Report of 93 autopsied cases with emphasis on diagnostic and surgical considerations. Am Heart J 1976;91:199.

37. McCartney FJ, Partridge JB, Scott O, Deverall PB. Common or single ventricle: an angiographic and haemodynamic study of 42 patients. Circulation 1976;53:543.

38. Soto B, Pacifico AD, Di Scascio G. Univentricular heart: an angiographic study. Am J Cardiol 1982;49:787.

39. Freedom RM, Harder J, Culham JAG, Trusler GD, Rowe RD. Ventricular hypoplasia: angiocardiography and surgical implications. In: Goodman MJ, Marquis R, eds. Pediatric cardiology. Vol. 4. Edinburgh: Churchill Livingstone, 1981.

40. Somerville J, Becu L, Ross D. Common ventricle with acquired subaortic obstruction. Am J Cardiol 1974;34:206.

41. Freedom RM, Fellows KE Jr. Radiographic visceral patterns in the asplenic syndrome. Radiology 1973;107:387.

42. Ivemark BI. Implications of agenesis of the spleen on the pathogenesis of cono-truncus anomalies in childhood: an analysis of the heart malformations in the splenic agenesis syndrome, with fourteen new cases. Acta Paediatr (Suppl 104) 1955;44:1.

43. Randall PA, Moller JH, Amplatz K. The spleen and congenital heart disease. Am J Roentgenol 1973;119:51.

44. Macartney FJ, Zuberbuhler JR, Anderson RH. Morphological considerations pertaining to recognition of atrial isomerism: consequences for sequential chamber localization. Br Heart J 1980;44:657.

45. Campbell M. Simple pulmonary stenosis: pulmonary valve stenosis with a closed ventricular septum. Br Heart J 1954;16:273.

46. Litwin SB, Williams WH, Freed MD, Bernhard WF. Critical pulmonary stenosis in infants: a surgical emergency. Surgery 1973;74:880.

47. Jeffry RF, Moller JH, Amplatz K. The dysplastic pulmonary valve: a new roentgenographic entity with a discussion of anatomy and radiology of other types of valvular pulmonary stenosis. Am J Roentgenol Rad Ther 1972;114:322.

48. Fellows KE, Martin EC, Rosenthal A. Angiocardiography of obstructing muscular bands of the right ventricle. Am J Roentgenol 1977;128:249.

49. Simon AL, Ross J Jr, Gault JH. Angiographic anatomy of the left ventricle and mitral valve in idiopathic hypertrophic subaortic stenosis. Circulation 1967;36:852.

50. Hastreeter AR, Van der Hurst RL, Dubrow IW, Eckner FO. Quantitative angiographic and morphologic aspects of aortic valve atresia. Am J Cardiol 1983;5:1705.

51. Keane JF, Fellows KE, LaFarge CG, Nadas AS, Bernhard WF. The surgical management of discrete and diffuse supravalvular aortic stenosis. Circulation 1976;54:112.

52. Kelley MJ, Higgins CB, Kirkpatrick SE. Axial left ventriculography in discrete subaortic stenosis. Radiology 1980;135:77.

53. Noonan JA, Nadas AS. The hypoplastic left heart syndrome: an analysis of 101 cases. Pediatr Clin North Am 1958;5:1029.

Chapter 6

Thoracic Aortic Disease

Charles B. Higgins

Suspected diseases of the thoracic aorta must be efficiently and thoroughly evaluated because some are immediately life threatening. Diagnosis or exclusion of thoracic aortic disease requires direct visualization of the aorta. This can now be attained with a number of techniques: contrast aortography; computed tomography; and magnetic resonance imaging. Transesophageal echocardiography can also visualize portions of the thoracic aorta.

Complete diagnostic evaluation of the thoracic aorta requires visualization of the lumen, aortic wall, and periaortic region in order to define intraluminal, mural, and extramural pathology. Primary aortic disease or its complications and secondary involvement of the aorta by mediastinal pathology can involve any or all of these three sites. Imaging modalities must be capable of evaluating the entire extent of the aorta and the origin of the arch vessels in order to define the extent of abnormalities. In some instances the status of the aortic valve and annulus must also be established.

Imaging studies are needed for the initial diagnosis of an abnormality and, in some instances, for monitoring the severity of the disease over time. Because of the latter requirement, a minimally invasive or noninvasive technique is desirable.

Diagnostic Tests: Advantages and Disadvantages

Contrast Aortography. This is the traditional definitive test. However, this test is invasive and expensive and has distinct limitations. The limitations are the inability to define a thrombosed false channel of an aortic dissection, strictly mural pathology, and periaortic pathology. The diagnosis of a thrombosed false channel can be inferred from angiography but cannot be directly demonstrated. Because it is invasive, it is not optimal for monitoring the course of aortic disease or for the postoperative evaluation of the thoracic aorta.

Computed Tomography. Computed tomography (CT) has now been shown to be at least as accurate as aortography for the diagnosis of thoracic aortic disease.[1-9] It provides visualization of the aortic lumen, aortic wall, and periaortic region. Because direct imaging is restricted to the transverse plane, it has some limitations in displaying the origin of the arch vessels. The need for contrast media may be undesirable in some patients; this is a consideration for patients with reduced renal function or those destined for emergent cardiopulmonary bypass surgery. At least theoretically, the latter event may adversely influence renal function and compound the effects of contrast media.

Magnetic Resonance Imaging. Magnetic resonance imaging (MRI) may be the ideal technique for the evaluation of these lesions.[1,10-15] It provides visualization of the lumen, wall, and periaortic region. It does not require contrast medium. Imaging in the sagittal, oblique sagittal, or coronal planes demonstrates the origin of the arch branches. The completely noninvasive nature of MRI renders it ideal for sequential monitoring of thoracic aortic diseases.[15] An occasional limitation is the requirement for immobility and strict cooperation by the patient; greater difficulty in monitoring of vital signs; and management of a hemodynamically unstable patient during MRI.

Transesophageal Echocardiography. Increasing experience is being acquired with transesophageal echocardiography (TEE), which is more invasive than standard echocardiography.[16,17] It requires the patient to swallow the transducer. The instrumentation is potentially portable, so the study can be done in the emergency room, the intensive care unit, or the operating room. It can visualize the aortic lumen, wall, and to a limited extent, the periaortic region. It has a very narrow field of view. Its limitations are inability to visualize the entire aorta and arch branches; incomplete visualization of the periaortic region; and invasiveness. Because of questionable reproduction of the imaging plane from study to study and its invasive nature, it is not ideal for sequential monitoring of thoracic aortic disease.

Comparison of Computed Tomography and Magnetic Resonance Imaging with Aortography

Aortography has been considered the gold standard and held as the verifying study for thoracic aortic disease during the past three decades. Consequently, new imaging modalities have been compared against it and many surgeons require that the results of noninvasive studies must be verified by aortography before surgery. Based upon a number of comparative studies conducted in the past ten years, this notion is not valid.[1,2,5–7] Indeed, for a variety of reasons, CT and MRI should be considered the procedure of choice for the diagnosis of thoracic aortic disease. However, situations do exist when aortography is preferable or even essential. An example of this is the evaluation of aortic trauma.

Compared to CT and MRI, aortography may be technically difficult in patients with tortuous and/or narrowed iliac arteries and has other risks associated with catheterization, such as contrast reactions. On the other hand, CT and MRI share the advantages of noninvasiveness, ease of performance, and selective visualization of structures. The latter attribute is due to the avoidance of superimposition of mediastinal shadows and spatial separation of the various portions of the aorta with CT and MRI, the aortic wall and periaortic regions are evaluated as well as the lumen of the vessel. The transverse tomographic techniques section the thoracic aorta perpendicular to the pathologic process, thus avoiding the need to select the optimal aortographic projection for each pathology. Computerized analysis and information storage provides the possibility for image reformation in a number of different planes and for quantitative analysis of the images. Finally, in some instances MRI can distinguish between various normal and pathologic tissues and fluids. The latter is especially useful for defining the presence of periaortic hematoma.

Unfortunately, the fixed and limited transaxial imaging plane of CT may hinder the evaluation of disease processes that are largely transaxial in orientation, such as traumatic aortic transection. This problem can also arise with MRI if the optimal plane for tomography is not chosen. This pitfall can be avoided by the MRI, which can image the thoracic aorta in two planes. It is recognized that MRI, for several reasons, is not advisable for the study of acute aortic trauma. As stated above, CT is limited in assessing the severity of aortic insufficiency and both MRI and CT cannot define the status of the coronary arteries.

Techniques

Aortography. Biplane aortography is ideal. The most useful projection is usually the 50° to 60° right posterior oblique. The projection separates the ascending and descending aorta and displays the origins of the arch branches. The second projection (at 90° angulation from the first) is necessary to detect pathology situated parallel to the right posterior oblique projection. Serial radiography is desirable because of its excellent spatial resolution and wide field of view. Digital angiography after direct aortic injection of contrast medium is now being used with increasing frequency.

For the assessment of the ascending aorta and arch, the catheter is placed approximately at the sinotubular junction for the injection. For evaluation of the descending thoracic aorta, the catheter is placed just beyond the aortic arch. A pigtail catheter is used. The injection volume and rate in the average adult is 45 to 50 ml and 25 to 30 ml/sec, respectively. This volume and rate may not be sufficient for the aneurysmal ascending aorta.

Computed Tomography (CT). Images are acquired in the transverse plane, extending from above the aorta to the diaphragm and sometimes into the abdomen as well. Section thickness is 10 mm. Dynamic scanning is preferable. A volume of 40 to 50 ml of iodinated 60% contrast media is injected into an arm vein at the rate of 2 to 5 ml/sec. Scans are acquired at several levels through the ascending aorta during the peak opacification caused by the "first pass" of the contrast media through the aorta (Fig. 6-1). After intravenous injection of contrast media, it arrives in the thoracic aorta about 12 to 15 sec later in normal subjects but may be much delayed in patients with low cardiac output and/or enlarged central blood volume. This is the circulation time, which can be defined exactly by giving a preliminary injection of indocyanine dye and recording the arrival time of the dye at some sites in the arterial circulation with a skin transducer–densitometer system. After the dynamic study, images of the entire thoracic aorta can be done during an intravenous infusion of contrast media. Another technique is the constant infusion, using a mechanical injector, at the rate of 2 ml/sec for a total volume of 80 to 100 ml, with the acquisition of scans commencing at 20 sec after the start of the injection.

Dynamic CT imaging of the thoracic aorta can be achieved optimally using the ultrafast CT scanner (Imatron). After the intravenous injection of 40 to 50 ml at the

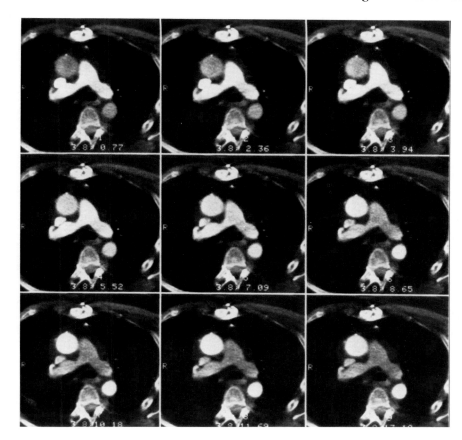

Figure 6-1. Series of CT scans obtained for sequential heartbeats during the passage of contrast media through the central circulation. The images in time are arranged from the upper left hand panel to the lower right hand panel. On the early images there was opacification of the superior vena cava and the pulmonary arteries, followed on later scans by opacification of the ascending and descending aorta. The exposure time for the cine CT scans is 50 msec, and scans can be obtained using the flow mode at sequential heartbeats during the period of opacification of the central cardiovascular structures.

rate of 3 to 5 ml/sec, scans are acquired at 8 to 10 levels within a 200-msec interval. Each series of scan is initiated by the R wave of the ECG. A total of 80 scans can be done, consisting of 10 scans at each of the 8 levels. The scanning procedure is initiated at the predicted time of arrival of the intravenously injected bolus of contrast media. This timing can be precisely defined by using a densitometric recording of the arrival time of indocyanine dye in the peripheral arterial circulation.

Magnetic Resonance Imaging. The standard imaging plane is transverse using electrocardiograph (ECG) gating. Multislice spin echo images (approximately 10 to 12 slices) are acquired from above the aortic arch to below the diaphragm. Slice thickness is usually 10 mm. The TR is equal to the RR interval of the ECG and the TE is 20 to 30 msec. Slices of 3 to 5 mm in thickness may be done at an area of particular interest. A series of images is sometimes also done in an oblique sagittal or sagittal plane. The oblique sagittal plane (similar to the right posterior oblique view) is produced by elevating the subject's right shoulder 20 to 30 degrees and imaging in the sagittal plane (Fig. 6-2). This plane can also be produced by applying oblique angulation of the slice-selective gradient. Signal from blood in the aorta and other thoracic

vessels is removed or decreased by using spatial presaturation of the protons in flowing blood; saturation pulses are applied superior and inferior to the imaged volume. Respiratory compensation is used to diminish breathing artifacts.

Several additional imaging techniques may be useful for the full assessment of thoracic aortic disease. Cine MR (ECG-referenced multiphase gradient echo technique) can be used to evaluate flow phenomenon and abnormal flow patterns in the aorta. On gradient echo (cine MR) images the blood pool generally has high signal intensity (Fig. 6-3A) under normal flow conditions. Abnormal flow conditions resulting in high-velocity turbulent flow or "jet" flow cause a signal void in the aorta. This signal void occurs at the site of and distal to an obstruction. It is observed in the ascending aorta in aortic stenosis (Fig. 6-3B) and the descending aorta in coarctation. It is also observed in the left ventricle in aortic regurgitation (see Fig. 6-3A). It is also useful in identifying thrombus in the aorta, as discussed later in this chapter. Velocity-encoded cine MRI and other phase mapping techniques can be used for distinguishing between flow signal and thrombus in the aorta and for measuring the velocity and flow rate of blood in the aorta (Fig. 6-4).

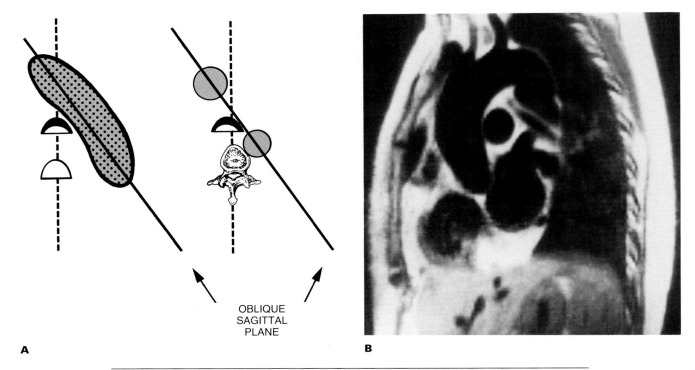

A

OBLIQUE
SAGITTAL
PLANE

B

Figure 6-2. The method for determining the angle of obliquity used for the oblique sagittal MRI plane. The diagram (*A*) depicts a line which passes through the mid-portion of the ascending and the mid-portion of the descending aorta or, alternately, passes through the middle of the aortic arch. This line prescribes the plane of the image, which optimally demonstrates the ascending aorta, aortic arch and descending aorta on a single tomographic image. The oblique sagittal MR image (*B*) demonstrates the ascending aorta, aortic arch and aortic arch branches and the proximal portion of the descending aorta.

Specific Diseases

Acquired diseases of the thoracic aorta are usually the result of degeneration of the aortic wall, but less frequently are caused by inflammation, infection, and trauma. The aorta can be involved by a number of systemic diseases including rheumatoid arthritis, ankylosing spondylitis, Reiter's syndrome, psoriatic arthritis, giant cell arteritis, and relapsing polychondritis and syphilis. Scleroderma and systemic lupus erythematosus may rarely involve the aorta. Takayasu's disease and Kawasaki's disease afflict the thoracic aorta and its branches. A number of diseases of the aorta also involve the aortic annulus or aortic valve and produce aortic regurgitation.

Congenital diseases of the thoracic aorta are hypoplasia, stenoses, dilatation, anomalous or double arch, and anomalous origin of arch branches. Stenoses are the following types: arch and/or isthmus hypoplasia, discrete juxtaductal coarctation of the aorta, or mid-thoracic or distal thoracic coarctation. Congenital dilatation occurs in Marfan's and Ehlers–Danlos syndromes. The types of anomalous arch are cervical arch, double arch, and right aortic arch.

Normal Dimensions

The aorta has sites of normal narrowing and widening. The aortic isthmus is sometimes a site of slight narrowing, especially in the infant. The diameter of the isthmus may be as small as 40% of the ascending aortic diameter and still be considered normal in infants.[18] This is the segment between the origin of the left subclavian artery and the point of attachment of the ligamentum arteriosus. Focal sites of slight dilatation are the aortic spindle and ductus diverticulum. Both are located at the site of the closed ductus. The spindle is a focal dilatation of the descending aorta, and the diverticulum is an outpocketing sometimes observed at the aortic end of the closed ductus arteriosus.

The normal dimensions of the thoracic aorta defined by CT as reported by Guthaner et al. are:[19]

$$\text{Aortic root} = 3.7 \pm 0.3 \text{ cm (SD)}$$
$$\text{Ascending aorta} = 3.3 \pm 0.6 \text{ cm}$$
$$\text{Descending aorta} = 2.4 \pm 0.3 \text{ cm}$$

The normal dimensions of the thoracic aorta defined by MRI as reported by Sommerhoff et al. are:[20]

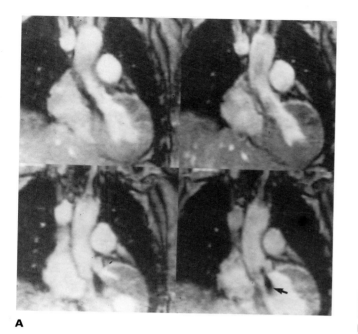

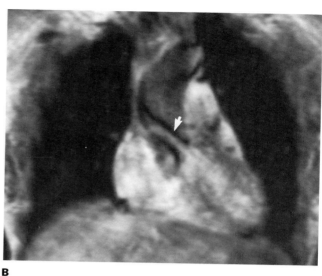

A   **B**

Figure 6-3. Cine MR images in patients with aortic regurgitation (*A*) and in a patient with aortic stenosis (*B*). Images in the coronal plane demonstrate that the signal intensity of the blood pool is bright on these images acquired with the gradient echo sequence (cine MRI) under normal flow conditions. In the presence of disturbed blood flow, which generally occurs at high velocities and frequently with turbulence, there appears a signal void within the blood pool. This signal void indicates the presence of disturbed blood flow patterns. The upper images in *A* demonstrate normal blood flow in the ascending aorta during systole. The lower images in *A* demonstrate a signal void emanating from the closed aortic valve (*arrow*) during diastole. This signal void indicates aortic regurgitation. *B* demonstrates the presence of signal void (*arrow*) during systole in the ascending aorta, which indicates aortic stenosis. There is also a general reduction in signal throughout the ascending aorta, which is caused by the eddy currents produced by aortic regurgitation.

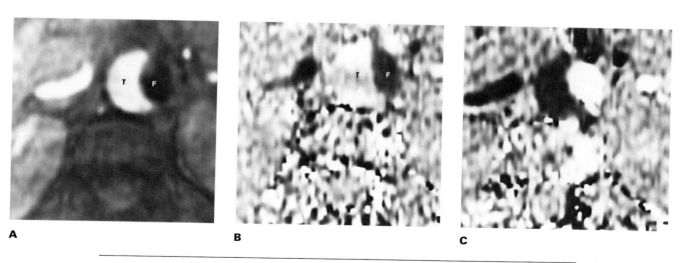

A   **B**   **C**

Figure 6-4. Cine MR intensity image (*A*) and phase images in systole (*B*) and diastole (*C*). The cine MR magnitude image demonstrates bright signal within the true channel (T) during the systolic phase of the cardiac cycle and absence of signal within the false channel (F). The phase image in systole demonstrates antegrade flow represented by bright coloration in the true channel (T) and retrograde flow in the false channel (F), as indicated by the dark coloration. The opposite coloration of the phase image appears in diastole, where there is retrograde flow in the true channel and antegrade flow in the false channel. On the phase images, the intensity of the gray scale is in proportion to the flow velocity. Directionality of flow is also represented by the gray-scale intensity, bright intensity representing antegrade flow and dark representing retrograde flow.

Aortic root = 3.3 ± 4 cm (SD)

Ascending aorta–mid = 3.0 ± 0.4 cm

Ascending aorta–pre-arch = 3.0 ± 0.4 cm

Aortic arch = 2.7 ± 0.4 cm

Descending aorta = 2.4 ± 0.4 cm

The normal dimensions of the thoracic aorta defined by angiography as reported by Dotter and Steinberg are:[21]

Ascending aorta = 28.6 mm (range = 16–38 mm)

Aortic arch = 24.8 mm (range = 13–34 mm)

Descending aorta = 22.9 mm (range = 12–32 mm)

An aortic diameter greater than 4 cm is generally considered dilated. However, many older patients, especially those with systemic hypertension, have aortic diameters greater than 4 cm and do not have primary aortic disease. Most authorities would agree that a localized dilatation exceeding 5 cm constitutes an aneurysm, whereas diffuse dilatation up to this dimension would be termed aneurysmal dilatation or a diffuse aneurysm.

The aorta has three layers: intima, media, and adventitia. The thick tunica media is composed predominantly of intertwined elastic tissue and little muscle. Nutrient vessels course in the aortic wall, the vaso vasorum.

Acquired Diseases

Aortic Dissection. The classification schemes for aortic dissection are shown in Figure 6-5.[22,23] The important clinical feature is whether the dissection involves the ascending aorta (DeBakey type I and II or Stanford type A) or is confined to the descending aorta and posterior aortic arch (DeBakey type III and Stanford type B).

Over 95% of dissections arise either in the ascending aorta within several centimeters of the aortic valve (type A), or in the descending thoracic aorta at a point just beyond the origin of the left subclavian artery at the site of the ligamentum arteriosum (type B).[24] Spontaneous dissection originating in the abdominal aorta or a major branch of the thoracic or abdominal aorta occurs, but is rare. Multiple entry and reentry points can be found frequently at autopsy and sometimes defined by angiography.[26,27] Two-thirds of dissections involve the ascending aorta. However, because the type A dissection can be rapidly lethal secondary to intrapericardial rupture and cardiac tamponade, many clinical series report a misleadingly high frequency of type B dissections. Without treatment, acute dissection of the ascending aorta is almost always rapidly fatal. Death will follow in more than 25% of patients with type A dissections within 24 hours and more than 75% within the first month after the acute event.[28]

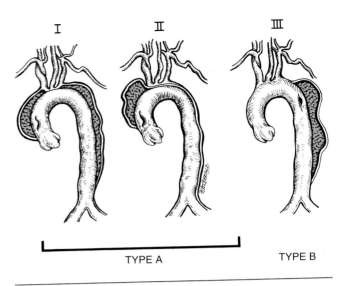

Figure 6-5. The types of aortic dissection. The DeBakey classification of aortic dissections recognizes types I, II, and III whereas the Stanford classification recognizes types A and B. Types I and II of DeBakey are equivalent to type A in the Stanford classification and type III is equivalent to type B.

The extent and site of the false channel is variable. Dissection usually involves the right anterior aspect of the ascending aorta and the posterior left lateral aspect of the descending aorta. Dissection of the left side of the abdominal aorta with ischemia of the left renal artery in the false channel is the most common version of a very variable pattern.[29]

Predisposing factors usually exist, of which the most common is hypertension. In young adults the predisposing factors are Marfan's or Ehlers–Danlos syndrome and pregnancy. Aortic valve disease is another predisposing factor. Giant cell arteritis may rarely be the predisposing factor. Dissection can also be caused by trauma during catheterization and surgery, especially coronary bypass graft operation.

It is unclear whether the primary event in spontaneous dissection is rupture of the intima with secondary extension into the media, or hemorrhage within a diseased media followed by disruption of the adjacent intima and subsequent propagation through the intimal tear. A recent report has demonstrated several cases of intramural hematoma of the thoracic aorta, of which some progressed to intimal rupture.[30] This finding suggests that a primary intramural hemorrhage is the initiating factor in at least some cases.

Goals of imaging studies are to identify:[31]

1. The intimal flap.
2. The extent of the dissection.
3. Involvement of aortic branches.
4. Patency of the false channel.
5. Periaortic hematoma or hemorrhagic pericardial effusion.

6. Significant aortic regurgitation.

7. Unusual complications.

Salient aortographic findings are:[25,26,27]

1. Intimal flap (Fig. 6-6). Biplane aortography is essential in order to ensure imaging perpendicular to the unpredictable position and course of the flap.

2. Delayed opacification and clearance of contrast medium from the false channel (Fig. 6-7).

3. Compression of the true lumen by a thrombosed false channel (Figs. 6-6; 6-7*D,E;* 6-8).

4. Extensive soft tissue shadow beyond the edge of the opacified aorta (see Fig. 6-7*D,E*).

5. Occlusion of the aortic branches. Asymmetric opacification of intercostal arteries may be a diagnostic clue.

6. Displacement of the catheter from the left lateral edge of the posterior aortic arch shadow (see Fig. 6-7*E*).

7. Aortic regurgitation associated with visualization of the flap in the sinus portion of the aorta (see Fig. 6-6*D*).

8. An ulcerlike projection from the opacified aorta may be an early sign of dissection or could be caused by nearly complete thrombosis of the false channel.[32]

Salient CT and MRI features are:

1. Intimal flap (Figs. 6-9 through 6-12).

2. Hematoma in the aortic wall. This has been detected with both CT and MRI and is probably the initial stage of some dissections.[30]

3. Differential blood flow in the true and false channel. CT shows different density of the two channels by the contrast medium and variable time-related enhancement and clearance of density of the two channels (see Fig. 6-11). Spin echo MRI may show signal in the false channel when the blood flow rate is below a threshold value (Figs. 6-4, 6-12, 6-13). Phase images can be calibrated in order to depict the difference in flow velocity in the two channels (see Figs. 6-4, 6-13) and have been used to distinguish between slow flow and thrombus.[33] The MR flow velocity maps display differences in flow velocity in the two channels and can even be used to measure the velocity or flow rate in the two channels (see Figs. 6-4, 6-13). These velocity maps are generated using a new MRI technique called velocity-encoded cine MRI.[34] The velocity map images can also be used to distinguish slow blood flow from thrombus in the false channels.[35,36] Velocity-encoded cine MRI scans have been used to plot simultaneously velocity-versus-time curves in the true and false channels.[36] With this technique peak velocity is shown to be lower in the false channel and a divergent phasic pattern is displayed in the two channels (see Figs. 6-4, 6-13).

4. Periaortic hematoma or pericardial hematoma. High-intensity fluid in CT indicates acute hemorrhage. High intensity of fluid on spin echo MRI scans with short

TR and TE intervals is characteristic for blood (Fig. 6-14), although the age of the blood is a variable, influencing its appearance.

5. Extent of dissection. Tomographic images can readily define the flap in the ascending aorta as well as the distal extent. The sagittal, oblique sagittal, and coronal MRI scans can display the position of the flap relative to the arch branches (Figs. 6-10, 6-15).

6. Compression of the true lumen by thrombosed false lumen (Fig. 6-16).

The potential pitfalls in the diagnosis of dissection by tomographic methods are:[37]

1. Linear artifacts coursing through the aorta can be mistaken for an intimal flap. High-density artifacts emanating from opacified venous structures on CT scans can cause this; artifacts originating from the edge of the opacified superior vena cava or brachiocephalic vein and from the pulmonary veins are the most common causes. Signal from slowly flowing blood can cause troublesome intraluminal signal on MRI scans (see Fig. 6-10*A*).

2. Periaortic structures can be misconstrued as the aortic wall. This problem has been caused by fluid in the superior pericardial recess on both CT and MRI (Fig. 6-17).

3. Inward projection of mural calcifications by partial volume errors caused by a tortuous aorta.

The differentiation of a dissection with thrombosed false channel from an aneurysm with extensive mural thrombus can be problematic for any imaging test. The CT and MRI features (see Fig. 6-8) that may aid in this differential diagnosis are:

1. A compressed as well as an eccentric or distorted contour of the aorta is consistent with dissection with clotted false channel, while a dilated and concentric lumen suggests an aneurysm with mural thrombus.

2. Eccentric wall thickening extending over more than 6 cm suggests dissection with thrombosed false channel.

Now that effective therapy has permitted the survival of many patients with dissection, long-term complications of dissection are emerging that can also be effectively evaluated by CT and MRI. Several studies have shown that the false lumen remains open in the majority of patients after surgical treatment of dissection (Fig. 6-18), with either increase or decrease in size of the false lumen over time. Such studies have also revealed the deposition and growth of thrombus in the false lumen.[15,38–42]

CT and MRI have now become well established and definitive imaging modalities for studying thoracic aortic disease, and have been employed widely for the evaluation of suspected dissection. A number of papers have shown that CT and MRI are at least as accurate for the

(*Text continues on page 188*)

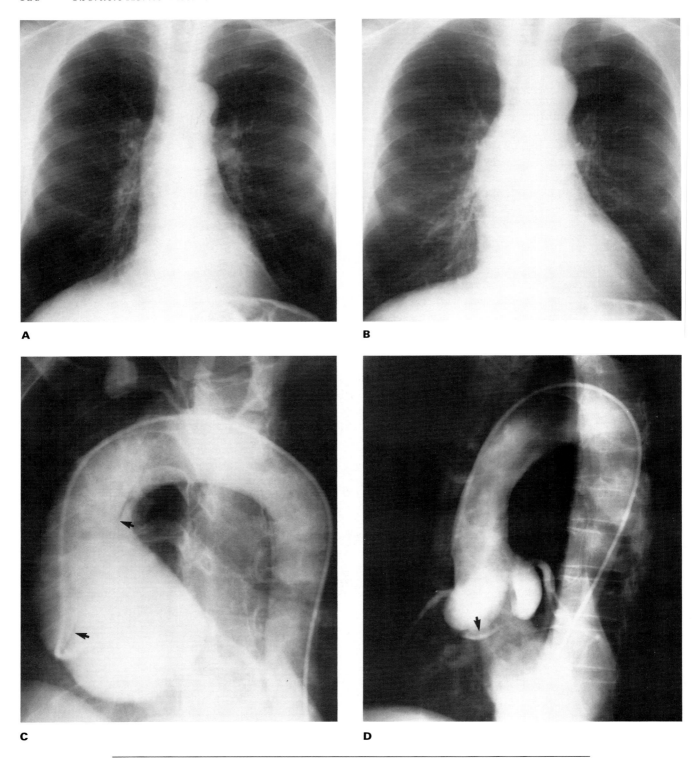

Figure 6-6. Thoracic radiographs and angiograms in aortic dissection. Comparison of an early (*A*) and later (*B*) radiograph in the same patient demonstrates interval increase in the size of the entire thoracic aorta and an interval increase in cardiac size. These findings suggest aortic dissection but are not diagnostic of this abnormality, since this pattern can occur in other abnormalities as well. Aortogram in the same patient (*C*) demonstrates an intimal flap (*arrow*) coursing through the ascending aorta. This indicates a type II or type A aortic dissection. Aortogram in another patient (*D*) demonstrates flattening of the contour of the ascending aorta and an intimal flap (*arrow*) visible only within the sinuses of Valsalva. Coronary arteries are shown to be patent.

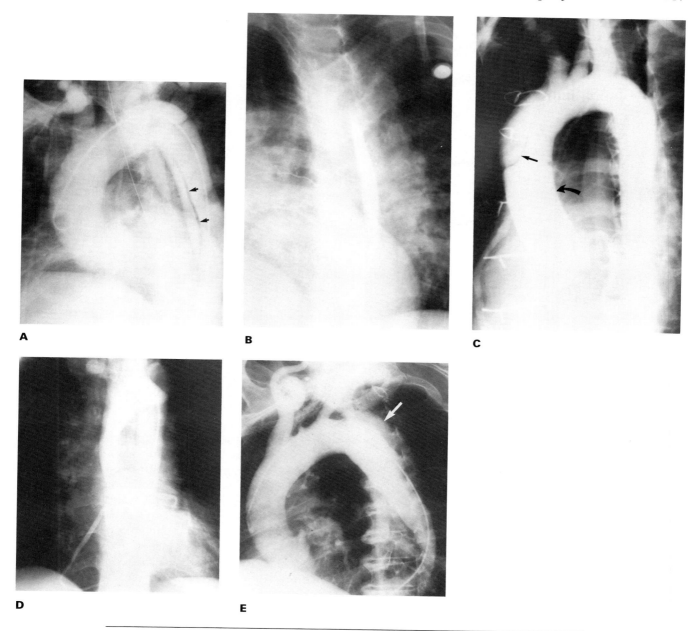

Figure 6-7. Aortograms in patients with type B aortic dissection (*A, B*) and a patient after repair of a type A dissection (*C*). The radiograph obtained during the early period of opacification of the thoracic aorta (*A*) demonstrates an intimal flap (*arrow*) coursing through the descending thoracic aorta. This indicates the presence of a type III or type B aortic dissection. A radiograph obtained later, after the injection of contrast medium, demonstrates persistence of the contrast medium within the false channel. Aortogram performed in another patient after repair of aortic dissection demonstrates the graft (*curved arrow*) in the proximal portion of the ascending aorta and demonstrates persistence of the intimal flap (*arrow*). This indicates that the false channel remains patent after surgical intervention. *D:* A frontal view of aortogram in another patient with type A (type II) shows compression of true channel. The false channel is not opacified. *E:* Right posterior oblique view of thoracic aortogram shows type B dissection with wide soft tissue shadow (*arrows*) extending beyond the opacified aortic lumen.

DISSECTION
- THROMBOSED
  FALSE
  CHANNEL

ANEURYSM
- MURAL
  THROMBUS

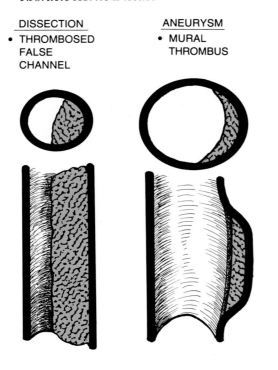

Figure 6-8. Diagram demonstrates the differential characteristics between thrombosis of a false channel of a type B dissection and thrombus laminated on the wall of a descending thoracic aortic aneurysm. In general, thrombosis of the false channel extends over a greater length and produces narrowing and compression of the opacified aortic lumen, and the aortic lumen is usually reduced rather than increased in size. In an aneurysm with thrombus, the length of the thrombus is less, the aortic lumen retains a concentric contour, and is increased in diameter.

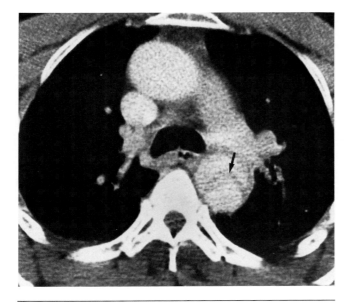

Figure 6-9. CT scan of the thoracic aorta in aortic dissection. Intimal flap (*arrow*) is visualized in the descending aorta. Intimal flap is outlined by contrast medium opacifying both the true and false lumen.

detection, determination of extent, and identification of complications of dissection as aortography.[1–4,7,14]

Thoracic Aortic Aneurysm. A true aneurysm of the thoracic aorta is an enlargement exceeding 4 cm in diameter and consisting of all three mural layers. The type, location, and extent of a thoracic aortic aneurysm is primarily determined by its etiology. Atherosclerosis is now the leading cause of such aneurysms. Since this process predominates in the arch and descending aorta, atherosclerotic aneurysms in the ascending aorta are less common. These aneurysms are often fusiform because atherosclerosis affects long segments of the aorta circumferentially. Many are actually thoracoabdominal aneurysms. Aneurysms developing in association with cystic medial necrosis and syphilis predominate in the ascending aorta. Aneurysm of the thoracic aorta can be caused by systemic connective tissue diseases such as relapsing polychondritis. Saccular aneurysms may be more prone to rupture and always raise the possibility of a false aneurysm (pseudoaneurysm). This appearance should suggest the possibility of mycotic aneurysm.

Aneurysms develop insidiously, the majority of patients being asymptomatic, and the aneurysms detected incidentally on chest radiograph.[43] A 27% five-year survival rate for patients with symptoms, as opposed to 58% in the absence of symptoms, has been reported in patients with thoracic aneurysms.[44] In the evaluation of aneurysms, size is important prognostically and in preoperative evaluation.[44–46] Overall, 30% to 50% of deaths from thoracic aortic aneurysm result from rupture. While less information is available in the natural history of thoracic aortic aneurysm compared to abdominal aortic aneurysms, it appears that rupture rarely occurs in aneurysms less than 5 cm in diameter, and ruptured aneurysms usually exceed 6 cm in diameter. The combination of chronic dissection and aneurysm of the descending aorta is occasionally encountered.

Aneurysms rupture into the pericardial or pleural space, trachea or bronchi, mediastinum, or adjacent vessels. An aortovascular fistula can form with a pulmonary artery or superior vena cava. Ascending aortic aneurysms usually rupture into the pericardium or right pleural space, and the descending aorta tends to rupture into the left pleural space.

The morphologic classification divides aneurysms into fusiform and saccular. Fusiform aneurysms involve the entire circumference of the aorta and tend to be more extensive. Saccular aneurysms involve only a portion of the circumference and are generally localized.

Salient aortographic findings are:[47,48]

1. Localized or diffuse dilatation of the thoracic aorta. Although a value of 4 cm is considered the upper

(*Text continues on page 192*)

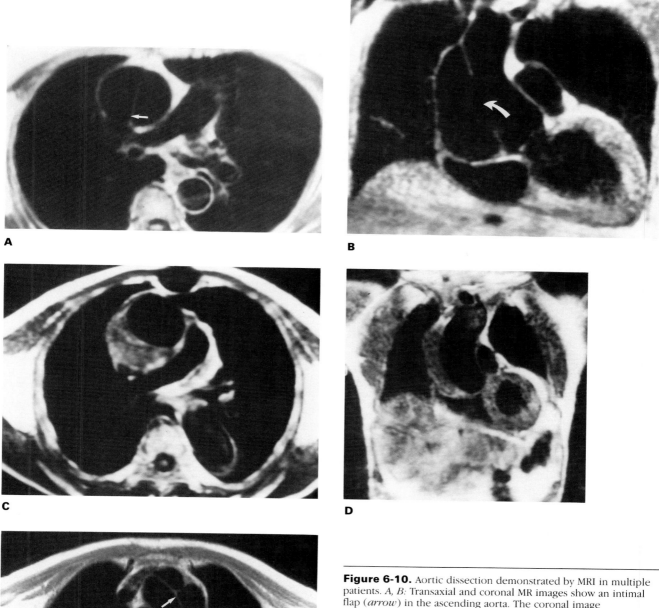

Figure 6-10. Aortic dissection demonstrated by MRI in multiple patients. *A, B:* Transaxial and coronal MR images show an intimal flap (*arrow*) in the ascending aorta. The coronal image demonstrates aneurysmal dilatation of the ascending aorta, a large entry point (*curved arrow*) between the true and false channel rendered visible by the flow void in both the true and false channels. *C, D:* Transverse and coronal images of type A aortic dissection. Images demonstrate a false channel filled with thrombus. Transverse image indicates loss of concentric contour of the ascending aorta. Coronal image demonstrates the extent of the thrombus, which begins at the level just above the aortic valve and extends to the aortic arch. *E:* Transaxial image demonstrates an intimal flap (*arrow*) extending across the aortic arch and into the descending aorta. The intimal flap is visible because of the signal void in both the true and false channels.

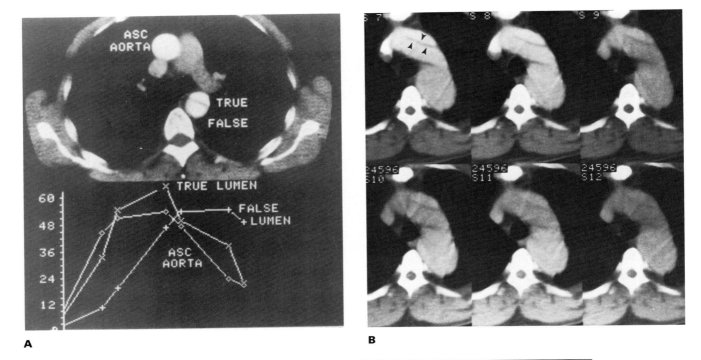

Figure 6-11. *A:* CT scan of the thorax demonstrates an intimal flap separating the true and false channels (*upper panel*). Opacification of both channels makes the intimal flap between the two readily visible. Time–density curve in the lower panel shows the CT numbers plotted on the vertical axis versus the time after injection of contrast media on the horizontal axis. The curves for the true and false lumen indicate disparate pattern of opacification with slower initial opacification of the false channel, causing it to reach peak density later than the true channel, and persistence of opacification of the false channel after clearance of contrast medium from the true lumen. *B:* Series of CT scans during the passage of contrast medium through the thoracic aorta demonstrates the intimal flap in the proximal portion of the aortic arch (*arrows*). After clearance of contrast medium from the true lumen there is persistent increased density in the false channel, indicating slower flow velocity in the false channel.

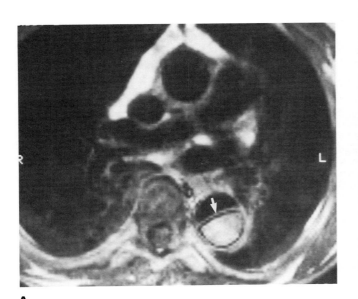

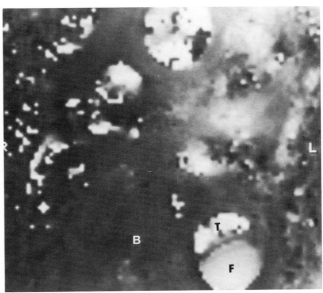

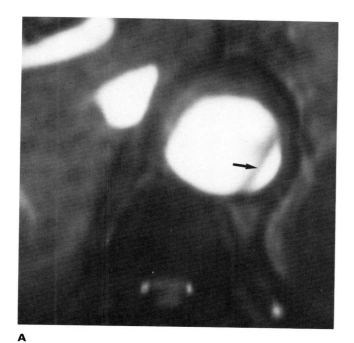

A

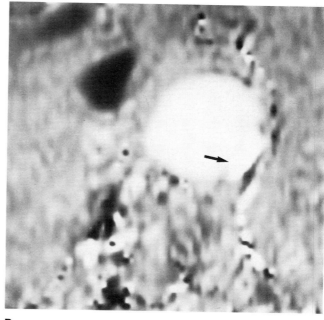

B

Average Velocity in True and False Channel

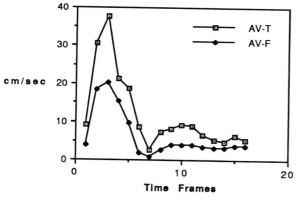

C

Figure 6-13. Cine MR intensity and phase images of a patient with aortic dissection. The MR intensity images (*A*) acquired with the gradient echo technique produces substantial contrast relative to the intimal flap (arrow) and renders the intimal flap readily visible. The phase image (*B*) displays the relative velocity of the two channels. Notice that the brightness of the two channels on the phase image is variable. This indicates variable velocity in the two channels, as would be expected with aortic dissection. *C:* Velocity versus time curve for the true and false lumen obtained from regions of interest placed within the true and false channel on the velocity-encoded cine MR phase image in the same patient. This plot was generated by measuring the velocities in the two channels on the phase images, which were acquired at multiple phases of the cardiac cycle using the cine MRI technique. The graph compares flow velocity in the false and true channels.

Figure 6-12. MR intensity (*A*) and phase image (*B*) MR images of the thorax demonstrate a dissection of the descending aorta. The intimal flap (*arrow*) is depicted separating the true and false channels. The true channel on the magnitude image demonstrates a normal signal void while the false channel demonstrates signal within the lumen. The phase image demonstrates that the signal within the false channel (F) is caused by slow blood flow. The phase image depicts voxels in which motion is absent as dark gray coloration. An example of this is the vertebral body (B). The voxels within the ascending and descending aorta, as well as other vessels, demonstrate either white or black signal, indicating movement of blood within these structures. Note that the signal of voxels representative of the true channel (T) is brighter than those for the false channel. This indicates a slower rate of blood flow within the false as compared to the true channel and the ascending aorta. The phase map was done using a technique that does not distinguish between antegrade and retrograde blood flow but merely distinguishes between voxels containing motion and indicates the relative velocity of this motion. (Reproduced with permission from Higgins EB, Hricak H. Magnetic Resonance Imaging of the Body. New York: Raven Press, 1987.)

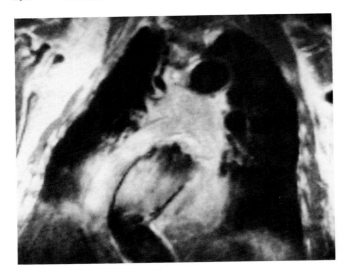

Figure 6-14. Coronal MR image. A patient with mediastinal hematoma caused by rupture of thoracic aortic aneurysm. The fluid surrounding the aorta on this T₁-weighted image has a signal intensity similar to or slightly less than subcutaneous fat. High signal intensity of fluid on a T₁-weighted image is characteristic for blood.

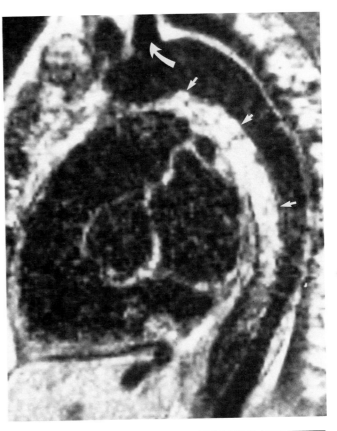

Figure 6-15. Sagittal MR image in type B aortic dissection. The false channel contains considerable signal due to slow blood flow and thrombus (*arrows*). The sagittal image shows the point of origin of the left subclavian artery (*curved arrow*) and indicates that the aortic dissection begins on the undersurface of the aortic arch just opposite the origin of the subclavian artery.

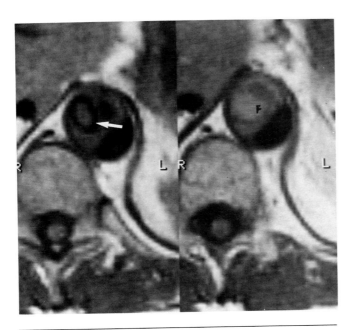

Figure 6-16. Aortic dissection with thrombus of most of the false channel. The image on the left was located approximately 1 cm proximal to the one on the right. The false channel (F) is nearly completely filled with thrombus. There is a small region within the center of the false channel in which a signal void (*arrow*) is produced by flowing blood. Note that the thrombus-filled false channel has caused eccentric contour and compression of the true channel. This appearance is characteristic for aortic dissection with thrombus of the false channel rather than thoracic aortic aneurysm with mural thrombus.

limit of aortic diameter, most diagnosticians would not invoke the term aneurysm until the aorta exceeds 5 cm in diameter. The fusiform aneurysm involves the full circumference of the aorta (Fig. 6-19). The saccular aneurysm involves only part of the circumference; it bulges from one side of the aorta (Fig. 6-20). Sometimes nearly the entire volume of the saccular aneurysm is filled with thrombus so that little contrast medium enters it; consequently, the true size and even the presence of saccular aneurysm may not be accurately defined by aortography (Fig. 6-21).

2. Extent of aneurysm and relationship to arch branches is depicted on the right posterior oblique view (see Fig. 6-20).

3. Relationship to surrounding structures such as bronchi, pulmonary arteries, and vertebral bodies (erosion). Rupture of the aneurysm into a pulmonary artery or superior vena cava is indicated by an aortovascular fistula.

4. Expanded soft-tissue shadow and calcification extending beyond the opacified lumen (Fig. 6-21). This may indicate extensive mural thrombus so that the diameter

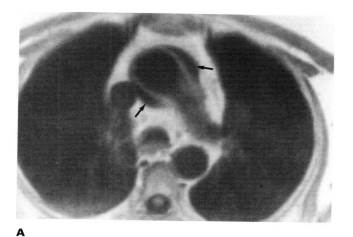

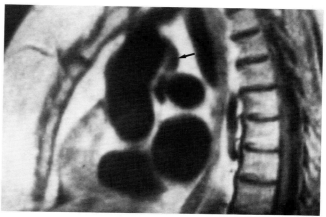

A

B

Figure 6-17. Diagnostic pitfall in the evaluation of aortic dissection with MRI. Transaxial (*A*) and sagittal (*B*) MR images demonstrate fluid within the superior pericardial recess (*arrow*) in a patient with acute pericarditis as the cause of chest pain. The low signal intensity of the superior pericardial recess surrounding the aorta must be recognized and distinguished from concentric intimal flap. The wall of the thoracic aorta separating the fluid-filled superior pericardial recess and the aortic lumen can be mistaken for an intimal flap. This pitfall can be avoided by recognizing the normal concentric appearance of the ascending aorta and by examining caudal slices at the level of the heart, which readily depict the pericardial effusion. The sagittal image demonstrates the fluid-filled sac (*arrow*) located between the right pulmonary and the ascending aorta.

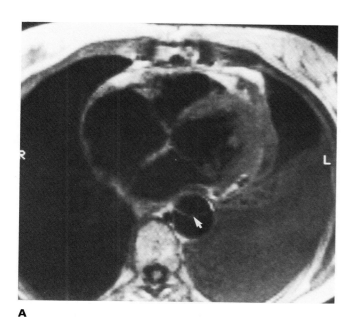

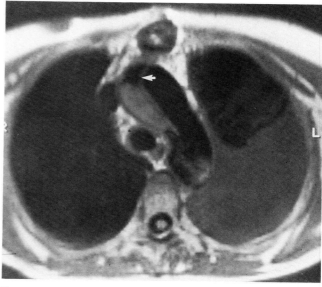

A

B

Figure 6-18. Transverse MR images through the region of the aortic arch (*A*) and descending aorta (*B*) in the early postoperative period after repair of aortic dissection. A persistent intimal flap (*arrows*) is recognized extending across the aortic arch and separating the true and false channels within the descending aorta. There is signal within the false channel due to slow blood flow. Note also the considerable thickening of the pericardium and the left pleural effusion.

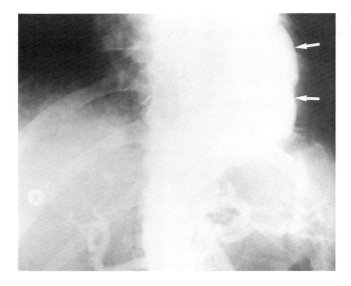

Figure 6-19. Angiographic frame shows fusiform thoracoabdominal aneurysm (*arrows*).

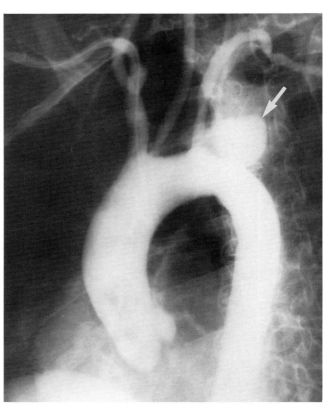

Figure 6-20. Angiographic frame demonstrates a saccular aneurysm (*arrow*) arising from the aortic arch just beyond the origin of the left subclavian artery. Because the ostium or neck of the aneurysm is small in diameter a mycotic aneurysm is suggested.

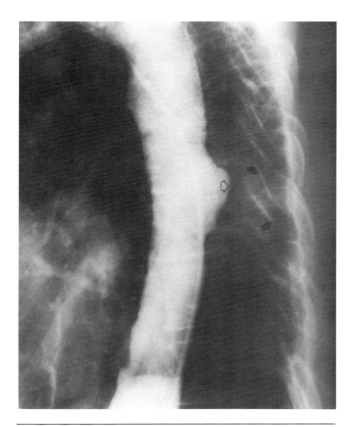

Figure 6-21. Angiographic frame shows a saccular aneurysm of the descending thoracic aorta. Note that the edge of the aneurysm is represented by soft tissue (*black arrows*), which extends considerably beyond the opacified lumen (*open arrow*) of the aneurysm. A substantial portion of the aneurysm has been obliterated by mural thrombus.

of the opacified aortic lumen underestimates the maximal diameter of the aneurysm.

5. Contrast medium extending beyond the wall of the aneurysm or recognition of disruption of the aneurysmal wall is a sign of rupture but is rarely observed because the active bleeding associated with it is rapidly fatal. A localized bulge on the aneurysm itself (aneurysm on aneurysm) has been taken as a sign of impending rupture. In a patient with acute chest pain, this finding must be considered a sign of leakage. Pleural effusion and displacement of mediastinal structures (i.e., trachea) may be indirect signs of leaking aneurysms.

6. Since about 50% of patients with an atherosclerotic thoracic aortic aneurysm also have an abdominal aortic aneurysm, aortography of the abdominal aorta is useful.

Salient CT and MRI findings are:[49–51]

1. Transverse diameter of the aorta exceeding 4 cm by definition and 5 cm by practicality. Fusiform aneurysms can be clearly distinguished from saccular aneurysms by demonstrating the presence (Fig. 6-22) or ab-

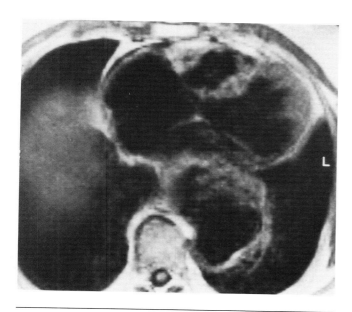

Figure 6-22. Transverse MR image of a fusiform aneurysm of the descending thoracic aorta. The large aneurysm produces compression of the left atrium. Signal within the lumen of the aneurysm is due to slow blood flow.

sence of involvement of the circumference of the aorta (Fig. 6-23). The approximately symmetrical dilatation of the aorta in fusiform aneurysms (Figs. 6-14, 6-22) and asymmetric bulging of the aorta in saccular aneurysms (Fig. 6-23) is very clearly depicted on sagittal and coronal MRI. Transverse CT and MRI tomograms are more accurate for determining the maximum diameter of the aneurysm than aortography, since they display the outer wall as well as the patent lumen within the aneurysm.

2. Extent of aneurysm and relationship to the arch branches can be defined from the stack of CT scans and MRI scans extending from above the arch to the diaphragm or below, if needed. The relationship of the aneurysm to the arch branches is effectively demonstrated on sagittal or oblique sagittal MRI (see Fig. 6-23).

3. Transverse tomograms are the most effective images for defining the relationship of the aneurysm to adjacent mediastinal structures such as the bronchi and pulmonary arteries and to the vertebral bodies and ribs (see Fig. 6-22). Transverse CT scans and MRI scans are far more effective for defining the effect on and relationship to adjacent structures than is aortography.

4. Mural thrombus in the aneurysm. Thrombus is displayed best on transverse tomograms. This is represented by a filling defect in the opacified channel on CT. MRI displays the mural thrombus as variable intensity depending upon its age (Figs. 6-24, 6-25). Subacute thrombus has high intensity on spin echo images, whereas chronic thrombus has low intensity on both T_1- and T_2-weighted images. A mural thrombus may be composed of both high- and low-intensity layers when it has two

vintages of thrombus (Figs. 6-24, 6-26). Imaging of a saccular aneurysm with thrombus could appear like a solid mass on coronal images (Fig. 6-26). Differentiation of slow blood flow in an aneurysm from mural thrombus can be accomplished using MR phase images or cine MRI (ECG-referenced repetitive gradient echo images). The thrombus has very low intensity on the cine MRI.[52]

5. Periaortic hematoma is recognized as high-density fluid on CT scan and high-intensity fluid on T_1-weighted MRI (Fig. 6-14). Fluid in the pleural or extrapleural spaces may also be discerned as blood on these scans. A localized bulge on the aneurysm is readily identified on transverse tomograms. Disruption of the aortic wall is not usually shown because the perforation is usually small and the tomographic thickness blurs this finding.

6. Calcification of the outer edge of the aneurysm is readily demonstrated on CT scans. Marginal calcification occurs in aneurysms, whereas inwardly displaced mural calcification may indicate dissection. Tortuosity of a segment, common in the aneurysmal aorta, may result in the erroneous appearance of inward displacement due to partial volume effects.

Thoracic Aortic Trauma. Aortic trauma can be caused by blunt or penetrating trauma. Blunt rupture of the thoracic aorta may result from a severe deceleration injury, and has been found in one-sixth of fatalities of automobile accidents.[53] Thoracic aortic injuries are also found in victims of falls from great heights and explosions. About one-third of patients with aortic injury also have a cardiac injury.[54] Although the thoracic aorta may be torn anywhere along its length, the most common point of rupture is in the aortic isthmus at the site of insertion of the ligamentum arteriosum just distal to the origin of the left subclavian artery. This is the site of approximately 90% of such injuries to the thoracic aorta.[54] At this point the more mobile ascending aorta and arch join the descending aorta, which is immobilized by the ligamentum arteriosus and the investing pleura. The next most common site is the proximal ascending aorta, where the intrapericardial location causes rapid death due to pericardial tamponade. A circumferential tear, constituting a complete transection, is found in 80% of cases of acute blunt aortic trauma.[55]

Approximately 80% of such patients will die immediately, although usually from other injuries, such as massive hemorrhage at other sites.[56] Of those who survive the initial event, death often occurs from progressive hemorrhage at the site of aortic tear within the first week. Accordingly, aggressive and expedient diagnosis of aortic transection followed by immediate surgical repair is essential. About 2% to 5% of patients with partially transected aorta will survive and develop pseudoaneurysms.

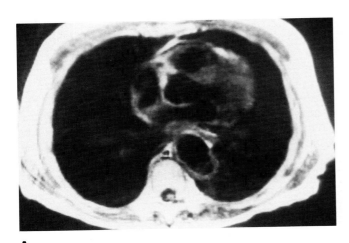

A

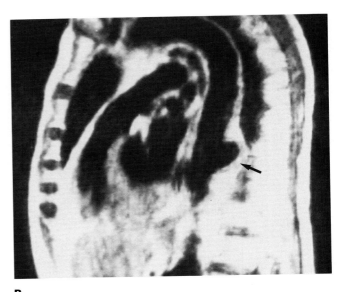

B

Figure 6-23. Transverse (*A*) and sagittal (*B*) MR images demonstrate a saccular aneurysm of the descending thoracic aorta. Sagittal image demonstrates the wide neck between the descending aorta and the aneurysm. A small amount of mural thrombus causes thickening of the posterior wall of the aneurysm (*arrow*). The maximum aneurysmal dimension is measured from the anterior aspect of the aorta to the posterior aspect of the aneurysm. Thus, the maximum diameter of the aorta at the site of the aneurysm is used to calculate the diameter of a saccular aneurysm. This measurement is important because the wall stress of the aneurysm is directly proportional to the maximum diameter of the aneurysm, and this parameter indicates the likelihood of aneurysmal rupture.

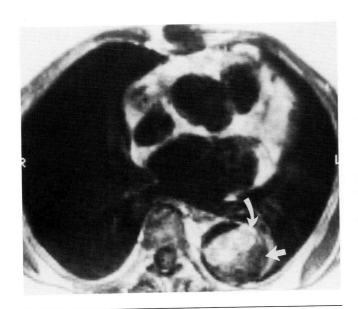

Figure 6-24. Transverse MR image in a patient with aortic dissection with obliteration of the false channel by subacute and old thrombus. The old thrombus produces a very low MR signal intensity (*arrow*), whereas the subacute thrombus has bright intensity (*curved arrow*). Note the compression of the true lumen by the thrombus-filled false lumen.

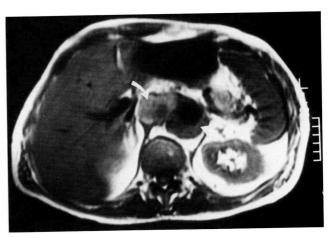

Figure 6-25. Transverse MR image shows a thoracoabdominal aneurysm with a considerable amount of thrombus (*arrow*) laminated on the wall of the aneurysm. The lumen is of normal or slightly increased dimension and retains a concentric contour. Note also the clotted hematoma (*curved arrow*) adjacent to the aortic aneurysm. The hematoma has split the fibers of the right crus of the diaphragm.

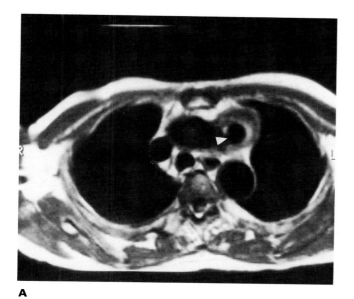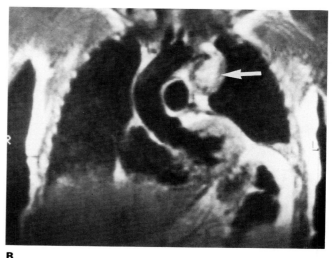

A **B**

Figure 6-26. Transverse (*A*) and coronal (*B*) MR images demonstrating a saccular aneurysm arising from the undersurface of the aortic arch. A considerable portion of the aneurysm has been obliterated by laminated mural thrombus. Note also that the ostium (*arrowhead*) connecting the aortic lumen and the aneurysm is small in diameter, suggesting a mycotic aneurysm. Coronal image demonstrates the mural thrombus and slow blood flow within the lumen of the aneurysm (*arrow*). The signal produced by the in-plane direction of blood flow at a slow velocity causes the aneurysm to have an appearance that could be mistaken for a solid structure on images done in a single plane. The coronal image demonstrates clearly that the aneurysm arises distal to the origin of the arch vessels.

Such aneurysms may remain small, but some expand progressively and may manifest delayed rupture.

Tomographic imaging modalities are suboptimal for detecting a tear in the transverse plane of the aorta because of imaging parallel to the tear and because the thickness of the tomogram may not identify the thin tear. For these reasons and because acute disruption is an emergency, aortography remains the imaging procedure of choice and should be performed immediately if such injury is suspected.[2,57] Additional problems with the evaluation of traumatic aortic disruption by CT, and presumably by MRI, are that subtle changes in aortic contour indicating transection with localized dilatation may be missed on a series of contiguous transaxial images because of the complicated anatomy of the distal arch and the difficulties in scanning traumatized patients. The sagittal MRI scan may obviate this pitfall but patients in the early period after trauma cannot be easily studied by MRI. Although CT and MRI are effective for identification of a mediastinal hematoma, this does not mean necessarily that the aorta is the site of hemorrhage. It may arise from damage to small mediastinal vessels that do not require surgical repair.

Penetrating trauma of the thoracic aorta or its branch arteries may be caused by puncture or laceration by foreign objects. Massive hemorrhage, often leading to rapidly fatal exsanguination, is common and requires im-

mediate surgical repair. Aortography remains the only proven reliable method for evaluating aortic trauma.

MRI and CT can be used effectively for the evaluation of chronic pseudoaneurysms caused by aortic trauma.

Salient aortographic findings are:

1. Discontinuity between the two components of the aorta may be observed in complete transection. A focal segment of dilatation and mural irregularity represents the disrupted segment between the two ends of the transected aorta (Fig. 6-27). The length of the disruption can be several centimeters due to retraction of the descending aorta after complete transection. The fusiform aneurysm between the separated parts of the aorta is a false aneurysm. Disruption of part of the aortic circumference produces a saccular false aneurysm.

2. Focal irregularity or a transverse lucent band across the aortic lumen is diagnostic. This abnormality usually occurs within a few centimeters of the origin of the left subclavian artery (site of ligamentum arteriosus).

3. Occlusion of the aorta at the site of transection is due to compression of the aorta by a periaortic hematoma.

4. Focal dissection is indicated by an intimal flap.[58] The flap may not be visible with intramural hematoma.

5. A large focal fusiform or saccular aneurysm at the

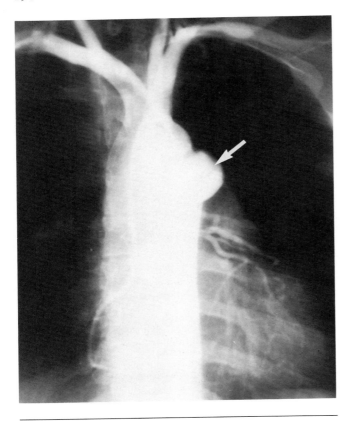

Figure 6-27. Frontal aortogram demonstrates traumatic disruption of the proximal portion of the descending thoracic aorta. Complete transection of the thoracic aorta has produced a pseudoaneurysm (*arrow*) between the two ends of the disruption. The pseudoaneurysm is located at the site of attachment of ligamentum arteriosus, which is the most common site of traumatic rupture of the aorta.

site of ligamentum arteriosus is observed in chronic pseudoaneurysm (Fig. 6-28). The saccular aneurysm usually extends anteriorly from the aorta.

Salient CT and MRI findings are:

1. Periaortic blood can be recognized on CT and MRI as discussed above (see Fig. 6-14).

2. Focal irregular dilatation may be observed in complete transection. CT has not been sufficiently accurate for use in the diagnosis or exclusion of acute traumatic rupture of the aorta.

3. Focal fusiform or saccular pseudoaneurysms are shown on transverse CT or MRI tomograms and are well demonstrated on sagittal MRI. The sagittal image demonstrates the relationship of the pseudoaneurysm to the arch branches.

Aortoanular Ectasia. Aortoanular ectasia is a degenerative disease that causes progressive dilatation of the aortic annulus, sinuses of Valsalva, and proximal ascending aorta.[59,60] It is frequently associated with

elongation and dilatation of the entire aorta, a disease sometimes called arteriomegaly. It frequently produces progressive aortic regurgitation. The pathologic process is cystic medial necrosis and among the complications of this disease are aortic dissection and aortic rupture. Dilatation of the aortic annulus causes separation of the cusps and results in aortic regurgitation. Silent as well as symptomatic dissection occurs in this disease. Although patients with Marfan's syndrome are afflicted with this pathology and this aortic morphology, only a minority of patients with aortoannular ectasia have a diagnosis of Marfan's syndrome or any somatic features of this syndrome. A rare cause of aortoannular ectasia is hemocystinuria. Aortoannular ectasia has a marked male predominance and the disease usually appears in the fourth to the sixth decade. This disease shows variable progression with increasing aortic dilatation and worsening aortic regurgitation. This disease is now recognized as the most common cause of descending aortic aneurysm and acquired aortic regurgitation in the middle-aged and elderly population.

The thoracic radiograph may reveal progressive enlargement of the thoracic aorta in an otherwise asymptomatic person. Even after aortic valve replacement, progressive ascending aortic enlargement is observed and may require subsequent graft replacement.[61]

Salient angiographic features are:

1. Dilatation of the sinuses of Valsalva and the ascending aorta (Fig. 6-29). Lemon and White in 1978 described three angiographic patterns consisting of pear-shaped enlargement of the aorta (56%), diffuse symmetrical dilatation (27%), and dilatation of the sinuses of Valsalva only (6%).[60] The pattern is not specific in the remaining percentage. The severity of the dilatation may be enormous. Sequential studies may reveal progressive enlargement.

2. Depiction of intimal flap when silent or symptomatic dissection is present.

3. Elongation and tortuosity of the entire aorta and its branches.

4. Aortic regurgitation. The report by Lemon and White showed that the aortic root diameter was a mean of 7.6 cm (range = 4.8–15 cm) in patients with aortic regurgitation due to aortoannular ectasia compared to a mean of 4.2 cm in patients with aortic regurgitation of other causes.

Salient CT and MRI features are:

1. Dilatation of the sinuses of Valsalva and the ascending aorta (Figs. 6-30, 6-31). The typical pattern can also be discerned on the transverse tomograms. However, the morphology of the aorta is depicted especially well on sagittal or oblique sagittal MRI. Both transverse and sagittal MRI scans are good for precisely measuring the aortic dimension and for monitoring the dimension

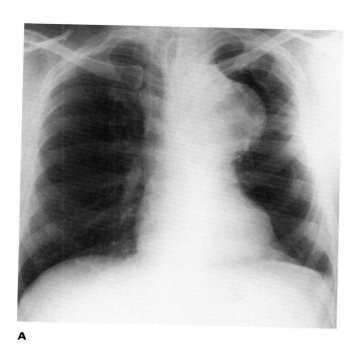

A

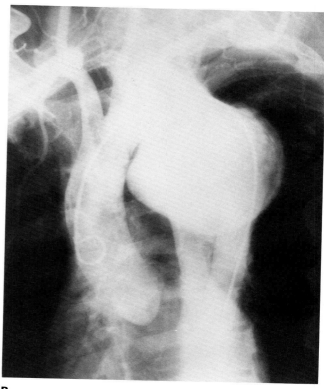

B

Figure 6-28. Frontal radiograph (*A*) and aortogram in the right posterior oblique view (*B*) demonstrate a calcified chronic pseudoaneurysm at the proximal descending thoracic aorta. This is the typical appearance and location of a chronic pseudoaneurysm caused by trauma.

over time. The completely noninvasive nature of MRI makes it ideal for monitoring the progressive disease.

2. Detection of intimal flap and false channel when this complication occurs (see Fig. 6-11).

3. Elongation and tortuosity of the entire aorta and its branches.

Aortic Inflammatory Disease (Aortitis). Aortitis is usually part of a systemic arteritis syndrome or generalized disease of connective tissue.[63] There are a large number of diseases that may involve the aorta or aortic annulus. These include Takayasu's arteritis, syphilis, giant cell arteritis, relapsing polychondritis, ankylosing spondylitis, Reiter's arthritis, psoriatic arthritis, and arthritis associated with ulcerative colitis. Only a few of these diseases occur with any frequency in North America. The end result of most etiologies of aortitis is aneurysm formation, saccular or fusiform. Takayasu's arteritis and radiation can cause stenoses.

Takayasu's arteritis is an inflammatory followed by fibrotic process involving the three layers of the aorta and its branches and the pulmonary artery.[63–67] Aortic involvement by this disease has been classified into three types of distribution (Fig. 6-32). The disease causes leatherlike

thickening of the aortic wall, sometimes with calcification (Fig. 6-33), resulting in coarctation of the aorta and occlusion or stenosis of any aortic branch, especially the subclavian arteries, and less frequently, aneurysms. Four patterns of vascular involvement have been described: (1) aortic arch and arch branches, (2) segmental involvement of the thoracoabdominal aorta and its branches, (3) combination of the first two patterns, and (4) pulmonary arterial involvement along with involvement at any other site.[64,65] The three patterns of aortic involvement are shown in Figure 6-32. About 75% of patients have systemic hypertension and some patients have aortic regurgitation. There is an 8:1 female predominance.

Coarctation of the aorta at an atypical site such as at the midthoracic aorta or thoracoabdominal aorta is an interesting differential diagnosis (see Fig. 6-33*B*). The most common cause is Takayasu's arteritis, and other possible causes are Williams' syndrome (supravalvular aortic stenosis), neurofibromatosis, rubella syndrome, and irradiation.

Giant cell arteritis is a disease of the elderly, with female predominance, and usually involves medium-size arteries but the aorta may be afflicted in some cases.[68]

(*Text continues on page 202*)

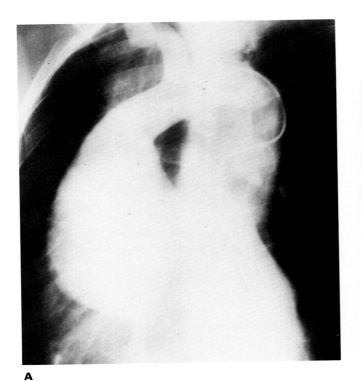
A

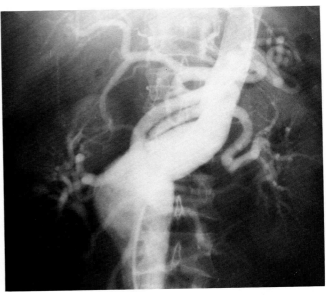
B

Figure 6-29. Thoracic aortogram in a shallow right posterior oblique view (A) and abdominal aortogram in the frontal view (B) in a patient with Marfan's syndrome. Thoracic aortogram demonstrates aortoanular ectasia. The dilatation of the proximal portion and midportion of the ascending aorta with normal diameter of the distal aorta produces the typical pear-shaped aorta characteristic of this abnormality. The abdominal aortogram demonstrates an infrarenal abdominal aortic aneurysm and marked elongation of the aortic branches. These are also characteristics of this syndrome.

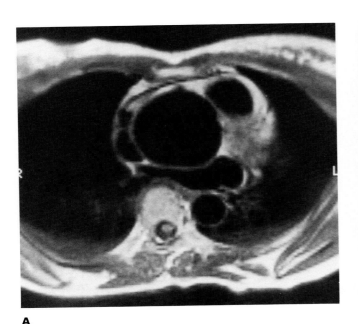
A

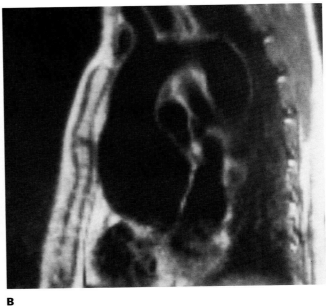
B

Figure 6-30. Transverse (A) and oblique sagittal (B) MR images demonstrate aortoannular ectasia. There is marked dilatation of the sinus portion and the proximal portion of the ascending aorta. The distal portion of the ascending aorta is of normal diameter. This appearance has been referred to as the Marfanoid aorta and is typical for aortoannular ectasia.

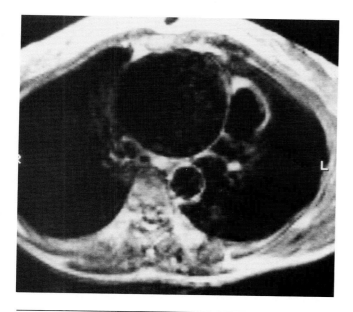

Figure 6-31. Transverse MR image at the proximal ascending aorta demonstrates large aneurysm of the proximal ascending aorta.

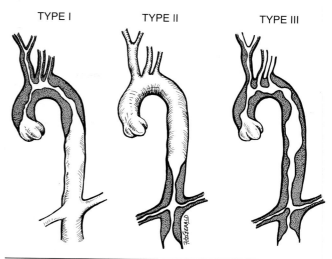

Figure 6-32. Diagram of three types of involvement of an aorta in Takayasu's disease. Type I consists of stenosis of the aortic arch and aortic arch branches. Type II consists of a long segment of stenosis involving the distal thoracic aorta and the proximal abdominal aorta. This variety frequently involves the renal arteries. Type III is a combination of types I and II with involvement of both the arch and arch vessels along with long-segment stenosis of the distal thoracic and proximal aorta.

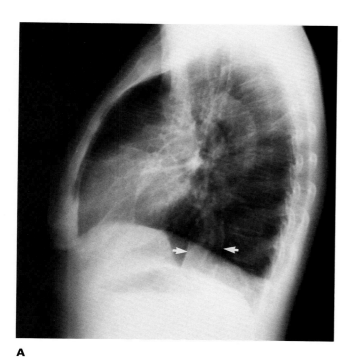

A

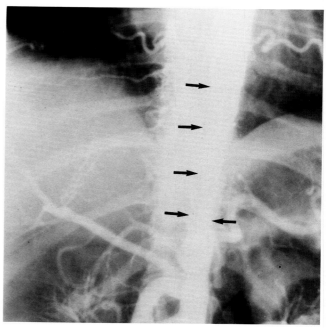

B

Figure 6-33. *A:* Lateral thoracic radiograph demonstrates heavy calcification (*arrows*) in the distal descending thoracic aorta. Calcification in this region of aorta is almost diagnostic of Takayasu's disease. *B:* Thoracoabdominal angiogram demonstrates a long segment of narrowing of the distal thoracic and proximal abdominal aorta (*arrows*). This type of midaortic coarctation is typical of Takayasu's arteritis, type II or type III.

The diagnosis is frequently established by biopsy of the temporal artery. The disease may cause aneurysm of the aorta and stenosis or occlusion of aortic branches, especially those of the arch.

Leutic aortitis is now rare. It produces ascending aortic aneurysm; heavy calcification of the ascending aorta; and aortic regurgitation. Aneurysms occur most frequently in the ascending aorta, followed by the arch, and descending thoracic and upper abdominal aorta. Heavy calcification of the ascending aorta suggests leutic aortitis, but calcification of lesser degrees is actually more common today in elderly patients with ascending aortic atherosclerosis, especially patients with aortic stenosis.[70] Takayasu's arteritis can also cause mild or heavy calcification at any site in the aorta.

Salient aortographic features in aortitis are:

1. Aortic coarctation. An atypical site such as the thoracoabdominal aorta is characteristic of Takayasu's aortitis (see Fig. 6-33*B*).

2. Occlusion or stenosis of arch branches.

3. Calcification of the thoracic aorta. Heavy calcification of the ascending aorta occurs with syphilis and heavy calcification at the coarctation site with Takayasu's arteritis (see Fig. 6-33*A*).

4. Diffuse or focal aneurysms.

5. Aortic regurgitation.

Salient CT and MRI features are:

1. Aortic coarctation at an atypical site.

2. Occlusion or stenosis of arch branches. These are generally depicted better by aortography than by tomographic techniques.

3. Calcification can be shown by CT but not by MRI.

4. The thickening of the aortic wall and adherent thrombus are demonstrated most effectively by MRI.

5. Diffuse or focal aneurysms. These are shown effectively by sagittal or oblique sagittal MRI.

Neoplasms. Primary tumors of the aorta are extremely rare. Case reports of angiosarcomas and spindle cell sarcomas are available. Secondary involvement of the aorta by mediastinal tumors and bronchogenic carcinoma renders these tumors inoperable. CT and MRI usually detect this during the staging of these tumors. Imaging studies are most frequently used to determine the vascular nature of a mediastinal mass.

Salient angiographic features are:

1. Filling defect in the aorta, which may be lobulated or otherwise display a distinctly irregular contour (Fig. 6-34).

2. Soft-tissue mass encasing or projecting from the aorta.

Salient CT and MRI features are:

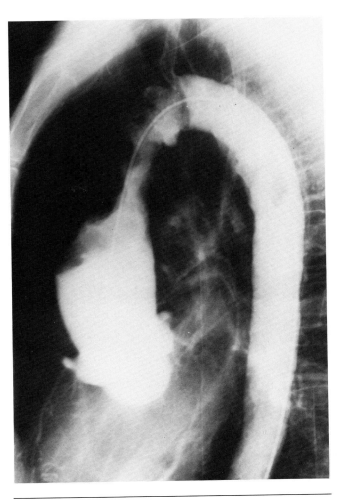

Figure 6-34. Lateral frame of abdominal aortogram demonstrates marked narrowing and lobulated contour abnormality of the distal ascending aorta caused by filling defects projecting into the opacified aortic lumen. This irregularly shaped long segment of narrowing was caused by an angiosarcoma of the thoracic aorta.

1. Tumor surrounding more than 180° of the circumference of the aorta is an indirect sign of likely involvement of the aorta by mediastinal or lung tumor.

2. Tumor projecting into the lumen of the aorta is the only definitive direct sign (Fig. 6-35).

3. Tumor projecting from the wall of the aorta (Fig. 6-36).

4. CT and especially MRI are the procedures of choice for establishing the vascular nature of a mediastinal mass (see Fig. 6-26).

Aortic Thromboembolic Disease. The source of peripheral arterial embolization is the left atrium and left ventricle in 90% of cases, and the aorta in about 5% to 10% of cases.[71] The sources in the aorta are thrombus on atherosclerotic plaques; ductus diverticulum; mural thrombus in an aneurysm; or aortic dissection.

The examination of the thoracic aorta for a site of the thrombus should be done with CT or MRI rather than

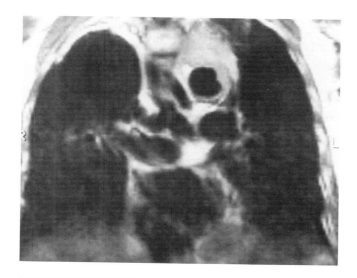

Figure 6-35. Coronal (ECG-gated) MR image demonstrates invasion of the posterior aortic arch by a lung carcinoma. Tumor surrounds the aorta and causes irregular thickening (*arrow*) of the aortic wall. The latter is a direct sign of aortic invasion.

aortography. After embolization, detection of the source necessitates that some residual thrombus is left at the originating site after the embolic episode. If all thrombotic material has embolized, it will not be detected by the imaging study.

Acquisition of MRI scans in planes perpendicular to each other has been quite effective in detecting an occult aortic source of emboli.[72] Images done in the transverse as well as the sagittal or coronary planes have detected

the thrombus, its extent, and its relationship to important arch branches (Fig. 6-37). Cine MRI is very useful for defining thrombus adherent to the aortic wall (Fig. 6-37). MRI has also been useful for monitoring dissolution of the thrombus during thrombolytic or anticoagulant therapy.

Septic Pseudoaneurysm and Periaortic Abscess. Septic pseudoaneurysm and periaortic abscess usually occurs as a complication of generalized sepsis or bacterial endocarditis.[73,74] The causative organs can be bacterial (*Staphyloccocus aureus, E. coli,* Salmonella) or fungal (Candida, Aspergillus). While the mycotic aneurysm is characteristically saccular, it can be fusiform. The mycotic aneurysm has a propensity for rupture since part of the wall is destroyed by the infection. Periaortic abscess or septic pseudoaneurysm may complicate infection of the aortic valve, especially staphylococcal infection. Predisposing aortic abnormalities include patent ductus arteriosus, coarctation, sinus of Valsalva aneurysm, damage to the aortic wall from indwelling catheter, or aortic incisions.

Salient aortographic findings are:

1. The aneurysm can be fusiform or saccular but the typical shape is saccular.[73,74] The most common site is the undersurface of the aortic arch near the attachment of the ligamentum arteriosum.

2. Contrast medium may enter irregular-shaped cavity adjacent to or below the aortic valve during ascending aortography or left ventriculography in the presence of infectious pseudoaneurysm of the aortic valve.

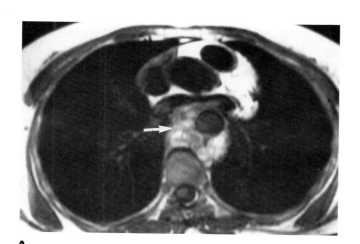

A

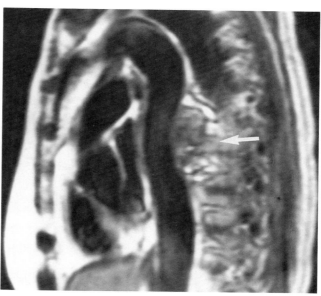

B

Figure 6-36. Transverse (*A*) and sagittal (*B*) MRI demonstrate a mass (*arrows*) arising from the aortic wall. This is a primary spindle-cell sarcoma of the aorta. (Courtesy of Clark Carroll, M.D., Houston, Texas.)

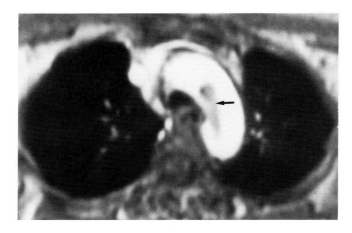

Figure 6-37. Transverse cine MR image at the level of the aortic arch demonstrates a filling defect (*arrow*) in the aortic arch. This represents a thrombus attached to the medial wall of the aortic arch. The blood has bright signal intensity on this gradient echo image, outlining the low-signal-intensity thrombus. Cine display of the images acquired at multiple phases of the cardiac cycle demonstrated mobility of this thrombus during the cardiac cycle.

Salient CT and MRI features are:

1. A tomographic technique may be preferred because it displays the periaortic region as well as the aorta (Fig. 6-38). CT or MRI show typically a saccular aneurysm.

2. The ostium of the aneurysm may be small (see Fig. 6-38*C*).

3. Inflammation of surrounding tissues or adjacent abscess may be demonstrated.

4. In recent years, MRI has been used to determine the extent of periaortic abscesses, complications such as bacterial endocarditis of the aortic valve, and their relationship to cardiac and extracardiac structures (see Fig. 6-38*A,B*).[75]

Echocardiography, especially transesophageal echocardiography, is probably now the most frequently employed technique for the detection of periaortic abscess complicating bacterial endocarditis of the aortic valve.

Congenital Diseases

Aortic Coarctation and Interruption. These congenital anomalies are described in detail elsewhere in this book. These exist in isolated forms and in association with other congenital anomalies. Only the isolated versions are discussed here.

Coarctation is usually discrete and is situated in the juxtaductal region of the aorta. Discrete juxtaductual coarctation may be associated with some degree of narrowing of the aortic isthmus. Tubular hypoplasia of the aorta consists of diffuse narrowing of the posterior aortic arch, isthmus, and proximal descending aorta. Interruption of the aortic arch can occur between any of the arch

vessels.[76,77] The isolated form nearly always occurs beyond the origin of the left subclavian artery in either the isthmus or the juxtaductal region.

The objectives of imaging studies are:

1. Identify the presence, site, and extent of the coarctation.

2. Define the severity of the coarctation. This is better done by measuring the gradient across it rather than the angiographic appearance.

3. Exclude associated anomalies.

4. Assess collateral circulation. No quantitative estimation of collateral circulation has ever been established for any imaging technique.

Angiography is the traditional method for evaluation of coarctation. MRI is now being used and has precluded the need for catheterization in some patients.

Salient angiographic features of coarctation[78] and interruption[76,77] of the aorta are:

1. Discrete coarctation in the juxtaductal region (Fig. 6-39).

2. Tubular hypoplasia of posterior aortic arch and isthmus. The isthmus region in the newborn is sometimes narrower than the arch and descending aorta. Isthmus hypoplasia may be defined when the diameter of the isthmus is less than 40% of the diameter of the distal ascending aorta (prearch portion).

3. Discrete coarctation and isthmus hypoplasia may both be displayed.

4. A severe coarctation is evident by the angiographic appearance; however, moderate and mild coarctation may not be accurately discerned by appearance alone. Precise gauging of severity is achieved by measuring the pressure gradient.

5. Poststenotic dilatation.

6. Collateral circulation. Collateral flow arising from intercostal arteries, intimal mammary arteries, long thoracic arteries, and other subclavian arterial branches is evident.

7. Relationship of origin of subclavian arteries to the coarctation. Discrete stenosis at the origin of a subclavian artery and subclavian steal syndrome are readily shown.

8. Discontinuity between the isthmus and the proximal descending aorta is shown for isolated interruption of the aorta. The distal aorta opacifies by collateral flow and shows a prolonged clearance period. Because of poor opacification of the distal aorta in some patients with both severe coarctation and interruption, it may be necessary to inject contrast medium into the aortic segment below the site of obstruction. Inability to maneuver the catheter into the ascending aorta from the femoral approach may require additional catheterization from the arm.

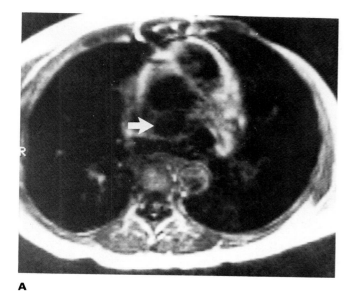

A

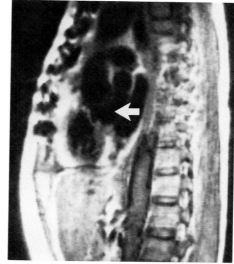

B

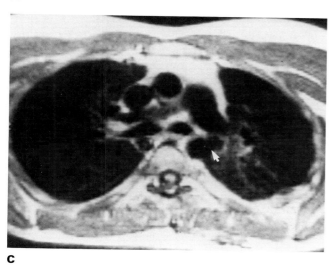

C

Figure 6-38. Pseudoaneurysms of the thoracic aorta demonstrated on transverse (*A*) and sagittal (*B*) MR images. The pseudoaneurysm is located between the base of the aorta and the anterior wall of the left atrium. The position of the pseudoaneurysm (*arrow*) is clearly indicated on both the transverse and the sagittal images. *C:* Pseudoaneurysm arising from the proximal portion of the descending aorta at the site of prior repair of coarctation of the aorta. The pseudoaneurysm has formed because of partial disruption of the anastomosis performed after resection of the coarctation. The connection (*arrow*) between the aortic lumen and the pseudoaneurysm is demonstrated on the transverse MR image.

Salient MRI findings in coarctation and interruption are:[79–81]

1. Narrow transverse diameter of the aorta on the MRI scans through the juxtaductal region is shown for discrete coarctation. In order to minimize overestimation of the diameter, thin-slice tomograms (3 mm thickness) should be done through this region. The presence, site, and diameter of the coarctation are depicted most effectively on sagittal or oblique sagittal tomograms using 3-mm thick slices (Fig. 6-40).

2. Diffuse tubular hypoplasia is indicated by reduced diameter on images through the arch, isthmus, and proximal descending aorta. Thin-slice sagittal or oblique sagittal tomograms display the extent of diffuse coarctation.

3. Collateral circulation can be displayed on MRI scans as a prominent vascular structure in the posterior mediastinum. These are usually situated in the periaortic region and adjacent to the vertebral bodies (see Fig. 6-40).

4. Poststenotic dilatation.

5. Relationship of arch branches to the coarctation is shown. However, discrete stenosis of the origin of the subclavian artery cannot be reliably defined by a tomographic image technique.

6. Interruption of the aorta can be shown by MRI. Furthermore, sagittal MRI is the best method available for defining the distance between the two ends of the interrupted aorta (Fig. 6-41).

Aortic Arch Anomalies. Some, but certainly not all, aortic arch anomalies cause a vascular and symptomatic compression of the airway and/or esophagus. The most frequently encountered types of aortic arch anom-

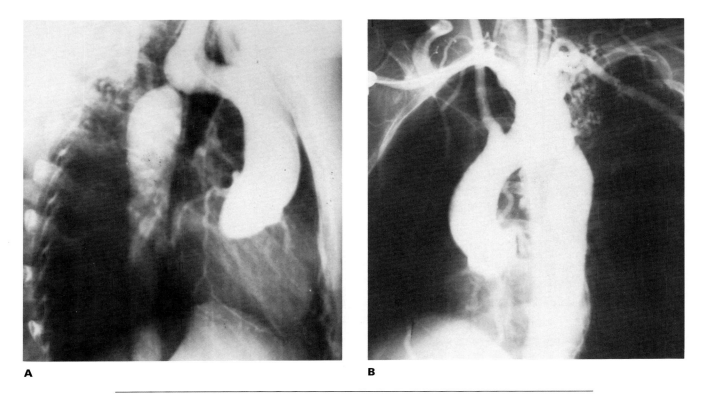

A

B

Figure 6-39. Lateral (*A*) and shallow right posterior oblique (*B*) frames of thoracic aortogram demonstrated juxtaductal coarctation of the aorta. There is severe coarctation with poststenotic dilatation of the proximal descending thoracic aorta. The coarctation is located in a typical site just beyond the origin of the left subclavian artery. Abundant collateral circulation from periscapular arteries is demonstrated.

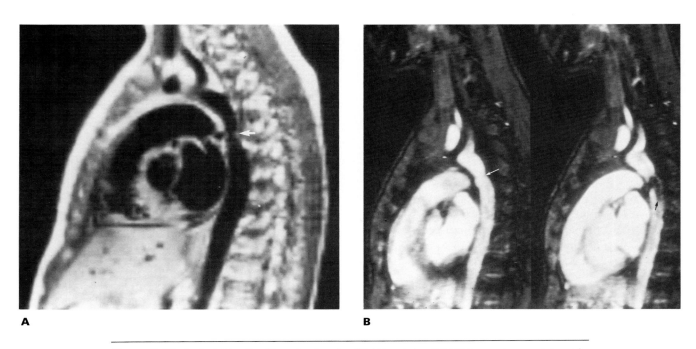

A

B

Figure 6-40. Sagittal thin slice (3 mm) spin echo MR (*A*) and cine MR (*B*) images in coarctation of the aorta. Spin echo image demonstrates a circumferential fibromuscular ring (*arrow*) which has produced narrowing of the aorta at a juxtaductal location. Cine MR images in diastole (*left*) and systole (*right*) demonstrate the turbulent blood flow at the site of the coarctation. Note that on the image in systole there is a signal void (*black arrow*) emanating from the coarctation site into the distal portion of the descending thoracic aorta. The signal void is caused by high-velocity turbulent blood flow occurring at the site of the coarctation. The diastolic image demonstrates a faint lucent line (*small white arrow*) extending across the proximal thoracic aorta.

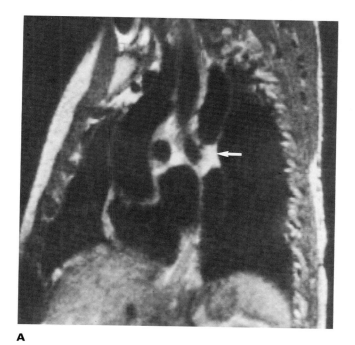

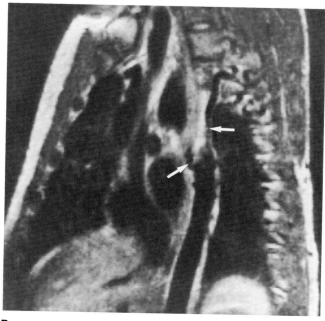

A   **B**

Figure 6-41. Sagittal MR images demonstrate interruption of the aortic arch beyond the origin of the left subclavian artery. The two segments of the interrupted aortic arch are separated by a segment of high signal intensity caused by interposed fatty tissue (*arrow*). Aortic branches are dilated (*B, arrows*) owing to collateral blood flow.

alies are diagramatically displayed in Figure 6-42 and have been described in detail by Shuford et al. and Steward et al.[82,83] A number of anomalies exist but some are very rare or only theoretically possible. Symptomatic airway compression may be caused by vascular anomalies other than those of the aortic arch, such as anomalous origin of the left pulmonary artery from the proximal right pulmonary artery with passage between the esophagus and trachea. The initial evaluation of aortic arch anomalies entails the thoracic radiograph, optimally with barium in the esophagus. All aortic arch anomalies cause an impression on the posterior aspect of the esophagus. The thoracic radiograph shows the side of the aortic arch and sometimes reveals portions of an anomalously coursing subclavian artery. It also may display anterior impression or displacement of the trachea.

The most frequently encountered aortic arch anomalies are:

1. Left aortic arch with retroesophageal right subclavian artery.
2. Right aortic arch with retroesophageal left subclavian artery (Fig. 6-43).
3. Complete double aortic arch (Figs. 6-43C, 6-44).
4. Incomplete double aortic arch, which is usually a patent right aortic arch with an atretic short segment in the posterior portion of the left arch.

The diagnosis of aortic arch anomalies can be done with angiographic and tomographic imaging tech-

COMMON ARCH ANOMALIES

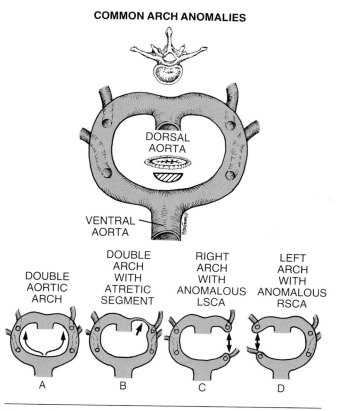

Figure 6-42. The primitive double aortic arch present in embryonic life. The four common types of aortic arch anomalies are shown and the manner in which they develop from the embryonic arch system is demonstrated.

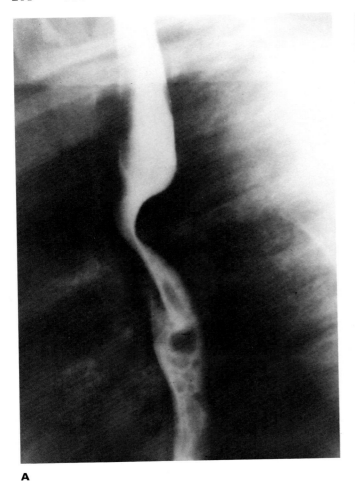

A

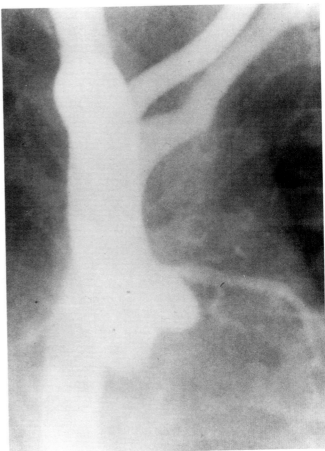

B

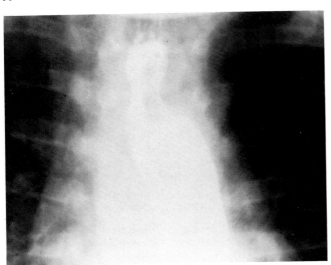

C

Figure 6-43. *A:* Lateral view of barium swallow demonstrates a large posterior impression on the barium-filled esophagus. This finding indicates the presence of an aortic arch anomaly but is usually nonspecific in indicating the precise type. *B:* Thoracic aortogram demonstrates a right aortic arch with anomalous origin of the left subclavian artery. Proximal portion of the left subclavian artery is typically dilated, as shown in this image. The vascular ring is completed because the ligamentum arteriosus has points of attachment to the base of this region of subclavian arterial dilatation and to the proximal portion of the left pulmonary artery. *C:* Frontal thoracic radiograph of barium-filled esophagus demonstrates impression on both sides of the esophagus. This finding is caused by a double aortic arch. The impression on the right side of the esophagus is located slightly more cranial than the impression on the left side of the esophagus. The impression on the left side of the esophagus is more prominent, which suggests that the left arch is the dominant of the two arches.

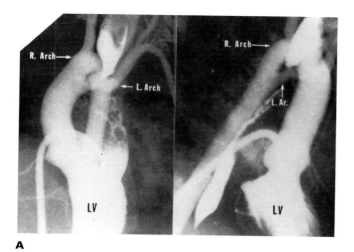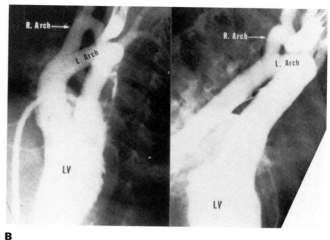

A   **B**

Figure 6-44. Angiograms demonstrate two types of double aortic arch in two separate patients. *A:* Cranial LAO view (*left*) and caudal RAO view (*right*) in a patient with double aortic arch in which the right-sided arch is dominant. This is the more common type of double arch, where the right arch is dominant. Note that the right arch occupies a more cranial position. Each arch provides the site of origin for one carotid and one subclavian artery. *B:* Cranial LAO (*left*) and caudal RAO (*right*) views of aortogram demonstrate double aortic arch in which the left arch is dominant. Each arch provides origin for one carotid and one subclavian artery. (From Tonkin IL, Elliot LP, Bargeron LM: Concomitant axial angiography in the evaluation of vascular rings. Radiology 1980;135:69. With permission of the Radiological Society of North America.)

niques.[83,84,85] The tomographic imaging techniques are now preferred because they display the vascular anomaly and also show its relationship to and effect upon the esophagus and airway.[85]

Salient angiographic features are:

1. Double arch. Cranial angulation in the left anterior oblique (right posterior oblique) view is optimal for separating the two arches (Fig. 6-44).[86] The right arch is the larger (and also higher) of the two arches in about 85% of cases. Ipsilateral carotid and subclavian arteries originate from each of the two arches.

2. Right arch provides origin to the left subclavian artery as its fourth (most distal) branch (Fig. 6-43). There is a dilatation at the origin of the subclavian artery. This dilatation marks the site of connection of the ligamentum arteriosum, which courses to the origin of the left pulmonary artery. The ligamentum completes the vascular ring.

3. Left aortic arch provides origin to the right subclavian artery as the fourth (most distal) branch. This anomaly usually does not cause a tight vascular ring.

Salient tomographic features of arch anomalies are:

1. Transverse images show two arches surrounding both sides of the esophagus and trachea. Transverse images above the arch display symmetrical arrangement of four arch branches at the base of the neck.

2. Transverse image shows the right arch coursing around the esophagus and trachea, while the left arch courses around these structures but is interrupted posteriorly (Fig. 6-45). The descending aorta shows an evagination on the left anterior aspect. This is the appearance of a double arch with an atretic posterior segment.

3. Retroesophageal aortic arch is identified on transverse images as a right aortic arch that passes from right to left behind the trachea in the superior mediastinum and produces compression and anterior displacement of the esophagus, trachea, or carina (Fig. 6-46).

4. Right or left arch with posterior origin of contralateral subclavian artery. The anomalous subclavian courses posterior to the esophagus. Anomalous subclavian is usually identified adjacent to the esophagus on a transverse image superior to the site of origin (Fig. 6-47).

5. Rare causes of vascular rings have also been identified on tomographic images (Fig. 6-48).

6. Transverse images demonstrate the focal decrease in diameter of the airway adjacent to the anomalous vascular structure (Figs. 6-45, 6-46).

7. Sagittal images demonstrate the vascular structure posterior to the esophagus and trachea along with the compression and displacement of these structures (Figs. 6-45, 6-46).

Cervical Arch. The cervical arch results from formation of the aortic arch by persistence of the third rather than the fourth primitive arch.[87] The cervical arch courses into the supraclavicular region and may be palpable at this site. Most cervical arches are right-sided. A

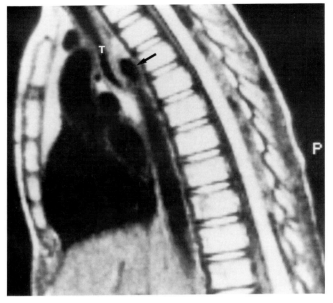

A

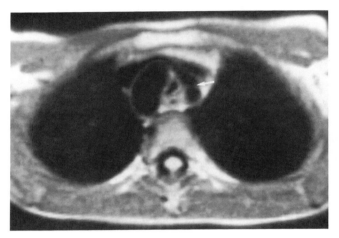

B

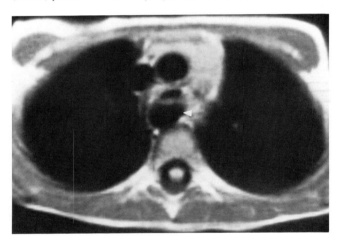

Figure 6-45. Sagittal (*A*) and transverse (*B, C*) MR images in a patient with double aortic arch with atresia of the posterior segment of the left arch. Transverse images are located adjacent to each other, with *B* situated 1 cm cranial to *C*. The right arch is dominant. The left arch (*arrow*) is smaller. Note the dilatation (*arrowhead*) of the descending aorta at the site where the short atretic segment attaches. Sagittal image shows the vascular segment (*arrow*) posterior to the esophagus and trachea (T).

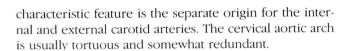

C

characteristic feature is the separate origin for the internal and external carotid arteries. The cervical aortic arch is usually tortuous and somewhat redundant.

Marfan's Syndrome. Some of the major cardiovascular manifestations of Marfan's syndrome afflict the thoracic aorta.[88] These include dilatation of the ascending aorta, aortic dissection, and ascending aortic aneurysm. These abnormalities may be asymptomatic and initially detected by thoracic radiography or may present acutely with chest pain or cardiovascular collapse. Detection of thoracic aortic abnormalities in asymptomatic patients with Marfan's syndrome or in members of their families can be conveniently done now using a completely noninvasive imaging technique such as MRI.[20] Moreover, patients with somatic characteristics suggesting Marfan's

syndrome may be candidates for MRI in order to fully exclude abnormal shape or abnormalities of the ascending aorta. This indication has occasionally arisen in very tall athletes, especially basketball players.

The angiographic features of Marfan's syndrome and its complications are:[89]

1. Dilatation of the sinuses of Valsalva and ascending aorta (see Fig. 6-29). The sinuses of Valsalva alone may be dilated; all three sinuses are enlarged. The dilatation of the ascending aorta usually is confined to the proximal ascending aorta (Marfanoid aorta); the pre-arch portion of the aorta has a normal diameter or is less dilated.

2. Aortic regurgitation.

3. Aortic dissection.

4. Ascending aortic aneurysm.

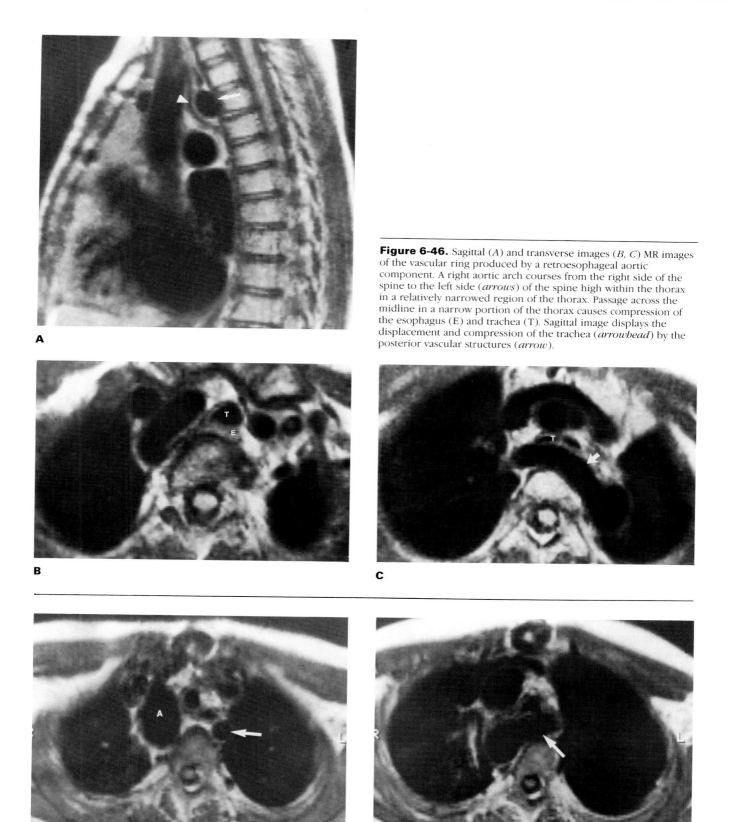

Figure 6-46. Sagittal (*A*) and transverse images (*B, C*) MR images of the vascular ring produced by a retroesophageal aortic component. A right aortic arch courses from the right side of the spine to the left side (*arrows*) of the spine high within the thorax in a relatively narrowed region of the thorax. Passage across the midline in a narrow portion of the thorax causes compression of the esophagus (E) and trachea (T). Sagittal image displays the displacement and compression of the trachea (*arrowhead*) by the posterior vascular structures (*arrow*).

Figure 6-47. Transverse MR images (*A, B*) show a right aortic arch with anomalous origin of the left subclavian artery. *A* is located 1 cm cranial to *B*. The left subclavian artery (*arrow*) passes behind the esophagus and trachea without causing significant narrowing of the trachea. Transverse images demonstrate the paraesophageal position of the left subclavian artery (*arrow*) at the level of the aortic arch (*A*), which is diagnostic for this anomaly on tomographic images.

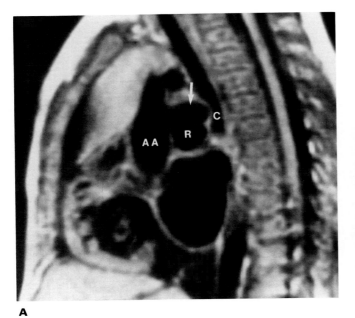

A

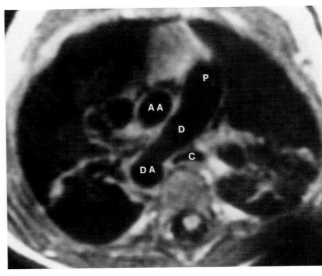

B

Figure 6-48. Sagittal (*A*) and transverse (*B*) MR images demonstrate a rare type of vascular compression of the airway caused by a mirror image type of right aortic arch with a right-sided patent ductus arteriosus. The dilated ductus arteriosus (*arrow*) produces narrowing of the carina (*C*) and right bronchus as it courses ventrally from the descending aorta on the right to the proximal left pulmonary artery on the left. (AA, ascending aorta; DA, descending aorta; D, ductus arteriosus; P, pulmonary artery; R, right pulmonary artery.)

The CT and MRI features are:[20]

1. Dilatation of the ascending aorta and/or the sinus of Valsalva (Figs. 6-30, 6-31). The diameter can be precisely measured on transverse or sagittal images. Because the dilatation usually involves only the proximal ascending aorta, the ratios of the diameter of the proximal ascending aorta to the distal ascending (prearch portion) and the descending aorta are significantly greater than for normal subjects (Table 6-1). These ratios can be useful for excluding Marfanoid characteristics in very tall individuals in whom the absolute diameter of segments of the aorta can exceed the limits recognized for the general population. MRI is an effective method for sequential quantitative monitoring of thoracic aortic dimensions in patients with Marfan's syndrome.

2. Aortic regurgitation is not identified by CT or standard spin echo MRI but can be recognized by cine MRI.

3. Aortic dissection in the Marfanoid aorta (see Fig. 6-10A,B).

4. Ascending aortic aneurysm (see Figs. 6-10, 6-31).

Table 6-1

Ratios of Aortic Segments

	Normal	Marfan's
$\dfrac{\text{Sinus}}{\text{Asc Ao}_d}$	1.1 ± 0.1	1.6 ± 0.2
$\dfrac{\text{Asc Ao}_p}{\text{Asc Ao}_d}$	1.0 ± 0.0	1.4 ± 0.3
$\dfrac{\text{Sinus}}{\text{Desc Ao}}$	1.4 ± 0.2	2.2 ± 0.4

Asc Ao$_p$, proximal ascending aorta (level of right pulmonary artery); Asc Ao$_d$, distal ascending aorta (pre arch level); Desc Ao, descending aorta; Sinus, sinuses of Valsalva.

References

1. White RD, Dooms GC, Higgins CB. Advances in imaging thoracic aortic disease. Invest Radiol 1986;21:761.
2. White RD, Lipton MJ, Higgins CB, Federle MP, Pogany AC, Kerlan RK, et al. Noninvasive evaluation of suspected thoracic aortic disease by contrast-enhanced computed tomography. Am J Cardiol 1986;57:282.
3. Egan TJ, Neiman HL, Herman RJ, et al. Computed tomography in the diagnosis of aortic aneurysm, dissection or traumatic injury. Radiology 1980;136:141.
4. Gross SC, Barr I, Eyler WR, et al. Computed tomography in dissection of the aorta. Radiology 1980;136:135.
5. Larde D, Belloir C, Vasile N, et al. Computed tomography of aortic dissection. Radiology 1980;136:147.
6. Heiberg E, Wolverson M, Sundaram M, et al. CT findings in thoracic aortic dissection. Am J Radiol 1981;136:13.
7. Thorsen MK, San Dretto MA, Lawson TL, et al. Dissecting aortic

aneurysms: accuracy of computed tomographic diagnosis. Radiology 1983;148:773.

8. Moncada R, Salinas M, Churchill R, et al. Diagnosis of dissecting aortic aneurysm by computed tomography. Lancet 1981;1:238.

9. Brundage BH, Rich S, Spiros D. Computed tomography of the heart and great vessels: Present and future. Ann Intern Med 1984;101:801.

10. Amparo EG, Higgins CB, Hricak H, et al. Aortic dissection: magnetic resonance imaging. Radiology 1985;155:399.

11. Geisinger MA, Risius B, O'Donnell JA, et al. Thoracic aortic dissections: magnetic resonance imaging. Radiology 1985;155:407.

12. Glazer HS, Gutierrez FR, Levitt G, et al. The thoracic aorta studied by MR imaging. Radiology 1985;157:149.

13. Pernes JM, Grenier P, Desbleds MT, de Brux JL. MR evaluation of chronic aortic dissection. J Comput Assist Tomogr 1987;11:975.

14. Kersting–Sommerhoff BA, Higgins CB, White RD, Sommerhoff CP, Lipton MJ. Aortic dissection: sensitivity and specificity of MR imaging. Radiology 1988;3:651.

15. White RD, Ullyot DJ, Higgins CB. MR imaging of the aorta after surgery for aortic dissection. Am J Radiol 1988;150:87.

16. Erbel R, Bomer N, Steller D, et al. Detection of aortic dissection by transesophageal echocardiography. Br Heart J 1987;58:45.

17. Erbel R, Daniel W, Visser C, Engberding R, Roelandt J, Rennollet H. Echocardiography in diagnosis of aortic dissection. Lancet 1989;1:457.

18. Monlaert AJ, Bruins CC, Oppenheimer R, Dekker A. Anomalies of the aortic arch and ventricular septal defects. Circulation 1976;53:1011.

19. Guthaner DF, Wexler L, Harrell G. CT demonstration of cardiac structures. Am J Radiol 1979;133:75.

20. Sommerhoff BA, Sechtem UP, Schiller NB, Lipton MJ, Higgins CB. MRI of the thoracic aorta in Marfan patients. J Comput Assist Tomogr 1987;11:633.

21. Dotter CT, Steinberg I. The angiographic measurement of the normal great vessels. Radiology 1949;52:353.

22. DeBakey ME, Henley WS, Cooley DA, et al. Surgical management of dissecting aneurysms of the aorta. J Thorac Cardiovasc Surg 1965;49:130.

23. Daily PO, Trueblood HW, Stinson EB, et al. Management of acute aortic dissection. Ann Thorac Surg 1970;10:237.

24. Roberts WC. Aortic dissection: anatomy, consequences, and causes. Am Heart J 1981;101:195.

25. McReynolds RA, Shin MS, Sims RD. Three channeled aortic dissection. Am J Radiol 1978;130:549.

26. Stein HL, Steinberg I. Selective aortography, the definitive technique, for diagnosis of dissecting aneurysm of the thoracic aorta. Am J Radiol 1968;102:333.

27. Shuford WH, Sybers RG, Weens HS. Problems in aortographic diagnosis of dissecting aneurysm of the aorta. N Engl J Med 1969;280:225.

28. Anagnostopoulos CE, Prabhakar MJS, Kittle CF. Aortic dissections and dissecting aneurysms. Am J Cardiol 1972;30:263.

29. Hayashi K, Meaney TF, Zelch JV, Tarar R. Aortographic analysis of aortic dissection. Am J Radiol 1974;122:769.

30. Yamada T, Tada S, Harada J. Aortic dissection without intimal rupture: diagnosis with MR imaging and CT. Radiology 1988;168:347.

31. Roberts WC. Aortic dissection: anatomy, consequences and causes. Am Heart J 1981;101:195.

32. Tisnado J, Cho S, Brochley MC, et al. Ulcerlike projections: a precursor angiographic sign to thoracic aortic dissection. Am J Radiol 1980;135:719.

33. Tavares NJ, Auffermann W, Brown JJ, Gilbert TJ, Sommerhoff C, Higgins CB. Detection of thrombus using phase-image MR scans: ROC curve analysis. Am J Radiol 1989;153:173.

34. Kondo C, Caputo GR, Semelka R, Higgins CB. Right and left ventricular stroke volume measurements with velocity encoded cine NMR imaging: *In vitro* and *in vivo* validation. Circulation 1990 (submitted).

35. Bogren HG, Underwood SR, Firmin DN, et al. Magnetic resonance velocity mapping in aortic dissection. Br J Radiol 1988;61:456.

36. Chang J-M, Friese K, Caputo GR, Kondo C, Higgins CB. MR measurement of blood flow in the true and false channel in chronic aortic dissection. Radiology 1990 (submitted).

37. Godwin JD, Breiman RS, Speckman JM. Problems and pitfalls in the evaluation of thoracic aortic dissection by computed tomography. J Comput Assist Tomogr 1982;6:750.

38. Guthaner DF, Miller DC, Silverman JF, et al. Fate of the false lumen following surgical repair of aortic dissections: an angiographic study. Radiology 1979;133:1.

39. Yamaguchi T, Naito H, Ohta M, et al. False lumens in type III aortic dissections: progress CT study. Radiology 1985;156:757.

40. Godwin JD, Turley K, Herfkens RJ, et al. Computed tomography for follow-up of chronic aortic dissections. Radiology 1981;139:655.

41. Yamaguchi T, Guthaner DF, Wexler L. Natural history of the false channel of type A aortic dissection after surgical repair: CT study. Radiology 1989;170:743.

42. Mathieu D, Keita K, Loisance D, et al. Postoperative CT followup of aortic dissection. J Comput Assist Tomogr 1986;10:216.

43. Pressler V, McNamara JJ. Thoracic aortic aneurysm: natural history and treatment. J Thorac Cardiovasc Surg 1980;79:489.

44. Joyce JW, Fairbairn JF, Kincaid OW, et al. Aneurysms of the thoracic aorta: a clinical study with special reference to prognosis. Circulation 1964;29:176.

45. Friedman SA. The evaluation and treatment of patients with arterial aneurysms. Med Clin North Am 1981;65:83.

46. Fomon JJ, Kurzweg FT, Broadaway RD. Aneurysms of the aorta: a review. Ann Surg 1967;165:557.

47. Lang EK. Aneurysms of the chest and neck. In: Teplick G, Haskins M, eds. Surgical Radiology. Philadelphia: WB Saunders, 1982.

48. Randall PA, Jarmalowski CR. Aneurysms of the thoracic aorta. In: Abrams HL, ed. Abrams Angiography. Vascular and Interventional Radiology. 3rd ed. Boston: Little Brown & Co., 1983.

49. Godwin JD, Herfkens RJ, Skioldebrand CG, et al. Evaluation of dissections and aneurysms of the thoracic aorta by conventional and dynamic CT scanning. Radiology 1980;136:125.

50. Amparo EG, Higgins CB, Hoddick W, et al. Magnetic resonance imaging of aortic disease: preliminary results. Am J Radiol 1984;143:1203.

51. Dinsmore RE, Liberthson RR, Wismer GL. Magnetic resonance imaging of thoracic aortic aneurysms. Am J Radiol 1986;146:309.

52. Seelos KC, Caputo GR, Hricak H, Higgins CB. Differentiation of tumor versus non-tumor thrombus using sequential gradient echo imaging (cine MRI). American Roentgen Ray Society 1990 Annual Meeting, 1990, Washington, DC (abstract).

53. Greendyke RM. Traumatic rupture of the aorta: special reference to automobile accidents. JAMA 1966;195:527.

54. Parmley LF, Mattingly TW, Manion WC, et al. Nonpenetrating traumatic injury of the aorta. Circulation 1958;17:1086.

55. Kirsh MM, Behrendt DM, Orringer MB, et al. The treatment of acute traumatic rupture of the aorta: a ten-year experience. Ann Surg 1976;184:308.

56. Strassman G. Traumatic rupture of the aorta. Am Heart J 1947;33:508.

57. Fisher RG, Hadlock F, Ben–Menachem YP. Laceration of the thoracic aorta and brachiocephalic arteries by blunt trauma. Radiol Clin North Am 1981;19:91.

58. Faraci RM, Westcott JL. Dissecting hematoma of the aorta secondary to blunt chest trauma. Radiology 1977;123:569.

59. Ellis PR, Cooley DA, DeBakey ME. Clinical considerations and surgical treatment of annulo-aortic ectasia. J Thorac Cardiovasc Surg 1961;43:363.

60. Lemon DK, White CW. Annulo-aortic ectasia: angiographic thermodynamic and clinical comparison with aortic insufficiency. Am J Cardiol 1978;41:482.

61. Chapman DW, Beazley HL, Peterson PK, et al. Annulo-aortic ectasia with cystic medial necrosis. Am J Cardiol 1965;16:679.

62. Nancarrow PA, Higgins CB. Progressive thoracic aortic dilation after aortic valve replacement. Am J Roentgen 1984;142:669.

63. Lande A, Beckman YM. Aortitis. Pathologic, clinical and arteriographic review. Radiol Clin North Am 1976;14:219.

64. Ishikawa K. Natural history and classification of occlusion thromboaortography (Takayasu's disease). Circulation 1978; 57:27.

65. Lupi–Herrera E, Sanchez–Torres G, Marcushamer J, et al. Takayasu's arteritis. Clinical study of 107 cases. Am Heart J 1977;93:94.

66. Lande A, LaPorta A. Takayasu arteritis: an arteriographic–pathological correlation. Arch Pathol Lab Med 1976;100:437.

67. Lande A, Bard R, Bole P, et al. Aortic arch syndrome (Takayasu's arteritis): arteriographic and surgical considerations. J Cardiovasc Surg 1978;19:507.

68. Ghose MK, Shensa S, Lerner PI. Arteritis of the aged (giant cell arteritis) and fever of unexplained origin. Am J Med 1976; 60:429.

69. Steinberg I, Dotter CT, Peabody G, et al. The angiographic diagnosis of syphilitic aortitis. Am J Radiol 1949;62:655.

70. Higgins CB, Reinke RT. Non-syphilitic etiology of linear calcification of the ascending aorta. Radiology 1974;113:606.

71. Heskell CA, Conn J. Aortoarterial emboli. Am J Surg 1976;132:4.

72. Seelos K, Funari M, Higgins CB. Identification of aortic source for peripheral embolization using MRI. Am J Radiol 1990 (submitted).

73. Weintraub RA, Abram HL. Mycotic aneurysm. Am J Radiol 1986;102:354.

74. Kaufman SL, White RI, Harrington DP, et al. Protean manifestations of mycotic aneurysms. Am J Radiol 1978;131:1019.

75. Winkler M, Higgins CB. Magnetic resonance imaging of the perivalvular infectious pseudoaneurysms. Am J Radiol 1986; 147:253.

76. Higgins CB, French JW, Silverman JF, et al. Interruption of the aortic arch: preoperative and postoperative clinical, hemodynamic, and angiographic features. Am J Cardiol 1977;39:563.

77. Jaffe RB. Complete interruption of the aortic arch: characteristic angiographic features with emphasis on collateral circulation to the descending aorta. Circulation 1976;53:161.

78. Figley MM. Accessory roentgen signs of coarctation of the aorta. Radiology 1954;62:671.

79. von Schulthess GK, Higashino SM, Higgins SS, Didier D, Fisher MR, Higgins CB. Coarctation of the aorta: MR imaging. Radiology 1986;158:469.

80. Simpson IA, Chung K, Glars RF, et al. Cine MRI for evaluation of anatomy and flow relations in infants and children with coarctation of the aorta. Circulation 1988;78:142.

81. Rees S, Sommerville J, Ward C, et al. Coarctation of the aorta: MR imaging in the late postoperative period. Radiology 1989; 173:499.

82. Shuford WH, Sybers RG. The aortic arch and its malformations. Springfield: Charles C. Thomas, 1974.

83. Stewart HR, Kincaid OW, Edwards JE. An atlas of vascular rings and related malformations of the aortic arch system. Springfield: Charles C. Thomas, 1964.

84. Baron RL, Guttierrez FR, McKnight RC. CT evaluation of the great arteries and aortic arch malformations. In: Friedman WE, Higgins CB, eds. Pediatric cardiac imaging. Philadelphia: WB Saunders, 1984.

85. Sommerhoff BK, Sechtem UP, Fisher MR, Higgins CB. MR imaging of congenital anomalies of the aortic arch. Am J Radiol 1987;149:9.

86. Tonkin IL, Elliott LP, Bargeron LM. Concomitant axial angiography in the evaluation of vascular rings. Radiology 1980;135:69.

87. Hyman RA, Stein HL. The cervical aortic arch anomaly. Angiology 1975;26:749.

88. Pyeritz RE, McKusick VA. The Marfan syndrome: diagnosis and management. N Engl J Med 1979;300:772.

89. Murlock JL, Walker BA, Halpern BL, et al. Life expectancy and causes of death in the Marfan syndrome. N Engl J Med 1972;286:804.

90. Soulen RL, Fishman EK, Pyeritz RE, et al. Marfan syndrome: evaluation with MR imaging vs CT. Radiology 1987;165:697.

91. Boxer RA, La Corte MA, Singh S, et al. Evaluation of the aorta in the Marfan syndrome by MRI. Am Heart J 1986;111:1001.

92. Schaefer S, Peshock RM, Mallory CR, et al. Nuclear magnetic resonance imaging in Marfan's syndrome. J Am Coll Cardiol 1987;9:70.

Chapter 7

Coronary Angiography

Hugo Spindola–Franco

Mark A. Greenberg

Bernard G. Fish

Coronary artery disease not only is the most common cause of mortality in the United States, but also results in considerable morbidity.[1] Fortunately, dramatic advances in the surgical and nonsurgical treatment of coronary disease have been made. The availability of these interventions mandate an exact knowledge of coronary anatomy and pathology.

Coronary atherosclerosis, which is almost synonymous with coronary artery disease, is a process that remains asymptomatic for many years in most persons and permanently so in many. Clinical manifestations occur because of luminal narrowing of a major coronary branch due to (1) progression of the atheromatous process, (2) coronary artery thrombosis, (3) intramural hemorrhage, (4) vasoconstriction, (5) coronary aneurysms (acquired or congenital), or (6) a combination thereof.

Atherosclerosis is a multifactorial process. Diet high in saturated fat and cholesterol, emotional stress, physical inactivity, hypertension, diabetes, gout, smoking, and inherited factors, including hyperlipidemia, are all considered possible risk factors for the development of atherosclerosis. The clinical manifestations can be divided into five groups: (1) stable angina pectoris, (2) unstable angina pectoris (preinfarction angina), (3) acute myocardial infarction, (4) heart failure induced by myocardial ischemia or infarction, and (5) sudden death.

Nonatherosclerotic causes of angina and myocardial infarction include aortic stenosis, subaortic stenosis, coronary embolism, and congenital anomalies of the coronary arteries. Furthermore, the small coronary vessels may be diseased with no involvement of the large epicardial coronary arteries.[2] Angina may occur in persons with normal coronary arteries due to anemia, metabolic abnormalities at the cellular or molecular level, or impaired coronary vasodilator reserve (syndrome X).[3]

Coronary artery disease, therefore, has a wide clinical spectrum that ranges from patients with critical coronary stenosis who are asymptomatic prior to a catastrophic event to highly symptomatic patients with angiographically normal coronary arteries. Thus, objective assessment for the presence and severity of coronary disease is necessary. Although noninvasive testing is important for initial assessment of patients with suspected ischemic heart disease, a definitive diagnosis can often be made only by coronary arteriography. Furthermore, selective coronary opacification is mandatory if surgery or angioplasty is contemplated, since angiography is the only available technique for delineation of the coronary arteries.

Coronary arteriography or angiography deals with the study of the anatomy of the coronary arteries, visualized radiologically by means of contrast medium that has been injected. Coronary arteriography is usually performed in conjunction with left ventriculography. Here the presence of contrast material within the left ventricle permits determination of the systolic and diastolic volumes of the left ventricle, the ejection fraction, the characteristics of the contractions of the left ventricle, and pathology of the mitral valve.

Indications

The indications for coronary arteriography are continuously evolving as newer noninvasive imaging techniques and therapeutic options emerge. Furthermore, not all practitioners may agree on each of the indications. Table

Special thanks to Michelle Keappock for her assistance in the preparation of this chapter.

7-1 lists Spindola–Franco's classification of indications for coronary angiography.[4] An American Heart Association/American College of Cardiology task force[5] has published a comprehensive report on indications for this procedure.

Not all patients with angina must have coronary angiography. Patients refractory to medical treatment, patients with unstable angina (new onset of severe angina, increase in frequency or severity of chronic angina, or angina at rest), and patients with markedly abnormal electrocardiogram (ECG), thallium or radionuclide ventriculography stress tests should be referred for angiographic study. Also patients with high-risk occupations such as airplane pilots and firefighters who are suspected of having coronary artery disease, as well as patients with known or suspected coronary artery disease undergoing high risk noncardiac surgical procedures, are often evaluated with selective coronary angiography.

Similarly, not all patients with myocardial infarction require catheterization. Early in the course of myocardial infarction (within six hours of onset), coronary angiograms are obtained in patients when percutaneous transluminal coronary angioplasty (PTCA) or intracoronary thrombolysis is considered. Later in the course of myocardial infarction, angiography is performed in patients who (a) demonstrate spontaneous or exercise-induced ischemia; (b) develop mechanical dysfunction such as mitral insufficiency or acute ventricular septal defect; (c) have congestive heart failure or severe left ventricular dysfunction; (d) were treated acutely with intravenous thrombolytic agents; (e) are younger than 50 years of age; or (f) exhibit refractory ventricular arrhythmias.

Table 7-1

Indications for Coronary Arteriography

Ischemic Heart Disease
Symptomatic patients
  Angina
    Clinical suspicion of angina but not conclusive
    Stable angina
      Inability to tolerate medication
      Reluctance to change life style
      For identification of patients with high-risk lesions
      To assess patency of bypass grafts
    Unstable angina
  Myocardial infarction
    Mechanical dysfunction
    Recurrent pain
    Elective for prognosis and therapy
Asymptomatic patients
  Abnormal ECG or stress test
  High-risk occupation

Heart Disease Other than Ischemic
Cardiomyopathy, arrhythmia
Suspected congenital anomaly of the coronary arteries
Preoperatively in valve surgery
Preoperatively in congenital heart disease

Contraindications

Coronary angiography is a relatively safe procedure in the hands of an experienced coronary angiographic team. The efficacy of this examination is considerable, as observed in the long list of indications. At present no absolute contraindication to coronary arteriography exists. However, relative contraindications must be kept in mind. These include all intercurrent disorders that could be treated and whose correction would improve the safety of the procedure (e.g., electrolyte disturbance, congestive heart failure, coagulation problems, digitalis toxicity).

Complications

The major complications of coronary arteriography are myocardial infarction, stroke, peripheral vascular embolization, thrombosis, and death. The incidence of such complications is less than 1% (0.33%–0.63%)[6,7] and is closely related to the experience of the angiographer, clinical status of the patient, and the extent of the disease as determined by coronary angiography and ventriculography.

Other complications of coronary angiography are ventricular fibrillation, complete heart block or asystole, vasovagal episode, pyrogen reaction, postnitroglycerin hypotension, allergic reaction to contrast media, and arterial complications at the puncture site (e.g., thrombosis, vessel wall damage, hematoma, pseudoaneurysm formation).

Technique

Selective opacification of the coronary arteries is mandatory for optimal visualization and for accurate interpretation. Nonselective studies (sinus of Valsalva injections) are important in those in which a diagnosis of coronary ostial stenosis is in question.

At present, two basic approaches exist for selective coronary arteriography: the Seldinger percutaneous technique[8] and the Sones cutdown brachial technique.[9] Several catheter designs (e.g., Judkins,[10] Amplatz[11]) are used with the percutaneous Seldinger approach for selective coronary arteriography. The technique of Judkins is the most widely used. It requires preformed separate catheters for the right and left coronary arteries and a pigtail catheter for ventriculography (Fig. 7-1). This technique has the advantage of the ease and speed of the transfemoral approach, permitting consistent selective coronary cannulation with minimal manipulation. The use of an introducer sheath facilitates catheter exchanges.

The Sones technique uses a flexible tapered-tipped

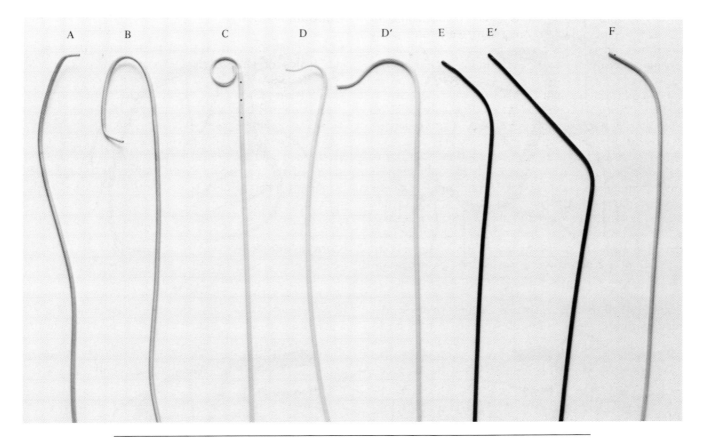

Figure 7-1. Catheters used in selective coronary arteriography and left ventriculography. *A:* Judkins right coronary; *B:* Judkins left coronary; *C:* pigtail catheter for left ventriculography; *D, D':* Amplatz (distal curves of right and left coronary catheters are similar); *E, E':* Sones B and A catheters (the same catheter is used for right and left coronary arteriography and for left ventriculography); *F:* Schoonmaker used for both coronary arteries. (Reproduced with permission from Spindola–Franco H, Fish BG. Radiology of the heart: cardiac imaging in infants, children and adults. New York: Springer–Verlag, 1985.)

catheter introduced by means of a brachial cutdown. Left ventriculography and hemodynamic recordings are obtained with the same catheter used for coronary angiography. A percutaneous technique with an introducer sheath can be used to avoid an arteriotomy when transbrachial access is required. Either the Sones catheter or the preformed coronary catheters can be used with this approach. Similar complication rates using either the percutaneous or cutdown brachial techniques have been reported.[12]

Despite improvements in digital subtraction angiography, 35 mm cine angiography remains the standard for filming coronary angiograms. Radiologic installations that allow rotation and angulation of the tube and image intensifier are necessary to avoid vascular superimposition and to optimally define proximal coronary artery lesions. The utility of these compound angulated views is illustrated below, following the discussion of normal coronary anatomy. Physiological monitors for continuous display of the ECG and pressure tracings are required.

Normal Coronary Anatomy

Thorough knowledge of the anatomic relationships of the coronary ostia to the root of the aorta and the sinuses of Valsalva is essential for successful coronary artery opacification. The sinuses of Valsalva are named to coincide with the origins of the coronary arteries: right, left, and noncoronary. The right sinus is anterior in location, the left sinus is posterior on the left, and the noncoronary sinus is posterior on the right.

Right Coronary Artery

The ostium of the right coronary artery (RCA) (Figs. 7-2, 7-3, see also Figs. 7-16, 7-17) is located in the right sinus of Valsalva at or about the level of the aortic ring; occasionally it may have a higher or lower position. The os-

(*Text continues on page 220*)

RIGHT DOMINANT SYSTEM

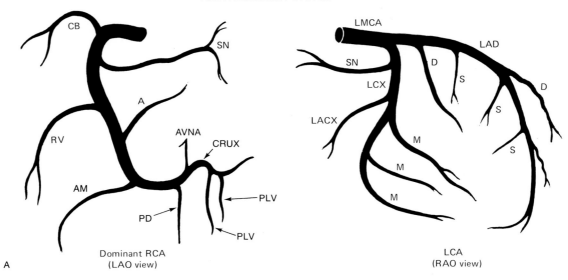

Dominant RCA
(LAO view)

LCA
(RAO view)

A

LEFT DOMINANT SYSTEM

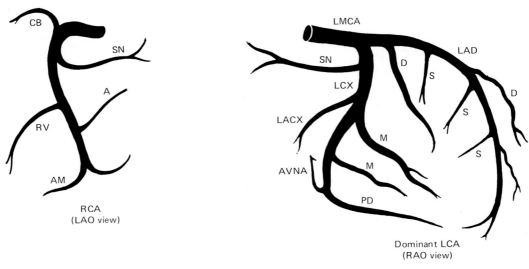

RCA
(LAO view)

Dominant LCA
(RAO view)

B

BALANCED CIRCULATION

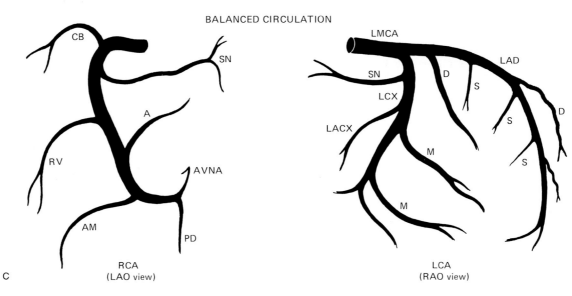

RCA
(LAO view)

LCA
(RAO view)

C

Figure 7-2. Normal coronary arteries and coronary artery dominance. Coronary dominance refers to the artery that supplies the diaphragmatic surface of the left ventricle and the posterior interventricular septum. The RCA is dominant in 80% of cases, the LCA in 9%. In about 11% of cases the circulation is balanced. *A:* Right coronary artery dominance. The RCA supplies the posterior interventricular septum by way of the descending artery (PD) and the diaphragmatic surface of the left ventricle by way of the crux artery and its posterolateral or posterior left ventricular branches (PLV). The crux artery also gives off a small branch to the left atrium. The atrioventricular node artery (AVNA) is usually the first branch of the crux artery and serves as a useful landmark to identify the PD in the LAO view. The PD is the branch just before the AVNA. *B:* Left coronary artery dominance. The LCA supplies the diaphragmatic wall of the left ventricle by marginal branches (M) of the left circumflex artery (LCX). It also supplies the posterior interventricular septum by way of the PD, which is now a branch of the LCX. With LCA dominance a crux artery is absent, and the RCA is small. The AVNA is a branch of the LCX, and the PD is distal to it. *C:* Balanced coronary arterial system. The diaphragmatic wall of the left ventricle is supplied by marginal branches of the LCX. The posterior interventricular septum is supplied by the RCA by way of the PD. The AVNA may be a branch of the RCA or a branch of the LCX. On occasion, two AVNAs exist, one from the distal RCA and one from the distal LCX. Note again that no crux artery is present in a balanced system and that the area normally perfused by it is supplied by marginal branches of the LCX. (A, atrial branch; AM, acute marginal branch; CB, conus branch or artery; CRUX, crux artery; D, diagonal branch; LACX, left atrial circumflex branch; LAD, left anterior descending artery; LCA, left coronary artery; LMCA, left main coronary artery; RCA, right coronary artery; RV, right ventricular, preventricular or muscular branch; S, septal perforator branch (septal artery); SN, sinus node artery.) (Although the sinus node artery is depicted here as a separate branch from the LCX, it usually occurs as a branch of the LACX.) (Modified from Spindola–Franco H. Coronary arteriography and left ventriculography. In: Goldberger E, ed. Textbook of clinical cardiology. St. Louis: CV Mosby, 1982;305.)

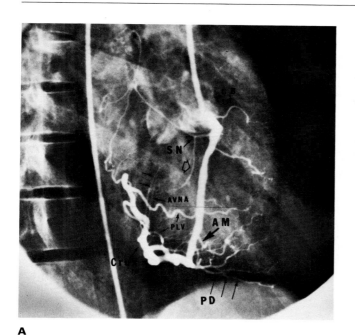

A

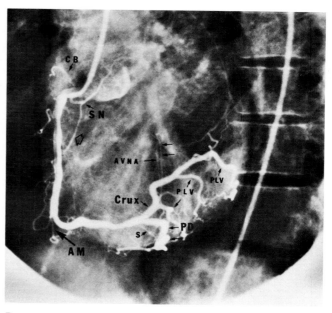

B

Figure 7-3. Dominant RCA. *A:* RAO view. *B:* LAO view. The first branch is the CB, which courses anteriorly and superiorly. The second branch is the sinus node artery (SN), which courses posteriorly and gives off two small branches, one to the sinus node and one to the posterior wall of the left atrium. In this case the SN also gives off a third branch, which descends around the atrial appendage (*open arrow*). The acute marginal branch (AM) is small in this patient. It originates at the acute margin of the right ventricle (compare AM here with Fig. 7-9). The RCA bifurcates distally into two branches, the posterior descending (PD) and the crux artery. The PD supplies the posterior interventricular septum (basal septum) via the septal arteries (S). The septal arteries from the PD are usually small compared to those from the left anterior descending artery. The crux artery supplies the diaphragmatic wall of the left ventricle by way of posterior left ventricular branches (PLV). It also gives off the atrioventricular node artery (AVNA), which has a straight vertical course. In this case two parallel AVNAs are noted (see also Fig. 7-5). The PD is recognized by its straight horizontal course along the posterior interventricular sulcus, whereas the crux artery, also known as the U-turn artery, loops superiorly. The looping course of the crux artery in the RAO view is very helpful in distinguishing it from the PD during interpretation of cine studies. In the LAO view the PD is identified because it usually precedes the AVNA. (Reproduced with permission from Spindola–Franco H, Fish BG. Radiology of the heart: cardiac imaging in infants, children and adults. New York: Springer–Verlag, 1985.)

tium is in front, either exactly in the center or slightly to the right of the center of the aortic root. Therefore, ostial lesions are best studied in the lateral and steep LAO projections.

The RCA, which takes origin from its ostium, passes for a short distance forward between the pulmonary artery and the right atrial appendage and then curves to the right, following the right atrioventricular groove toward the crux cordis (the intersection of the atrioventricular and interventricular sulci posteriorly). There the RCA terminates in various ways. If it is dominant (Figs. 7-2, 7-3) it will supply the diaphragmatic and free walls of the right ventricle (right ventricular branches) and almost half of the diaphragmatic surface of the left ventricle by way of the crux artery through its posterior left ventricular branches. The basal (posterior) interventricular septum is supplied by the posterior descending artery. The RCA also gives off branches to the right atrium and to the root of the pulmonary artery and aorta.

The conus branch (CB), the first branch of the RCA, runs anteriorly and superiorly, encircling the outflow tract of the right ventricle at the level of the pulmonic valve. There the CB may anastomose with branches of the left coronary artery (LCA), to form the anastomotic circle of Vieussens. This collateral pathway is of considerable significance in occlusions of either the RCA or the left anterior descending (LAD) artery, as a source of blood distal to the occlusion. The CB may originate from an ostium separate from that of the RCA and is then known as the third coronary artery (preinfundibular artery of Crainicianu or arteria accessoria of Banchi).[13]

The second branch of the RCA, the sinoatrial node (SA node) artery, originates from the proximal RCA about 60% of the time and from the left circumflex artery 40% of the time.[13] The SA node artery passes superiorly, dorsally, and to the right, between the atrial appendage and aorta to encircle the ostium of the superior vena cava. The SA node artery usually bifurcates into a branch to the SA node artery proper and a branch to the posterior wall of the left atrium. Either branch can provide a collateral pathway in the event of occlusion of the left circumflex or right coronary artery.

The right superior septal artery (RSSA) (Fig. 7-4) is an uncommon but important branch of the RCA, occurring in 1% to 3% of cases.[14] It may arise directly from the proximal RCA, or it may be a branch of the conus artery. The RSSA penetrates the myocardium to run in the parietal band of the crista supraventricularis, supplying the area of the septum normally perfused by the first septal perforator from the LAD. The RSSA is an important collateral pathway in instances of occlusion of the LAD or posterior descending artery or both.

Right ventricular (also known as muscular or preventricular) branches arise from the RCA, course anteriorly, and supply the right ventricular myocardium. The acute marginal (AM) branch is usually a large right ven-

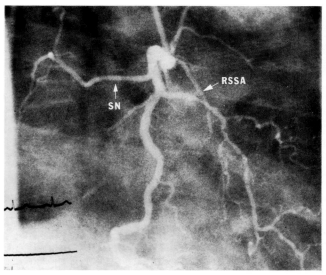

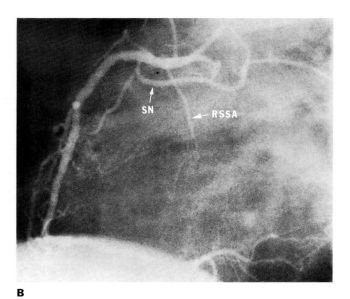

A   **B**

Figure 7-4. Right superior septal artery. *A:* RAO view; *B:* LAO view of right coronary artery. The right superior septal artery (RSSA) arises from the proximal right coronary artery after the conus branch and before the sinus node artery (SN). The RSSA perforates the myocardium in the vicinity of the crista supraventricularis to reach the interventricular septum. (Reproduced with permission from Spindola–Franco H, Fish BG. Radiology of the heart: cardiac imaging in infants, children and adults. New York: Springer–Verlag, 1985.)

tricular vessel arising from the RCA at the level of the acute margin of the heart. These right ventricular vessels may provide intercoronary and intracoronary collateral flow when coronary occlusion occurs.

At or near the crux of the heart the RCA divides into the posterior descending (PD) artery and crux artery. The PD courses in the posterior interventricular sulcus to anastomose with branches of the left anterior descending artery near the apex of the heart. The PD supplies primarily the basal (posterior) septum and to a small degree the inferior surface of both ventricles. Important variations of the PD exist in 25% of persons with a dominant RCA.[15] These variations include multiple posterior descending arteries, early origin of the PD, and partial supply of the distribution of the PD by the acute marginal or posterior right ventricular branches of the RCA (dual supply).

The crux artery (on occasion called the U-turn artery) continues past the interventricular sulcus (Fig. 7-5).

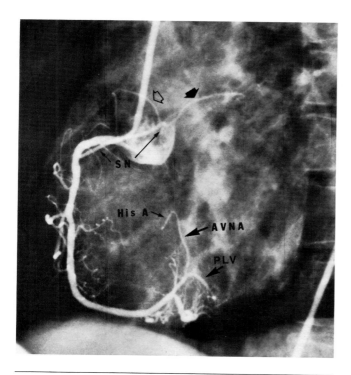

Figure 7-5. Atrioventricular node artery (AVNA), LAO view. A particularly excellent image of the AVNA is illustrated. The bundle of His artery (His A) is also clearly noted to branch off from the AVNA at an acute angle. Note that the posterior descending precedes the AVNA. This right coronary artery is dominant because it supplies the posterior interventricular septum by way of the posterior descending artery and the diaphragmatic wall of the left ventricle by way of the crux artery and its posterior left ventricular branch (PLV). The crux artery and its single PLV are small in this patient. Note also that the sinus node artery (SN) bifurcates into a branch to the sinus node (*open arrow*) and a branch to the left atrium (*closed arrow*). (Reproduced with permission from Spindola–Franco H, Fish BG. Radiology of the heart: cardiac imaging in infants, children and adults. New York: Springer–Verlag, 1985.)

It first gives rise to the atrioventricular node artery (AVNA) prior to giving off the usually large posterior left ventricular (PLV) branches. The PLV branches supply most of the posterior diaphragmatic wall and part of the posterior lateral wall of the left ventricle. The bundle of His artery, which is a branch of the atrioventricular node artery, may also be visualized on arteriography.

The foregoing describes a dominant RCA system that occurs in the majority of persons. Coronary dominance[4,16] refers to the vessel that supplies the diaphragmatic surface of the left ventricle and the posterior interventricular septum by way of the crux artery and PD artery, respectively. In a dominant LCA system, the RCA is small and terminates before the crux of the heart (Fig. 7-6). In such instances the crux artery does not exist. The area ordinarily supplied by the crux artery is perfused by distal marginal branches of the left circumflex (LCX) artery. The PD also arises from the LCX. Similarly, in the balanced coronary arterial system, the crux artery does not exist. The RCA terminates after giving origin to the PD and occasionally the AVNA, while the diaphragmatic wall of the left ventricle is supplied by marginal branches as in a dominant left coronary system. In a previous study of 2333 coronary angiograms, 1856 (80%) had a dominant RCA, 207 (9%) had a dominant LCA, and 270 (11%) had a balanced coronary arterial system.[4]

Left Coronary Artery

The left main coronary artery (LMCA) passes forward for a short distance between the base of the pulmonary artery and the left atrial appendage and then divides into two major branches, the left anterior descending (LAD) and the left circumflex artery (LCX) (Figs. 7-2, 7-7, 7-8, and 7-11–7-15). Often the LMCA trifurcates and gives rise to a third branch termed the ramus medianus (Fig. 7-9*C,D*; see also Fig. 7-21).

The LAD runs in the anterior interventricular sulcus to the apex of the heart, often encircling the apex and terminating in the anterior third of the posterior interventricular sulcus. The LAD supplies branches to the interventricular septum (septal perforators), muscular branches to the anterolateral left ventricular wall (diagonal vessels) and small branches to the anterior surface of the right ventricle. The septal arteries vary in number and size; the first septal perforator usually is the largest and most important. Severe lesions of the LAD before the origin of the first septal artery are more life threatening than lesions located distal to the origin of the first septal vessel.[17] Angiographically, septal arteries usually are observed to arise from the LAD at a 90° angle and to run a straight course, usually ending in a characteristic forklike configuration. The vessels of the septum represent an

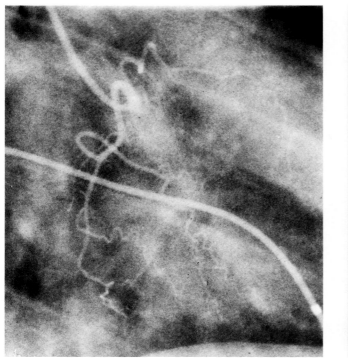

A

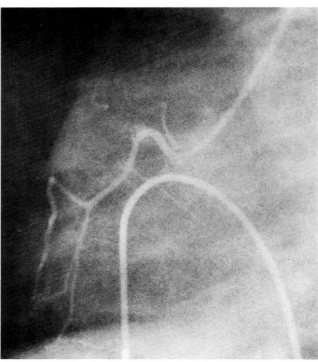

B

Figure 7-6. Nondominant right coronary artery. *A:* RAO view; *B:* LAO view. In contrast to the dominant right coronary artery (Fig. 7-3) the nondominant vessel is small and terminates before the crux of the heart. Therefore it does not give off a posterior descending or crux artery. The posterior descending artery is a branch of the left circumflex artery. The area supplied by the crux artery is supplied instead by marginal branches of the left circumflex. See also Figure 7-2. (Reproduced with permission from Spindola–Franco H, Fish BG. Radiology of the heart: cardiac imaging in infants, children and adults. New York: Springer–Verlag, 1985.)

important collateral pathway between the RCA and LCA (Fig. 7-9).

The diagonal arteries are branches from the LAD, supplying the left ventricular wall, with an oblique course toward the apex. The caliber of these diagonal arteries and their number are variable, on occasion being even longer and larger than the LAD or LCX. Angiographically the diagonal arteries have a motion opposite from the LAD (crisscross or seesaw motion).

The LCX is a branch from the LMCA, running posteriorly along the atrioventricular groove toward the crux of the heart. In the majority of instances the LCX ends before reaching the posterior interventricular septum. With a dominant LCA system the LCX reaches the crux area and supplies the distribution of the posterior descending artery, the PLVs and the atrioventricular node artery (see Fig. 7-8).

The LCX gives off marginal (muscular; see Fig. 7-7) and atrial branches. The marginal branches supply the lateral and posterolateral surface of the left ventricle, varying in size, length, and number. The left atrial circumflex artery (LACX) commonly originates from the proximal LCX to supply the left atrium. In some other cases when the LACX does not exist, the left atrium is supplied by multiple small branches from the LCX. In about 40% of cases, the SA node artery is a branch of the LCA, usually arising from the LCX, and on occasion from the LMCA.

Kugel's artery (arteria anastomotica auricularis magna)[18] is a branch from the proximal LCX, which runs in the atrioventricular plane at the base of the interatrial septum; it may anastomose with the SA node artery and AVNA. Kugel's artery is usually observed as a collateral pathway in occlusions of either the right or left coronary arteries. In practice a collateral pathway noted frequently on angiography between the SA node artery (from the RCA) and the AVNA (from the crux artery) is also called Kugel's artery (Fig. 7-10).

The ramus medianus (RM) (see Fig. 7-9*C,D*) is a branch of the LMCA, running diagonally across the midportion of the anterior left ventricular wall. Unless the origin of the RM is identified it may be confused with a proximal marginal branch of the LCX (obtuse marginal) or proximal diagonal branch of the LAD.

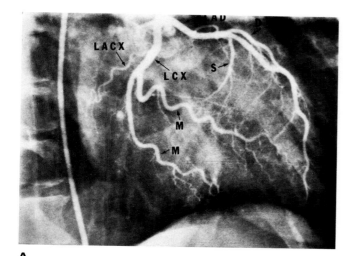

A

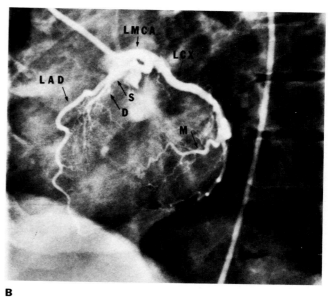

B

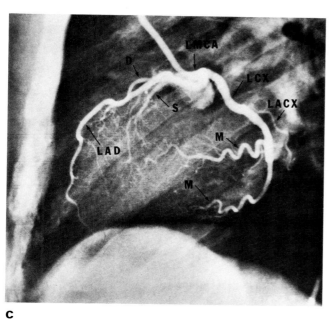
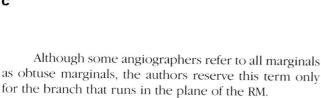

C

Figure 7-7. Normal nondominant left coronary artery. *A:* RAO view; *B:* LAO view; *C:* lateral view. The left main coronary artery (LMCA) usually bifurcates into two branches, the left anterior descending artery (LAD), and the left circumflex artery (LCX). Not infrequently the LMCA divides into three branches, the third branch being designated the ramus medianus (see Fig. 7-9*C, D*). The LAD courses in the anterior interventricular sulcus and supplies branches to the anterior interventricular septum (septal perforators or septal arteries (S), and diagonal branches (D) to the anterolateral left ventricular wall. Note the rather straight courses and forked terminations of the septal arteries. The LCX runs posteriorly along the atrioventricular groove toward the crux of the heart and gives off marginal branches (M) to the posterolateral wall of the left ventricle. The LCX also supplies the left atrium via the left atrial circumflex branch (LACX). (Reproduced with permission from Spindola–Franco H, Fish BG. Radiology of the heart: cardiac imaging in infants, children and adults. New York: Springer–Verlag, 1985.)

Although some angiographers refer to all marginals as obtuse marginals, the authors reserve this term only for the branch that runs in the plane of the RM.

Compound Angulated Views

The above description of the normal anatomy uses standard right anterior oblique and left anterior oblique views (Figs. 7-2–7-9) or lateral views (Figs. 7-7*C,* 7-9*C*). Although these familiar views for coronary imaging facilitate identification of the coronary artery, in practice, compound angulated views are necessary to completely delineate the coronary arterial tree. Because of tortuosity of vessels and superimposition of the vessels on the stan-

dard views, cranial and caudal angulated views are mandatory.

The terms cranial and caudal refer to the position of the image intensifier in relation to the patient. Although technical terminology that describes the direction of the x-ray beam such as caudal–cranial or cranial–caudal is more precise, it is cumbersome and is not commonly used. Several systems are available from various manufacturers to obtain these angulated views. Figures 7-11–7-15 illustrate the C-arm position and corresponding left coronary anatomy for standard and angulated views. Figures 7-16 and 7-17 illustrate the angulated views for the RCA.

Each view is helpful in visualizing specific portions of the coronary arterial tree. The caudal–RAO view of the

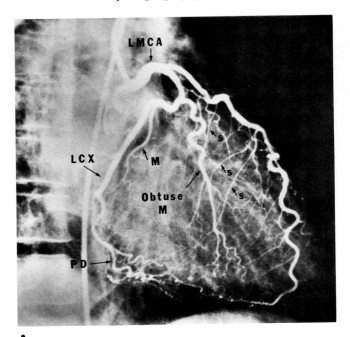

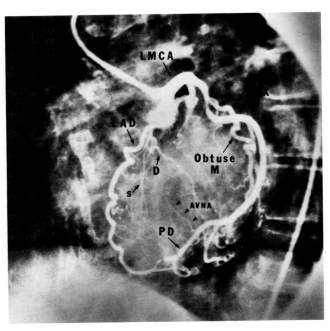

A　　　　　　　　　　　　　　　　　　　　　　**B**

Figure 7-8. Dominant left coronary artery. *A:* RAO view; *B:* LAO view. The posterior left ventricular wall is supplied by the left circumflex artery (LCX) by way of the marginal branches (M). The LCX supplies the posterior interventricular septum by way of the posterior descending artery (PD). Note that the atrioventricular node artery (AVNA; *arrowheads*) antecedes the PD. The first marginal branch is called an obtuse marginal because it courses in the plane of the ramus medianus (see Fig. 7-9C, D). (D, diagonal branch; LAD, left anterior descending artery; LMCA, left main coronary artery; S, septal perforator branch.) (Reproduced with permission from Spindola–Franco H, Fish BG. Radiology of the heart: cardiac imaging in infants, children and adults. New York: Springer–Verlag, 1985.)

LCA (see Fig. 7-12) widely separates the LAD from the LCX and differentiates the ramus medianus, when present, from either a proximal diagonal or a marginal branch. This view is particularly helpful for visualizing the LCX and marginal branches as well as the proximal portion of the LAD. The cranial–RAO view of the LCA (see Fig. 7-13) is an excellent view to delineate the LAD and the origins of its diagonal and septal branches. The cranial–LAO view is also very good for visualizing the LAD and diagonal arteries (see Fig. 7-14); however, the septal arteries frquently overlap the LAD. The caudal–LAO view of the LCA (see Fig. 7-15) is particularly helpful for visualizing the left main coronary artery and the origins of the LAD, LCX, and ramus medianus as well as the LCX and its marginal branches. Each of the angulated views of the RCA (Figs. 7-16, 7-17) may be helpful for visualizing the distal bifurcation of the RCA into the PD and crux artery as well as the branches of the crux artery (posterior left ventricular branches). Despite these basic principles, no view is ideal for every individual study. Furthermore, all the visualized coronary segments must be critically assessed in each view obtained, since one cannot always predict which view will best demonstrate the coronary pathology.

A diagnostic coronary angiogram generally consists of the following views: cranial and caudal angulation in both the RAO and LAO views in addition to the standard projections for the LCA; standard RAO and cranial LAO views of the RCA, although other angulated views are frequently necessary. In patients with suspicion of coronary artery disease, a full diagnostic study is necessary even if the vessels appear normal on the initial standard views.

Coronary Anomalies

In addition to a thorough knowledge of the normal coronary anatomy, one must also have a clear understanding of the congenital abnormalities of the coronary arteries. Although less common than acquired coronary disease, these anomalies may cause morbidity and mortality, including sudden death. They may also present considerable difficulties in interpretation of coronary arteriograms and may cause errors in surgical approach if not recognized. Our classification divides these lesions into three major categories: anomalies of origin, anomalies of course, and anomalies of termination.[20]

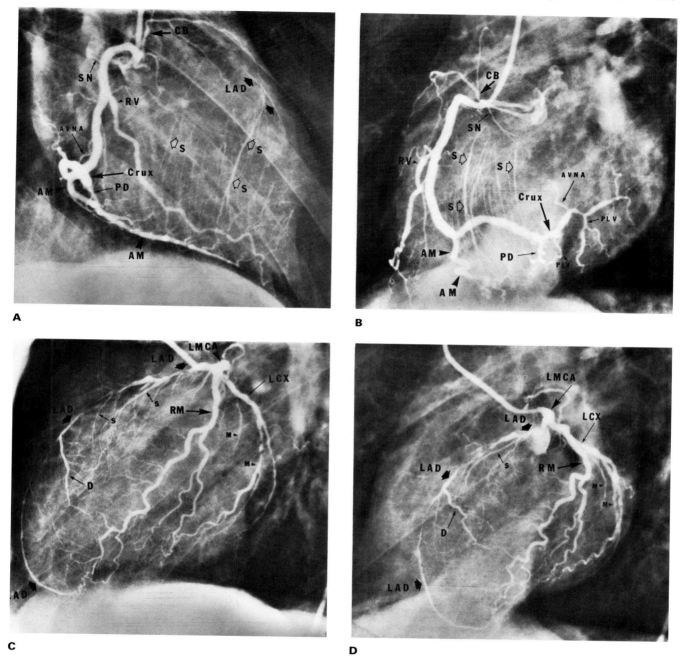

Figure 7-9. Septal collateral flow. *A:* RAO and *B:* LAO views of right coronary artery; *C:* lateral and *D:* LAO views of left coronary artery. The right coronary artery gives off numerous large septal arteries (S) which provide collateral flow to the left anterior descending artery (LAD). There is dual supply to the posterior interventricular septum because the acute marginal branch (AM) is large and gives off branches to the posterior ventricular septum. The posterior descending artery (PD) is small. The LAD is severely stenosed in its proximal portion and opacifies segmentally because of dilution from unopacified blood from septal collaterals seen in frames *A* and *B.* The marginal branches (M) of the LCX are also severely stenosed. Note that the LMCA trifurcates in this patient. The third branch is called the ramus medianus (RM). If the ramus medianus arises from the LCX it becomes the obtuse marginal branch (see Fig. 7-8). If the ramus medianus takes its origin from the LAD it becomes a diagonal branch. (AVNA, atrioventricular node artery; CB, conus branch or conus artery; CRUX, crux artery; D, diagonal branch; LMCA, left main coronary artery; LCX, left circumflex artery; M, marginal branch; PLV, posterolateral or posterior left ventricular branch; RV, right ventricular, preventricular, or muscular branch; SN, sinus node artery. (Reproduced with permission from Spindola–Franco H. In: Goldberger E, ed. Textbook of clinical cardiology. St. Louis: CV Mosby, 1982;305.)

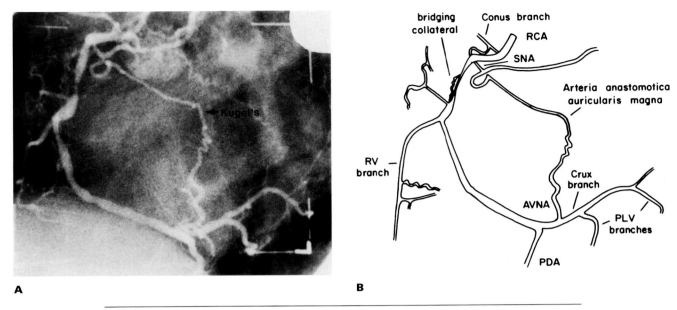

A   **B**

Figure 7-10. Kugel's artery (arteria anastomotica auricularis magna). LAO view of right coronary angiogram *A* and diagram *B.* The Kugel's artery is a collateral pathway connecting the sinus node artery (SNA) to the atrioventricular node artery (AVNA). It serves as a collateral pathway to the distal RCA. Note also that the RCA is occluded distal to the conus artery and reconstitutes by way of multiple bridging collaterals. (RV branch, right ventricular branch; PDA, posterior descending coronary artery; PLV branches, posterior left ventricular branches. (Reproduced with permission from Spindola–Franco H, Fish BG. Radiology of the heart: cardiac imaging in infants, children and adults. New York: Springer–Verlag, 1985.)

Anomalies of Origin

As previously discussed, the RCA normally arises from the right (anterior) sinus of Valsalva and the LCA arises from the left sinus of Valsalva, which is on the left and posterior. The noncoronary sinus normally gives off no coronary artery. The coronary ostia are at or near the level of the aortic ring.[19] Our classification of variations from this normal pattern follows:[20]

   I. Position and number of ostia.
     A. High and low take-off.
     B. Multiple ostia.
     C. Origin of a coronary artery or branch from the opposite sinus of Valsalva or from the noncoronary sinus.
  II. Single coronary artery.
 III. Anomalous origin from the pulmonary artery.
     A. LCA or branch.
     B. RCA.
     C. Both coronary arteries.
 IV. Origin from systemic vessels.

High or Low Take-Off. When the coronary arteries arise from the proper sinus, variation in the height in the aortic sinus may cause difficulty in cannulating the vessels during coronary angiography. A low take-off oc-

curs when the coronary ostium lies below the aortic ring and a high take-off may occur when the ostium is more than 1 cm above it.

Multiple Ostia. The usual cause of multiple ostia is that the RCA and the conus branch arise separately or that the LAD and the LCX arise separately with no left main coronary artery (LMCA). Separate ostia of the LAD and left circumflex from the left aortic sinus occurs in 0.5% to 1% of patients.[13]

Origin of a Coronary Artery from the Opposite Sinus of Valsalva or from the Posterior Sinus of Valsalva. The four patterns that have been recognized are as follows: (1) both coronary arteries may arise from the left coronary sinus; (2) both coronary arteries may arise from the right coronary sinus; (3) the LAD or the LCX may arise from the right sinus of Valsalva; and (4) the LCA or RCA, or a branch of either one, may arise from the posterior sinus. In any of these patterns the coronary ostia may be at the normal level, or may have a high or low take-off.

Symptoms seldom result when both coronary arteries arise from the left aortic sinus. In contrast, the patient is at increased risk for sudden death when both coronary arteries arise from the right sinus. In the latter

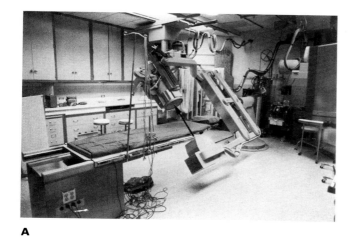

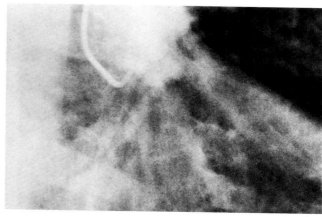

A

B

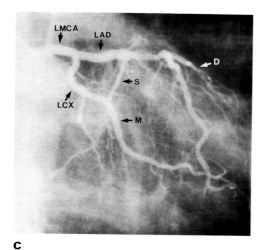

C

Figure 7-11. RAO view of the left coronary artery. In *A* the x-ray tube is below the table on the left. The image intensifier is above the table and on the right. The direction of the x-ray beam is indicated by the arrow. *B* presents the typical appearance of catheter tip in the left coronary artery. *C* shows the typical appearance of the left coronary artery in the RAO view. (Reproduced with permission from Spindola–Franco H, Fish BG. Radiology of the heart: cardiac imaging in infants, children and adults. New York: Springer–Verlag, 1985.)

variation the left main coronary artery courses either between the aorta and the pulmonary artery or anterior to the pulmonary artery. Rarely, it may have a retroaortic course. The course between the aorta and the pulmonary artery carries the highest risk for sudden death.[21,22]

The LAD may arise from the right coronary sinus either as a branch of the RCA or from a separate ostium. This abnormality is commonly associated with congenital abnormalities (tetralogy of Fallot, double-outlet right ventricle, and transposition complexes).[23–25] The LAD may travel either anterior to the pulmonary artery or between the aorta and main pulmonary artery. This latter variation is associated with angina and sudden death.

The LCX may also arise from the right sinus of Valsalva. Origin of the LCX from either the RCA itself (Fig. 7-18) or the right aortic sinus is the most common coronary anomaly that occurs in otherwise normal patients.[25,26] Fortunately, this anomaly has not been associated with death; however, proper identification of this pattern is important for patients undergoing coronary bypass surgery or valvular surgery.

Although either the LCA or the RCA may arise in the posterior aortic sinus, both these anomalies are unusual in otherwise normal hearts. Origin of the LCA from the posterior aortic sinus may be found rarely in complete transposition of the great arteries. Origin of the right coronary from the posterior aortic sinus is quite common in complete transposition of the great vessels, being present in approximately 60% of the cases.[23,24]

Single Coronary Artery. Various anatomic classifications of single coronary artery have been suggested.[27–29] Smith proposes the following categorization: (1) the single coronary artery may follow the pattern of a normal RCA or a LCA; (2) the single coronary artery may divide into two branches with distributions of the RCA and LCA; (3) a single coronary artery may have a distribution different from the normal coronary arterial tree.[29]

Lipton's classification, based on coronary angiograms, modified the classification of Smith as well as others[28] by using the letters R and L to signify whether the coronary ostium is in the right or left aortic sinus as

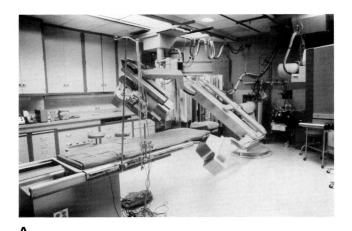

A

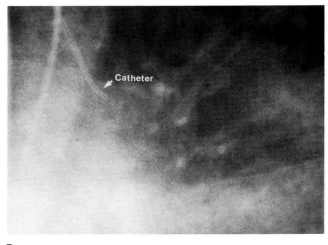

B

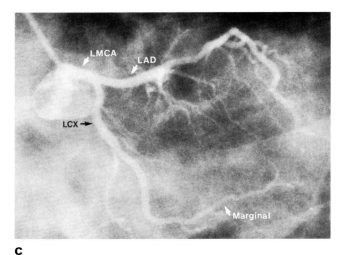

C

Figure 7-12. Compound RAO view of the left coronary artery with caudal tilt (also known as footward RAO or RAO with craniocaudal angulation). *A* shows the position of the x-ray tube and image intensifier. In *B* the catheter tip points down to enter the LCA. *C* shows the appearance of the LCA in the RAO view with caudal tilt. The LAD and LCX are widely separated without overlap of the origins so that each origin can be examined separately. In addition, this view allows differentiation of a ramus medianus, a branch of the distal LMCA, from an obtuse marginal, a branch of the LCX (see also Fig. 7-13*H*). The middle portion of the LAD forms an angle pointing superiorly reminiscent of the top of a tent, while the LCX and its marginal branch form a similar angle pointing inferiorly (this same patient is the same as that shown in Figs. 7-11*B, C* and 7-13*B, C*). (Reproduced with permission from Spindola–Franco H, Fish BG. Radiology of the heart: cardiac imaging in infants, children and adults. New York: Springer–Verlag, 1985.)

well as the letters A, B, and P to signify whether the artery courses anterior to, between, or posterior to the great vessels. Figure 7-19 demonstrates Lipton's classification of single coronary artery.

Although a single coronary artery may be compatible with a normal life expectancy, patients are at increased risk of sudden death if a major coronary branch crosses between the pulmonary artery and the aorta. Furthermore, some patients may develop angina pectoris during childhood or adolescence. Even though a single coronary artery may not predispose a person to atherosclerosis, certainly a proximal stenosis of a single coronary artery may be devastating because of the inability to develop collateral channels.

Coronary Arteries Arising from the Pulmonary Artery. Coronary arteries arising from the pulmonary artery (Bland–White–Garland syndrome) is one of the most serious congenital coronary artery defects.[30] It

usually results in death during infancy, and only a few patients survive to adulthood[31–34] (Fig. 7-20). Either the LCA or the RCA, both major coronary arteries, or rarely, the LAD or LCX may originate from the pulmonary artery. The usual presentation is an anomalous LCA arising from the pulmonary artery and the RCA arising from the aorta.[34] The RCA arising from the pulmonary artery is unusual, but when it does occur, it is a relatively benign anomaly. Rarely, both coronary arteries originate from the pulmonary artery.[35] This variety is not compatible with life except in the presence of an associated defect such as a ventricular septal defect, which allows increased oxygenation and systemic level pressure in the pulmonary artery.[36]

Origin from Systemic Vessels. Anastomoses between the coronary arteries and extracardiac vessels have

(*Text continues on page 235*)

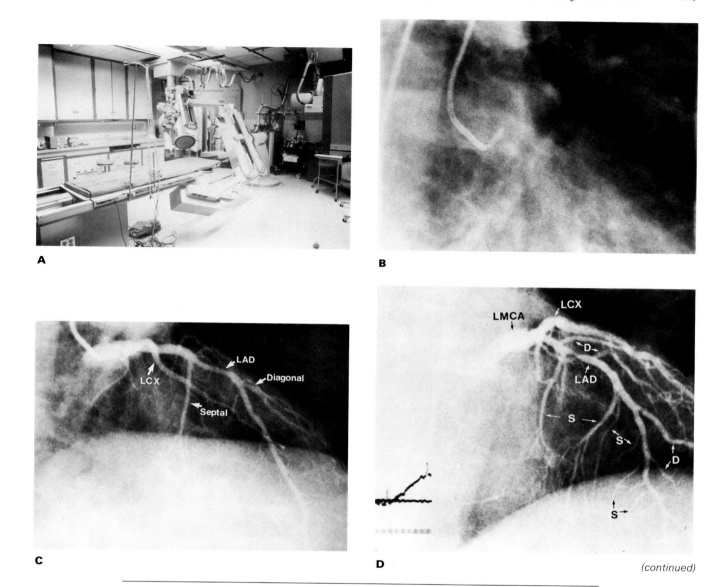

A

B

C

D

(continued)

Figure 7-13. RAO view of the left coronary artery with cranial tilt, also known as headward RAO or RAO with caudocranial angulation. In *A* the C-arm is positioned for the RAO with 20°–25° cranial tilt. In *B* the catheter tip in the LCA points superiorly. In *C* the LAD and LCX tend to be close to one another and may be superimposed, or the LCX may cross the LAD to appear above the LAD in contrast to the appearance in the RAO with caudal tilt Figure 7-12. The RAO with cranial tilt is useful in delineating the entire course of the LAD, and the origins of the diagonal and septal arteries. Further headward angulation (>25°) exaggerates the superior position of the LCX and inferior position of the LAD allowing better delineation of the origins of the diagonal and septal branches; however, increased angulation impairs resolution, especially in heavy patients. *D* is from a different patient and illustrates the effect of a 30° cranial angulation, giving the LAD the appearance of a denuded spine of a fish with the septal arteries pointing inferiorly and the diagonal branches superiorly. The origin of the septal (S) and diagonal (D) branches are clearly delineated.

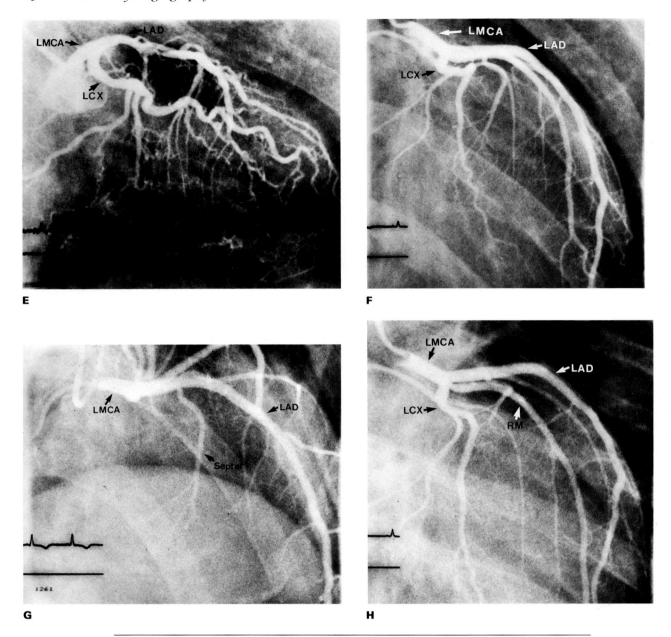

Figure 7-13 (continued). *E* is the standard RAO view in the same patient for comparison. In patients with dilated cardiomyopathy the same effect can be achieved without increasing the headward angulation. *F, G,* and *H* are from a different patient with dilated cardiomyopathy. In *F,* the standard RAO view, the LAD, the diagonals, and a third vessel are superimposed. It is not possible to determine in this view whether the third vessel is a ramus medianus, an obtuse marginal branch, or a large proximal diagonal vessel. In *G,* the RAO view with cranial tilt, the LCX and the third vessel are superior to the LAD. The entire LAD and the origins of the septals and diagonals can now be assessed individually. *H* is an RAO view with caudal tilt in the same patient showing the opposite effect, with the LCX being inferior and widely separated from the LAD. In this view the third vessel is recognized as a ramus medianus (RM) because it takes origin from the distal left main coronary artery (trifurcation). This view allows separation of the origins of the LAD, the LCX, and the ramus medianus if present. In addition the entire left main coronary artery is visible. (Reproduced with permission from Spindola–Franco H, Fish BG. Radiology of the heart: cardiac imaging in infants, children and adults. New York: Springer–Verlag, 1985.)

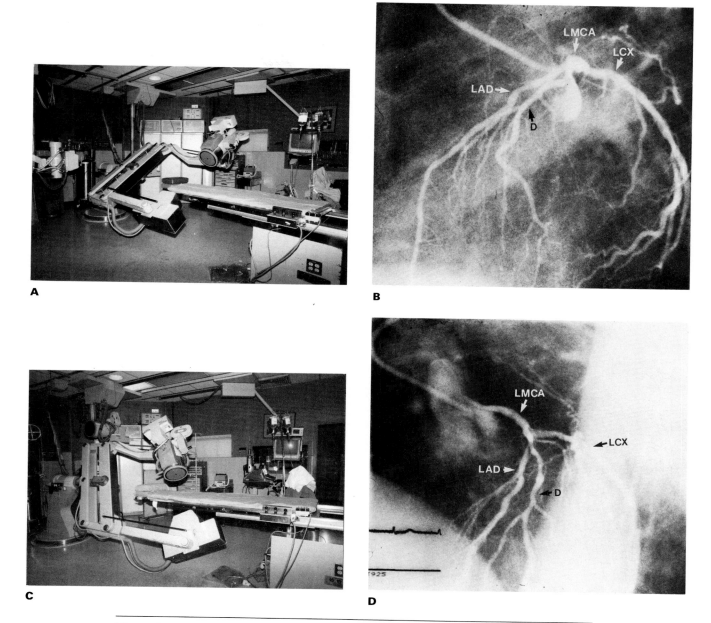

Figure 7-14. Standard LAO view, and LAO view of the left coronary artery with cranial tilt. The LAO view with cranial tilt is also known as headward LAO, LAO with caudocranial angulation, hepatoclavicular view, and four-chamber view. *A* shows the position of the C-arm for a standard LAO view. In *B* the left coronary angiogram in the LAO view shows the left main coronary artery (LMCA) on end. The proximal portions of the LAD and the large diagonal branch (D) are foreshortened. No stenosis is apparent in this view. In *C* the C-arm is positioned for an LAO view with cranial tilt. In *D* the corresponding angiogram of the left coronary artery in the same patient. The LMCA is visualized in its entirety and the proximal portion of the LAD and large diagonal branch are delineated. A significant stenosis of the LAD is now evident just distal to the origin of the large diagonal branch. (Reproduced with permission from Spindola–Franco H, Fish BG. Radiology of the heart: cardiac imaging in infants, children and adults. New York: Springer–Verlag, 1985.)

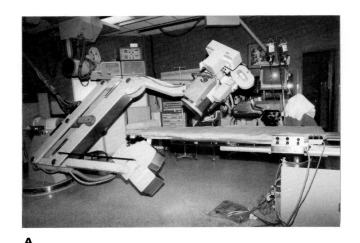

A

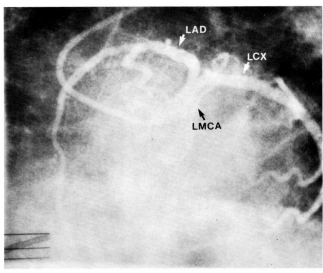

B

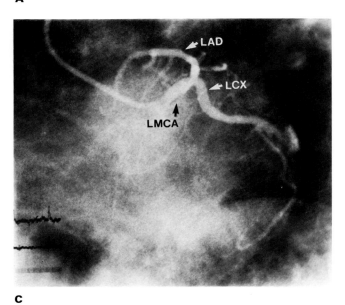

C

Figure 7-15. LAO view with caudal tilt. This view is also known as footward LAO or LAO with craniocaudal angulation. In *A,* the C-arm is positioned for the LAO view with caudal tilt. In *B,* the LAO view of the left coronary artery with caudal tilt, the left main coronary artery points superiorly and the LAD and LCX diverge, so that the origins and proximal portions are separate. The appearance of the LAD and LCX in this view is reminiscent of a bat flying, the left main coronary artery (LMCA) being the head and the LAD and LCX being the wings. *C* is an illustration of the same view in a different patient with a short LAD. The right wing of the bat is shorter. The appearance of the LMCA and branches in this view is strikingly different from that observed in the LAO with cranial tilt (Fig. 7-14*C,* *D*). (Reproduced with permission from Spindola–Franco H, Fish BG. Radiology of the heart: cardiac imaging in infants, children and adults. New York: Springer–Verlag, 1985.)

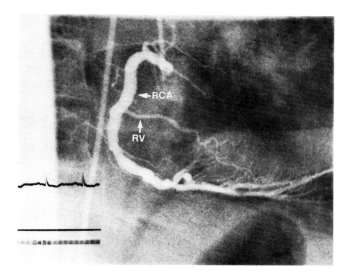
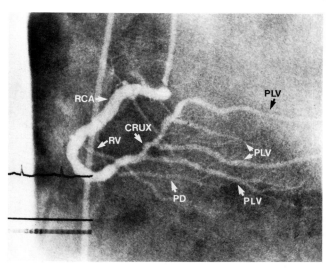

A   **B**

Figure 7-16. Standard and cranial-tilt RAO views of the right coronary artery. *A* shows the standard RAO view of the right coronary artery (see also Fig. 7-3). In the standard RAO view, the posterior descending artery (PD) and the crux artery and its branches (the posterior left ventricular branches, or PLVs) are superimposed. *B* shows the RAO view of the RCA with cranial angulation. In this view the crux artery becomes nearly vertical pointing superiorly. The PD and PVLs are separated so that they appear as parallel horizontal lines similar to the steps of a ladder. The PD is at the bottom, with the PVLs above it. The origins are all clearly visualized. (RV, right ventricular branch arising from the midportion of the right coronary artery.) (Reproduced with permission from Spindola–Franco H, Fish BG. Radiology of the heart: cardiac imaging in infants, children and adults. New York: Springer–Verlag, 1985.)

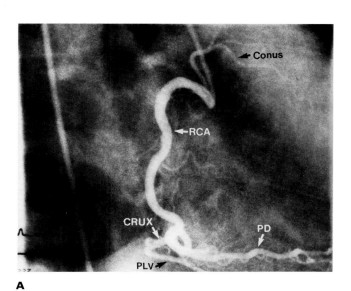
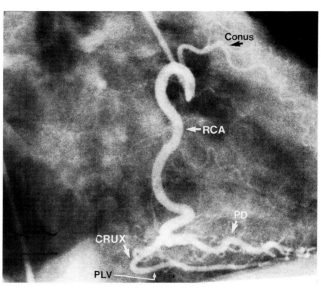

A   **B**

Figure 7-17. Standard RAO view of the right coronary artery (RCA) (*A*) and RAO view with caudal tile (*B*). As in Figure 7-16, the angulated view (*B*) causes the crux artery to become vertical. The posterior descending artery (PD) is now at the top with the posterior left ventricular branches (PLV) projecting below in a manner similar to the steps of a ladder. This patient has only one PLV. The distal portion of the RCA, and the origins of the PD and PLV are separated in this view. (Reproduced with permission from Spindola–Franco H, Fish BG. Radiology of the heart: cardiac imaging in infants, children and adults. New York: Springer–Verlag, 1985.)

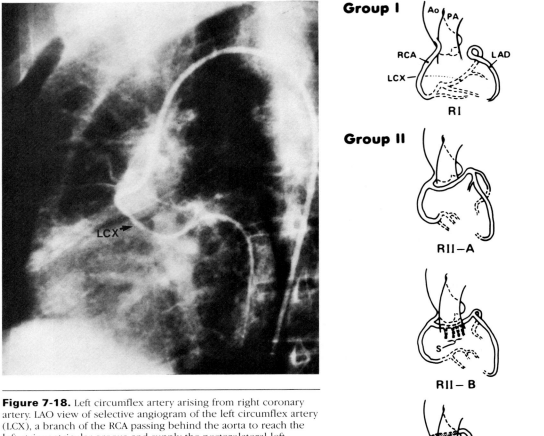

Figure 7-18. Left circumflex artery arising from right coronary artery. LAO view of selective angiogram of the left circumflex artery (LCX), a branch of the RCA passing behind the aorta to reach the left atrioventricular groove and supply the posterolateral left ventricular wall. The RCA proper is not visualized because the catheter is selectively in the left circumflex artery. (Reproduced with permission from Spindola–Franco H, Fish BG. Radiology of the heart: cardiac imaging in infants, children and adults. New York: Springer–Verlag, 1985.)

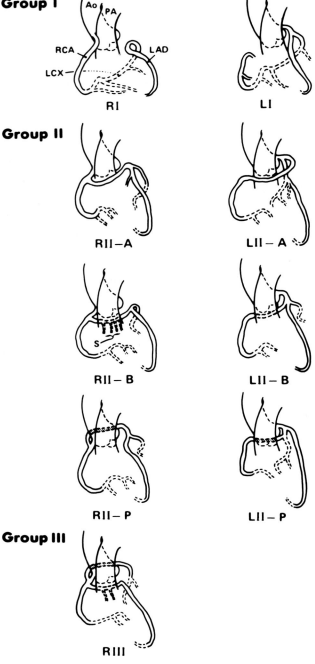

Figure 7-19. Single coronary artery. A single coronary artery may arise from the left or right sinus of Valsalva. In group I the right or left single coronary artery continues past the crux of the heart within the atrioventricular groove to supply the area normally perfused by the contralateral artery distribution. In group II-A a large branch of the single coronary artery crosses anterior to the pulmonary artery. In group II-B the large trunk passes between the aorta and the pulmonary artery, whereas in group II-P the large trunk crosses posterior to the aorta. Group III includes subtypes with two smaller vessels that supply the contralateral distribution. One branch crosses between the great vessels, and one crosses behind the great vessels. Group II-B, in which the trunk passes between the great vessels, may be a cause of sudden death as a result of compression of the artery by the aorta and pulmonary artery. (R, right; L, left; Ao, aorta; PA, main pulmonary artery; LAD, left anterior descending coronary artery; LCX, left circumflex coronary artery; RCA, right coronary artery; A, anterior; B, between; and P, posterior to the great vessels.) Shading of the transverse trunk indicates that this artery crosses posterior to the aorta. (Reproduced with permission from Lipton MJ, et al. Isolated single coronary artery: diagnosis, angiographic classifications and clinical significance. Radiology 1979;130:39.)

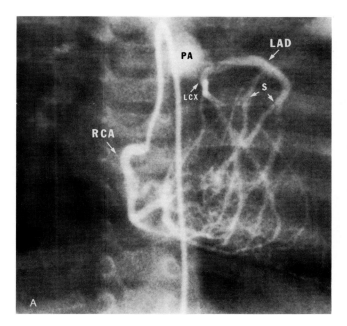
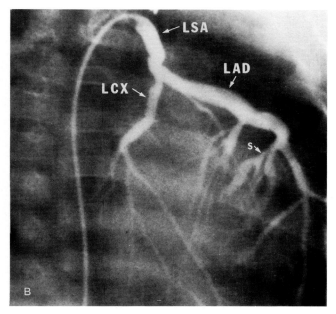

Figure 7-20. Anomalous origin of the LCA from the pulmonary artery in a 2-year-old child. *A:* Frontal view of right coronary (RCA) angiogram demonstrating retrograde opacification of the left anterior descending (LAD), left circumflex (LCX), and the left main coronary arteries by way of septal (S) and epicardial collaterals. There is a small left-to-right shunt with visualization of the main pulmonary artery (PA). The septal arteries are markedly dilated. *B:* RAO view of the left subclavian artery (LSA) angiogram obtained postoperatively, demonstrating the anastomosis of the LSA to the left main coronary artery. The septal arteries remain markedly dilated 9 months after surgery. (Reproduced with permission from Greenberg MA, et al. Congenital anomalies of the coronary arteries: classification and significance. Radiol Clin North Am 1989;27:1127.)

been recognized since the beginning of the 19th century.[37] These include anastomosis with bronchial, internal mammary, pericardial, and anterior mediastinal arteries as well as superior and inferior phrenic, intercostal, and esophageal branches of the aorta.

Anomalies of Course

Although the origin of the major coronary arteries may be in the normal sinus and position, the course of the blood vessels may be unusual and lead to confusion both in interpretation of the coronary angiogram and in identification of the blood vessels at the time of surgery.

Our classification of anomalies of the course of the coronary arteries follows:[20]

  I. Normal pattern with an intramyocardial segment (myocardial bridge).
  II. Duplication of arteries.
    A. Multiple posterior descending arteries.
    B. Dual LAD.
    C. Parallel LAD.
  III. Coronary artery passing between the pulmonary trunk and the aorta (discussed with anomalies of origin).

Myocardial Bridge. Myocardial bridging is caused by a coronary artery being embedded in the myocardium for a variable distance and reemerging on the surface thereafter. This creates a phenomenon of "milking" whereby the artery is constricted only in systole and returns to a normal caliber in diastole (Fig. 7-21). Functionally, no stenosis is present, and myocardial bridging should not be confused with a long segment of stenosis.

Duplication of Arteries. Normal variations in the right coronary artery are common and are usually easily recognized.[15] Conversely, the left anterior descending coronary artery is the vessel in the human heart that has the most constant origin, course, and distribution. Thus, when the LAD displays unusual anatomy, confusion often results.

Spindola–Franco and colleagues previously described four variants of dual LAD.[38] A dual LAD system consists of an early bifurcation of the LAD into one early terminating branch, which remains in the anterior interventricular sulcus (AIVS) and is termed the short LAD, and a second branch, which has a variable course outside the AIVS and is the long LAD. Figure 7-22 demonstrates these four anatomic variants. Type I, the most common variant of dual LAD, is characterized by a short and a long

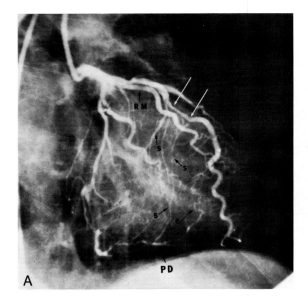
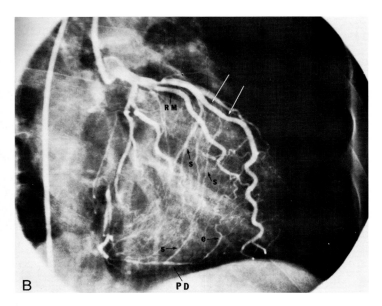

Figure 7-21. Myocardial bridging or "milking" of a coronary artery. RAO view of LCA; *A:* Systole; *B:* diastole. Note the long segment of marked narrowing of the left anterior descending artery during systole, which completely disappears during diastole. This segment is embedded in the myocardium with an overlying myocardial bridge (*long arrows*). Observe also reconstitution of the posterior descending artery (PD) by septal (S), and epicardial (e) collaterals. The left atrial circumflex branch provides flow to the crux artery by way of the atrioventricular node artery. The right coronary angiogram showed occlusion of that vessel. (RM, ramus medianus.) (Reproduced with permission from Spindola–Franco H, Fish BG. Radiology of the heart: cardiac imaging in infants, children and adults. New York: Springer–Verlag, 1985.)

LAD, both of which originate from the LAD proper. The short LAD runs in the AIVS and terminates well before reaching the apex. The long LAD leaves the AIVS and runs on the anterior epicardial surface of the left ventricle for two-thirds of its course. The distal third of the long LAD reenters the sulcus and continues to the apex (Fig. 7-23). Type II is similar, but the long LAD runs on the anterior wall of the right ventricle for the first two-thirds of its course instead of on the anterior wall of the left ventricle, as in type I. Type III is characterized by an intramyocardial long LAD. This long LAD has its proximal course deep within the interventricular septum and then makes an abrupt turn towards the AIVS, emerging on the epicardial surface, and turning to run in the apical portion of the AIVS (Fig. 7-24). Type IV differs in that the long LAD originates from the RCA. The long LAD crosses anterior to the infundibulum of the right ventricle and makes a sharp turn to descend on the anterior interventricular sulcus, giving off septal and left ventricular diagonal vessels. The LAD proper and the short LAD form a single very short vessel from which the major septal perforators and left ventricular diagonal branches originate (Fig. 7-25).

It is important to be familiar with these variations in patients undergoing coronary artery bypass surgery to prevent bypass to the wrong vessel. At the time of surgery the two left anterior descending vessels may be mistaken for one another unless the surgeon is forewarned. Furthermore, in patients with atherosclerotic disease in whom part or all of the dual LAD system fills through collaterals, the proper interpretation of the angiogram may be difficult.

These four variants of the dual LAD should not be confused with parallel LAD, in which a diagonal branch runs parallel to the LAD (Fig. 7-26). The parallel diagonal branch does not reenter the AIVS to take over the course of the distal LAD, as does the long LAD.[13]

Anomalies of Termination

I. Abnormal termination into a cardiac chamber, great vessel, or systemic vein (coronary arteriovenous fistula)
II. Thebesian vein drainage
III. Termination outside the heart (pulmonary steal syndrome)
IV. Coronary arcade of Spindola–Franco

Congenital coronary arteriovenous fistula is an uncommon cardiac lesion in which communication exists

(*Text continues on page 240*)

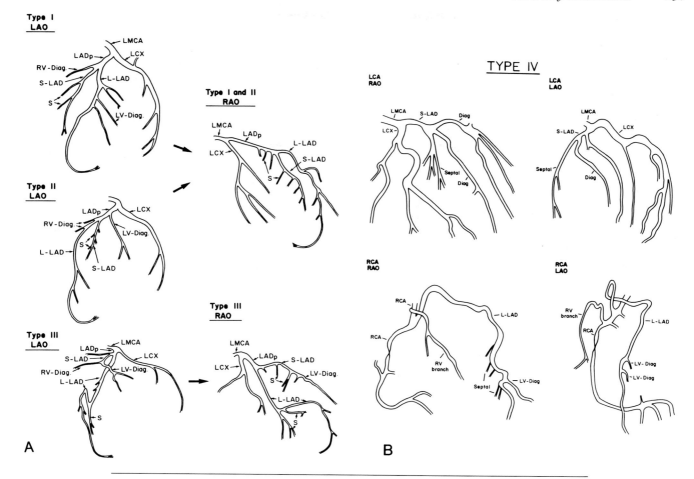

Figure 7-22. Dual left anterior descending artery (LAD) variants. *A:* In types I, II, and III the LAD proper (LAD_p) divides into two branches: the short LAD (S-LAD) and the long LAD (L-LAD). The S-LAD runs within the interventricular sulcus, but terminates well before the apex. The L-LAD runs initially outside the interventricular sulcus but reenters the sulcus to assume the course of the LAD distally. In type I the L-LAD runs along the left ventricular surface. In type II the L-LAD runs along the right ventricular surface. In type III the L-LAD runs within the interventricular septum. *B:* In type IV the LAD_p and S-LAD form a single very short vessel situated high in the interventricular sulcus. The first septal perforator and proximal diagonal branches are given off by this vessel. The L-LAD is a branch of the right coronary artery (RCA). The first portion of the L-LAD is formed by a transverse trunk that courses anteriorly to the infundibulum and makes a sharp turn to descend along the anterior interventricular sulcus, while giving off septal and left ventricular diagonal branches. (LCA, left coronary artery; LMCA, left main coronary artery; LCX, left circumflex artery; LV-Diag, diagonal branch to the wall of the left ventricle; S, septal artery; RV-Diag, diagonal branch to the wall of the right ventricle; Diag, diagonal branch; septal, septal artery; RV-branch, right ventricular branch.) (Reproduced with permission from Spindola–Franco H, et al. Dual left anterior descending coronary artery: angiographic description of important variants and surgical implications. Am Heart J 1983;105:445.)

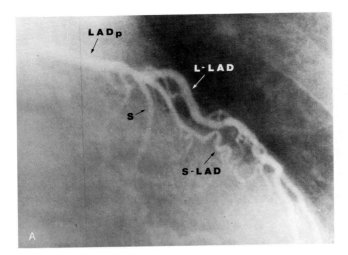
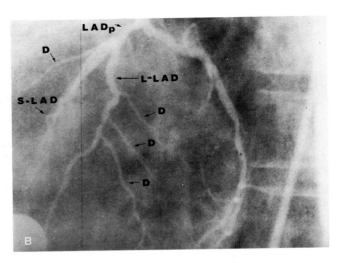

Figure 7-23. Dual left anterior descending artery (LAD) type I. *A:* RAO view; *B:* LAO view. The LAD proper (LAD$_p$) divides into a short LAD (S-LAD) and a long LAD (L-LAD). The S-LAD gives off the major septal perforators, and a diagonal branch to the right ventricle (D). The undulating course of the S-LAD is evidence that it represents an epicardial vessel. The L-LAD courses initially on the epicardial surface of the left ventricle and then returns to the anterior interventricular sulcus distally to occupy the course of the LAD. The L-LAD gives off the diagonal branches to the left ventricle. Note the apparent "avascular" area between the S-LAD and L-LAD and the gap between the S-LAD and the L-LAD within the interventricular sulcus. In the RAO view the LCX is not included in the area filmed. (Reproduced with permission from Spindola–Franco H, et al. Dual left anterior descending coronary artery: angiographic description of important variants and surgical implications. Am Heart J 1983;105:445.)

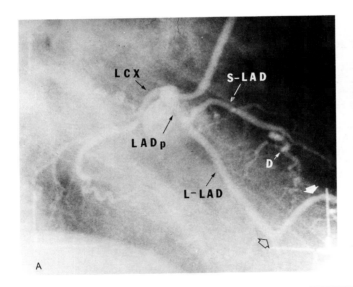
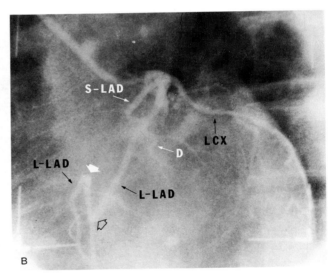

Figure 7-24. Dual LAD type III. RAO (*A*) and LAO (*B*) views of left coronary angiogram. The LAD proper (LAD$_p$) gives off two branches: the long LAD (L-LAD) and the short LAD (S-LAD). The S-LAD runs along the anterior interventricular sulcus and gives off diagonals (D). The L-LAD runs initially within the interventricular septum. The L-LAD makes a sharp turn (*open arrow*) to emerge beyond the termination of the S-LAD and takes over its course distally (*white arrow*). Note the long gap in the interventricular sulcus between the S-LAD and the L-LAD. (Reproduced with permission from Spindola–Franco H, et al. Dual left anterior descending coronary artery: angiographic description of important variants and surgical implications. Am Heart J 1983;105:445.)

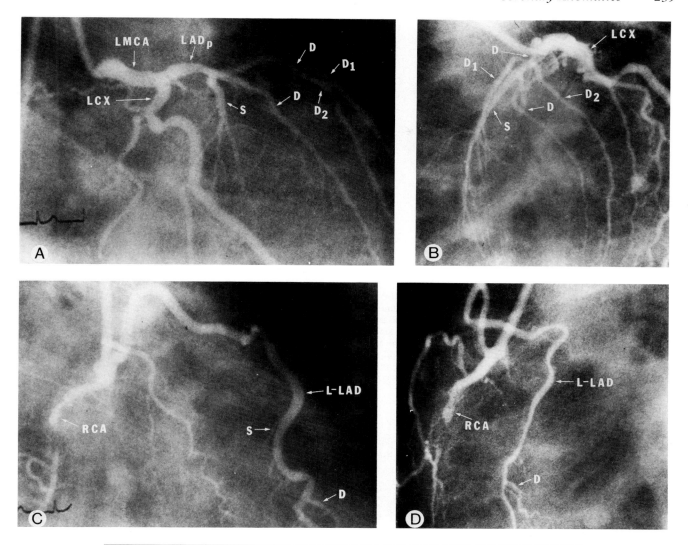

Figure 7-25. Dual left anterior descending artery (LAD) type IV. RAO (*A*) and LAO (*B*) views of LCA; RAO (*C*) and LAO (*D*) view of right coronary artery (RCA). The LAD proper (LAD$_p$) and short LAD form a single very short vessel situated high in the anterior interventricular sulcus. The major septal (S) and left ventricular diagonal (D) branches originate from this short vessel. The long LAD (L-LAD) is a branch of the RCA. The first portion of the L-LAD is formed by a transverse trunk that courses anteriorly to the infundibulum of the right ventricle and makes a sharp turn to descend on the anterior interventricular sulcus. The L-LAD gives off septal (S) and left ventricular diagonal branches (D). (LMCA, left main coronary artery; LCX, left circumflex artery; D$_1$ and D$_2$, superior and inferior branches of the first diagonal.) (Reproduced with permission from Spindola–Franco H, et al. Dual left anterior descending coronary artery: angiographic description of important variants and surgical implications. Am Heart J 1983;105:445.)

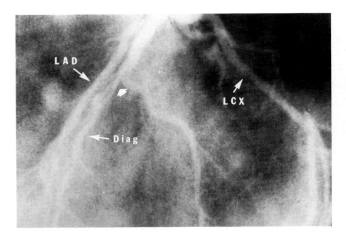

Figure 7-26. Parallel diagonal vessel. LAO view of left coronary angiogram. A large diagonal vessel (Diag) runs parallel to the left anterior descending (LAD) but does not take over the course of the LAD. Both vessels extend to the apex. This variation should be differentiated from dual LAD type I. There is severe stenosis in the parallel diagonal (*arrow*). It will be important to distinguish the two vessels at surgery so that the correct one is grafted. (LCX, left circumflex artery.) (Reproduced with permission from Spindola–Franco H, et al. Dual left anterior descending coronary artery: angiographic description of important variants and surgical implications. Am Heart J 1983;105:445.)

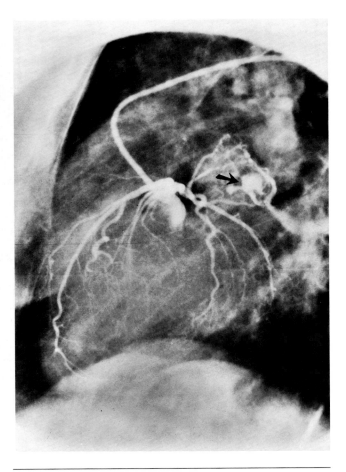

Figure 7-27. Neovascularity and direct intracavitary drainage into the left atrial appendage in a 63-year-old woman with mitral stenosis. Lateral view of selective LCA injection. Branches of the left atrial circumflex artery shows numerous distal vessels (neovascularity) and direct drainage into the cavity of the left atrial appendage. The arrow points toward a momentary concentration or "puddle" of contrast medium within the left atrial appendage. This contrast material is quickly diluted and carried away by unopacified blood. No left atrial thrombus or neoplasm was observed at operation. (Reproduced with permission from Spindola–Franco H, Fish BG. Radiology of the heart: cardiac imaging in infants, children and adults. New York: Springer–Verlag, 1985.)

between the coronary artery and a cardiac chamber, the coronary sinus, the superior vena cava, or the pulmonary artery. This disorder must be differentiated from anomalous origin of a coronary artery from the pulmonary artery, which is discussed above. Most commonly the coronary arteriovenous fistula involves the RCA alone. This occurs in 60% of the cases, as compared to 40% for the LCA.[39,40] The fistula may terminate either in single or multiple entry sites, or may terminate in an aneurysmal dilatation.[41] The most common site of drainage is the right ventricle, followed by the right atrium and the pulmonary artery. Drainage into the left atrium and left ventricle is less common.

An incidental finding in association with severe mitral stenosis is an acquired fistulous connection between the left circumflex artery (left atrial circumflex) and the left atrial appendage, ending in a network of fistulous tracts (Fig. 7-27). These fistulae may result from erosion or neovascularity secondary to a thrombus.[42,43] In our experience this type of neovascularity and fistulous drainage may also occur in patients with mitral stenosis in the absence of thrombus.[4] These vessels may have formed in response to a thrombus that subsequently dissolved or embolized or may be due to a local atrial wall abnormality.

An artifact that should not be mistaken for a coronary arteriovenous fistula is a pseudocoronary arteriovenous fistula resulting from occlusion of a coronary artery by the catheter during coronary arteriography (Fig.

7-28). Several characteristic patterns of coronary occlusion arteriography have been reported by Spindola–Franco and colleagues.[44]

Thebesian Vein Drainage. An occasional finding on coronary arteriography is drainage from the coronary arteries directly into the ventricular cavities without opacification of the coronary sinus. We have observed this finding in normal patients and in those with cardiomyopathy, rheumatic heart disease, and prolapse of the mitral valve.[4] This finding probably represents the Thebesian connections known to exist as part of the deep venous drainage system of the heart.[44]

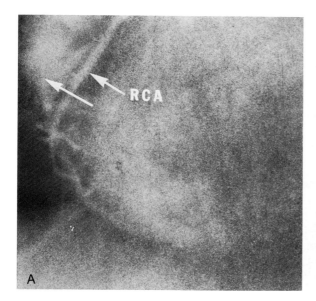 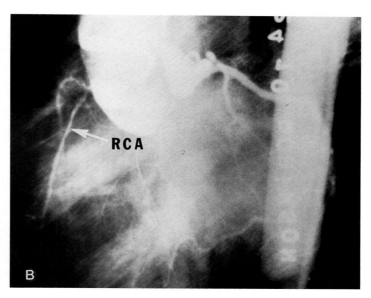

Figure 7-28. Occlusion arteriography causing pseudocoronary arteriovenious fistula. *A:* LAO view of right coronary artery (RCA) angiogram; *B:* flush aortogram, same case. Note in *A* opacification of the right atrium (*long arrow*) by way of the anterior cardiac veins before the coronary sinus fills, simulating an arteriovenous fistula from RCA to right atrium. The flush aortogram shows that the RCA is small and that no arteriovenous fistula is present. (Reproduced with permission from Spindola–Franco H, et al. Coronary vascular patterns during occlusion arteriography. Radiology 1975;114:59.)

Extracardiac Terminations. As described in the section on systemic origin of cardiac vessels, connections exist between bronchial and coronary arteries regardless of age or pathology. These connections, however, become functional only when a pressure gradient exists. In patients with pulmonary disease such as tumor or inflammation that decreases perfusion in the bronchial vascular bed, flow from coronary to bronchial arteries may occur.[45,46]

Spindola–Franco and others have reported a patient with angina pectoris in whom the pulmonary artery branch to an apical lung segment was supplied by a bronchial collateral vessel, which in turn originated from the LACX (Pulmonary steal syndrome)[47] (Fig. 7-29). The patient's angina was cured by ligation of the apical pulmonary artery branch. Although one cannot exclude previous pulmonary inflammatory disease as a stimulus to formation of this collateral pathway, it is also possible that this may represent a true congenital anomaly.

Coronary Arcade. Rarely, a communication can exist between the RCA and the LCX in the absence of coronary artery stenosis[20] (Fig. 7-30). Although these intercoronary communications between normal vessels are rare in the coronary circulation, they are common in other vascular systems. Examples of such arterial–arterial communications include (1) superficial volar arch of the hand, which is a communication between the ulnar and radial arteries, (2) intestinal branches of the superior

mesenteric artery from multiple arches, (3) the gastric artery which extends from the right to the left gastroepiploic artery, (4) the circle of Willis. Such an intercoronary communication in the heart would protect the myocardium from acute occlusion of either coronary artery and would be more effective than coronary collateral vessels, which develop only in response to chronic coronary vascular disease.

Roentgen Pathology of Coronary Artery Disease

Once the coronary anatomy has been determined, each of the coronary arteries should then be individually assessed for (1) extent of the disease; (2) location (i.e., proximal or distal); (3) degree of obstruction (less or greater than 75% of the arterial lumen); (4) length of the coronary occlusive lesions; (5) anatomy of the vessel distal to the obstruction; and (6) presence or absence of coronary dilatation or ectasia. Arteriomegaly is present when the dilatation is secondary to atherosclerosis (Fig. 7-31). It is usually localized to the proximal segments. Characteristically the dilatation is not uniform and often it is associated with stasis of contrast material along the arterial wall. Calcification, ulceration (Fig. 7-32), and aneurysm (Fig. 7-33) should also be identified and reported.

Fixed coronary artery stenosis is hemodynamically significant if it impairs maximal coronary flow reserve.

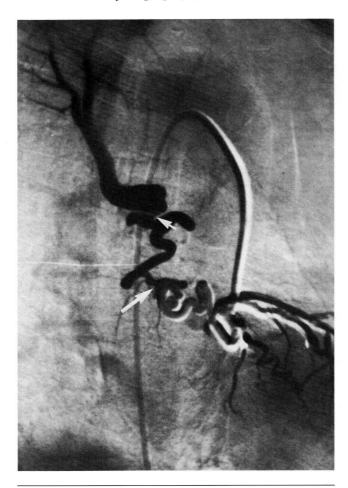

Figure 7-29. Pulmonary steal syndrome in a 53-year-old male with angina. RAO view of a left coronary angiogram (subtraction film). This syndrome consists of an unusual connection between a coronary artery and a pulmonary artery by way of a bronchial artery, allowing blood to be diverted away from the myocardium to the pulmonary circulation. The white arrows demonstrate the anastomosis between the left atrial circumflex and the bronchial artery and between the bronchial artery and the pulmonary artery. The caliber of the left atrial circumflex artery is larger than that of the major branches of the left coronary artery. (Reproduced with permission from Spindola–Franco H, et al. Pulmonary steal syndrome: an unusual case of coronary-bronchial-pulmonary artery communication. Radiology 1978;126:25.)

This usually occurs if the diameter of the vessel is diminished by more than 75%, when reciprocating flow is present, or when collateral vessels are apparent. Reciprocating flow (Figs. 7-34, 7-35) refers to the phasic alternation of the direction of movement of blood in a coronary artery so that in some phases of the cardiac cycle it is antegrade and in others retrograde.[48] This flow pattern represents competitive flow between opacified antegrade and the unopacified collateral blood. Visualization of reciprocating flow in epicardial vessels is associated with more than 85% of coronary stenosis or with occlusion

with collateral pathways and a perfusable (viable) capillary bed. Reciprocating flow is not detected in diffusely diseased coronary arteries. The presence of reciprocating flow should, therefore, be considered a favorable sign if coronary artery bypass surgery is contemplated. Furthermore, caution must be exercised to avoid misdiagnosis of a coronary stenosis in a vessel exhibiting reciprocating flow.

Spasm of the Coronary Arteries

Spasm of a coronary artery can be the cause of chest pain and ST-segment elevation in patients with Prinzmetal variant angina (PVA). Spasm also occurs in patients with typical and preinfarctional angina. It is important to differentiate spasm from fixed stenosis because spasm may be managed medically, whereas fixed stenosis may require surgery or angioplasty. Symptomatic (spontaneous) spasm of a coronary artery must also be differentiated from catheter-induced spasm, which requires no treatment.[49] Catheter-induced spasm (Fig. 7-36) is asymptomatic and is almost exclusively confined to the RCA. Characteristically, catheter-induced spasm has the appearance of a smooth, concentric, 1- to 2-mm narrowing at the site of the tip of the catheter. This form of spasm disappears after administration of nitroglycerin or after repositioning of the catheter. On the other hand, in patients with PVA, spasm (Fig. 7-37) can occur in any coronary artery, being frequently associated with transient ST-segment changes, angina, hypotension, cardiac dysrhythmias, and even cardiac standstill. PVA-induced spasm begins 1 to 4 mm beyond the tip of the catheter, involving a fairly long segment with an irregular or eccentric appearance, which may simulate fixed obstruction.

In patients with PVA the coronary angiogram should be obtained again after administration of nitroglycerin or calcium channel blockers (e.g., nifedipine, verapamil, diltiazem) to differentiate spasm from fixed obstruction. In some instances spasm in PVA is refractory to pharmacologic manipulation (Fig. 7-38). If the presence of spasm is suspected because of the clinical findings, it may be necessary to obtain another coronary arteriogram later to substantiate the diagnosis.

In patients with ischemic symptoms, but with normal coronary arteries on angiography, ergonovine can be given intravenously to provoke spasm to determine a cause for the symptoms.[50]

Unusual Coronary Artery Pathology

Kawasaki disease (which seems to be identical to polyarteritis nodosa) is the most common inflammatory disease that affects the coronary arteries. Lupus erythema-

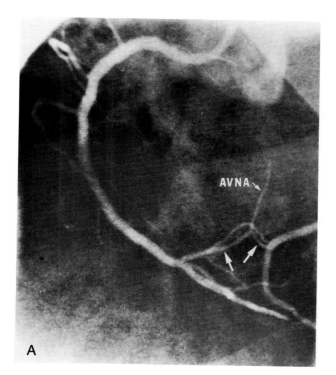

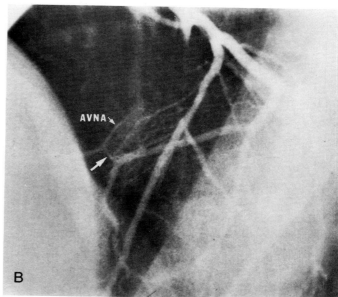

Figure 7-30. Coronary arcade (intercoronary anastomosis without obstructive coronary disease). LAO views with cranial angulation of the right (*A*) and left (*B*) selective coronary angiograms. The right and left coronary arteries interconnect at the crux, forming a vascular arcade (*arrows*) with the atrioventricular nodal artery (AVNA) arising from this connecting vessel. There is free flow into the contralateral vessel from either coronary injection through the interconnecting vessel. No areas of narrowing are observed in either the coronary ostia or the vessels themselves. (Reproduced with permission from Greenberg, et al. Congenital anomalies of the coronary arteries. Radiol Clin North Am 1989;27:1127.)

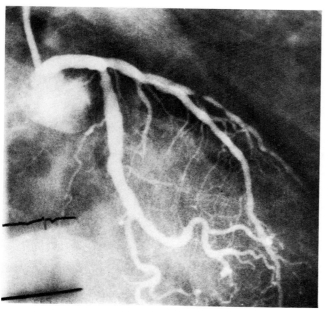

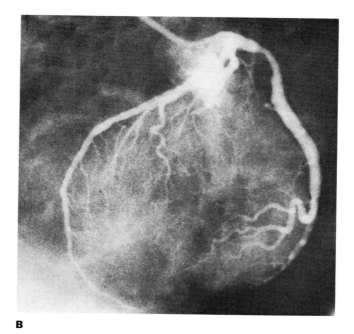

Figure 7-31. Coronary artery ectasia or arteriomegaly. RAO (*A*) and LAO (*B*) views of LCA. The LCX displays diffuse ectasia in its proximal and middle segments. Diffuse ectasia (arteriomegaly) predisposes to coronary artery thrombosis. Note also diffuse atherosclerotic change in the LAD and diagonal vessels. (Reproduced with permission from Spindola–Franco H, Fish BG. Radiology of the heart: cardiac imaging in infants, children and adults. New York: Springer–Verlag, 1985.)

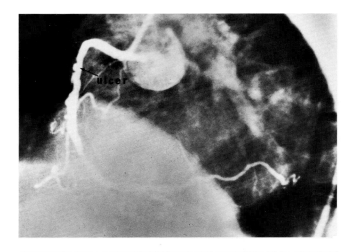

Figure 7-32. Atherosclerotic ulcer. The LAO view of the RCA shows an atherosclerotic ulcer. (Reproduced with permission from Spindola–Franco H, Fish BG. Radiology of the heart: cardiac imaging in infants, children and adults. New York: Springer–Verlag, 1985.)

tosus and other collagen vascular diseases also produce vasculitis that occasionally affects the coronary arteries. Degos syndrome is a rare disease that produces atrophic papular lesions of the skin, gastrointestinal ulcerations, and on occasion coronary arteriolar stenosis. In some metabolic disorders abnormal deposits may obliterate the coronary arteries. Among these are the mucopolysaccharidoses (e.g., Hurler disease), homocystinuria, Fabry disease, and pseudoxanthoma elasticum. Progeria produces accelerated atherosclerotic changes. Ehlers–Danlos syndrome may cause aneurysms of multiple arteries, including the coronaries.

Percutaneous Transluminal Coronary Angioplasty

Percutaneous transluminal coronary angioplasty (PTCA) is a nonoperative catheterization method designed for the relief of coronary artery obstruction. The angioplasty technique is derived from early work by Dotter and Judkins[51] and was first successfully utilized in the treatment of coronary disease by Gruntzig in 1977.[52] Since the early experience of Gruntzig in which PTCA was used only in single-vessel and single-lesion coronary disease, PTCA has been extended to the treatment of multilesion,

(*Text continues on page 251*)

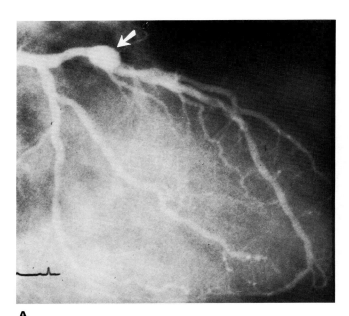

A

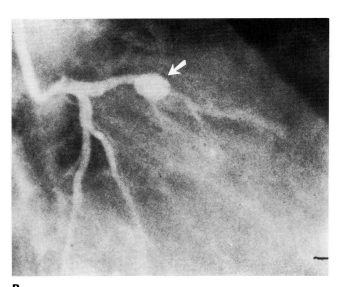

B

Figure 7-33. Coronary artery aneurysm. RAO view of LCA *A:* Early film; *B:* later film. The aneurysm (*arrow*) and the LCX fill immediately. The LAD opacifies after the aneurysm is visualized. On later films (not shown here) the aneurysm remains opacified after the coronary arteries empty. Congenital aneurysms of the coronary arteries characteristically occur at sites of bifurcations and are characterized by the presence of a narrow neck and smooth walls. The tendency exists for thrombosis to occur in the coronary artery so affected. (Reproduced with permission from Spindola–Franco H, Fish BG. Radiology of the heart: cardiac imaging in infants, children and adults. New York: Springer–Verlag, 1985.)

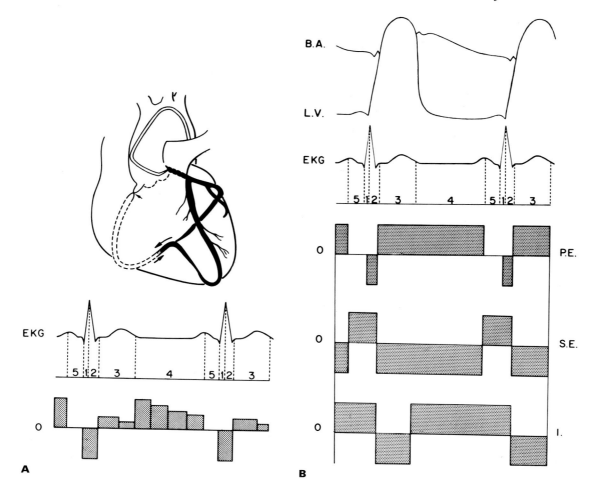

Figure 7-34. Patterns of reciprocating flow. *A:* The direction of reciprocating flow related to the events of the cardiac cycle. Primary epicardial flow is noted in the distal portion of the occluded vessel from collateral flow. During most of the cardiac cycle, blood can be observed to flow toward the lesion (positive direction on the bar graph). During isovolumic contraction the blood may cease to flow or may reverse its direction (negative direction on the bar graph). This flow pattern is identical to the normal pattern of flow in the coronary circulation. The reversal of direction probably reflects both increased intramyocardial resistance to flow and compression of the intramyocardial capillary bed. Reciprocating flow in epicardial vessels is associated with significant localized coronary artery obstruction with a perfusable coronary arterial bed. Reciprocating flow is not present in diffusely diseased vessels. Thus, its presence should be construed as a favorable sign if coronary bypass surgery is contemplated. *B:* Secondary epicardial flow pattern (SE) represents the reverse of the primary epicardial flow pattern (PE), apparent after injection into the diseased artery. Antegrade flow occurs in the diseased vessel only during isovolumic contraction. At other times, retrograde motion of the column of opacified blood is present because of collateral flow. In intramyocardial vessels (I) retrograde flow is noted during the ejection period and antegrade flow during the rest of the cardiac cycle. (Reproduced with permission from Spindola–Franco H, et al. Reciprocating flow in the coronary circulation. Radiology 1973;107:497.)

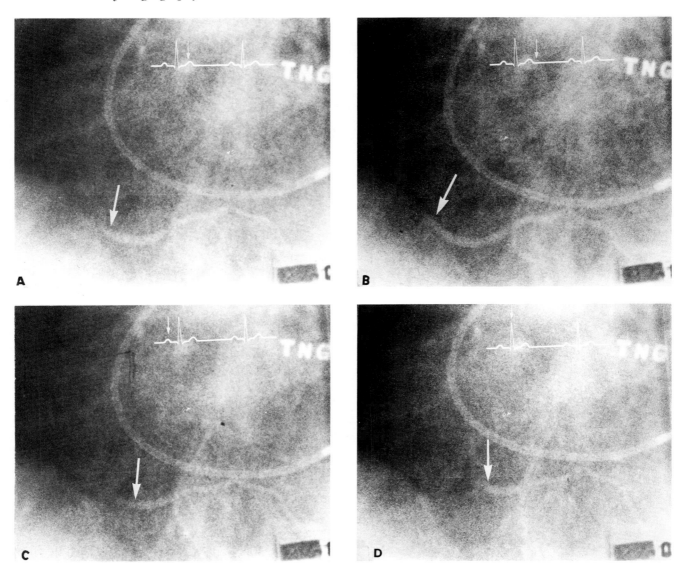

Figure 7-35. Reciprocating flow (primary epicardial flow pattern). Cine frames after LCA injection in a patient with occlusion of the proximal RCA. The timing of each frame relative to the cardiac cycle is indicated by small arrow above the ECG. The distal RCA is indicated by the large arrow. Note the antegrade flow (toward the lesion) during *A* (ventricular systole), which is maximal during *B* (ventricular diastole). Flow ceases in *C* (atrial systole) and reverses during *D* (isovolumic contraction). (Reproduced with permission from Spindola–Franco H, et al. Reciprocating flow in the coronary circulation. Radiology 1973;107:497.)

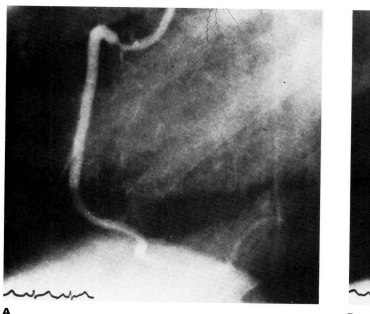

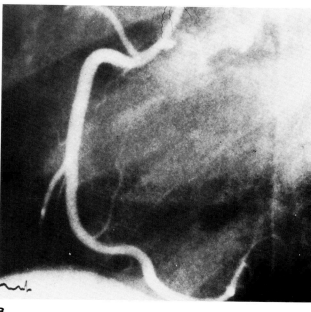

A

B

Figure 7-36. Catheter-induced spasm. LAO view of RCA. *A:* Note the spasm identified as a very short segment of narrowing just at the catheter tip. Symptoms and ECG changes were absent. *B* shows resolution after administration of nitroglycerin. (Reproduced with permission from Friedman AC, et al. Coronary spasm: Prinzmetal's variant angina vs catheter-induced spasm: refractory spasm vs fixed stenosis. Am J Roentgenol 1979;132:897.)

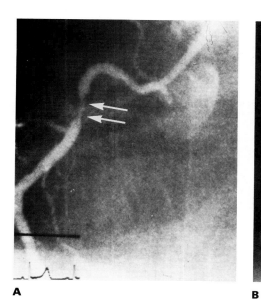

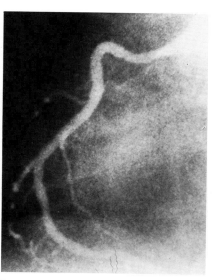

A

B

Figure 7-37. Prinzmetal variant angina spasm in the RCA. *A:* LAO view. Observe the long segment of narrowing (*arrows*) with irregular walls 2 cm distal to the catheter tip. Pain in the chest and elevation of the ST segments were associated. After sublingual administration of nitroglycerin the pain and elevation of the ST segment cleared, as did the spasm (*B*). (Reproduced with permission from Friedman AC, et al. Coronary spasm: Prinzmetal's variant angina vs catheter-induced spasm; refractory spasm vs fixed stenosis. Am J Roentgenol 1979;132:897.)

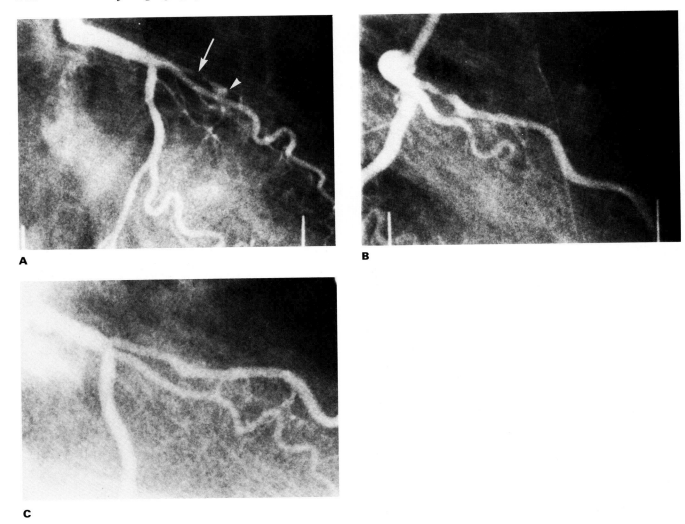

Figure 7-38. Refractory spasm. RAO view. *A* shows 99% stenosis of the left anterior descending coronary artery before the first septal perforator (*arrow*). Just beyond the first septal perforator the left anterior descending coronary artery is occluded (*arrowhead*). *B,* following administration of nitroglycerin, shows resolution of the occlusion but persistence of the severe stenosis. In *C,* during recatheterization because of suspicion of spasm, the left anterior descending artery is normal.

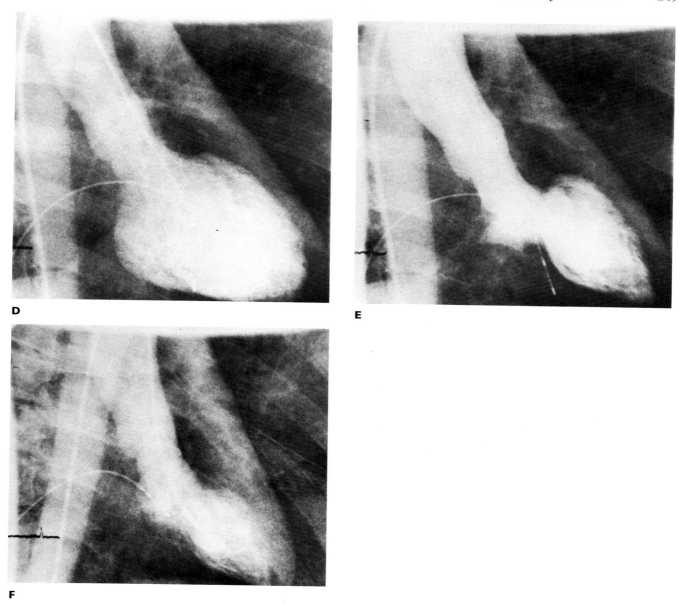

D

E

F

Figure 7-38 (*continued*). *D* and *E* represent diastolic and systolic frames of the left ventriculogram in the RAO view at the time of spasm of the left anterior descending coronary artery. The ventricle is slightly dilated during diastole. During systole the apex and the anterolateral wall are akinetic. Apical dyskinesis was noted on the LAO view (not shown). *F* is a systolic frame from the same patient after resolution of the coronary artery spasm. The contractions of the ventricle have reverted to normal. (Reproduced with permission from Friedman AC, et al. Coronary spasm: Prinzmetal's variant angina vs catheter-induced spasm: refractory spasm vs fixed stenosis. Am J Roentgenol 1979;132:897.)

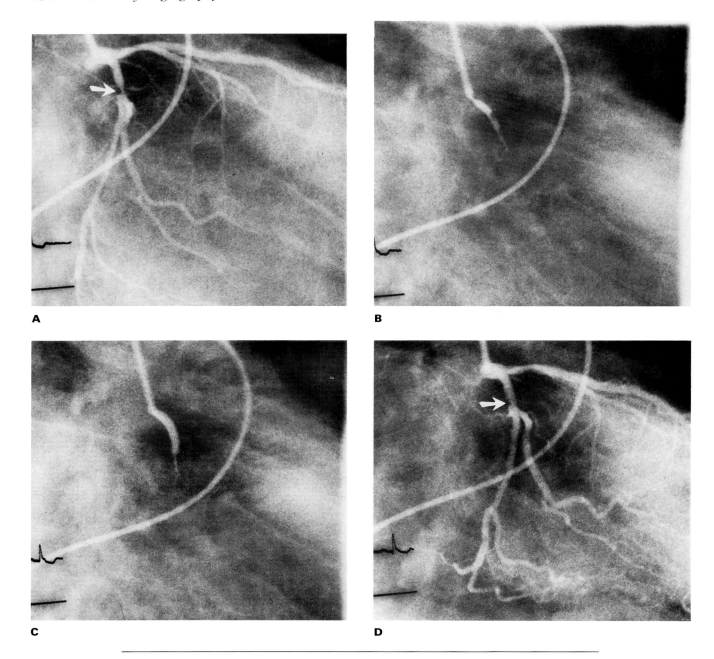

Figure 7-39. Percutaneous transluminal coronary angioplasty. *A:* Left coronary angiogram RAO view shows 99% stenosis (*arrow*) of the proximal left circumflex artery. *B:* The guiding and the dilating catheters are in place, and the balloon is distended. Note the lucent notch produced by the stenosis. *C:* With further distention the lucent defect has disappeared. *D:* Postdilatation angiogram demonstrates minimal residual stenosis (*arrow*). (Reproduced with permission from Spindola–Franco H, Fish BG. Radiology of the heart: cardiac imaging in infants, children and adults. New York: Springer–Verlag, 1985.)

multivessel disease, including lesions in coronary artery bypass grafts. Technologic advances in guidewire and balloon design have facilitated the ability of the angiographer to cross and dilate coronary lesions that were previously considered unapproachable.[53] Both over-the-wire and fixed-wire systems are available for performing PTCA. The over-the-wire system offers the greatest flexibility in choice of guidewires and exchange of balloon catheters and is therefore the most commonly used. Fixed-wire systems, on the other hand, are usually lower in profile and are useful in crossing complex lesions.

Coronary angiography following successful PTCA should demonstrate reduction in the stenosis of the vessel to less than 50% luminal diameter narrowing (Fig. 7-39). However, reducing the stenosis below 30% may decrease the incidence of restenosis. Small intimal tears are often noted after PTCA and do not represent a risk for either vessel closure or restenosis. A large intimal flap, especially with compression of the true lumen, may result in acute closure of the vessel in 3% to 5% of angioplasties, thus necessitating operative back-up whenever PTCA is performed. These intimal flaps may, however, completely heal. A restenosis rate of 25% to 35% represents a persistent major problem for PTCA. When restenosis occurs, it typically presents within the first 6 months and can often be treated with a second PTCA. A second restenosis may occur in 10% to 15% of patients undergoing angioplasty and may be treated either surgically, medically, or by repeat PTCA with or without an intracoronary stent.[53]

References

1. U.S. Department of Health. A frequently updated report presenting national data on morbidity and mortality, health delivery costs, and prevention programs with detailed tables. U.S. Department of Health and Human Service Center for Health Statistics. DHHS Publication No. (PHS) 85–1232, December 1985.
2. James TN. Pathology of small coronary arteries. Am J Cardiol 1967;20:679.
3. Greenberg MA, Grose RM, Neuburger N, et al. Impaired coronary vasodilator responsiveness as a cause of lactate production during pacing-induced ischemia in patients with angina and normal coronary arteries. J Am Coll Cardiol 1987;9:743.
4. Spindola–Franco H, Fish BG. Radiology of the heart: cardiac imaging in infants, children and adults. New York: Springer–Verlag, 1985.
5. Ross J Jr, Brandenburg RO, Dinsmore RE, et al. Guidelines for coronary angiography: a report of the American College of Cardiology/American Heart Association task force on assessment of diagnostic and therapeutic cardiovascular procedures (subcommittee on coronary angiography). Circulation 1987;76:963A.
6. Adams DF, Fraser DB, Abrams HL. The complications of coronary arteriography. Circulation 1973;48:609.
7. Davis K, Kennedy JW, Kemp HG, et al. Complications of coronary arteriography from the collaborative study of coronary artery surgery (CASS). Circulation 1979;59:1105.
8. Seldinger SI. Catheter replacement of the needle in percutaneous arteriography. A new technique. Acta Radiol 1953;39:368.
9. Sones FM Jr, Shirery EK. Cine coronary arteriography. Mod Concepts Cardiovasc Dis 1962;31:735.
10. Judkins MP. Percutaneous transfemoral selective coronary arteriography. Radiol Clin North Am 1968;6:467.
11. Amplatz K, Formanek G, Stanger P, Wilson W. Mechanics of selective coronary artery catheterization via femoral approach. Radiology 1967;89:1040.
12. Cohen M, Rentrop KP, Cohen BM. Safety and efficacy of percutaneous entry of the brachial artery versus cutdown and arteriotomy for left-sided cardiac catheterization. Am J Cardiol 1986;57:682.
13. Paulin S. Coronary angiography: a technical, anatomic and clinical study. Acta Radiol (Suppl) 1964;233:11.
14. Bream PR, Souza AS Jr, Elliot LP, et al. Right superior septal perforator artery: its angiographic description and clinical significance. Am J Roentgenol 1979;133:67.
15. Levin DC, Baltaxe HA. Angiographic demonstration of important anatomic variations of the posterior descending coronary artery. Am J Roentgenol 1972;116:41.
16. Spindola–Franco H. Coronary arteriography and left ventriculography. In: Goldberger E, ed. Textbook of clinical cardiology. St. Louis: CV Mosby, 1982:305.
17. Schuster EH, Griffith LS, Bulkley BH. Preponderance of acute proximal left anterior descending coronary arterial lesions in fatal myocardial infarction: a clinicopathologic study. Am J Cardiol 1981;47:1189.
18. Kugel MA. Anatomical studies on the coronary arteries and their branches. I. Arteria anastomotica auricularis magna. Am Heart J 1927;3:260.
19. Abrams HL, Adams DF. The coronary arteriogram: structural and functional aspects. N Eng J Med 1969;28:1336.
20. Greenberg MA, Fish B, Spindola–Franco H. Congenital anomalies of the coronary arteries: classification and significance. Radiolog Clin North Am 1989;27:1127.
21. Benson PA. Anomalous aortic origin of coronary artery with sudden death: case report and review. Am Heart J 1970;79:254.
22. Cheitlin MD, DeCastro CM, McAllister HA. Sudden death as a complication of anomalous left coronary origin from the anterior sinus of valsalva: a not-so-minor congenital anomaly. Circulation 1974;50:780.
23. Elliot LP, Amplatz K, Edwards JE. Coronary arterial patterns in transposition complexes: anatomic and angiographic studies. Am J Cardiol 1966;17:362.
24. Elliot LP, Neufeld HN, Anderson RC, et al. Complete transposition of the great vessel. I. An anatomic study of sixty cases. Circulation 1963;27:1105.
25. Kimbiris D, Iskandrian AS, Segal BL, et al. Anomalous aortic origin of coronary arteries. Circulation 1978;58:606.
26. Chaitman BR, Lesperance J, Saltiel J, et al. Clinical, angiographic, and hemodynamic findings in patients with anomalous origin of the coronary arteries. Circulation 1976;53:122.
27. Lipton MJ, Barry WH, Obrez I, et al. Isolated single coronary artery: diagnosis, angiographic classifications, and clinical significance. Radiology 1979;130:39.
28. Ogden JA, Goodyer AVN. Patterns of distribution of the single coronary artery. Yale J Biol Med 1970;43:11.
29. Smith JC. Review of single coronary artery with report of two cases. Circulation 1950;1:1168.
30. Bland EF, White PD, Garland J. Congenital anomalies of the coronary arteries: report of an unusual case associated with cardiac hypertrophy. Am Heart J 1933;8:787.
31. Askenazi J, Nadas AS. Anomalous left coronary artery originating from the pulmonary artery: report on 15 cases. Circulation 1975;51:976.

32. Talner NS, Halloran KH, Mahdavy M, et al. Anomalous origin of the left coronary artery from the pulmonary artery: a clinical spectrum. Am J Cardiol 1965;15:689.

33. Wesselhoeft H, Fawcett JS, Johnson AL. Anomalous origin of the left coronary artery from the pulmonary trunk: its clinical spectrum, pathology, and pathophysiology. Based on review of 140 cases with seven further cases. Circulation 1968;38:403.

34. Roberts WC. Major anomalies of coronary arterial origin seen in adulthood. Am Heart J 1986;111:941.

35. Roberts WC. Anomalous origin of both coronary arteries from the pulmonary artery. Am J Cardiol 1962;10:595.

36. Feldt RH, Ongley PA, Titus JL. Total coronary arterial circulation from the pulmonary artery with survival to age seven: report of a case. Mayo Clin Proc 1965;40:539.

37. VonHaller A. First lines of physiology. 1st Am ed, p 35, 1803. Wearn JT. Harvey Lecture. 1939–1940:243 (cited by Moberg A. Anastomoses between extracardiac vessels and coronary arteries). Acta Med Scand (Suppl) 1968;485:5.

38. Spindola–Franco H, Grose R, Solomon N. Dual left anterior descending artery: angiographic description of important variants and surgical implications. Am Heart J 1983;105:445.

39. McNamara JJ, Grose RE. Congenital coronary artery fistula. Surgery 1969;65:59.

40. Neufeld HN, Lester RG, Adams P Jr, et al. Congenital communication of a coronary artery with a cardiac chamber or the pulmonary trunk ("coronary artery fistula"). Circulation 1961;24:171.

41. Goor DA, Lillehei CW. Congenital malformations of the heart. New York: Grune & Stratton, 1975:372.

42. Standen JR. "Tumor vascularity" in left atrial thrombus demonstrated by selective coronary arteriography. Radiology 1975;116:549.

43. Soulen RL, Grollman JH, Paglia D, Kreulen T. Coronary neovascularity and fistula formation: a sign of mural thrombus. Circulation 1977;56:663.

44. Spindola–Franco H, Eldh, P, Adams DF, et al. Coronary vascular patterns during occlusion arteriography. Radiology 1975;114:59.

45. Smith SC, Adams DF, Herman MV, et al. Coronary-to-bronchial anastomoses: an *in vivo* demonstration by selective coronary arteriography. Radiology 1972;104:289.

46. Viamonte M Jr, Parks RE, Smeak WM III. Guided catheterization of the bronchial arteries. Radiology 1965;85:205.

47. Spindola–Franco H, Weisel A, Delman AJ. Pulmonary steal syndrome: an unusual case of coronary-brachial-pulmonary artery communication. Radiology 1978;126:25.

48. Spindola–Franco H, Adams DF, Herman MV, Abrams HL. Reciprocating flow in the coronary circulation. Radiology 1973;107:497.

49. Friedman AC, Spindola–Franco H, Nivatpumin T. Coronary spasm: Prinzmetal's variant angina (PVA) versus catheter-induced spasm, refractory spasm versus fixed stenosis. Am J Roentgenol 1979;132:897.

50. Pepine CJ, Feldman RL, Conti CR, et al. Recommendations for use of ergonovine to provoke coronary artery spasm. Cathet Cardiovasc Diagn 1980;16:423.

51. Dotter CT, Judkins MP. Transluminal treatment of arteriosclerotic obstruction: description of a new technique and a preliminary report of its application. Circulation 1964;30:654.

52. Gruntzig AR, Senning A, Siegenthaler WE. Nonoperative dilatation of coronary artery stenosis: percutaneous transluminal coronary angioplasty. N Engl J Med 1979;301:61.

53. Greenberg MA, Menegus MA, Issenberg H, Spindola–Franco H. Advances in interventional cardiology: coronary balloon angioplasty and alternative techniques. Current Opinion in Radiology 1990;2:602.

Chapter 8

Magnetic Resonance Imaging of Acquired Heart Disease

Charles B. Higgins

Magnetic resonance imaging (MRI) has three important attributes that make it advantageous for evaluation of the heart. First, a high natural contrast exists between the blood pool and the cardiovascular structures because of the lack of signal from flowing blood on spin-echo MRI pulse sequences, or a bright signal intensity from blood on gradient echo sequences. When the spin-echo technique is used blood appears black on images (Fig. 8-1). Therefore, internal structures of the heart can be visualized within the signal void of the cardiac chambers. When the gradient-echo technique (cine MRI) is used blood has bright signal intensity, which causes it to be clearly discerned from the cardiac and vascular walls (Fig. 8-2). Consequently, contrast media are not required for discrimination of the blood pool on either the spin-echo or the gradient-echo techniques. Second, a wide range of soft-tissue contrast provides potential for characterization of myocardial tissue. This contrast among tissues depends on proton (hydrogen nuclei) density and magnetic resonance relaxation times of the protons. Third, MRI is essentially a three-dimensional imaging technique, that allows precise quantification of cardiac mass and volumes. When tomographic images are acquired that entirely encompass the heart, the technique is essentially three-dimensional. This three-dimensional set of data provides a method for direct measurement of cardiac mass and volumes without the use of any assumed formulas or geometric models. Moreover, such volume imaging provides the possibility for reproducibility of measurements from one study to the next.

Effects of Moving Blood on MRI

The motion of nuclei through the region that is being imaged greatly influences signal intensity. The movement of protons in flowing blood during the application of radiofrequency (RF) pulses and the selective or nonselective nature of those pulses determines the MRI signal received from the blood pool. For spin-echo images, there are two pulses, a 90° initiation pulse and a 180° refocusing pulse. Both the 90° and 180° pulses are selectively applied and influence a single tomographic slice. Because multiple sets of these pulses are applied during an imaging sequence, the protons in the selected slice are partially saturated, which causes some reduction in the signal recovered from them. The influence of the repetitive set of RF pulses on flowing blood is complex and depends on the velocity of the blood flow. Two factors to be considered are inflow enhancement and high-velocity signal loss. Inflow enhancement dictates that blood flowing into a slice in the TR (repetition time) interval replenishes protons that have been partially saturated by the previous set of RF pulses. Consequently, the signal of blood is augmented by the percentage of intravascular protons replaced in the TR interval, which depends on the blood flow rate. This effect is generally overwhelmed by the factor of high-velocity signal loss, or the slice transition effect, which occurs when the flow velocity is such that the moving protons pass through the slice during the pulse sequence and fail to experience both the 90° and 180° pulses, and consequently no signal can be detected

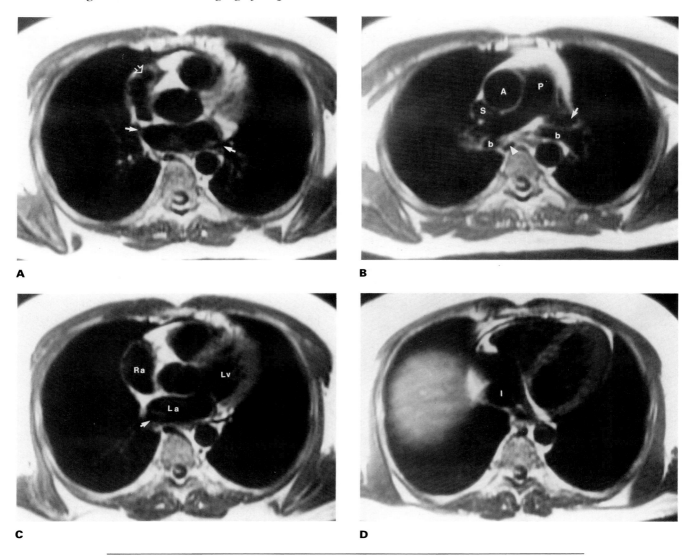

Figure 8-1. Series of ECG gated spin-echo images extending from cranial (*A*) to caudal (*D*). Blood pool is black with the spin-echo technique, providing good contrast between the blood and myocardium. (A, aorta; b, bronchus; I, inferior vena cava; La, left atrium; Lv, left ventricle; P, pulmonary artery; Ra, right atrium; S, superior vena cava; open arrow, right atrial appendage; closed arrow, pulmonary veins; arrowhead, azygous vein.)

from them. For spin-echo images both the 90° and 180° pulses are selective for the slice being imaged. Because the 180° pulse is applied at the middle of a TE (echo delay time), high velocity signal loss occurs when the flow velocity exceeds a value equal to slice thickness divided by ½TE. In most arteries and veins, the flow velocity is such that little or no signal is recovered from the blood pool on the spin echo sequence.

For gradient-echo images, the inflow enhancement effect is exaggerated and unopposed by the slice transition effect. Because the TR is even shorter and repeated more frequently per unit time, the protons of stationary tissue are even more saturated than with the spin-echo technique. This causes a relatively higher signal from flowing blood relative to stationary tissues on the gradient-echo (cine MRI) compared with the spin-echo technique. The slice transition effect is not operative for the gradient-echo technique because the 180° refocusing pulse is not used and the 90° pulse is applied for the entire image volume (nonselective pulse). Consequently, even if the blood traverses a particular tomographic slice rapidly, signal is still recovered from the blood.

Flowing blood causes bright signal on the gradient-echo technique (cine MRI). In this circumstance, blood appears substantially brighter (white) than the cardiac walls (see Fig. 8-2). The signal from flowing blood also

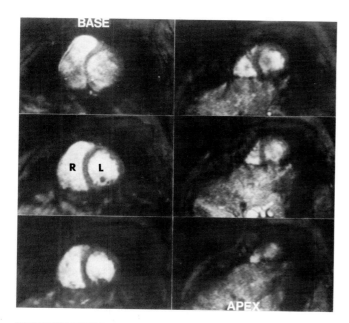

Figure 8-2. Cine (gradient-echo) images extending from the base to the apex of the ventricles. Blood pool is white, providing good contrast between the blood and myocardium. (L, left ventricle; R, right ventricle.)

depends on the pattern of flow; distorted flow associated with high-velocity jets and turbulence cause loss of signal in the blood pool on gradient-echo images. High-velocity jets produced by flow across stenotic or regurgitant valves can be recognized as a signal void within the signal-filled cardiac chambers.

Technique of MRI of the Heart

Cardiac imaging requires some form of physiologic gating of the imaging sequence. Acquisition of MRI signals of the thorax without gating results in poor cardiac images because of loss of signal from moving structures and the variable position of the cardiac structure relative to imaging voxels when data are acquired indiscriminately throughout the cardiac cycle.

Gating with MRI

Gating is associated with unique problems. Sensors, wire leads, and transducers are usually composed of ferromagnetic materials, which can generate noise or may grossly distort the images within the radiofrequency-shielded room containing the MRI device. Consequently, gating with MRI requires the use of a nonferromagnetic physiologic signal-sensing circuit. Electronically isolated electrocardiogram (ECG) electrode-lead circuits contain-

ing very little metal have been used for repetitive synchronization, i.e., ECG gating, of pulse sequences to fixed segments of the cardiac cycle.

Prospective gating consists of initiation of the RF pulse sequences at a fixed time in the cardiac cycle at each anatomic level; the data acquisition is guided by the ECG signal. Retrospective gating consists of continuous application of the RF pulse sequences and simultaneous recording of the ECG signal. Later the data acquired at specific phases of the cardiac cycle, as indicated by the recorded ECG signal, are reconstructed into images corresponding to the specific interval of the cycle.

Multislice Techniques

Several imaging strategies are used depending on the information desired.[1] For anatomic diagnosis, the *ECG-gated multislice technique* is used (Fig. 8-3). This technique is economical in time, requiring less than 10 min-

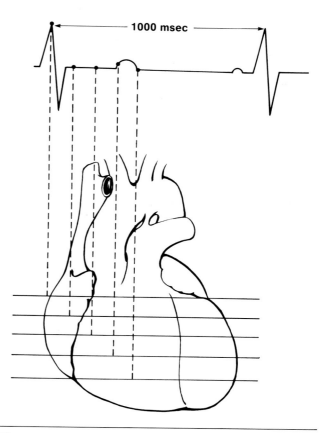

Figure 8-3. Diagram showing the sequence of acquisition of spin-echo images in relation to the ECG. During an imaging sequence, images are acquired at several anatomical levels. The cranial image is acquired at the R wave of the ECG, whereas each subsequent image is acquired at a delay relative to the adjacent image; the delay between adjacent images is usually 30 to 50 msec.

utes for the acquisition of tomograms at 10 anatomic levels, which usually encompasses the entire heart and root of the great vessels. A time difference of 30 to 100 msec exists between each adjacent level, so the images are obtained at different phases of the cardiac cycle. The reason why images can be obtained at multiple anatomic levels during a single imaging sequence is that the time required to complete a set of RF pulses and sample the emitted signal for each line on that image is usually 20 to 60 msec (TE interval), whereas the time duration between the application of repetitive sets of pulses is approximately 500 to 1000 msec (TR interval). Consequently, the inactive time for each cycle is long, frequently over 90% of the cycle. Efficiency is improved by applying the set of spin-echo pulses at other levels during the magnetization recovery period. Therefore, after completion of a 50-ms duty cycle at one level, the full set of pulses is selectively applied at the next adjacent tomographic level and then the next, and so forth. With this multislice technique, the total number of tomographic levels that can be imaged is approximately TR/TE. As indicated earlier, TR equals the length of the cardiac cycle (R–R interval) when using ECG gating.

The *multiphasic multislice technique* is used for the evaluation of cardiac dimensions and function.[2] With this technique, each anatomic section is imaged at five phases of the cardiac cycle (Fig. 8-4). Using end diastolic and end (late) systolic images of each anatomic level, measurement can be made of diastolic and systolic volumes, stroke volume, ejection fraction, myocardial mass, and extent of left ventricular regional wall thickening. With this technique, wall-thickening dynamics have been measured for various regions of the left ventricle in healthy subjects and patients with global and regional myocardial dysfunction and in patients with focal and generalized hypertrophy.

The *biphasic spin-echo technique* is performed by acquiring images at multiple anatomic locations at end diastole (R curve of the ECG) and end systole (down slope of the T wave of the ECG).[3] Images of four levels are obtained in 77 msec at the R wave and repeated at the down slope of the T wave (Figs. 8-5 and 8-6). To fully encompass the heart, the four sets of images are repeated at four additional levels in alternate heart beats or at every third heart beat if 12 anatomic levels are required. The time required for acquiring images at end diastole and end systole for 1 cm tomograms encompassing the entire heart is only 11 to 20 minutes.

Cine MRI

Cine MRI is accomplished by ECG referencing of fast imaging sequences (Fig. 8-7). This approach can produce approximately 16 to 30 images (20 to 30 msec in dura-

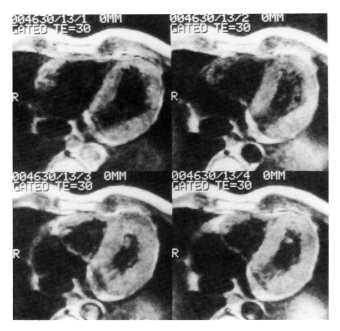

Figure 8-4. Series of images at four phases of the cardiac cycle. Images proceed from end diastole (*upper left*) to the early part of the next diastole (*lower right*). The multislice, multiphasic technique provides images at multiple anatomic levels acquired at multiple phases of the cardiac cycle. During each imaging sequence the temporal order of acquisition of images at anatomic levels are varied so that after five acquisitions, images are produced at five phases of the cardiac cycle at each of the five anatomic levels.

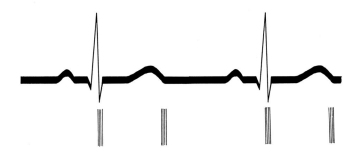

Figure 8-5. ECG gated biphasic spin-echo technique. The ECG is shown in relation to a vertical line which indicated the time of acquisition of tomograms. As shown here, data for four tomograms at different anatomic levels are cyclically acquired during a 77-msec interval at the R wave (end diastole) and down slope of the T wave (end systole). The duration of end diastole and end systole is approximately 66 msec.

tion) during the cardiac cycle. These images are laced together in a cinematic display so wall motion of the ventricles, valve motion, and blood flow patterns in the heart and great vessels can be visualized.[4] The gradient-echo technique is used with short TR (20 to 30 msec) and TE (4 to 17 msec) values.

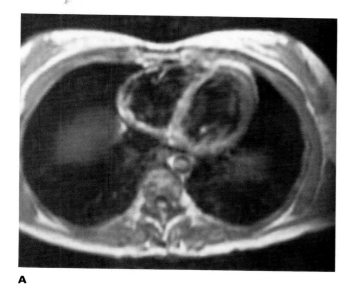 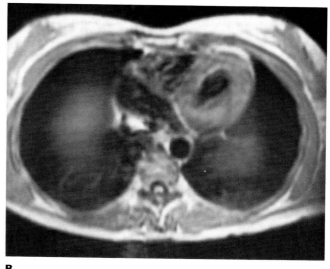

A   **B**

Figure 8-6. Images at end diastole (*A*) and end systole (*B*) acquired with the biphasic spin-echo technique.

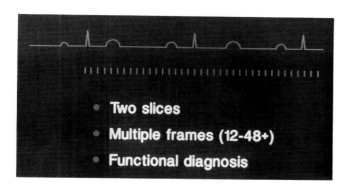

Figure 8-7. Diagram of the cine (gradient-echo) MRI acquisition technique. Images at one to four anatomic levels (slices) are acquired at multiple phases of the cardiac cycle. Each vertical line represents the time of acquisition of an image at a single anatomic level. The number of images that can be acquired at the various anatomic levels (slices) is defined by the quotient of the RR interval of the ECG and the TR interval (usually 21 msec). The total number of images available is divided among the anatomic levels. Acquisition of images at two levels only is frequently done to provide sufficient temporal resolution so that images close to end diastole and end systole are obtained.

Volume or three-dimensional data acquisition has also been achieved with an ECG-gated sequence. With this technique, images of any desired plane can be reconstructed later, and all reconstructed planes are in the same phase of the cardiac cycle (in contrast to the multislice technique). The time cost of volume imaging is considerable; the acquisition time for volume imaging of an equal portion of the heart is longer for this technique than for the multislice technique.

Information Derived from MRI of the Heart

Morphology of Cardiac Abnormalities. The tomographic images in various planes depict variations in structure caused by cardiac disease states and provide anatomic diagnosis. Spin-echo images are usually used for displaying morphologic abnormalities.

Identification of Functional Abnormalities. The cine MRI technique demonstrates abnormalities of valves and abnormal flow patterns in the heart and great vessels.

Quantification of Cardiac Dimensions and Function. Quantification of ventricular volumes and mass can be achieved in a precise and accurate manner using sets of images that encompass the entire heart acquired at end diastole and end systole. This can be done using either the cine MRI technique or the biphasic spin-echo technique.[3]

Tissue Characterization. Abnormal myocardial tissue may be manifested as a regional difference in myocardial intensity, such as the increased intensity of acutely infarcted myocardium compared with normal myocardium.[5,6] Tissue characterization by MRI is achieved by measurements of relative signal intensity and relaxation times of the tissue. Tissue characterization using this means is still somewhat imprecise because of motion-related artifactual variations in the magnetic relaxation times of myocardial tissue. Signal intensity on spin-echo images increases with increase in hydrogen density and

T_2 relaxation time and decreases with T_1 relaxation time. The contrast in intensity between tissues can be augmented by varying the technical factors used in acquiring the MR images. Decreasing the TR and TE factors produces greater contrast-related differences in T_1 relaxation times among tissues (T_1-weighted images). An increase in TR and TE causes greater contrast primarily on the basis of differences in T_2 relaxation times between tissues (T_2-weighted images). The contrast relationship between tissues on gradient-echo (cine MRI) images is somewhat different, but these images can also be T_1- and T_2-weighted. An additional important factor that affects contrast on these images is the magnetic susceptibility effect, however.[7] Magnetic susceptibility effect results in a severe decrease or a complete loss of signal intensity within a tissue. These magnetic susceptibility effects result from local variations in magnetic field from adjacent foci within the tissue. They can be due to the compartmentalization of paramagnetic substances within the tissue. An example of this is hemosiderin compartmentalized within the cell and existing in either a lower or no concentration within the extracellular space. The magnetic susceptibility effect becomes particularly evident in the presence of paramagnetic substances within hemorrhage. MRI contrast media can be used to improve the T_1 or T_2 differences between normal and pathologic myocardium.

Cardiac Imaging Planes and Cardiac Anatomy

The planes generally used for cardiac imaging are the transverse, sagittal, and coronal planes. These are orthogonal to the thorax but oblique to the heart (Fig. 8-8). MRI of the heart is most often performed with the patient supine. The Z-axis imaging plane is aligned with the patient in a head-to-toe orientation, which uses the patient as a frame of reference for imaging (i.e., coronal, sagittal, and transaxial image orientations). MRI planes parallel to the long and short axis of the heart but actually oblique to the thorax can be acquired (Fig. 8-9).[8] These planes should theoretically improve the precision of measurement of linear dimensions such as wall thickness and internal diameters. Anatomic diagnosis and volume measurements (ventricular mass and volume) should be equally accurate using either orthogonal or oblique imaging planes when the multiple tomograms fully encompass the entire heart, however.[9] The orientation of the slice-selective gradient to achieve cardiac short- and long-axis images is easily performed; however, achieving these imaging planes does require preliminary imaging in other planes. The transverse image is initially acquired; from it the coordinates for the long-axis image are defined (see Fig. 8-9). A coordinate marking the midportion of the anterior apical region of the left ventricle and an-

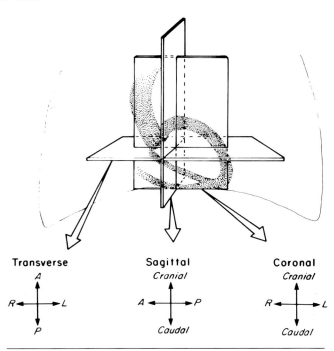

Figure 8-8. Diagram shows the orientation of the heart in relation to imaging planes orthogonal to the axis of the body. Because the heart lies obliquely in the thorax, these orthogonal planes cut the heart obliquely. (Reproduced with permission from Higgins CB, Byrd BF III, Stark D, et al. Magnetic resonance imaging in hypertrophic cardiomyopathy. Am J Cardiol 1985;55:1121.)

other coordinate marking the midportion of the mitral valve are defined. A line between these two points represents the long axis of the left ventricle. Images acquired parallel to this line are designated long-axis images. Using the long-axis image, which displays the mitral valve and the left ventricular apex, a point is marked in the middle of the mitral valve and another in the middle of the apex (see Fig. 8-9). A line between these two points is constructed. An imaging plane perpendicular to this line is the short-axis plane.

Ischemic Heart Disease

The following are several of the ways MRI can be used in the evaluation of ischemic heart disease.

1. To define the site and extent of previous myocardial infarctions (Fig. 8-10).[10]
2. To determine the presence of residual myocardium in a region under consideration for revascularization (Fig. 8-11).
3. To demonstrate complications of previous myocardial infarction (Figs. 8-11, 8-12 and 8-13).
4. To demonstrate alterations in signal intensity and tissue characteristics of acute and chronic myocardial infarction.[5,6,10]

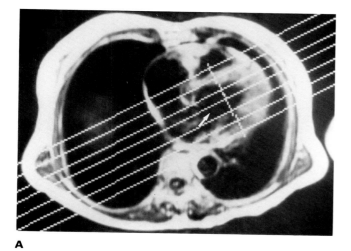

A

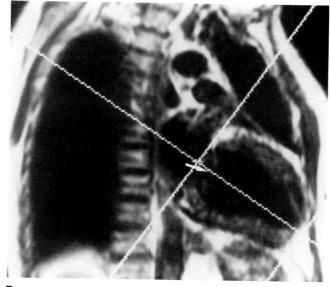

B

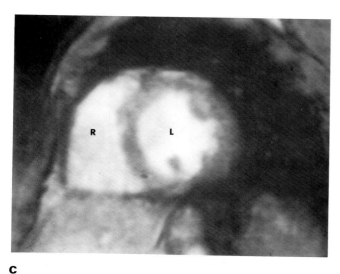

C

Figure 8-9. Method for defining the cardiac vertical long- and short-axis planes. Using the transverse plane (*A*), a line is drawn through the middle of the mitral valve (*arrow*) to the anterior wall of the left ventricle. Images acquired parallel to this line are the vertical long-axis images (*B*). Using the long-axis image, a line extending from the middle of the mitral valve to the left ventricular apex is the long axis of the left ventricle. Images acquired perpendicular to this line are short-axis images (*C*). (L, left ventricle; R, right ventricle.)

5. To demonstrate regional myocardial function.[11]
6. To demonstrate regional myocardial perfusion.

The demonstration of regional myocardial perfusion requires the use of magnetic resonance contrast media. This potential use of the technique has not achieved clinical popularity but a number of new contrast media are under experimental evaluation for this purpose.[12] The demonstration of the coronary arteries using MRI is an elusive but highly desirable goal that has not been achieved.

Acute Myocardial Infarction

Gated MR images from patients studied within the 7 to 10 days after the onset of acute myocardial infarction have revealed high signal intensity from the infarcted region (see Fig. 8-10).[5,13] This increased signal intensity of the infarcted region has been observed within the initial 24 hours after onset of symptoms.[13] The differential contrast between infarcted and normal myocardium is improved with greater T_2 weighting of the images. The high signal intensity of the infarcted region is demonstrated well on images with a TE value of 60 to 90 msec. This pattern of contrast change with increasing TE value is consistent with myocardial edema and has been observed both in experimental animals and in humans.

Signal from blood in the left ventricular chamber is also observed on systolic images from some patients with acute infarcts. Although such signal from nearly stationary blood is observed in healthy people during late diastole, intrachamber signal occurring during systole suggests left ventricular regional dysfunction. It is important to distinguish between the intense signal arising from blood lying stagnant along the ventricular walls and signal from

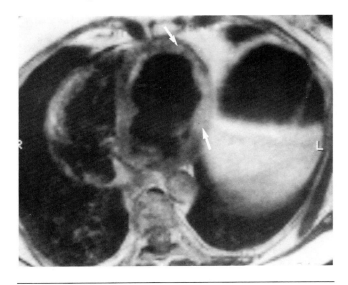

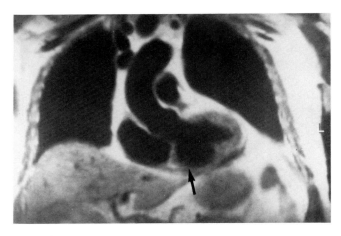

Figure 8-11. Ventricular aneurysm. ECG gated spin-echo coronal image shows a region devoid of myocardium (*arrow*) in the diaphragmatic wall of the left ventricle.

Figure 8-10. Acute myocardial infarction. ECG gated spin-echo transverse image displays a region of high signal intensity (*arrow*) in the anterolateral region of the left ventricle.

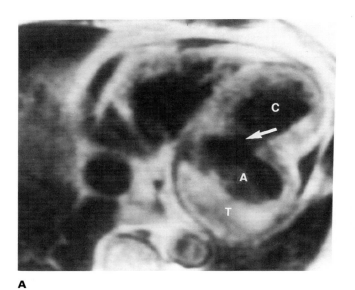

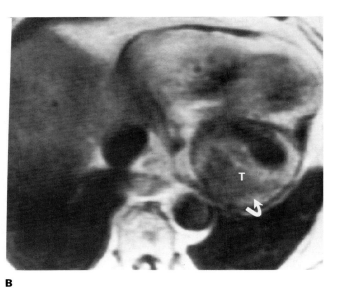

A

B

Figure 8-12. False aneurysm of the left ventricle. Panel *A* is located 1 cm cranial to the one on the right. ECG gated spin-echo transverse images show a narrow ostium (*arrow*) communicating between the false aneurysm (A) and the ventricular chamber (C). The more caudal image (*B*) shows the portion of the aneurysm (*curved arrow*) that extends posterior to the cardiac apex. The aneurysm is partially filled with thrombus (T).

a subendocardial acute infarction. Such a distinction can be facilitated by using a long TE value on a single-echo sequence. With this type of imaging sequence, greater T_2 contrast is achieved, but without the even-echo rephasing of slowly moving protons in blood. Infarction delineation can also be achieved with a calculated T_2 image on which the density window is set to the anticipated range of infarcted myocardium. The T_2 for the infarct is usually greater than 50 but less than 100 msec.[5]

There are some pitfalls to the recognition of high signal intensity within regions of the left ventricular myocardium. Motion artifacts can cause variation in signal intensity within one or another region of the myocardium. Such regions can be erroneously interpreted as sites of acute myocardial infarction. In addition, displacement of high-intensity flow signal into the ventricular wall as a consequence of the temporal and spatial discordance that occurs as a result of the difference in time between application of phase encoding and readout gradients can mimic signal from a subendocardial myocardial infarction. Finally, increase in signal in the diaphragmatic wall of the left ventricle can be caused by partial volume effect from epicardial fat. Differentiation between increased signal intensity from an actual infarct because of prolonged T_2 relaxation time and artifactual variation in myocardial signal intensity can be done by comparing contrast differences for the first and second spin-echo images. The percentage contrast between infarcted and normal myocardium increases from the first to the second echo image.[5] The difference in signals observed for different regions in healthy people changes little or may even decrease on the second echo image. Thus, the effect of a long T_2 relaxation time is not evident when comparing first and second echo images when the increased signal intensity is artifactual in nature.

MRI seems to be capable of demonstrating ischemically injured myocardium soon after acute coronary occlusion. Such observations have been made in dogs studied by MRI at frequent intervals during the first 6 hours after coronary occlusion.[14] Gated MRI was performed in dogs with acute myocardial infarction immediately after coronary occlusion and serially up to 5 hours. MRI and measurements from it indicated that the signal intensity from the infarcted myocardium was significantly greater than that from normal myocardium at 3 hours after coronary occlusion and there was a significant prolongation of T_2 relaxation time at this point. MRI has also shown considerable accuracy in determining the size of acute myocardial infarction in dogs.[15]

Complications of Acute Myocardial Infarctions. Left ventricular aneurysms have been recognized on MRI as severe wall thinning (less than 2 mm in thickness) and diastolic bulging of the left ventricular wall (see Fig. 8-11). MRI can clearly localize the site of the aneurysm in the various segments of the left ventricle;

most true aneurysms are situated in the anterior lateral region or apical region of the left ventricle. True aneurysms less frequently involve the diaphragmatic or posterior region of the left ventricle.

False aneurysms can also be readily identified on gated MRI. The false aneurysm is larger than the average true aneurysm, is located on the posterior or diaphragmatic region of the left ventricle, and has a relatively small ostium connecting to the aneurysm (see Fig. 8-12). MRI is especially effective in demonstrating the diameter of the ostium of the aneurysm. When the ostium is less than one half of the diameter of the widest point of the aneurysm, this suggests the presence of a pseudoaneurysm.

Left ventricular thrombus has been demonstrated by MRI.[16] Mural thrombus is demonstrated on spin-echo images as a mass adherent to the ventricular wall or a mass filling a left ventricular aneurysm (Figs. 8-12 and 8-13). The signal intensity of the thrombus varies depending on its age. The subacute thrombus usually has medium to high signal intensity on T_1-weighted images and bright signal intensity on T_2-weighted images. Chronic organized thrombus may have low signal intensity on both T_1- and T_2-weighted spin-echo images, however. The differentiation of a clot from a tumor within the cardiac chambers may not always be possible using spin-echo images; however, this distinction seems to be more easily achieved with cine MRI.[17] The gradient-echo (cine MRI) images are highly sensitive to magnetic susceptibility effects. The paramagnetic substances within clotted blood, such as deoxyhemoglobin, methemoglobin, and iron, induce a magnetic susceptibility effect. This magnetic susceptibility effect causes loss of signal on gradient-echo images; thus, the clot has low signal intensity on such images. Conversely, tumor thrombus has a signal intensity similar to other types of solid tissue and is shown as a medium signal intensity on gradient-echo images. An example of the difference in signal intensity of clot and tumor within the cardiac chambers is shown in Figure 8-14.

MRI in patients with ischemic cardiomyopathy usually demonstrates multiple regions of wall thinning and substantial left ventricular enlargement. Regional wall thinning in ischemic cardiomyopathy can be clearly defined by MRI, thereby usually distinguishing these patients from those with more uniform wall thinning caused by idiopathic congestive (dilated) cardiomyopathy.

Chronic Myocardial Infarction

Previous myocardial infarctions are demonstrated as regions of wall thinning on MRI.[10] Such regional wall thinning has been observed in nearly all patients with documented infarctions. There is usually an abrupt transition

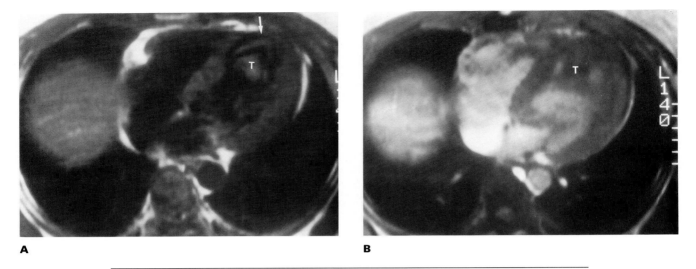

A   **B**

Figure 8-13. Left ventricular thrombus and chronic myocardial infarction. *A:* Spin-echo transverse image shows wall thinning at the infarction site (*arrow*) and thrombus (T) laminated on the infarcted wall. *B:* Cine MR image shows the thrombus (T) causing a low signal intensity filling defect in the ventricular blood pool.

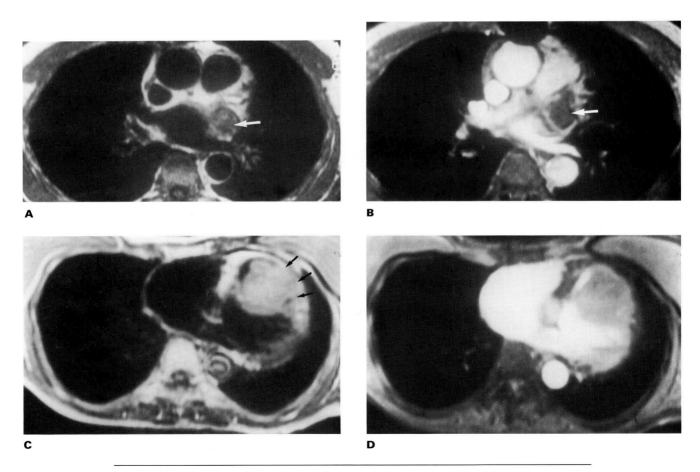

A   **B**

C   **D**

Figure 8-14. Thrombus of left atrial appendage and metastatic tumor of the right ventricle. *A:* Spin-echo transverse image shows thrombus in the left atrial appendage (*arrow*). *B:* Cine MR image shows the thrombus within the high signal blood pool. *C:* Spin-echo MR image shows a tumor of the right ventricle. The site of attachment to the right ventricular wall is shown (*arrows*). *D:* Cine MR image demonstrates that the mass has medium signal intensity.

in thickness from normal myocardium to the scar at the site of a transmural infarction (see Fig. 8-11). Transverse MRI displays anterolateral or anteroseptal wall thinning after occlusion of the left anterior descending artery and posterolateral or diaphragmatic wall thinning after occlusion of the right coronary artery.

Because MRI provides direct visualization of the myocardium on multislice images encompassing the entire heart, it is possible to estimate the volume of muscle lost because of a previous infarction. Measurements of the spatial distribution of the thin myocardium on multiple slices allows estimation of infarct volume. MRI can also be used to indicate residual myocardium in a region in which myocardial revascularization surgery is being considered; failure to demonstrate residual myocardium might be used to indicate the futility of revascularization of a region. Correlation of MRI with angiography and two-dimensional echocardiography has shown the accuracy of MRI for defining the sites of previous myocardial infarctions. In some patients who have had a previous infarction, low signal has been observed in the ventricular wall at the site of the infarction; presumably this represents replacement of the myocardium with fibrous scar.[10]

In many patients who have had a previous infarction, bright MRI signal has been identified within the left ventricular chamber adjacent to the site of infarction. Presumably this signal represents stasis of blood flow within the region and is demonstrated best on second-echo (even-echo) images. This even-echo rephasing of flowing spins is consistent with slow blood flow during systole in the presence of regional ventricular dysfunction.

Regional Function in Ischemic Heart Disease

Cine MRI and multiphasic spin-echo images can be used to demonstrate the extent of wall thickening during the cardiac cycle.[11,18] The normal range for the percent wall thickening and the absolute extent of wall thickening during systole in the various regions of the left ventricle have been defined using MRI. These studies have demonstrated that the percent wall thickening is generally in the range of 60% and the absolute wall thickening is greater than 2 mm in normal myocardium. A decrease in the percent wall thickening and the absolute extent of wall thickening has been observed at sites of previous myocardial infarctions. The identification of regional myocardial dysfunction in ischemic heart disease as shown by MRI has correlated well with the same observations made by angiography.

MRI Contrast Media in Ischemic Heart Disease

The role of MRI in ischemic heart disease has been relatively minor until now and has been limited primarily to the demonstration of complications of acute myocardial infarction. The reason for this is that a major goal of noninvasive imaging studies in ischemic heart disease is to identify the presence of ischemic myocardium. MRI does not demonstrate ischemic but not yet infarcted myocardium using standard techniques. The differentiation of normal from ischemic myocardium using MRI has been accomplished by demonstrating the differential distribution of contrast media.[12,19,20] Although some experience exists with the use of MRI contrast media in patients with ischemic heart disease, most information has been obtained in experimental models. Both T_1 relaxation-enhancing and magnetic susceptibility contrast media have been used to identify ischemic myocardium.[19,20] The paramagnetic contrast media enhance the signal intensity of the myocardium on T_1-weighted images. The magnetic susceptibility agents decrease the signal intensity of the myocardium on T_2-weighted or gradient-echo images. Both of these agents can be used to demonstrate the jeopardy zone produced by an acute coronary occlusion. The jeopardy zone is seen as a region of decreased signal intensity (cold spot) when paramagnetic contrast media are used and a region of increased (hot spot) signal intensity when magnetic susceptibility agents are used.

Paramagnetic contrast media have also been shown to differentiate between occlusive and reperfused myocardial infarctions.[19] Thus, in patients whose myocardial infarction is treated with thrombolytic therapy these agents may be able to document the occurrence of reperfusion of the infarct.

In humans, a paramagnetic contrast medium (gadolinium diethylenetriamine pentaacetic acid [Gd DTPA]) has been used to increase the differential contrast between normal and infarcted myocardium.[21,22] Reports from several institutions have shown varied results for a contrast medium used in this circumstance. There is evidence that the contrast medium does improve the discrimination of the infarcted myocardium during the acute and subacute phase, but is less effective in chronic infarctions.[22] The contrast medium has been shown to increase the signal intensity of the periphery of the infarction during the acute and subacute phases. Chronic myocardial infarctions have not shown enhancement by contrast media, however, presumably because the injured myocardium is replaced by scar.

Cardiomyopathies

MRI has been used for the evaluation of congestive cardiomyopathy, hypertrophic cardiomyopathy, and restrictive cardiomyopathy.[9,23,24] The spin-echo technique has been used to demonstrate the morphologic abnormalities in these diseases and cine MRI has been used to demonstrate the functional abnormality. It has not been possible to demonstrate a consistent abnormality in the signal intensity or relaxation times of myocardium in any of the cardiomyopathies.

Congestive Cardiomyopathy

In congestive cardiomyopathy, MRI has demonstrated dilatation of the left ventricle and, in many cases, dilatation of the right ventricle as well.[9] The thickness of the left ventricular wall has usually been normal, resulting in an overall substantial increase in left ventricular mass. Wall thickness is usually uniform around the circumference of the left ventricle in idiopathic congestive cardiomyopathy, but nonuniform with regions of extreme wall thinning as a consequence of previous myocardial infarction in patients with ischemic cardiomyopathy. In many patients a pericardial effusion of some degree is also demonstrated.

MRI has been used for quantifying the ventricular volumes and the wall thickness and mass in patients with congestive cardiomyopathy.[9,25] When patients are studied on two separate occasions the variability of measurements is small. The percent variability in ventricular volume and mass is generally less than 5%, which makes the technique sufficiently reproducible from one time to the next so that it is useful for documenting the effect of therapeutic interventions.[25]

Cine MRI has been used to assess left ventricular and, to some degree, right ventricular function in patients with cardiomyopathy.[9] With this technique the extent of wall thickening, ejection fraction, stroke volume, and left ventricular end-systolic wall stress can be measured (Fig. 8-15). This technique has been used to monitor the functional status of the left ventricle over time and to evaluate the effect of various interventions. Cine MRI has demonstrated that in spite of a substantial increase in left ventricular mass in patients with congestive cardiomyopathy, the left ventricular end- and peak-systolic wall stress are markedly increased.

Hypertrophic Cardiomyopathy

MRI has provided accurate definitions of the extent, location, and severity of hypertrophy in patients with hypertrophic cardiomyopathy (Figs. 8-16 and 8-17).[23] Echocardiography is generally used for the diagnosis and assessment of the severity of hypertrophic cardiomyopathy. The major role of MRI has been to document the presence of unusual forms of hypertrophic cardiomyopathy. There is considerable variability in ventricular morphology in these patients. In some patients hypertrophy exists only in the outflow septum, whereas in others the entire septum is hypertrophied. The midventricular and apical forms of hypertrophic cardiomyopathy have focal hypertrophy in these regions of the left ventricle. MRI has been especially effective in demonstrating these variant forms of hypertrophic cardiomyopathy.

Cine MRI can be used to demonstrate the functional characteristics of the left ventricle and to document and

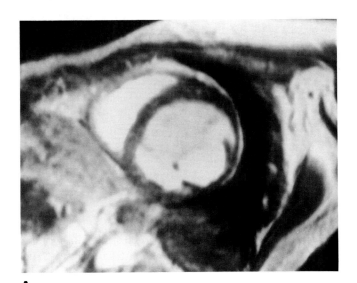
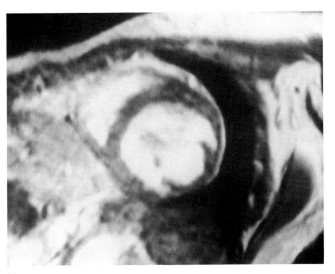

A   **B**

Figure 8-15. Congestive cardiomyopathy. Cine MRI through the middle of the ventricle in the short-axis plane acquired at end diastole (*A*) and end systole (*B*) in a patient with dilated (congestive) cardiomyopathy. The area of the ventricular chamber shows little change from diastole to systole, indicating a low ejection fraction. The left ventricle is considerably dilated.

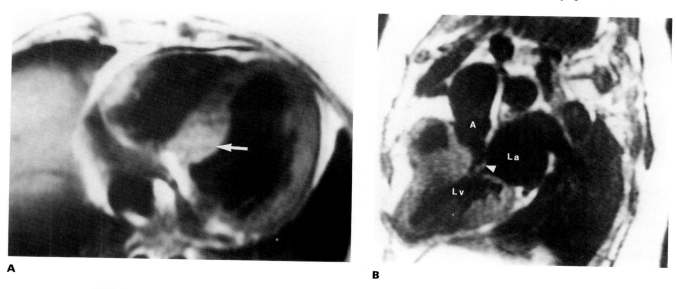

Figure 8-16. Hypertrophic cardiomyopathy. ECG gated spin-echo transverse (*A*) and coronal (*B*) images of a patient with the asymmetric form of hypertrophic cardiomyopathy. Note the thickening of the cranial portion of the ventricular septum (*arrow*). In the sagittal view the anterior leaflet of the mitral valve (*arrowhead*) is opposed to the hypertrophied septum in systole. (A, aorta; Lv, left ventricle; La, left atrium.)

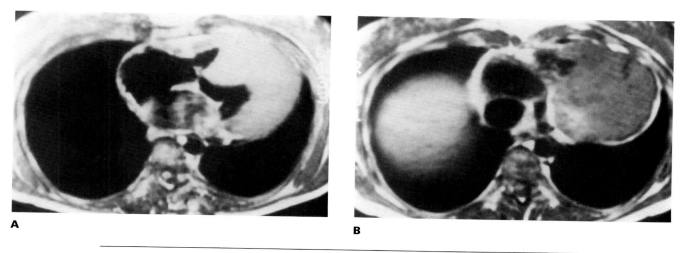

Figure 8-17. Hypertrophic cardiomyopathy. ECG gated spin-echo transverse images at the level of the mitral valve (*A*) and the apical region of the left ventricle (*B*) in a patient with the symmetrical form of hypertrophic cardiomyopathy. Note the extreme thickening of myocardium in all regions of the left ventricle. Because of the hypertrophy, the cavity at the apex is obliterated. There is also thickening of the free wall of the right ventricle.

assess the severity of the frequently associated mitral regurgitation. Cine MRI has also been used to quantify the left ventricular mass, ventricular volume, and ejection fraction in these patients. It has also been used to determine the increase in right ventricular mass that frequently occurs in patients with hypertrophic cardiomyopathy (Fig. 8-18). Similarly, cine MRI has been used to demonstrate a decrease in the diastolic filling pattern of

the right ventricle. Abnormalities in diastolic filling of the left ventricle are well known from ventriculographic and echocardiographic studies in patients with hypertrophic cardiomyopathy. Cine MRI in diastole can be used to measure the peak filling rate and time-to-peak filling rate of the right as well as the left ventricle. A recent report has indicated that diastolic filling parameters of the right ventricle are abnormal, indicating reduced compliance of

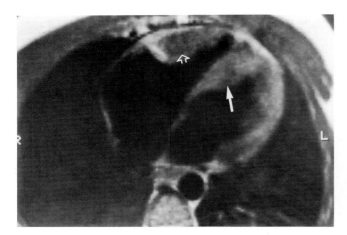

Figure 8-18. Hypertrophic cardiomyopathy. ECG gated spin-echo transverse images at the middle of the ventricle in a patient with hypertrophic cardiomyopathy. Note the thickened septum (*arrow*) and the thickened free wall of the right ventricle (*open arrow*).

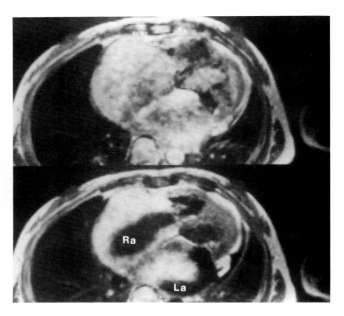

Figure 8-19. Restrictive cardiomyopathy. ECG gated spin-echo images at the midventricular level. *Top:* The first echo images (TE = 30 msec). *Bottom:* Second echo image (TE = 60 msec). Considerable signal is present in the atrial chambers because of stasis of blood caused by severely reduced compliance of the ventricles. Note the marked enlargement of the left (La) and right (Ra) atria, and normal size of the ventricles. (Reproduced with permission from Sechtem U, Higgins CB, Sommerhoff BA, Lipton MJ, Huycke EC. Magnetic resonance imaging of restrictive cardiomyopathy. Am J Cardiol 1987;59:480.)

this ventricle in patients with hypertrophic cardiomyopathy.[26]

Restrictive Cardiomyopathy

The diagnosis of restrictive cardiomyopathy is difficult to confirm with imaging techniques. This diagnosis is suspected from catheterization data indicating elevated diastolic pressure in both ventricles. The diastolic pressures are nearly equal in the two ventricles but may show some separation with physiologic maneuvers. Imaging studies are usually done to differentiate between constrictive pericarditis and restrictive cardiomyopathy. MRI is useful for distinguishing between the two; the major distinguishing feature is thickened pericardium (> 4 mm thickness) in constrictive pericarditis, and normal thickness in restrictive cardiomyopathy.

Other but less specific features of restrictive cardiomyopathy are enlarged atria with usually normal ventricular volumes and a markedly dilated inferior vena cava and hepatic veins (Fig. 8-19).[24] The wall thickness of either or both ventricles is usually increased in the restrictive cardiomyopathy associated with amyloidosis. Although the wall thickness of amyloid heart disease may be suggestive of hypertrophic cardiomyopathy, the systolic ventricular function of the two diseases is different. Systolic function as measured by ejection fraction and wall motion is normal or increased in hypertrophic cardiomyopathy but decreased in amyloidosis. Other infiltrative diseases also cause restrictive cardiomyopathy. One, sarcoidosis, causes high intensity nodules within the myocardial wall on T_2-weighted images.[27]

Because of blood stasis in the atria in restrictive cardiomyopathy, bright signal appears in the atria on spin-

echo images. Restrictive cardiomyopathy is frequently complicated by mitral or tricuspid regurgitation; this regurgitation can be demonstrated and even quantified using cine MRI.[28]

Pericardial Disease

MRI is effective for the evaluation of pericardial diseases. Its role in this regard is supplementary to echocardiography at this time. MRI should be considered for the evaluation of the following pericardial abnormalities:

1. Pericardial effusions, especially loculated effusions.
2. Differentiation of hemorrhagic versus nonhemorrhagic pericardial effusions.
3. Detection of pericardial metastasis or direct extension of tumors through the pericardium.[29]
4. Diagnosis of constrictive pericarditis.[30,31]
5. Evaluation of primary pericardial cysts or tumors.
6. Diagnosis of partial or complete absence of the pericardium (Higgins CB, personal communication, 1991).

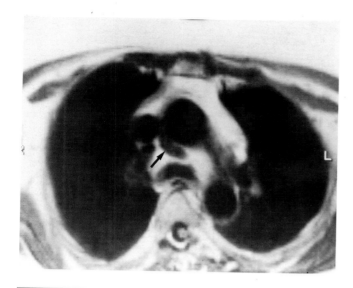

Figure 8-20. Superior pericardial recess. ECG gated spin-echo image at the level of the distal ascending aorta shows fluid in the superior pericardial recess (*arrow*).

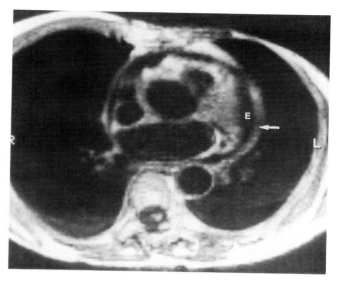

Figure 8-21. Pericardial effusion. ECG gated spin-echo images show low-intensity fluid surrounding the heart. The parietal pericardium is thickened (*arrow*). Nonhemorrhagic effusion (E) produces low intensity on T$_1$-weighted spin-echo image.

Pericardial Effusion. MRI demonstrates small volumes of pericardial fluid in healthy subjects.[32] Fluid in the superior pericardial recess is observed in many healthy subjects (Fig. 8-20). The technique is sensitive for identifying generalized or loculated pericardial effusions (Figs. 8-21 and 8-22). The wide field-of-view of MRI makes it effective for defining and depicting the size of loculated effusions (see Figs. 8-21 and 8-22).

Hemorrhagic effusion is characterized by high intensity on T$_1$-weighted spin-echo images (see Fig. 8-22). Conversely, the nonhemorrhagic effusion has low intensity on T$_1$-weighted spin-echo images (see Fig. 8-22) and high intensity on cine MRI-weighted images.

Constrictive Pericarditis. The pericardium is directly visualized on MRI; consequently, MRI is an ideal technique for the diagnosis of constrictive pericarditis.[30,31] The normal pericardial thickness is less than 4 mm. A thickness of 4 mm or greater indicates pericardial thickening, and in the proper clinical setting is a diagnostic finding in constrictive pericarditis. Pericardial thickening can be observed in the absence of constrictive pericarditis. The pericardium can be thickened for weeks or months after cardiac surgery; pericardial thickening is persistent in patients with the postpericardiotomy syndrome (Dressler's syndrome). It is also thickened during inflammatory processes of the pericardium, such as acute pericarditis (Fig. 8-23) and uremic pericarditis (Fig. 8-24). The central cardiovascular structures have a characteristic appearance in constrictive pericarditis; the inferior vena cava, hepatic veins, and right atrium are substantially dilated, whereas the right ventricle has normal or reduced

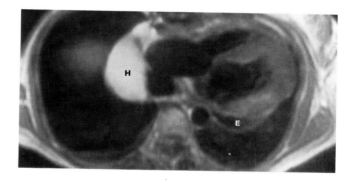

Figure 8-22. Loculated effusions. ECG gated spin-echo image at the midventricular level shows hemorrhagic (H) and nonhemorrhagic (E) effusions. On T$_1$-weighted images these two types of effusions have a different signal intensity, which permits differentiation.

volume (Fig. 8-25). An elongated, narrow-shaped right ventricle and a sigmoid-shaped ventricular septum are sometimes observed in this disease.

Constriction is sometimes localized to the right side of the heart or to the right atrioventricular groove alone. In many circumstances, pericardial thickening is observed only over the right atrium and right ventricle (Fig. 8-25). Transverse MRI has displayed pericardial thickening of the right atrioventricular groove, causing narrowing of the tricuspid valve orifice (Fig. 8-26).

MRI can distinguish between constrictive pericarditis and restrictive cardiomyopathy. Both diseases cause dilated atria and nearly normal volumes of the ventricles;

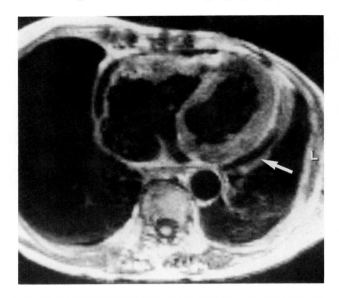

Figure 8-23. Acute pericarditis. ECG gated spin-echo image shows markedly thickened pericardium (*arrow*) and pericardial effusion with low signal intensity.

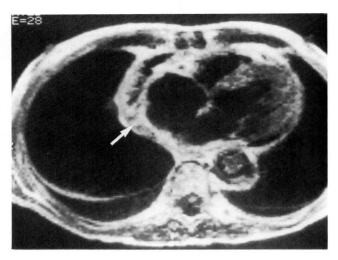

Figure 8-24. Uremic pericarditis. ECG gated spin-echo image shows pericardial fluid and thickening of visceral and parietal pleura. Inflammatory adhesions and exudate (*arrow*) extend between the two pericardial layers. The high signal of the pericardium suggests acute inflammatory alterations.

however, the recognition of pericardial thickening indicates the presence of constrictive pericarditis.

Pericardial Masses and Cysts. MRI, with its wide field-of-view, has been effective for demonstrating pericardial tumors and pericardial cysts.[29,33] The pericardial cyst in its typical form is recognized by low signal intensity on a T_1-weighted image and homogeneous high signal intensity on T_2-weighted images. With prolongation of the TE interval there is generally a progressive increase in signal intensity of fluid within the pericardial cyst. The pericardial cyst is typically located in the right cardiophrenic angle but may be located anywhere within the pericardium. When situated in an unusual location, the pericardial cyst may be indistinguishable from a bronchogenic cyst or a thymic cyst. Any cyst containing simple fluid (low protein concentration and nonhemorrhagic) has low intensity on T_1-weighted images and high, homogeneous intensity on T_2-weighted images.

Pericardial tumors generally occur by extension from mediastinal or lung tumors or by metastasis. Pericardial tumors are much more frequently secondary rather than primary tumors. A tumor extending to the pericardium but not through the pericardium can be recognized by the presence of an intact pericardial line (Fig. 8-27). Those tumors that have extended through the pericardium may be recognized by focal obliteration of the pericardial line (Fig. 8-28) and the presence of a pericardial effusion. Many tumors metastatic to the heart or extending through the pericardium induce a hemorrhagic pericardial effusion. Because of the high signal intensity of the blood within the pericardial sac on spin-echo im-

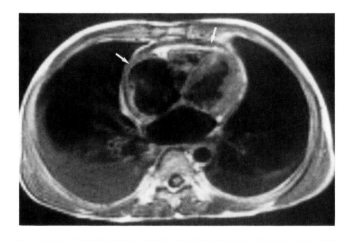

Figure 8-25. Constrictive pericarditis. ECG gated spin-echo image shows thickened pericardium (*arrows*) over right and ventral regions of the heart. Thickened pericardial line produces low intensity and is recognized between the high signal of the subepicardial and pericardial fat layers. Note the marked enlargement of the right atrium and normal size of the right ventricle.

ages, it may not be possible to recognize the tumor separate from the high signal intensity of blood within the pericardial sac (Fig. 8-29).

The most frequent paracardiac masses are pericardial cysts and pseudocysts, enlarged pericardial fat pad, lymphoma, teratoma, diaphragmatic eventration and hernia, bronchogenic and metastatic carcinoma, and inferior extension of anterior thoracic tumors (thymoma and teratoma). An intrapericardial pheochromocytoma is one of the unusual extra-adrenal sites of this tumor (Fig. 8-30).

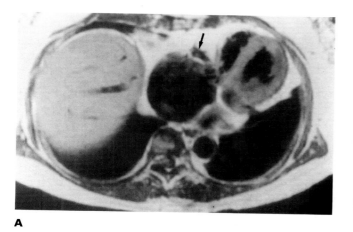

A

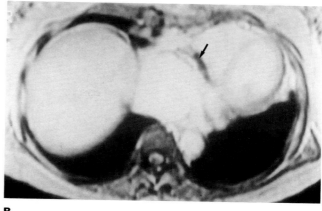

B

Figure 8-26. Focal pericardial constriction. ECG gated spin-echo (*A*) and cine (*B*) MR images show focal pericardial thickening (*arrow*) in the right atrioventricular groove. The focal pericardial constriction compresses the tricuspid annulus (arrow).

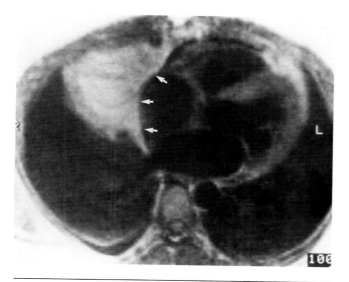

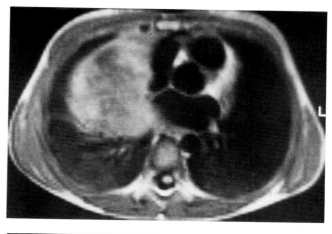

Figure 8-28. Paracardiac mass. ECG gated spin-echo image indicates obliteration of the pericardial line, consistent with extension of the tumor through the pericardium. The mass cannot be separated from the right or left atrial wall.

Figure 8-27. Paracardiac mass. ECG gated spin-echo image shows a mass adjacent to the right side of the heart. The mass extends to, but not through, the pericardium, as indicated by the intact pericardial line (*arrows*).

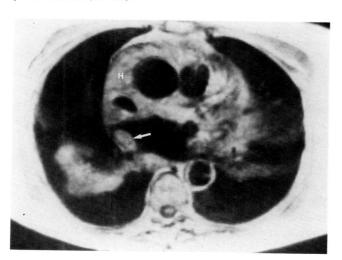

Figure 8-29. Pericardial and cardiac metastasis with pericardial hemorrhage. ECG gated spin-echo image shows high signal intensity of pericardial effusion (hemorrhagic effusion [H]). A metastatic nodule is attached to the left atrial wall (*arrow*). The signal intensities of this nodule and the effusion are similar.

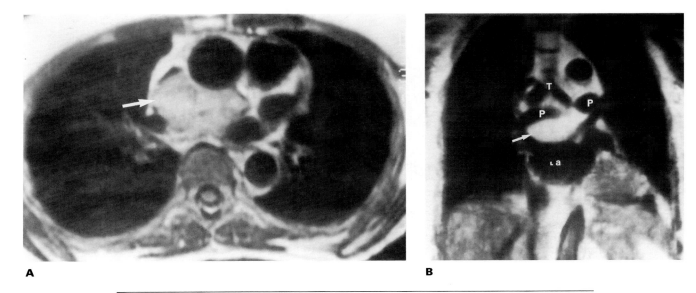

A   **B**

Figure 8-30. Intrapericardial pheochromocytoma. ECG gated spin-echo transverse image at the base of the heart (*A*) and coronal image (*B*) show a mass (*arrow*) posterior to the ascending aorta. The mass is located just above the roof of the left atrium. Coronal image shows that the mass indents the roof of the left atrium (La). (P, pulmonary artery; T, trachea.)

Intracardiac Masses

Gated spin-echo MRI has been effective for demonstrating the presence, location, extent, and in some instances, nature of intracardiac masses.[33] The most frequent intracardiac mass is thrombus, which is usually located within the left atrium (see Figs. 8-12 to 8-14) or left ventricle. The most frequent benign tumors are myxoma and lipoma. The former is usually located in the left atrium and the latter in the right atrium. MRI has demonstrated the various configurations of the myxoma (Figs. 8-31, 8-32, and 8-33), from a spherically shaped tumor with a narrow pedicle attached to the region of the fossa ovalis of the atrial septum (see Fig. 8-32) to a filiform-shaped tumor with a wide base of attachment to the lower atrial septum or the atrial side of the mitral valve (see Fig. 8-33). A broad point of attachment to the atrial septum is considered by many to raise the possibility of a malignant tumor (Fig. 8-34). The lipoma may be observed as a mass with high signal intensity lying within the right atrial cavity or, more frequently, consists of broad, generalized fatty thickening of the atrial septum, with components projecting into the right atrial cavity. The lipoma can be definitely demonstrated using a fat saturation image. This type of sequence causes similar attenuation of the signal in the subcutaneous fat and lipoma (Fig. 8-34).

The most common malignant intracardiac tumor is an angiosarcoma, usually involving the right atrium. The most frequent tumor in children is a rhabdomyoma. Rhabdomyomas may vary in size and frequently are mul-

tiple. Some of these have demonstrated higher signal intensity than the myocardium. These tumors may be difficult to recognize because of their small size and entirely intramural location; however, many cause a focal distortion of the myocardial wall or project into the chamber. The larger tumors distort the myocardial wall and because of their large size, may also distort the external configuration of the heart as well as the cavities.

Some tumors have a characteristic signal intensity, such as the low signal intensity on T_2-weighted images of fibromas of the ventricular wall. One case of proven fibroma showed no enhancement after administration of Gd-DTPA. Lipoma of the right atrium, or lipomatous degeneration of the atrial septum, is recognized by a high-signal-intensity mass on T_1-weighted images. These masses demonstrate nearly the same signal intensity characteristics of subcutaneous fat on all imaging sequences (see Fig. 8-34). The use of a fat saturation technique that reduces or eliminates the signal intensity from subcutaneous fat also eliminates or greatly reduces the signal intensity from the lipoma. With this technique it is possible to recognize the lipomatous nature of some right atrial tumors.

Secondary Tumors of the Heart

Secondary tumors of the heart are 40 to 50 times more frequent than primary tumors of the heart. The involvement of the heart by tumors may occur by direct spread

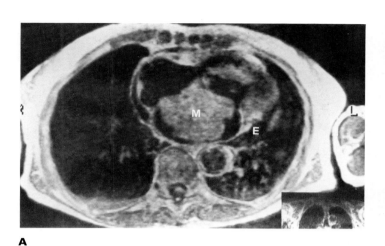

A

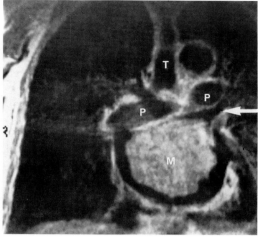

B

Figure 8-31. Left atrial myxoma. ECG gated spin-echo transverse (*A*) and coronal (*B*) images demonstrate a large mass (M) with a broad interface with the atrial septum and filling most of the left atrial cavity. (E, pericardial effusion; P, pulmonary artery, left and right; T, trachea; arrow, pulmonary vein.) (Courtesy of A. Lomonaco, MD, Tucson, Arizona.)

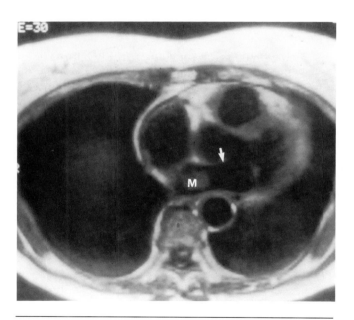

Figure 8-32. Left atrial myxoma. ECG gated spin-echo image shows a small mass (M) attached by a pedicle (*arrowhead*) to the atrial septum. Mitral valve leaflet is indicated by an arrow.

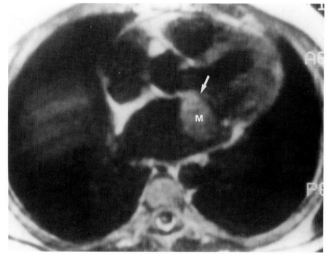

Figure 8-33. Left atrial myxoma. ECG gated spin-echo image demonstrates a myxoma (M) attached by a broad pedicle to the base of the anterior leaflet (*arrow*) of the mitral valve.

from mediastinal and lung tumors; by extension of tumors of the upper abdomen through the inferior vena cava and into the right atrium, and by metastases to the pericardium, myocardium, or cardiac chambers. MRI has been effective for depicting each of these types of secondary tumors of the heart.[29] It has demonstrated the extension of mediastinal and lung tumors to the heart (Fig. 8-35). Extension of tumors through the inferior vena cava

from primary tumors of the kidneys, adrenals, and liver has been demonstrated by MRI (Fig. 8-36). An important observation in this regard is the extent of attachment of such tumors to the right atrial wall. Extension through the inferior vena cava without invasion of the right atrial wall may permit removal of the tumors at the time of surgery. Metastases to the cardiac chambers are effectively demonstrated by MRI, which also displays the extent of the tumor attachment to the cardiac walls (Figs. 8-14 and 8-37). Tumors are readily recognized within the

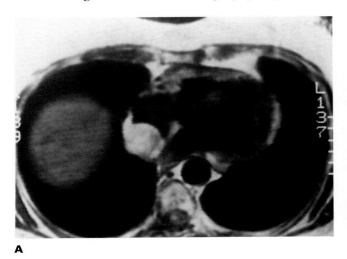

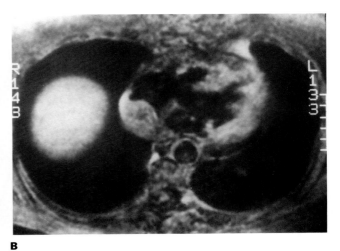

A   **B**

Figure 8-34. Right atrial lipoma. ECG gated spin-echo (*A*) and fat-saturated spin-echo images (*B*) show the mass in the right atrium. The fat saturation sequence is produced by applying a preliminary radiofrequency pulse at the specific frequency of protons in lipids so that their signal is reduced on the subsequent spin-echo sequences. The signal of the tumor is reduced to a degree similar to that imposed on subcutaneous fat.

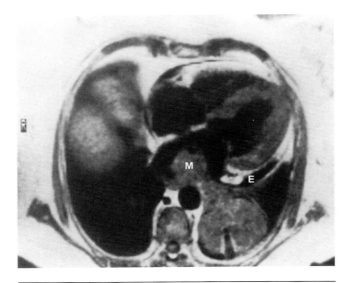

Figure 8-35. Tumor of the lung extending into the left atrium. ECG gated spin-echo image depicts a tumor (M) of the left lung extending into the left atrium. There is a small posterior pericardial effusion (E).

Differentiation of Tumor Thrombus Versus Clot

It has become possible in some cases to distinguish a tumor thrombus from a blood clot. On spin-echo images, the signal intensity of blood clot can vary depending on its age (see Figs. 8-12 to 8-14). The relatively fresh clot causes bright signal intensity whereas the old clot tends to produce low signal intensity, especially on T_2-weighted sequences. Similarly, tumors can have variable signal intensity, although most tumors have high signal intensity on T_2-weighted images. The differentiation between tumor and clot is accomplished most effectively using gradient-echo images rather than spin-echo images.[17] On gradient-echo images tumor thrombus has medium signal intensity (see Figs. 8-14 and 8-38). The signal intensity is similar to other types of tissues; the signal of tumors of the inferior vena cava is similar to that of the liver and the signal of intracardiac tumors is similar to or higher than that of ventricular myocardium. Conversely, the blood clot usually has low signal intensity on gradient-echo images; the signal is less than that of skeletal muscle. The clot has lower signal intensity than solid organs such as the liver or the myocardium on gradient-echo images. Atrial myxomas may have a signal intensity indistinguishable from clot on cine MRI; they may have very low signal intensity because of the presence of considerable fibrosis, calcification, or inspissation of iron within the tumor. Iron within the tumor has the effect of decreasing signal intensity on gradient-echo images and causing them to appear as dark as clots. Because of the low signal intensity of some left atrial myxomas, these tumors are not visible on spin-echo images but are read-

low signal intensity of the blood pool on spin-echo images and within the high signal intensity of the blood pool on gradient-echo images (Figs. 8-14 and 8-38).

The most frequent mass within the heart is the clot, which most frequently involves the left ventricle or the left atrium. Clots are readily demonstrated by echocardiography. Clots within the atrial appendage and on the lateral wall of the left atrium may be difficult to demonstrate with two-dimensional echocardiography, however. These regions are readily examined with MRI (see Fig. 8-14).

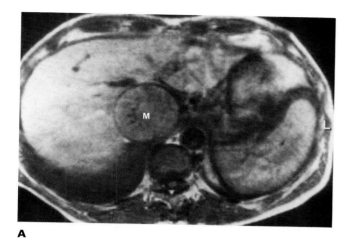

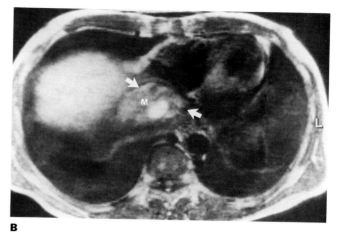

Figure 8-36. Adrenal tumor extending through the inferior vena cava and into the right atrium. Spin-echo images at the level of the liver (*A*) and right atrium (*B*) show tumor (M) expanding the inferior vena cava and extending into the right atrium (*arrows*).

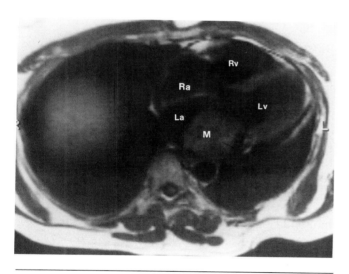

Figure 8-37. Metastatic tumor in the left atrium. ECG gated spin-echo image shows a mass in the left atrial cavity and indicates a narrow point of attachment to the left atrial wall. (La, left atrium; Lv, left ventricle; M, mass; Ra, right atrium; Rv, right ventricle.)

ily recognized as very low signal intensity masses within the high signal intensity of the blood pool on the gradient-echo images (Fig. 8-39).

Valvular Heart Disease

Repetitive gradient refocused MRI (cine MRI) has been found to be useful for evaluating ventricular and valvular function in valvular heart disease.[4,28,35,36] Studies in patients with mitral and aortic regurgitation have shown that the regurgitant jet can be visualized on cine MRI as an area of signal void extending from the incompetent valve into the recipient cardiac chamber (Figs. 8-40 and 8-41). Abnormal signal has also been noted at the site of valvular stenosis and extending into the chamber or great artery distal to the stenosis (Fig. 8-42).

On cine MRI mitral regurgitation can be identified by a circumscript area of signal loss emanating from the insufficient mitral valve into the left atrium during ventricular systole (see Fig. 8-41).[4,28,36] This area of signal loss can be clearly differentiated from the high signal intensity of the cardiac blood pool. Aortic regurgitation can be identified by an area of signal loss extending from the incompetent aortic valve into the left ventricle during ventricular diastole (see Fig. 8-40).[4,28,36]

Cine MRI can also be used for quantification of the volume of regurgitation. The regurgitant volume in patients with regurgitation of only one valve can be assessed by the difference between right and left ventricular stroke volumes as calculated from the stack of MR images acquired at end diastole and end systole.[37] The stroke volume is the difference between end-diastolic and end-systolic volumes. In healthy subjects the stroke volume is equal for the right and left ventricles. The regurgitant volume is the difference in stroke volumes between the two ventricles. This calculation is invalidated if valves on both sides of the heart are regurgitant. This value provides a measure of the total regurgitant volume on one side of the heart. Measurements of the volume of signal loss can also be used to estimate the severity of regurgitation.[28,35,36] This calculation has been shown to differentiate between mild, moderate, and severe lesions in both aortic and mitral regurgitation and has correlated with the echocardiographic or angiographic gradings. In groups of patients with mitral regurgitation and aortic re-

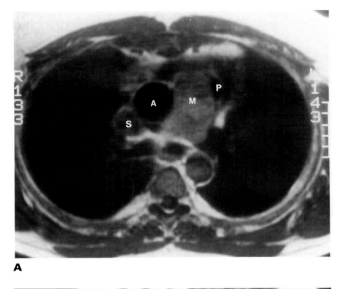

A

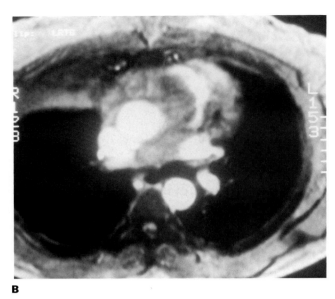

B

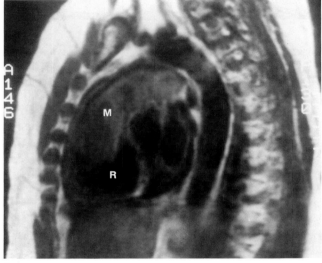

C

Figure 8-38. Liposarcoma of the right ventricle extending into the main pulmonary artery. ECG gated spin-echo (*A*) and cine (*B*) images in the transverse plane and spin-echo image in the sagittal plane (*C*). Note that the tumor extends from the right ventricle and almost completely occludes the pulmonary artery. Cine MR images show the high signal intensity of flowing blood in the narrow channel around the mass. Sagittal image demonstrates the longitudinal extent of the mass. (A, ascending aorta; P, pulmonary artery; M, mass; R, right ventricle; S, superior vena cava.)

gurgitation, the regurgitant volume was determined by the difference of left and right ventricular stroke volume and then correlated to the volume of signal void.[28] The correlation between the two methods for measuring regurgitation was good for patients with isolated aortic or mitral regurgitation. It should be noted that the volume of this signal void is significantly altered by changes in imaging and image display parameters. Shortening of the echo delay time can cause reduction in the volume of the regurgitant signal void.

Another method for quantification of aortic regurgitation is velocity-encoded cine MRI. With this technique the phase shifts of protons within various voxels of the image are displayed in the gray level, corresponding to the degree of phase shift.[38,39] The major factor causing such phase shift is motion and the phase shift is directly

proportional to motion over time, and hence velocity. A measurement of average velocity is made for the proximal aorta and pulmonary artery in each velocity-encoded cine MR image. Usually, the cardiac cycle is segmented into 15 to 30 images equally spaced throughout the cycle. Average velocity and the cross-sectional area for the aorta and pulmonary artery are measured for each image. Instantaneous blood flow is calculated as the product of average flow velocity and cross-sectional area of the great artery. Integration of the blood flow values from images in systole estimates stroke volume for the left and right ventricles. The technique can distinguish between antegrade and retrograde flow so that retrograde flow in diastole can be measured to directly quantify aortic regurgitation. Aortic regurgitation can be estimated in two ways with this technique. For isolated aortic regurgitation

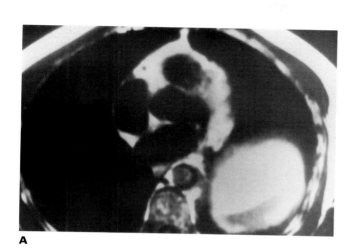

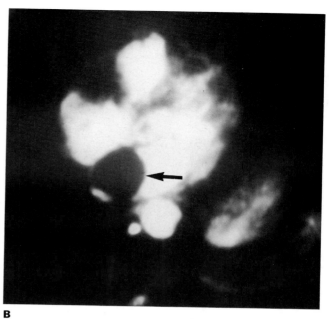

A

B

Figure 8-39. Left atrial myxoma. ECG gated spin-echo (*A*) and cine (*B*) MR images in a patient with left atrial myxoma. The myxoma contained considerable iron, which caused very low signal intensity due to the magnetic susceptibility effect; consequently, it is not visible on the spin-echo image. On the cine MR image, it is recognized as a large filling defect (*arrow*) in the left atrial blood pool.

the difference in calculated stroke volume between the two ventricles is the regurgitation volume. The retrograde flow in the aorta during diastole is a direct measurement of regurgitation and should be valid even in the presence of pulmonic regurgitation. In some patients with a large stroke volume, however, signal loss occurs in the ascending aorta during systole. In such instances, measurements using velocity-encoded cine MRI could be inaccurate unless the flow void can be eliminated by using a very short TE value for imaging.

The high-velocity turbulent flow across valvular stenosis causes a signal void projected into the downstream chamber or great artery (see Fig. 8-42). Quantitative phase imaging (velocity-encoded cine MRI) can be used as a method for determining peak gradient across the aortic valve using theories and formulas currently in vogue for Doppler echocardiography.[40] Measurement of velocity across the stenotic valve is complicated by the presence of high-velocity turbulent flow, however, causing loss of signal across beyond the valve. Although the signal void on cine MRI caused by turbulence permits recognition of stenosis and regurgitation and even estimation of the severity of regurgitation, the signal loss can invalidate measures of velocity at such sites. It has now been shown that velocities as great as 6 m/sec can be measured by lowering the TE value; a TE value of 7 msec allows measurement of flow velocities in this range for

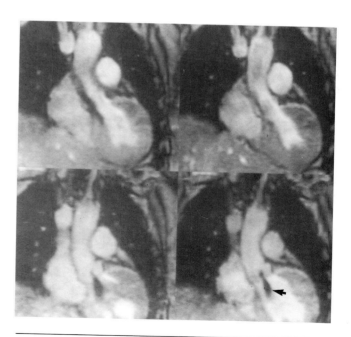

Figure 8-40. Aortic regurgitation. Series of cine MR coronal images in systole (*upper panels*) and diastole (*lower panels*). A single void (*arrow*) emanates from the closed aortic valve, indicating aortic regurgitation.

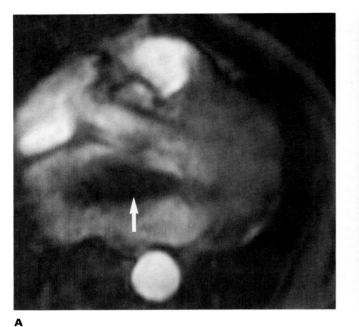

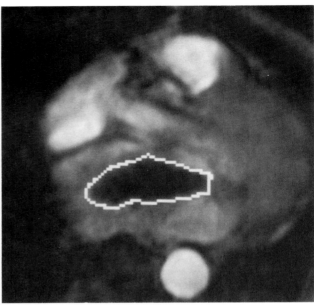

A   **B**

Figure 8-41. Mitral regurgitation. Cine MR image at the level of the mitral valve during early systole. The signal void (*arrow*) emanating from the mitral valve during systole represents mitral regurgitation. The area of the signal void is outlined and measured; this measurement provides a semiquantitative estimate of the regurgitant volume.

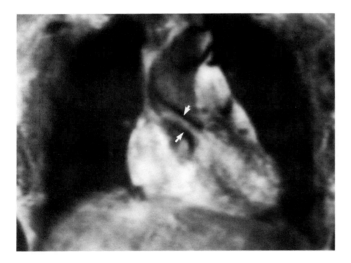

Figure 8-42. Aortic stenosis. Cine MR image in coronal plane during systole shows a narrow jet surrounded by a signal void in the ascending aorta. The signal void (*arrows*) is caused by the turbulence induced by the aortic jet.

images acquired at 1.5 T. A recent study has shown the feasibility of measuring peak velocity across valvular and vascular stenoses using a velocity-encoded gradient echo technique.[41]

Cardiac Function

Ventricular function can be assessed using MRI techniques that acquire multiple images for each cardiac cycle. Division of the cardiac cycle into numerous phases is necessary to effectively acquire an image that corresponds to end diastole and end systole. Techniques for this purpose include multiphasic, multislice spin-echo imaging; biphasic spin-echo imaging; and cine MRI. Biphasic MRI is a technique for acquiring images at multiple anatomic levels at two phases of the cardiac cycle, near end diastole and end systole. Cine MRI is probably the most effective technique for functional evaluation of the heart. With this technique, images are acquired at a rate of 16 to about 30 frames per cardiac cycle. These images can be laced together and displayed in a cinematic format. The cinematic format allows assessment of global right ventricular and left ventricular function and regional wall thickening to define regional myocardial function. After obtaining 10 to 12 tomograms encompassing the entire heart from the apex to the bifurcation of the pulmonary artery, left and right ventricular volumes can be calculated as the sum of the cavity area times slice thickness (Fig. 8-43). On cine MRI, blood flowing at normal velocities produces high signal intensity (white coloration) and can be clearly differentiated from the myo-

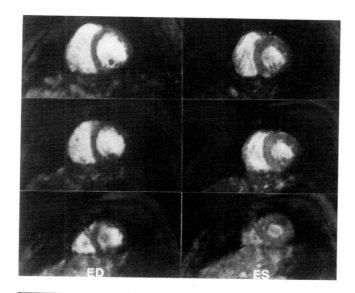

Figure 8-43. Cine MR images at end diastole (*left column*) and end systole (*right column*), which were acquired near the base of the ventricles (*upper panels*), in the middle of the ventricles (*middle panels*), and near the apex of the ventricles (*lower panels*). These images can be used to calculate stroke volume, ejection fraction, and the extent of wall thickening during the cardiac cycle.

cardium. End systole and end diastole are defined as the smallest and largest cavity areas. Images at the valvular level are used to confirm the correct timing of end diastole (last image before opening of the aortic valve) and end systole (last image before opening of the mitral valve). With the time resolution of cine MRI, changes in volume can be shown at 16 to 30 points during the cardiac cycle. The measurements done with these images are end diastole, end systole, and stroke volumes for the right and left ventricles. Ejection fraction as an indicator of ventricular function is calculated as the stroke volume of the left or right ventricle divided by the respective end-diastolic volume.

Cine MRI provides accurate measurements of left ventricular mass, determined as the summation of myocardial areas on each slice encompassing the left ventricle multiplied by the myocardial specific gravity (1.05). Measurements of ventricular volumes and mass in transverse and left ventricular long-axis planes have been shown to correlate well with values obtained by cine angiography and two-dimensional cardiography.

Because of potential angulation errors and partial volume effects in the transverse plane, a higher accuracy for the assessment of left ventricular geometry and function was expected in the short-axis plane. Actual experiments have not confirmed this supposition. A recent study has demonstrated excellent correlation between the transverse and short-axis plane in healthy subjects and in patients with dilated cardiomyopathy.[9] The mea-

surements of left ventricular volumes and stroke volume were nearly identical for studies assessed in the short-axis plane compared with the transverse plane.

Regional Myocardial Function

The use of the short-axis plane is essential for the measurement of left ventricular wall thickening during the cardiac cycle. Since both the endocardial and epicardial borders are well-defined by cine MRI, it is possible to assess wall thickening during the cardiac cycle and to detect regional myocardial dysfunction. The cinematic display of MRI facilitates identification of abnormal wall motion during the cardiac cycle. The percentage wall thickening can be expressed by the formula:

$$\text{Wall thickening (\%)} = \frac{T_{es} - T_{ed}}{T_{ed}}$$

where T_{es} is end-systolic wall thickness (mm) and T_{ed} is end-diastolic wall thickness (mm). In healthy subjects, the percentage of wall thickening and absolute extent of wall thickening can vary among regions of the left ventricle. In patients with previous infarction, the region involved by the infarction has a demonstrated wall thickening of less than 2 mm, whereas normal myocardial regions show a wall thickening of 2 mm or greater.

Three-dimensional functional geometry can be evaluated with cine MRI by determining the systolic wall thickening at multiple levels from base to apex (see Fig. 8-43). Healthy subjects and patients with dilated cardiomyopathy were imaged in the left ventricular short-axis plane with images encompassing the entire heart from base to apex. The healthy left ventricle showed an increasing gradient in wall thickening from base to apex (Fig. 8-44). This gradient was absent in patients with dilated cardiomyopathy. Cine MRI can provide noninvasive three-dimensional evaluaton of global and regional function of the normal and diseased left ventricle. These measurements have been shown to be highly reproducible on sequential studies in healthy, dilated, and hypertrophied ventricles.[25,42]

Measurement of Blood Flow

Several techniques have been devised for measuring blood flow. One of these techniques is called the time of flight technique, in which protons are tagged at one anatomic level and then this tag is imaged at another level further downstream within the blood vessel (Fig. 8-45).[43] Since the time between measurement and tagging of the protons within flowing blood and the distance between

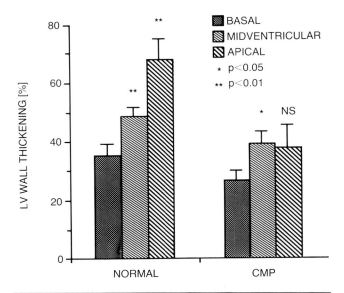

Figure 8-44. Diagram shows the extent of wall thickening at the basal, mid, and apical levels of the left ventricle, measured on cine MR images in healthy (normal) subjects and patients with dilated (congestive) cardiomyopathy. In healthy subjects a gradient in the extent wall thickening (end-systolic–end-diastolic wall thickness) was observed, whereas the gradient was not present in the patients with dilated cardiomyopathy. (Reproduced with permission from Buser PT, Auffermann W, Holt WW, et al. Noninvasive evaluation of the global left ventricular function using cine MR imaging. J Am Coll Cardiol 1989;13:1294.)

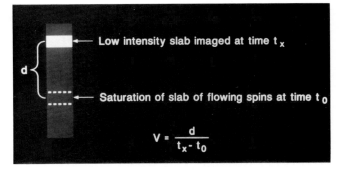

Figure 8-45. Diagram shows the salient concept associated with the measurement of blood flow velocity by the time of flight technique. A slab of blood is tagged by applying a selective saturation pulse at one tomographic level and then the tagged slice is detected at a downstream level. (V, velocity; d, distance; t_x, time of imaging; t_0, time of saturation pulse.)

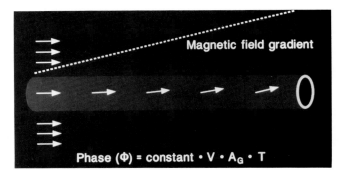

Figure 8-46. Diagram shows the salient concept associated with the measurement of blood flow velocity by the phase change technique. This technique depends on the principle that spins flowing along a magnetic gradient change their phase relative to stationary spins depending on the distance moved in a unit of time. (A_G, strength of magnetic gradient; T, time; V, velocity.)

the two sites is known, it is possible to calculate the velocity of blood flow. Another technique measures the change in phase of protons that are in motion relative to nonmobile protons (Fig. 8-46), which maintain the same phase during the MRI sequence. It is based on the proportionality of the phase change to the velocity of motion of spins that flow along a magnetic gradient during the imaging sequence. This technique is referred to as the velocity-encoded cine MRI technique and is perhaps the most effective technique for measuring blood flow.[38,39] Using this technique, it is possible to measure peak flow, blood flow at any site across the lumen of the vessel, and mean blood flow in the vessel. This imaging technique provides a magnitude image on which the cross-sectional area of the vessel is measured and a phase image on which flow velocity is measured for any voxel in the lumen (Fig. 8-47).

The quantitative phase technique has been verified in three ways. First, a flow phantom in which blood flow velocity and volume are precisely controlled has been compared to velocity-encoded cine MRI. These measurements have been found to correlate precisely over a flow range from 10 to 600 cm/sec when using a TE value of 7 msec for imaging at 1.5 Te.[39] In vivo validation has been done by comparing the measurement of left ventricular stroke volume as defined by the quantitative phase tech-

nique with left ventricular stroke volume as measured by volume calculations from a stack of cine MR images.[39] Correlation between these measurements has been excellent, with a correlation coefficient of 0.95 and a standard error of the estimate of 4.8 mm/sec. The third method of verification has been comparison to echo Doppler measurements. Echo Doppler measurements have been found to provide almost the same value as the quantitative phase technique for the measurement of peak velocity in the pulmonary artery.[44] As expected, the values for peak velocity are nearly identical, but the values for the mean blood flow rate by velocity-encoded cine MRI and the Doppler measurement have not been the same.

The velocity-encoded cine MRI technique has been used to measure blood flow separately in the right and left pulmonary arteries.[45] The precision of this technique is indicated by the finding that the sum of the blood flow

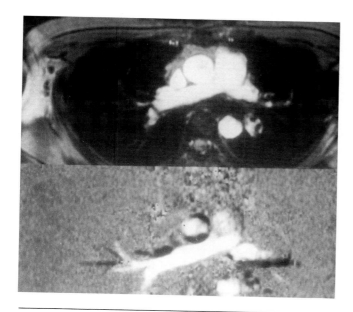

Figure 8-47. Cine MR magnitude (*above*) and phase (*below*) images at the level of the right pulmonary artery. The phase image displays blood vessels only; the intensity of the signal in each voxel is proportional to the blood flow velocity. Velocity can be measured at any site in the vascular lamina or can be calculated as the spatial average velocity for the entire cross-section of the vessel.

within the right and left pulmonary arteries correlated nearly precisely with the measurement of blood flow in the main pulmonary artery. The technique can also be used to demonstrate the blood flow pattern. An example of this is the comparison of blood flow patterns in healthy people with those from patients with pulmonary arterial hypertension.[44] It was recognized that the flow pattern in the normal pulmonary artery shows almost no retrograde flow during diastole or systole. In pulmonary arterial hypertension, the peak velocity of blood flow is achieved earlier during the systolic period and there is retrograde flow during portions of systole as well as diastole. Also of note is that the direction of blood flow in the pulmonary artery during systole is antegrade in some regions and retrograde in other regions in patients with pulmonary arterial hypertension.

There are numerous applications for blood flow measurements in cardiovascular diagnosis. These include the measurement of right and left ventricular stroke volume and the calculation of cardiac output. The technique can be used to compare right and left ventricular stroke volumes to quantitate the volumes of intracardiac shunts. It can also be used for the quantitation of aortic regurgitation, whereby the antegrade blood flow is measured during systole and retrograde blood flow is measured during diastole in the aorta (Figs. 8-48 and 8-49). Aortic regurgitation can be quantified as:

1. The difference in the integrated systolic flow values measured on the phase images for the aorta and pulmonary artery (difference in stroke volume between two ventricles).
2. The integrated retrograde flow values acquired during diastole for the aorta (direct measure of regurgitant flow volume).

Comparison of Cine MRI and Other Cardiac Imaging Techniques

Like standard MRI, cine MRI represents inherently a three-dimensional imaging technique, so that volume measurements necessary for determination of global ventricular function can be accomplished without the need for geometric assumption, as it is done for cine ventriculography or echocardiography. Furthermore, cine MRI combines good anatomic resolution with high temporal resolution for defining intracardiac function. These attributes are attained by only one other imaging technique, cine computed tomography (CT). The advantage of cine MRI compared with cine CT is that MRI requires no ionizing radiation or injection of contrast agents to depict the blood pool. Moreover, cine CT does not detect a unique signal indicative of the high-velocity jet caused by valvular stenosis, valvular regurgitation, or atrial and ventricular septal defects.

In comparison with the known attributes of echocardiography, Doppler and two-dimensional cardiography, cine MRI can also define intracardiac anatomy, global and regional ventricular contraction, and high-velocity flow associated with stenosis, regurgitation, and shunts. Both cine MRI and Doppler color flow mapping can provide a semiquantitative assessment of the severity of regurgitant lesions. Advantages compared with echocardiography are better edge definition of the ventricular walls, a wider field-of-view for defining cardiac anatomy and especially for showing vascular anatomy, and the independence of image quality from operator finesse and body habitus of patients. The advantages of echocardiography are universal availability, portability, and lower expense.

The greater temporal and spatial resolutions of cine MRI are decided advantages over radionuclide imaging for the evaluation of cardiovascular anatomy and function. Additionally, radionuclide studies cannot demonstrate the intracardiac flow patterns caused by shunt and regurgitant flow. MRI has not yet been shown to be effective for demonstrating regional myocardial perfusion necessary for the detection of myocardial ischemia, however, as is possible with thallium scintigraphy. Experimental results using new MRI contrast media and fast MRI techniques suggest that this will be possible in the future.

MRI has progressed to the extent that it is now possible to provide both anatomic and functional diagnoses in acquired heart disease. It has also become apparent

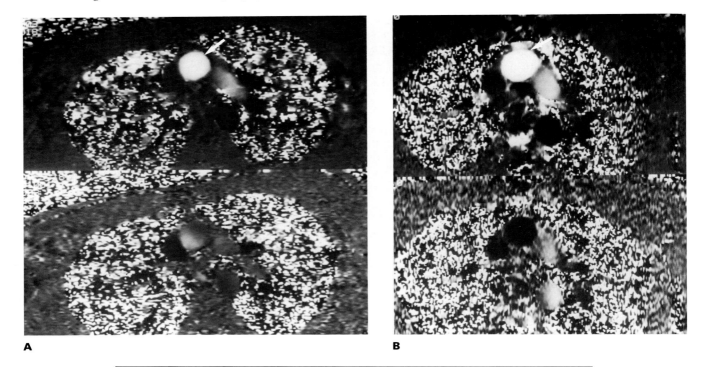

A   **B**

Figure 8-48. Phase images in aortic regurgitation and measurement of aortic regurgitation from the phase images. Phase images in systole (*top*) and diastole (*bottom*) in healthy subject (*A*) and patient with aortic regurgitation (*B*). In the healthy subject, the white intensity in the ascending aorta (*arrow*) in systole indicates forward flow. In diastole, the aorta shows an intensity similar to the relatively immobile tissues, such as the spine, indicating cessation of flow in diastole. In the patient with aortic regurgitation, the lumen of the aorta is white in systole, indicating forward flow, whereas it is black in diastole, indicating retrograde flow (aortic regurgitation).

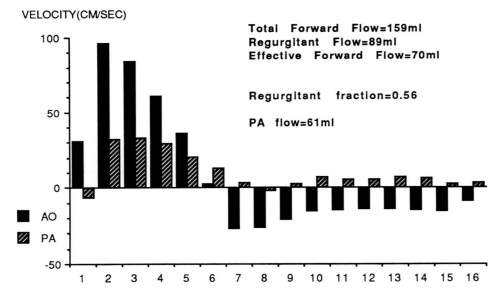

Figure 8-49. Diagram displays the flow velocity calculated from each of the 16 images acquired at evenly spaced intervals during the cardiac cycle. Values are shown in the aorta and pulmonary artery. Because of the increased stroke volume caused by aortic regurgitation, velocity is greater in the aorta compared with the pulmonary artery. Note the retrograde flow velocity in the aorta during diastole. Integration of the flow values during diastole provides a direct measurement of the volume of aortic regurgitation.

that this technique is the most precise one for the quantification of ventricular dimensions and function. The high reproducibility of measurements between studies indicates that MRI is useful for the assessment of response to therapeutic interventions in a variety of cardiac disease states.

Acknowledgment. Portions of the text in this chapter and many of the illustrations have been used with permission from *Magnetic Resonance Imaging of the Body,* 2nd edition, Higgins CB, Hricak H, eds., published by Raven Press, Ltd., New York, 1991.

References

1. Crooks LE, Barker B, Chang H, et al. Magnetic resonance imaging strategies for heart studies. Radiology 1984;153:459.

2. Fisher MR, von Schulthess GK, Higgins CB. Multiphasic cardiac magnetic resonance imaging: normal regional left ventricular wall thickening. AJR 1985;145:27.

3. Caputo GR, Suzuki J-I, Kondo C, et al. Determination of left ventricular volume and mass with use of biphasic spin-echo MR imaging: comparison with cine MR. Radiology 1990;177:773.

4. Sechtem U, Pflugfelder PW, White RD, et al. Cine MRI: potential for the evaluation of cardiovascular function. AJR 1987;148:239.

5. McNamara MT, Higgins CB, Schechtmann N, et al. Detection and characterization of acute myocardial infarctions in man with the use of gated magnetic resonance imaging. Circulation 1985; 71:717.

6. Wesbey G, Higgins CB, Lanzer P, Botvinick E, Lipton MJ. Imaging and characterization of acute myocardial infarction *in vivo* by gated nuclear magnetic resonance. Circulation 1984;69:125.

7. Renshaw PF, Owen CS, McLaughlin AC, Frey TG, Leigh JS. Ferromagnetic contrast agents: a new approach. Magn Reson Med 1986;3:217.

8. Dinsmore RE, Wismer GL, Levine RA, Okada RD, Brady T. MRI of the heart: positioning and gradient angle selection for optimal imaging planes. AJR 1984;143:1135.

9. Buser PT, Auffermann W, Holt WW, et al. Noninvasive evaluation of the global left ventricular function using cine MR imaging. J Am Coll Cardiol 1989;13:1294.

10. McNamara MT, Higgins CB. Magnetic resonance imaging of chronic myocardial infarcts in man. AJR 1986;146:315.

11. Pflugfelder PW, Sechtem UP, White RD, Higgins CB. Quantification of regional myocardial function by rapid (cine) magnetic resonance imaging. AJR 1988;150:523.

12. Brown JJ, Higgins CB. Myocardial contrast agents for magnetic resonance imaging. AJR 1988;151:865.

13. Johnson DC, Mulvagh SC, Cashion RW, O'Neil PG, Roberts R, Rokey R. NMR imaging of acute myocardial infarction within 24 hours of chest pain onset. Am J Cardiol 1989;64:172.

14. Tscholakoff D, Higgins CB, McNamara MT, Derugin N. Early phase myocardial infarction: evaluation by magnetic resonance imaging. Radiology 1986;159:667.

15. Caputo GR, Sechtem U, Tscholakoff D, Higgins CB. Measurement of myocardial infarct size at early and late time intervals using MR imaging: an experimental study in dogs. AJR 1987; 149:237.

16. Dooms GC, Higgins CB. MR imaging of cardiac thrombi. J Comput Assist Tomogr 1986;10:415.

17. Seelos K, Caputo GR, Carrol CL, Hricak H, Higgins CB. Sequential gradient echo imaging (cine MRI) of intravascular masses: differentiation between tumor and non-tumor thrombus (clot). Radiology 1991 (submitted).

18. Sechtem U, Sommerhoff BA, Markiewicz W, White RD, Cheitlin MD, Higgins CB. Assessment of regional left ventricular wall thickening by magnetic resonance imaging: evaluation of normal persons and patients with global and regional dysfunction. Am J Cardiol 1987;59:145.

19. Saeed M, Wagner S, Wendland MF, Derugin N, Finkbeiner WE, Higgins CB. Occlusive and reperfused myocardial infarcts: differentiation with Mn-DPDP-enhanced MR imaging. Radiology 1989;172:59.

20. Saeed M, Wendland MF, Tomei E, et al. Demarcation of myocardial ischemia: magnetic susceptibility effect of contrast medium in MR imaging. Radiology 1989;173:763.

21. de Roos A, van Rossum AC, van der Wall E, et al. Reperfused and nonreperfused myocardial infarctions: diagnostic potential of Gd-DTPA-enhanced MRI. Radiology 1989;172:717.

22. Nishimura T, Kobayashi H, Ohara Y, et al. Serial assessment of myocardial infarction by using gated MRI and Gd-DTPA. AJR 1990;153:715.

23. Higgins CB, Byrd BF III, Stark D, et al. Magnetic resonance imaging in hypertrophic cardiomyopathy. Am J Cardiol 1985;55:1121.

24. Sechtem U, Higgins CB, Sommerhoff BA, Lipton MJ, Huycke EC. Magnetic resonance imaging of restrictive cardiomyopathy. Am J Cardiol 1987;59:480.

25. Semelka RC, Tomei E, Wagner S, et al. Interstudy reproducibility of dimensional and functional measurements between cine magnetic resonance studies in the morphologically abnormal left ventricle. Am Heart J 1990;119:1367.

26. Suzuki J-I, Chang J-M, Caputo GR, Higgins CB. Evaluation of right ventricular early diastolic filling by cine nuclear magnetic resonance imaging in patients with hypertrophic cardiomyopathy. J Am Coll Cardiol 1991 (in press).

27. Riedy K, Fisher MS, Belic N, Koenigsberg DI. MR imaging of myocardial sarcoidosis. AJR 1988;151:915.

28. Wagner S, Auffermann W, Buser P, et al. Diagnostic accuracy and estimation of the severity of valvular regurgitation from the signal void in cine MR. Am Heart J 1989;118:760.

29. Barakos JA, Brown JJ, Higgins CB. Magnetic resonance imaging of secondary cardiac and paracardiac masses: pictorial essay. AJR 1989;153:47.

30. Sechtem U, Tscholakoff D, Higgins CB. MRI of the abnormal pericardium. AJR 1986;147:245.

31. Soulen RL, Stark DD, Higgins CB. Magnetic resonance imaging of constrictive pericardial heart disease. Am J Cardiol 1985; 55:480.

32. Sechtem U, Tscholakoff D, Higgins CB. MRI of the normal pericardium. AJR 1986;147:239.

33. Amparo EG, Higgins CB, Farmer K, Gamsu G, McNamara M. Gated magnetic resonance imaging (MRI) of cardiac and paracardiac masses. AJR 1984;143:1151.

34. Freedberg RS, Kronzon I, Rumanik WM, Liebeskind D. The contribution of MRI to the evaluation of intracardiac tumors diagnosed by echocardiography. Circulation 1988;77:94.

35. Pflugfelder PW, Landzberg JS, Cassidy MM, et al. Comparison of cine MR imaging with Doppler echocardiography for the evaluation of aortic regurgitation. AJR 1989;152:729.

36. Pflugfelder PW, Sechtem UP, White RD, Cassidy MM, Schiller NB, Higgins CB. Noninvasive evaluation of mitral regurgitation by analysis of left atrial signal loss in cine magnetic resonance. Am Heart J 1989;117:1113.

37. Sechtem U, Pflugfelder PW, Cassidy MM, et al. Mitral or aortic regurgitation: quantification of regurgitant volumes with cine MR imaging. Radiology 1988;167:425.

38. Nayler GL, Firmin DN, Longmore DB. Blood flow imaging by

cine magnetic resonance. J Comput Assist Tomogr 1986;10:715.

39. Kondo C, Caputo GR, Semelka R, Foster E, Shimakawa S, Higgins CB. Right and left ventricular stroke volume measurements with velocity encoded cine NMR imaging: in vitro and in vivo validation. AJR 1991 (in press).

40. Sahn DJ. Instrumentation and physical factors related to visualization of stenotic and regurgitant jets by Doppler color flow mapping. J Am Coll Cardiol 1988;12:1354.

41. Mohiaddin RH, Kilner MB, Amanuma M, Pennel DJ, Longmore DB. MR flow imaging of healthy and diseased mitral valves. Radiology 1990;177(P):100.

42. Semelka RC, Tomei E, Wagner S, et al. Normal left ventricular dimensions and function: interstudy reproducibility of measurements with cine MR imaging. Radiology 1990;174:763.

43. Edelman RR, Shaw B, Lim C, et al. MR angiography and dynamic flow evaluation of the portal venous system. AJR 1989;153:755.

44. Kondo C, Caputo GR, Masui T, et al. Pulmonary flow quantification and flow profile analysis in patients with pulmonary hypertension by using MRI phase velocity mapping. Radiology 1991 (in press).

45. Caputo GR, Kondo C, Masui T, et al. Determination of right and left lung perfusion with oblique angle velocity encoded cine MR imaging: in vitro and in vivo validation. Radiology 1991 (in press).

Chapter 9

MRI of Congenital Heart Disease

Charles B. Higgins

This chapter describes the MRI appearance of the cardiovascular anatomy in a segmental fashion, which is the most effective approach for the analysis of complex CHD. The depiction of congenital cardiovascular lesions is organized into abnormalities situated at four segmental cardiovascular levels: great arteries, atria, ventricles, and visceroatrial sites. The reader is referred to Chapter 2 for a review of the salient anatomic features of specific congenital anomalies.

Major attention will be directed toward lesions which are most frequently evaluated by MRI at the current time. These include evaluation of the presence and size of central pulmonary arteries in pulmonary atresia, definition of great vessel anatomy and intracardiac anatomy in complex anomalies, identification of visceroatrial situs and splenic syndromes, definition of thoracic aortic anomalies, and depiction of the anatomy of the extracardiac as well as the intracardiac component of the altered anatomy after various corrective surgical procedures.

MRI Techniques for CHD

MRI for CHD utilizes primarily the electrocardiogram (ECG) gated spin-echo multislice technique. Respiratory compensation sequences are used to remove data acquired during the instant of maximum respiratory extension and thereby reduce the respiratory motion artifacts. Equipment limitations prevent the use of the respiratory compensation technique in small children. Respiratory gating is not necessary and is generally unrealistic. For the evaluation of CHD, diagnostic-quality studies can be expected in over 90% of patients.[1] The cause of nondiagnostic studies is usually patient motion; consequently, MRI cannot be accomplished in uncooperative children. Image quality is also degraded by exaggerated respiratory motion such as that caused by tachypnea and excessive chest wall motion occurring in patients with diaphragmatic paralysis.

Children older than 6 or 7 years usually can be studied without sedation. Cooperation can be greatly facilitated by careful explanation of the procedure to the child and parent(s). For younger children, sedation is necessary. Because of the length of time during which motion must be suspended, effective sedation requires larger doses than usually used for computed tomography and echocardiography. The most effective sedation has been achieved with chloral hydrate, 75 to 100 mg/kg, administered orally approximately 45 minutes before entry into the magnet, or pentobarbital 1.5 mg/kg given intravenously. To minimize disturbance of the sleeping child, the ECG leads are attached before sedation. The ECG signal is monitored and respiration is observed during the imaging procedure. A finger tip oximeter is used to monitor oxygen saturation during the imaging procedure. A capnograph is sometimes employed to monitor expired CO_2 and respiratory rate.

Multislice transverse images are obtained from the top of the aorta to the diaphragm (Fig. 9-1). The time required to obtain a 10-slice, single-echo sequence varies from 6 to 10 minutes. Such images may also be obtained in the true short axis of the heart using electronic angulation of the slice-selective gradient. Precise determination of the short axis for each patient necessitates preliminary coronal or transverse images from which the cardiac long axis is defined. From the long-axis image, the short-axis plane is determined. The transverse or short-axis images are supplemented by coronal, sagittal, or oblique images depending on the pathoanatomy to be evaluated. A useful view for visualization of coarctation of the aorta is the left anterior oblique equivalent (LAO-equivalent) view, achieved by elevating the right side of

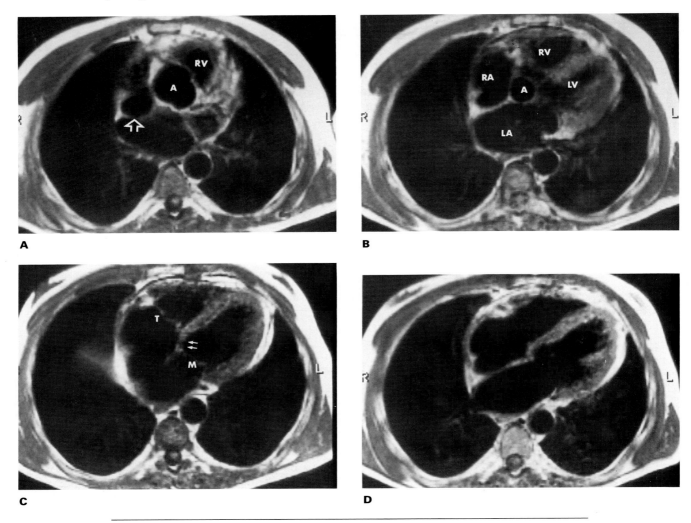

Figure 9-1. Transverse spin-echo images (*A* to *D*) extending from the base of the heart (*A*) to the middle of the ventricles (*D*). The portion of the atrial septum separating the superior vena cava from the left atrium is the sinus venosus portion of the atrial septum (*open arrow* in *A*). The portion of the atrial septum at the level of the atrioventricular valves (*C*) is considered the primum portion of the septum. The remainder of the atrial septum is essentially the secundum portion. The outlet portion of the ventricular septum separates the aorta from the right ventricle. The inlet portion of the ventricular septum is that portion located at the level of the tricuspid and mitral valves. The atrioventricular septum separates the left ventricle from the right atrium (*small arrows* in *C*). On panel C, the thin fossa ovalis region produces very little signal, causing an apparent defect in the atrial septum. (A, base of aorta; LA, left atrium; LV, left ventricle; M, mitral valve; RA, right atrium; RV, right ventricle; T, tricuspid valve.)

the supine patient by 20° to 30° and imaging in the sagittal plane or by oblique angulation of the slice-selective gradient in an orientation parallel to the aortic arch.

For the evaluation of morphology, ECG gated spin-echo images are optimal. Since the prime purpose of imaging in congenital heart disease is the precise depiction of the abnormal anatomy, the multislice spin-echo technique is the mainstay of the study. The cine magnetic resonance (MR) technique, consisting of gradient echo images at multiple phases of the cardiac cycle, can demonstrate abnormal flow in the cardiac chambers and great vessels.[2,3] This technique can be used to detect abnormal flow across septal defects (Fig. 9-2) and stenotic valves (Fig. 9-3) or ventricular outlet regions. Abnormal flow is also shown with valvular regurgitation. The high velocity flow associated with these lesions causes a signal void in the normally high signal intensity of the blood pool on cine MR images. A cine MR sequence is frequently done after the spin-echo sequences have been completed. The cine MR sequence is done at anatomic levels where ab-

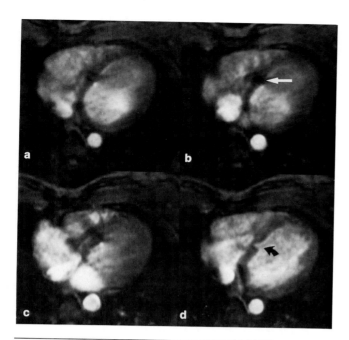

Figure 9-2. Cine MR images through the middle of the ventricles demonstrate a muscular ventricular septal defect. Images were acquired in systole (*A, B*) and diastole (*D*). During systole a flow void (*white arrow*) is demonstrated at the site of the VSD due to high-velocity blood flow across the defect. The defect is filled with high signal intensity blood during diastole (*curved black arrow*). On cine MR images the blood pool has a bright signal intensity. Turbulent high-velocity blood flow causes a signal void, as is evident at the site of the VSD.

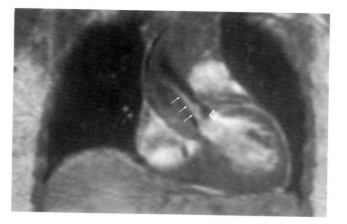

Figure 9-3. Cine MR image in the coronal plane in patient with aortic stenosis. There is a high signal intensity jet across the aortic valve (*small arrows*). At the margin of the jet there is a signal void caused by eddies of turbulent blood flow. Because of the turbulent blood flow there is generalized reduction of signal intensity within the ascending aorta. The blood pool within the left ventricle has a bright signal intensity. The level of the aortic valve is marked by the open arrow.

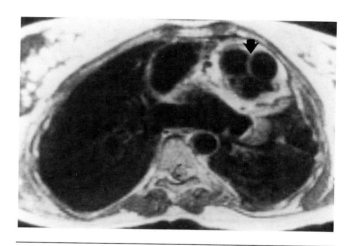

Figure 9-4. Transverse ECG gated image at the level of the aortic valve in a patient with *l*-transposition of the great arteries and pulmonary atresia. Note the tricuspid nature of the enlarged aortic valve (*arrow*). (Reproduced with permission from Sechtem U, Pflugfelder P, Cassidy MC, Holt W, Wolfe C, Higgins CB. Ventricular septal defect: visualization of shunt flow and determination of shunt size by cine magnetic resonance imaging. AJR 1987;149:689.)

normal flow patterns are suspected. A cine MR sequence is also done at levels in the middle of the ventricles for the qualitative assessment of ventricular function, or is performed at all tomographic levels encompassing the heart to precisely measure ventricular volumes and ejection fraction.

The slice thickness employed for the evaluation of congenital heart disease is usually 5 mm; however, 3 mm sections are employed for the study of small infants and for the assessment of small structures such as the central pulmonary arterial segments in patients with pulmonary atresia. Thin slices are also acquired in the sagittal plane, with the slice placed on the center of the descending aorta in patients with coarctation of the aorta. Thin slices and precise centering of the image volumes is necessary to minimize partial volume errors when measuring the luminal diameter of the coarctation.

Segmental Anatomy

Transverse sections extending from the base of the heart to the cranial portion of the liver depict segmental cardiovascular anatomy. The normal relationships and nearly equivalent sizes of the great vessels are depicted

on images at the base of the heart; the aorta is observed to the right and posterior to the pulmonary artery or the right ventricular outflow tract. This anatomic relationship is clearly depicted in healthy subjects (see Fig. 9-1). The aortic and pulmonary valves are sometimes seen and the tricuspid nature of the valve may be recognized (Fig. 9-4). In normal situs, the right pulmonary artery is ventral to the right bronchus and the left pulmonary artery passes over (cranial) the left bronchus at the level of the pulmonary arterial bifurcation (Fig. 9-5). Reversal of this relationship is seen with situs inversus. Bilateral right pulmonary arterial morphology indicates right-sided iso-merism and bilateral left pulmonary arterial morphology indicates left-sided isomerism.

Both the lower lobe and the right upper lobe pulmonary veins are readily recognized in all patients (Figs. 9-1 and 9-6). On transverse images the left upper lobe pulmonary vein is seen ventral to the bifurcation of the left bronchus and must be distinguished from the nearby left atrial appendage (see Fig. 9-6). The proximal portion of the vein can usually be followed to the vicinity of the roof of the left atrium, and even if not seen, a normal position of the proximal portion of the vein can be construed as normal connection. Recognition of normal connections is possible in nearly all patients with abnormal pulmonary venous connections.

Images through the middle of the right and left ventricles usually define the ventricular loop. The anatomic right ventricle is recognized by a location anteriorly and to the right, a triangular configuration, and a coarse trabecular pattern of the apical septum with the moderator band at its apex and the right atrioventricular (AV) valve located closer to the cardiac apex compared with the left

ventricle (Fig. 9-7). Transverse images also clearly disclose the presence of an infundibulum separating the semilunar and AV valves; in the presence of complex ventricular anomalies, this may be the only reliable discerning characteristic permitting ventricular assignment. The morphologic left ventricle is characterized by a location posteriorly and to the left, an elliptical configuration, and a smooth trabecular pattern of the apical septum, and the left AV valve is situated farther from the cardiac apex. There is direct continuity between the atrioventricular and semilunar valves (see Fig. 9-7).

On MRI the distinctive anatomic characteristics of the right and left atria are the shapes of the appendages.[4] The morphologic systemic venous atrium (right-sided in situs solitus) has an appendage with a wide ostium and triangular configuration whereas the pulmonary venous atrium (left-sided in situs solitus) has an appendage with a narrower ostium and a tubular configuration (Fig. 9-8).

The different portions of the atrial and ventricular septa are clearly identified on transverse MR images (Fig. 9-9). In 31 of 32 patients without defects in the atrial or ventricular septum and imaged through the full extent of

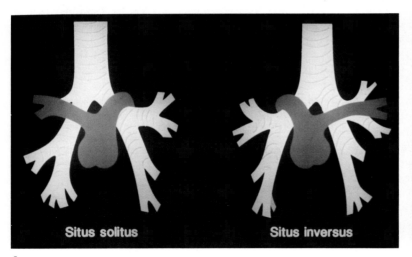

A

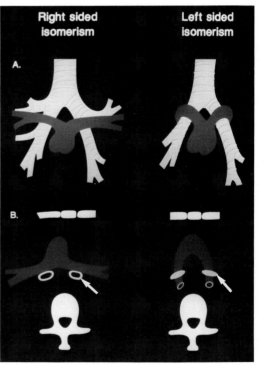

B

Figure 9-5. Diagrams depict the relationship of the pulmonary arteries to the bronchi in situs solitus, situs inversus, right-sided isomerism, and left-sided isomerism. For right-sided and left-sided isomerism the diagram demonstrates the relationship in the coronal plane (*A*) and transaxial plane (*B*). Note that in right-sided isomerism both pulmonary arteries are located ventral to the bronchi (*arrows*). Conversely, in left-sided isomerism both pulmonary arteries are cranial to (pass over) the bronchi (*arrow*).

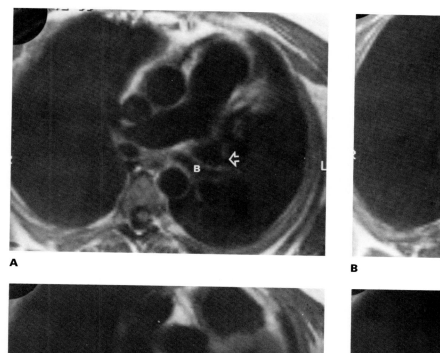

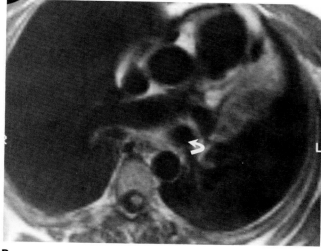

A

B

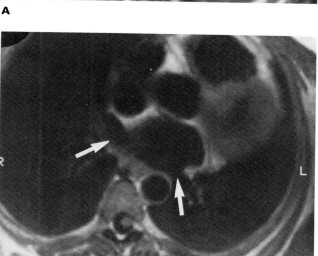

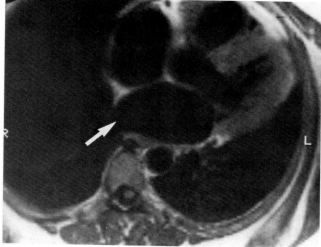

C

D

Detection of the Connections of the Normal Pulmonary Veins by MR Imaging

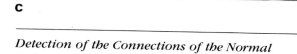

Pulmonary Vein	*No. (%)*
Right upper	54 (96)
Right lower	55 (98)
Left upper	52 (93)
Left lower	56 (100)
Four	49 (88)
At least three	56 (100)

n = 56

E

Figure 9-6. Transaxial images (*A* to *D*) extend from cranial (*A*) to caudal (*D*) show the normal pulmonary venous anatomy. Note that the left upper lobe pulmonary vein (*open arrow*) is located directly ventral to the left bronchus (B). Although the point of connection of the left upper lobe pulmonary vein to the top of the left atrium may not always be visualized, its location directly ventral to the left bronchus indicates a normal connection. Curved arrow shows site of connection of left upper pulmonary vein to the left atrium. The sites of connection of the other pulmonary veins to the left atrium are indicated (*closed arrow*). The chart indicates the frequency in which the connection of the pulmonary veins to the left atrium could be visualized on transverse images in a series of 50 subjects with congenital heart disease.

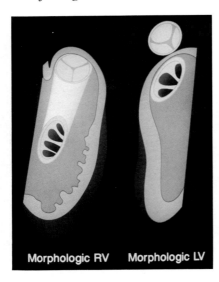

Figure 9-7. Diagram demonstrating the characteristics of the morphologic right ventricle and morphologic left ventricle. The morphologic right ventricle is characterized by muscle separating the atrioventricular valve from the semilunar valve and a roughly trabeculated contour to the right ventricular aspect of the apical portion of the ventricular septum. The morphologic left ventricle is characterized by direct continuity between the atrioventricular valve and the semilunar valve and a smooth contour to the left ventricular aspect of the apical portion of the ventricular septum.

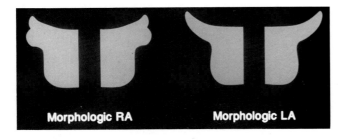

Figure 9-8. Morphologic characteristics of the right and left atrium. The characteristic morphologic appearance of the atria can be recognized whether the right atrium is located on the right or left side of the body, and the same holds for the left atrium. The characteristic features of the right atrium are a rectangularly or triangularly-shaped right atrial appendage with a wide ostium connecting the appendage to the atrial body. The morphologic left atrium is characterized by a more cylindrical appearance and a narrow ostium connecting it to the left atrial body.

the heart, the atrial and ventricular septa were identified as intact.[5] The various portions of the atrial septum (sinus venosus, secundum, and primum regions) are discernible on the transverse and short-axis images (see Figs. 9-1 and 9-6). A thin fossa ovalis may result in signal dropout at this site and thereby simulate an atrial septal defect (Fig. 9-10). Similarly, the several distinct regions of the ventricular septum can be assigned on the basis of im-

ages in the transverse and sagittal planes (see Fig. 9-9). It is even possible to visualize the short AV septum separating the right atrium and left ventricle (see Fig. 9-9).

The identification of a right-sided inferior vena cava and coronary sinus entering the right atrium as well as the right-sided liver allows determination of a viscero-atrial situs solitus. Transverse images in the upper abdomen also identify the spleen.

Sagittal sections demonstrate the right ventricular outflow tract and the main pulmonary artery. The connection of the vena cava with the right atrium can also be displayed on a single section in this plane. The tomographic sections similar to the angiographic LAO view depict the ascending aorta, arch, and proximal descending aorta on a single image (Fig. 9-11).

The reliability of gated MRI for defining normal segmental cardiovascular anatomy was reported in 74 patients suspected of having CHD.[6,7] Determination of the relationships among great vessels, visceroatrial situs, and type of ventricular loop was possible in all patients in whom images encompassed a sufficient portion of the heart. In all instances the MRI findings correlated with corroborative studies.

Congenital Cardiovascular Lesions

Situs Determination and Isomerism

Isomerism is nearly always associated with complex CHD. Left-sided isomerism is usually seen with polysplenia and right-sided isomerism with asplenia. The most reliable sign of isomerism is demonstration of symmetry of the bronchi and pulmonary arteries. This has been clearly depicted by MRI, which shows bilateral epiarterial bronchi in right-sided isomerism (Fig. 9-12) and bilateral hyparterial bronchi in left-sided isomerism (Fig. 9-13).

Situs solitus is characterized by a morphologic right (systemic venous) atrium positioned to the right of the spine and morphologic left (pulmonary venous) atrium to the left of the spine. The normal ventricular relationship is a D-ventricular loop, with the anatomic right ventricle located to the right of the left ventricle. Situs inversus has the anatomic right atrium (systemic venous) on the left and the anatomic left (pulmonary venous) atrium on the right. There is an L-ventricular loop with the anatomic right ventricle located to the left of the left ventricle.

The distinguishing features of the ventricles and atria from which they can be identified as morphologically "right" and "left" were described earlier. In mirror-image dextrocardia as well as in nonmirror-image dextrocardia, these features must be used to identify the

(*Text continues on page 291*)

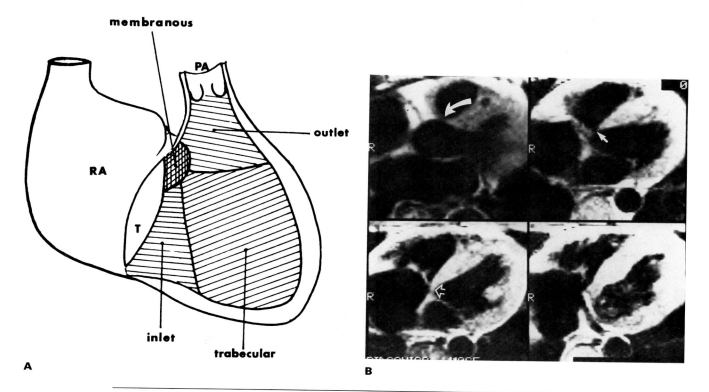

Figure 9-9. Diagram (*A*) demonstrates the various portions of the ventricular septum. Multislice transverse images (*B*) demonstrate the various portions of the ventricular septum. The images extend from cranial (*upper left*) to caudal (*lower right*). Note that the outlet septum (*curved arrow*) separates the right ventricular outflow region from the base of the aorta. The membranous or perimembranous portion of the ventricular septum is the thin portion located between the inlet and outlet portions of the ventricular septum (*solid arrow*). The inlet portion of the ventricular septum is located between the tricuspid and mitral valves (*open arrow*). The muscular or trabecular portion of the ventricular septum constitutes the major component of the ventricular septum. Parts of the trabecular septum are observed on each of the four transverse slices. (Reproduced with permission from Didier D, Higgins CB. Identification and localization of ventricular septal defects by gated magnetic resonance imaging. Am J Cardiol 1986;57:1363.)

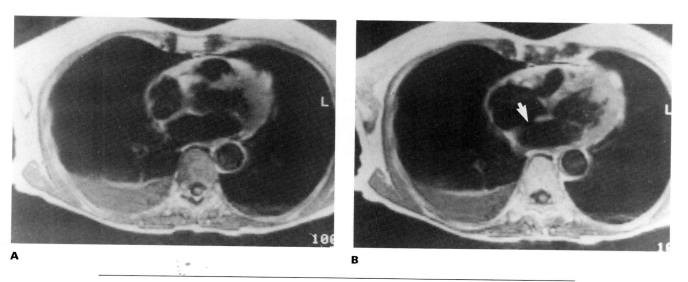

Figure 9-10. Transverse images through the atria. The image on the left is located 1 cm cranial to the one on the right. Note that the atrial septum appears to be intact on the more cranial image and shows a small defect in the more caudal image. This small defect (*arrow*), observed on only a single transverse slice, suggests the possibility of a thin fossa ovalis or patent foramen ovale rather than a true ASD.

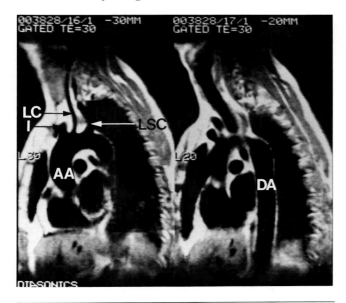

Figure 9-11. Oblique sagittal view demonstrating the ascending aorta, aortic arch, and proximal descending aorta on a single tomographic image. The image on the left is located 1 cm to the left of the image on the right. (AA, ascending aorta; DA, descending aorta; I, innominate artery; LC, left carotid artery; LSC, left subclavian artery.) (Reproduced with permission from Higgins CB, Silverman NH, Kerstig-Sommerhoff BA, Schmidt KG. Congenital heart disease: echocardiography and magnetic resonance imaging. New York, Raven Press, 1990.)

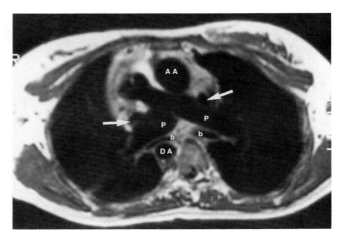

Figure 9-12. Transverse MR image in a patient with right-sided isomerism. The pulmonary artery is located to the right of the aorta. Both pulmonary arteries are located ventral to the bronchi. Note the bilateral superior vena cavae (*arrows*). (AA, ascending aorta; b, bronchi; DA, descending aorta; P, pulmonary arteries.)

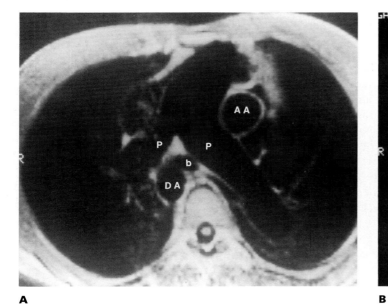

A

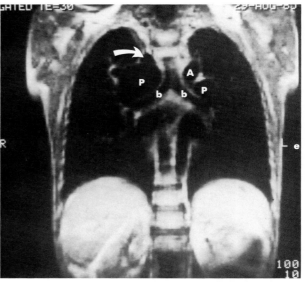

B

Figure 9-13. Left-sided isomerism. Transverse (*A*) and coronal (*B*) images in two patients with left-sided isomerism. The transverse image demonstrates that both pulmonary arteries pass cranial to the bronchi. The coronal image demonstrates that both the large right pulmonary artery and the smaller left pulmonary artery are located cranial to the bronchi. There is an enlarged azygous vein (*curved arrow*) because the inferior vena cava is interrupted. (A, aortic arch; AA, ascending aorta; b, bronchus; DA, descending aorta; P, pulmonary artery.)

various chambers correctly. In atrial isomerism, which is frequently but not always associated with isomerism of the bronchi, the two atria are not distinguishable.

Abnormalities of Arterioventricular Connections

Arterioventricular (ventriculoarterial) connection abnormalities are a diverse group in which the great arteries are not connected to their appropriate ventricle (transposition), or both great arteries are predominantly connected to one ventricle (double-outlet left and double-outlet right ventricle), or only a single large trunk connects to the ventricle (truncus arteriosus) (Fig. 9-14). Spatial relationship of the great arteries to each other at the base of the heart and the connections to the ventricles are clearly depicted on transverse images through the base of the heart. The arterial relationships are also depicted on sagittal and coronal images.

Arterioventricular connections can be concordant or discordant. Concordant connections are aorta with left ventricle and pulmonary artery with right ventricle. Discordant connections are pulmonary artery with left ventricle and aorta with right ventricle (complete transposition). Corrected transposition has discordant arterioventricular relationships and discordant atrioventricular relationships (see Fig. 9-14).

Transposition of Great Arteries

Several reports have indicated the effectiveness of MRI for defining the pathoanatomy of transposition and other positional anomalies of the great vessels.[1,6,7,8] Transverse images at the base of the heart demonstrate the aorta anterior to the pulmonary artery; it is to the right of the pulmonary artery in *d*-transposition (see Fig. 9-14) and to the left of the pulmonary artery in *l*-transposition (Figs. 9-14 and 9-15). When examining transverse images in great-vessel anomalies, one must distinguish the aorta and pulmonary artery; the pulmonary artery is identified by examining transverse images extending to the level of the pulmonary arterial bifurcation. The aorta can be recognized by identifying the arch and following the ascending aorta caudally to the base of the heart. Transverse or sagittal scans at the base of the heart reveal the origin of the aorta from the right ventricle and the pulmonary artery from the left ventricle in transposition (Fig. 9-16). In complete transposition, sequential transverse images show the right-sided aorta arising from a normally positioned right ventricle (to the right in relation to the left ventricle, D-bulboventricular loop) (see Fig. 9-14). In corrected transposition, the aorta is to the left and arises from the right ventricle, inverted to a position to the left

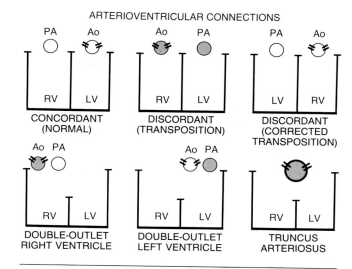

Figure 9-14. Diagram showing the various types of arterioventricular connections. Concordant connection is the aorta connected to the left ventricle and pulmonary artery to the right ventricle. (Ao, aorta; LV, left ventricle; PA, pulmonary artery; RV, right ventricle.)

of the morphologic left ventricle (L-bulboventricular loop) (Figs. 9-14, 9-15, and 9-17).[9]

The anomalies associated with transposition are also depicted by MRI. Transverse images can define the presence and severity of atrial and ventricular septal defects and valvular and subvalvular pulmonic stenosis. In transposition with severe pulmonary stenosis or pulmonary atresia, MRI is indicated to determine and measure the size of the central pulmonary arteries (Fig. 9-18). MRI can also precisely define the size of the interatrial communication after either balloon or blade septostomy or after partial surgical excision of the atrial septum. MRI reveals reversal in shape and muscle thickness of the right ventricle in relation to the left ventricle, which is characteristic for transposition of the great arteries (TGA). When the mural thickness of the left ventricle is equal to that of the right ventricle, this should suggest severe pulmonary arterial hypertension or pulmonary outflow obstruction in patients with complete transposition.

Double-Outlet Right Ventricle (DORV)

The side-by-side relationship of the great vessels at the semilunar valve level characterizes this anomaly on transverse MR images (see Fig. 9-14). Sequential transverse images reveal the origins of both vessels from the anteriorly located right ventricular outflow tract (Fig. 9-19). The site of a ventricular septal defect in relation to the semilunar valves can be defined by transverse MRI (Fig. 9-19). Coronal images confirm the side-by-side relation-

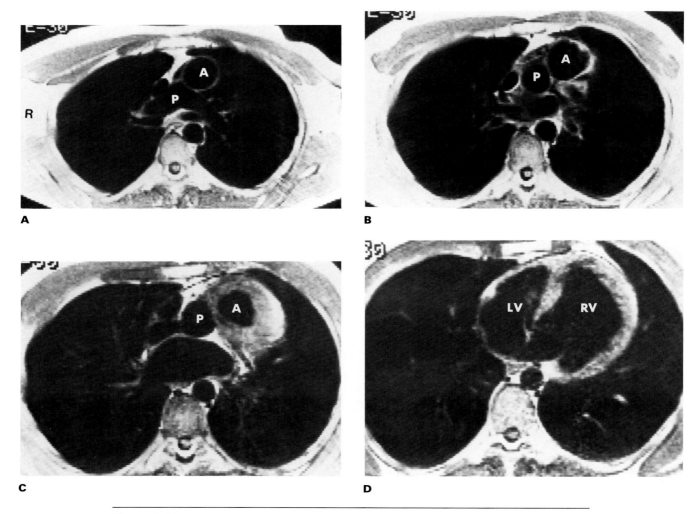

Figure 9-15. Transverse images (*A* to *D*) in a patient with *l*-transposition of the great arteries. Note that the aorta is located anterior and to the left of the pulmonary artery. The pulmonary artery is recognized by its bifurcation. The right ventricle is located to the left side of the left ventricle, indicating inversion of the ventricles. Inversion of the ventricles and *l*-transposition of the great arteries are indicative of corrected transposition. (A, aorta; LV, left ventricle; P, pulmonary artery; RV, right ventricle.) (Reproduced with permission from Higgins CB, Silverman NH, Kerstig-Sommerhoff BA, Schmidt KG. Congenital heart disease: echocardiography and magnetic resonance imaging. New York, Raven Press, 1990.)

ship of the semilunar valves, the origins of both great vessels from the right ventricle, and isolation of the left ventricle from the site of the semilunar valves (Fig. 9-20). The anatomic features of double-outlet right ventricle (DORV) on MR images have been reported.[10]

The position of the great arteries is not always side by side at the base of the heart. In some cases the aorta is anterior to the pulmonary artery and located either to the left anterior or right anterior aspect of the pulmonary artery.

A critical finding on transverse images is that neither semilunar valve is in direct fibrous continuity with the mitral valve. A complete rim of muscle intervening between both semilunar valves and the anterior leaflet of

the mitral valve is a diagnostic feature (see Fig. 9-19). Side-by-side circles of myocardium in the outflow region of the right ventricle may be observed on transverse MR images acquired at the base of the heart (see Figs. 9-19 and 9-20).

The relationship of the ventricular septal defect (VSD) to either or both of the great arteries can usually be defined by transverse images. The defect may lie immediately beneath the aortic valve (subaortic VSD), pulmonic valve (subpulmonic VSD), both semilunar valves (doubly committed VSD), or displaced from both semilunar valves (noncommitted VSD).

Subvalvular or valvular stenosis of the pulmonary artery occurs in some patients with DORV, especially in

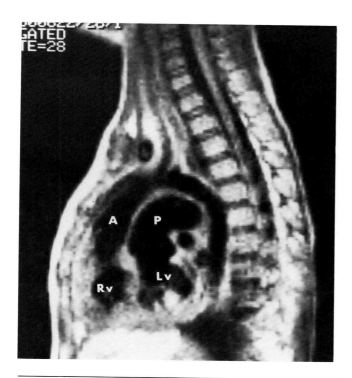

Figure 9-16. Sagittal image in a patient with transposition of the great arteries. Note that the aorta arises from the anterior ventricle and can be followed into the aortic arch. The pulmonary artery arises from the posterior ventricle, which is the left ventricle. (A, aorta; Lv, left ventricle; P, pulmonary artery; Rv, right ventricle.)

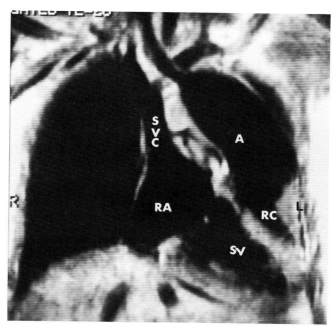

Figure 9-17. Coronal image in a patient with *l*-transposition of the great arteries. The aorta arises from an inverted right ventricular outlet chamber, which is connected to the single ventricle. (A, aorta; RA, right atrium; RC, right ventricular outlet chamber; SV, single ventricle; SVC, superior vena cava.) (Reproduced with permission from Higgins CB, Byrd BF III, Farmer D, Silverman N, Cheitlin M. Magnetic resonance imaging in patients with congenital heart disease. Circulation 1984;70:851.)

those with a subaortic VSD. The angiographic and clinical features of this type of DORV may be difficult to distinguish from tetralogy of Fallot. Transverse MR tomograms readily establish the diagnosis of this type of DORV by showing a complete circle of muscle separating the aortic from the mitral valve. The advantage of MRI is that it provides direct visualization of the myocardium rather than inferring its presence by the distance separating the aortic and mitral valves, as shown on left ventriculography.

Truncus Arteriosus

Transverse and sagittal images at the base of the heart can demonstrate a large truncus arising above the VSD and aligned over both the right and left ventricles (Fig. 9-21). In type I truncus, the origin of a main pulmonary artery from the truncus can be defind (see Fig. 9-21). Transverse scans can reveal the relative sizes of the two ventricles. A large single vessel arising from the base of the heart can also be observed on sagittal images in pulmonary atresia. Differentiation between truncus and pulmonary atresia is done by showing a small infundibular chamber on transverse images in the latter anomaly. Sagittal images are useful for depicting the truncus and demonstrating the

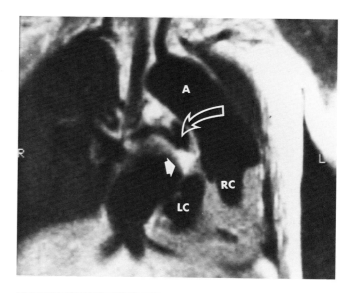

Figure 9-18. Transposition of the great arteries with pulmonary atresia and single ventricle. Note that the aorta is located to the left of the pulmonary artery, indicating *l*-transposition of the great arteries. The confluence of the right and left pulmonary arteries is indicated (*open arrow*). Note the fat separating the pulmonary artery from the ventricular chamber (*closed arrow*). (A, aorta; LC, left ventricular chamber; RC, right ventricular outlet chamber.)

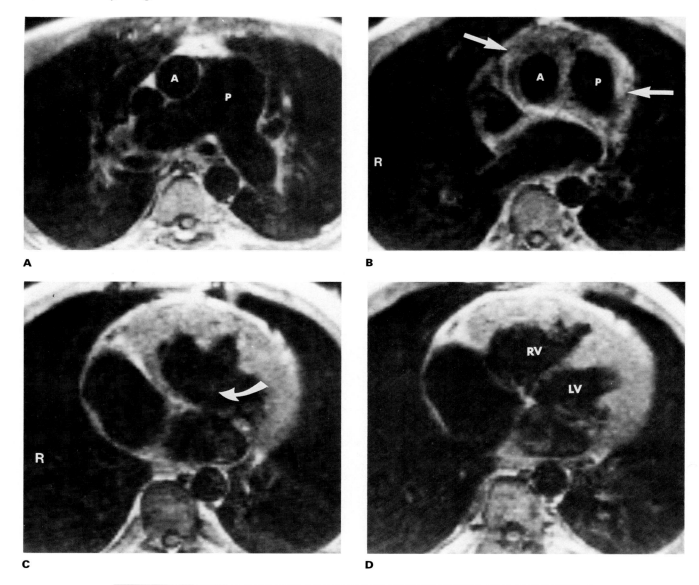

Figure 9-19. Series of transverse images (*A* to *D*) in a patient with double outlet right ventricle. Images extend from cranial (*A*) to caudal (*D*). The most cranial image demonstrates that the pulmonary artery and the aorta lie side by side. This finding suggests the presence of double outlet right ventricle. The next level demonstrates that there is infundibular tissue (*arrows*) beneath both the aorta (A) and pulmonary artery (P). Note that there is muscular tissue separating both atrioventricular valves from the pulmonary artery and the aorta. This finding is indicative of double outlet right ventricle. Note also that the VSD is large and is located beneath both the aorta and the pulmonary artery. (A, aorta; curved arrow, ventricular septal defect; LV, left ventricle; P, pulmonary artery; RV, right ventricle.)

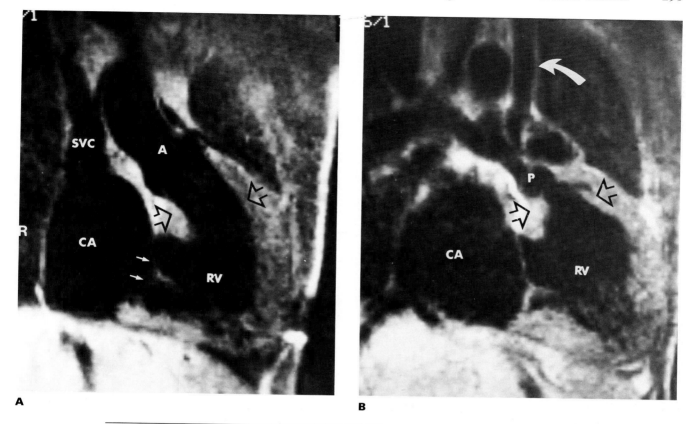

Figure 9-20. Coronal images (*A, B*) in a patient with single ventricle of the right ventricular type. Both great arteries arise from the right ventricle. The coronal image demonstrates infundibular or muscular tissue beneath the aorta (*open arrows*) and beneath the pulmonary artery (*open arrows*). The presence of muscular tissue beneath both the aorta and the pulmonary artery is consistent with the diagnosis of a double-outlet right ventricle. There are bilateral superior vena cavae; the curved arrow indicates the left superior vena cava. (A, aorta; CA, common atrium; P, pulmonary artery; RV, right ventricle; SVC, superior vena cava.)

origin of the pulmonary arteries from the truncus. MR images, usually thin (3 mm) tomograms, are used to assess the size of the right and left pulmonary arteries. MRI in transverse and sagittal planes is also used to evaluate the caliber of anastomoses after placement of a Rastelli conduit for the repair of truncus (Fig. 9-22). Demonstration of focal stenosis of the distal anastomosis or of the central pulmonary artery requires thin transverse tomograms.

Tetralogy of Fallot

Sagittal and transverse tomograms are used to assess tetralogy.[1,11] Sagittal images demonstrate the narrowing of the right ventricular outflow region (see Fig. 9-23). Transverse tomograms depict the VSD and the infundibular, annular, and pulmonary arterial stenosis (Figs. 9-23 and 9-24).

Transverse MR images can reveal disparity in the sizes of the aorta and pulmonary artery in tetralogy (see Figs. 9-23 and 9-24); there tends to be a reciprocal relationship in the sizes of the great vessels in this anomaly. Sequential transverse images can be used to determine stenosis of the main pulmonary artery and pulmonary annulus and obstruction of the infundibulum (Figs. 9-24 and 9-25). This can also be depicted on sagittal images. On MR images, tetralogy of Fallot is characterized by an enlarged anteriorly displaced aorta, small pulmonic annulus, multilevel narrowing of the infundibulum, and perimembranous VSD.

Important information provided by MRI concerns the sizes of the main and central pulmonary vessels in patients with severe stenosis or pulmonary atresia (Figs. 9-25 to 9-29). Depiction of the size of the right and left pulmonary arteries requires very thin tomograms (2 to 3 mm slice thickness). Usually an initial series of 5-mm thick tomograms is obtained through the entire heart and

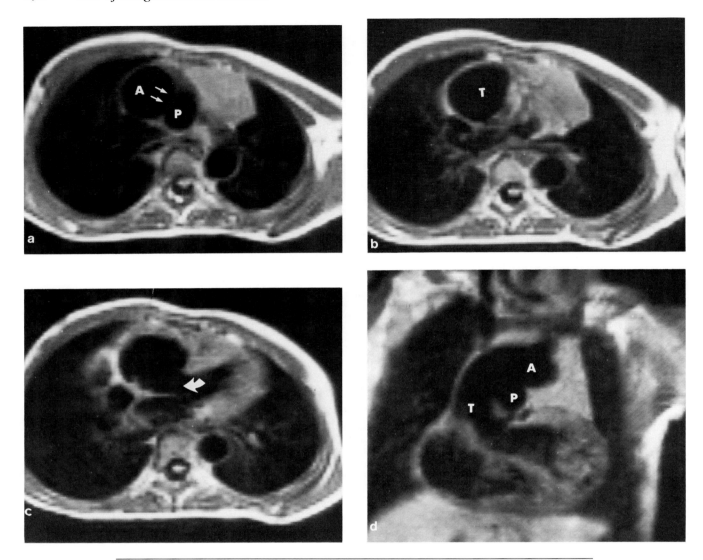

Figure 9-21. Series of transverse images (*A* to *D*) extending from cranial (*A*) to caudal (*D*) in a patient with truncus arteriosus, type 1. The most cranial image demonstrates the septum dividing the aortic (A) and pulmonary (P) arterial components of the truncus arteriosus. At the next cranial level the truncus arteriosus (T) is indicated. Note the large VSD located beneath the truncus arteriosus (*curved arrow*). Coronal image demonstrates the pulmonary artery arising from the truncus arteriosus and the truncus continuing into the aortic arch (A). (Reproduced with permission from Higgins CB, Silverman NH, Kerstig-Sommerhoff BA, Schmidt KG. Congenital heart disease: echocardiography and magnetic resonance imaging. New York, Raven Press, 1990.)

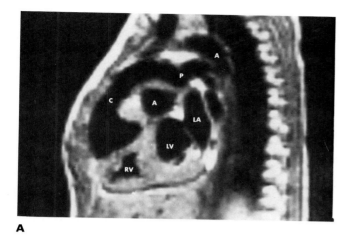

A

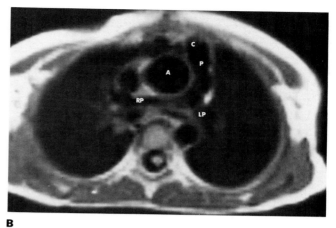

B

Figure 9-22. Coronal (*A*) and transaxial (*B*) images in a patient with truncus arteriosus repaired with a conduit from the right ventricle to the pulmonary artery. The conduit extending from the anterior aspect of the right ventricle to the distal pulmonary artery is indicated on the sagittal and transaxial images. The anastomoses are widely patent. (A, aorta; C, conduit; LA, left atrium; LP, left pulmonary artery; LV, left ventricle; P, pulmonary artery; RP, right pulmonary artery; RV, right ventricle.)

then 2- to 3-mm thick tomograms at the pulmonary arterial level. Because it is not necessary to opacify the pulmonary arteries for visualization by MRI, determination of the presence of central pulmonary arteries and a central confluence of the right and left pulmonary arteries is a unique capability of MRI. Assessment of blood supply to the lungs is achieved on both transverse and coronal images. On transverse images at the level of the carina and immediately below, it is usually possible to distinguish between pulmonary and bronchial arteries. Pulmonary arteries are situated ventral to the bronchi, whereas bronchial arteries are located posterior to the bronchi (see Figs. 9-25 and 9-26). Occasionally, a bronchial artery arising from subclavian arteries may be located ventral to the bronchi. The origin of bronchial arteries from the descending aorta can be observed on transverse and coronal images (Figs. 9-26, 9-27, and 9-30).

Pulmonary Atresia

Pulmonary atresia is depicted on transverse MR images as a solid layer of muscle in the region of the right ventricular outflow tract at the base of the heart; this represents the blind-ended infundibulum (see Fig. 9-28). Continuity of the lumen of the right ventricle cannot be traced into the main pulmonary artery on sequential transverse MR images. The length of atresia may be shown to be extensive or focal at the value level. Focal membranous valvular atresia may not always be discern-

ible as such on transverse tomograms because of partial volume inclusion of the patent lumen above or below the focal atresia on 5- or 10-mm sections. Consequently, valvular atresia and severe stenosis may not be distinguishable on spin-echo images. The presence or absence of flow across the valve can be determined on cine MR images in the transverse or sagittal planes, however. The length of the atresia of the main pulmonary artery as well as the infundibulum is demonstrated on sequential transverse tomograms.

In pulmonary atresia the aorta is usually markedly enlarged. There is generally a reciprocal relationship between the diameters of the aorta and pulmonary artery in patients with right ventricular outflow tract obstruction.

The aortic valve straddles a large VSD in pulmonary atresia with VSD (severe form of tetralogy of Fallot). A VSD is not observed in the form of pulmonary atresia with an intact ventricular septum. In the latter, MRI is effective for determining the size of the right ventricle, which varies from severely hypoplastic to enlarged.

The most useful information provided by MRI in patients with pulmonary atresia is the determination of the status of the main and central pulmonary arteries distal to the atresia (Figs. 9-28 to 9-31). The right pulmonary artery is sought in the image containing the right main bronchus; it courses in front of the right bronchus (Figs. 9-28, 9-29, 9-31, and 9-32). The left pulmonary artery courses over the left bronchus and is observed on the same tomogram as the proximal left bronchus or the one

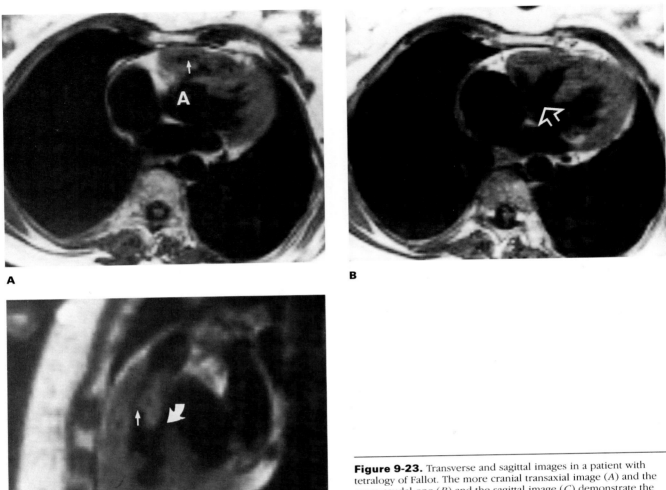

A

B

C

Figure 9-23. Transverse and sagittal images in a patient with tetralogy of Fallot. The more cranial transaxial image (*A*) and the more caudal one (*B*) and the sagittal image (*C*) demonstrate the severe narrowing (*arrow*) of the right ventricular outflow tract and the VSD (*open arrow*). Note on both the transaxial and especially the sagittal image, the severe narrowing of the right ventricular outflow region. The VSD is indicated on the transaxial image (*open arrow*) and on the sagittal image (*closed curved arrow*).

just cranial to the left bronchus. It is useful to determine if a main pulmonary artery or a central confluence between the pulmonary arteries exists (see Figs. 9-29 and 9-32). A recent report indicated that MRI is at least as accurate as angiography in defining the presence of main and central pulmonary arterial segments in patients with pulmonary atresia.[12] The pulmonary arteries frequently are hypoplastic to varying degrees or contain stenoses at the origin of the right, left, or segmental pulmonary arterial segments in patients with pulmonary atresia and VSD. The pulmonary arteries are usually normal or nearly normal in diameter and usually do not contain stenoses in patients with pulmonary atresia with an intact ventricular septum.

The presence of both right and left pulmonary arteries, their diameter, and whether there is a central confluence can be accurately defined by MRI.[12,13] Adequate diameters of the central pulmonary arteries and the presence of a central confluence identifies a patient as a good candidate for a Rastelli procedure, whereas the opposite finding indicates a poor candidate.

MRI also effectively displays the bronchial arterial supply to the lungs. MRI can be used to monitor the size of the surgically constructed systemic-to-pulmonary shunts, either by direct anastomosis or through an interposed graft (see Fig. 9-32). Distortion or stenosis of the pulmonary arteries caused by construction of these shunts is also depicted on images (see Fig. 9-32). The

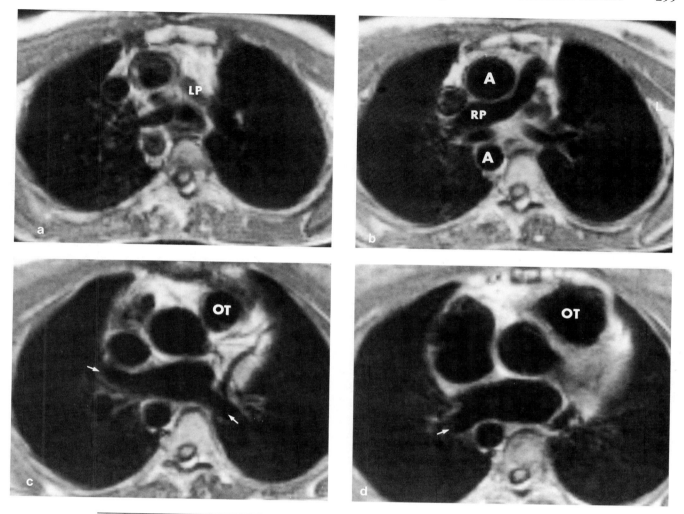

Figure 9-24. Transaxial images (*A* to *D*) extending from cranial (*A*) to caudal (*D*) in a patient with tetralogy of Fallot. There is substantial narrowing of the left pulmonary artery (LP) and a small main pulmonary artery. Note the moderate narrowing of the right ventricular outflow tract (OT). Note the decrease in diameter of the outflow tract in the distal portion compared with the more proximal portion. The connection of the pulmonary veins to the left atrium is indicated (*arrows*). (A, aorta; RP, right pulmonary artery.)

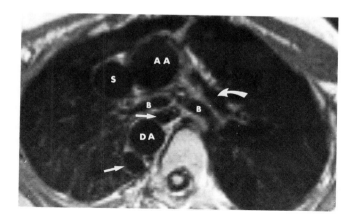

Figure 9-25. Pulmonary atresia with VSD. The transverse image demonstrates that the bronchial arteries (*arrows*) are located posterior to the bronchi (B), whereas the pulmonary artery (*curved arrow*) is located ventral to the bronchi. (AA, ascending aorta; DA, descending aorta; S, superior vena cava.)

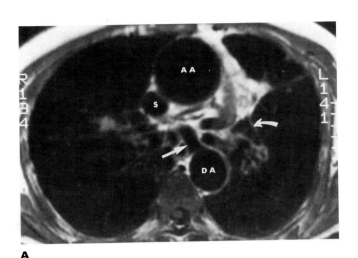

A

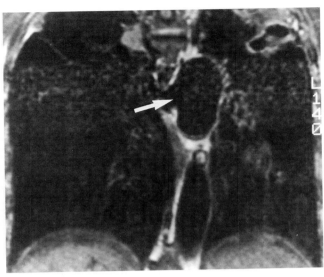

B

Figure 9-26. Transaxial (*A*) and coronal (*B*) images demonstrate enlarged bronchial arteries in a patient with pulmonary atresia with VSD. The large bronchial arteries originating from the descending aorta are evident on both images (*arrow*). A portion of the hilar left pulmonary artery (*curved arrow*) is also recognized. (AA, ascending aorta; DA, descending aorta; S, superior vena cava.)

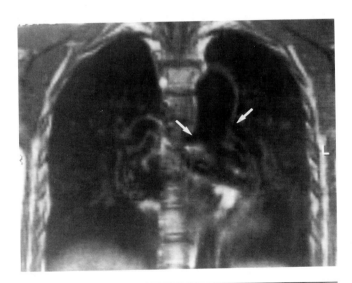

Figure 9-27. Coronal image demonstrates several enlarged bronchial arteries arising from the descending aorta in a patient with pulmonary atresia. The bronchial arteries (*arrows*) originate from both sides of the descending aorta.

evaluation of the main and central pulmonary arterial segments is accomplished by transverse and coronal MR images, generally using the spin-echo sequence. Oblique coronal images ("sit-up view") can be used to depict the length of the main pulmonary artery and bifurcation.[14] The region of the main and central pulmonary arterial segments is usually studied with 3-mm thick tomograms, frequently using four excitations (averages) to minimize partial volume averaging and enhance the accuracy of quantification of arterial diameter.

MRI is an effective method for monitoring the size and growth of the pulmonary arteries after surgical procedures intended to augment blood flow into them.[15,16] Stenoses in pulmonary artery segments distal to surgical shunts, conduits, and anastomoses have been shown by MRI.

Ventricular Septal Defect

MRI can identify the presence and site of VSD.[5] Transverse images are the most useful for this purpose because they separate the inflow and outflow portions of the ventricular septum. In our initial group of patients with CHD evaluated by MRI, VSD was identified in 20 of 22 patients.[5]

The various locations where defects occur in the ventricular septum are shown graphically in Fig. 9-33. Using adjacent transverse images, the various components of the ventricular septum can be identified. The segmental transverse images transect the specific components of the septum (Fig. 9-34).

The most frequently encountered defect is the perimembranous VSD. These can be clearly identified on transverse scans just below the aortic cusps. A transverse

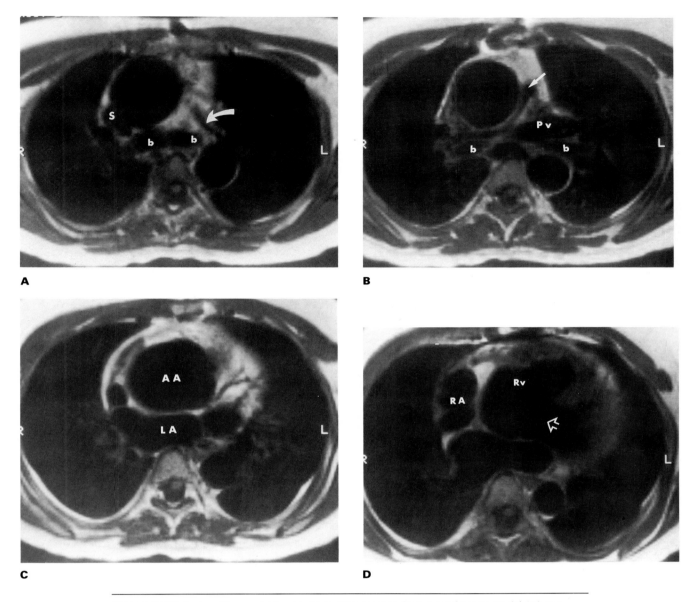

Figure 9-28. Series of transaxial images (*A* to *D*) extending from cranial (*A*) to caudal (*D*) in a patient with pulmonary atresia and VSD. The main (*closed arrow*), right, and left pulmonary arteries (*curved arrow*) are small in size. Note that the central pulmonary arteries are located ventral to the bronchi (b). There is a large VSD (*open arrow*). (AA, ascending aorta; B, bronchus; LA, left atrium; Pv, left upper pulmonary vein; RA, right atrium; Rv, right ventricle; S, superior vena cava.)

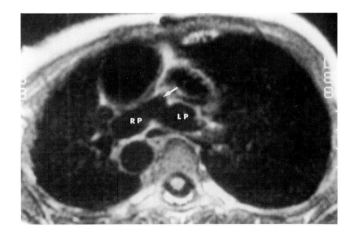

Figure 9-29. Transverse image at the level of the pulmonary arteries in a patient with right-sided isomerism, asplenia, and pulmonary atresia. There is a central confluence (*arrow*) between the right (RP) and left pulmonary (LP) arteries. The right and left pulmonary arteries are normal in size. No significant stenoses are recognized along the course of the right pulmonary artery.

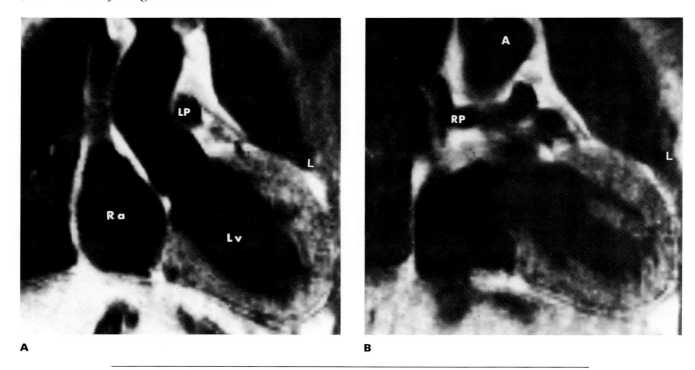

A   **B**

Figure 9-30. Coronal images (*A* is anterior to *B*) demonstrate the diameters of the left (LP) and right (RP) pulmonary arteries. Although smaller than normal, the central pulmonary arteries are not severely hypoplastic. (A, aortic arch; Lv, left ventricle; Ra, right atrium.)

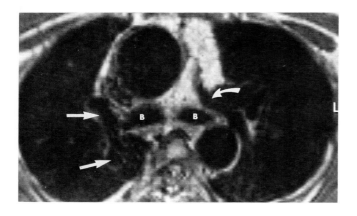

Figure 9-31. Transverse image at the level of the pulmonary arteries in a patient with pulmonary atresia. There is a small left pulmonary artery (*curved arrow*) but virtually no central right pulmonary artery. Segments of the right pulmonary artery are visualized in the right hilum (*arrows*). (B, bronchi.)

section located 1 cm caudal to the base of the aorta demonstrates perimembranous VSD (Fig. 9-35). The extensiveness of large perimembranous VSDs extending into the inlet or the outlet septa can be defined by adjacent transverse MR images (see Fig. 9-35). The position of

perimembranous VSDs below the crista supraventricularis of the right ventricle can be discerned on both transverse and sagittal images. Aneurysm of the ventricular septum associated with a membranous VSD can also be demonstrated on transverse scans (Fig. 9-36A).

VSDs involving the inlet septum (AV-canal-type VSD) have been demonstrated in patients with complete endocardial cushion defects (Fig. 9-36B).[17] The other components of the endocardial cushion defect, that is, ostium primum atrial septal defect and common AV valve, can also be visualized on transverse images positioned at a level to include all four chambers. Endocardial cushion defect is usually called the atrioventricular septal defect.

Defects involving the outlet septum can be identified on transverse, sagittal, and coronal images. These defects include subpulmonic VSDs and malalignment VSDs associated with truncus arteriosus, tetralogy of Fallot, and DORV. Most malalignment VSDs studied by MRI have been large and associated with dilation of the overlying great vessel. They have been demonstrated effectively on both transverse and sagittal images (see Fig. 9-24).

Another way of describing the location of VSDs relates to their location in relation to the crista supraventricularis. Distinction between infracristal and supracristal locations can be established on transverse or short-

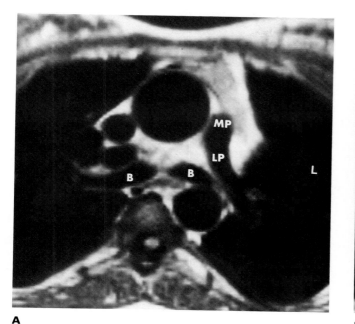

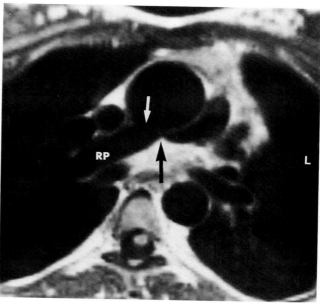

A

B

Figure 9-32. Transaxial images at the level of the left (*A*) and right pulmonary artery (*B*). An ascending aorta to the right pulmonary artery anastomosis is demonstrated (white arrow). There is a severe stenosis (*black arrow*) located just proximal to the aortopulmonary anastomosis. (B, bronchi; LP, left pulmonary artery; MP, main pulmonary artery; RP, right pulmonary artery.)

axis images through the right ventricular outflow tract. These images define cristal muscle between the pulmonary valve and the defect, indicating an infracristal VSD (see Fig. 9-35). Absence of muscle between the pulmonary valve and the defect is observed with a supracristal VSD (Fig. 9-37). In the latter anomaly, the defect appears to directly connect the right ventricular outflow tract to the aorta. Cine MRI assists in locating the site of the VSD by showing a signal void at the defect that extends into the right ventricle in left-to-right shunts.

Bulboventricular foramina connecting the predominant ventricular chamber with the hypoplastic outflow chamber in the left ventricular type of single ventricle have also been identified and their dimensions assessed by MRI (Fig. 9-38). The ideal imaging plane for demonstrating the foramina depends on their orientation, which can vary considerably. Sometimes the septum in cases of single ventricle is oriented in the sagittal plane, so that the foramen is depicted best on a coronal image (see Fig. 9-38).

Abnormalities of Atrioventricular Connections

Normal atrioventricular connections consist of the right atrium to the right ventricle and the left atrium to the left

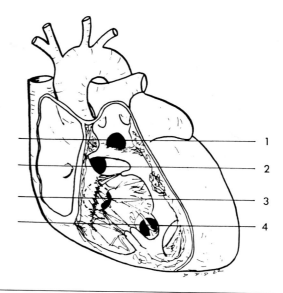

Figure 9-33. Diagram showing the various sites of VSD. The VSDs are viewed through opening of the right ventricular free wall. (1, outlet VSD; 2, perimembranous VSD; 3, inlet VSD; 4, trabecular (muscular) VSD.) (Reproduced with permission from Didier D, Higgins CB. Identification and localization of ventricular septal defects by gated magnetic resonance imaging. Am J Cardiol 1986;57:1363.)

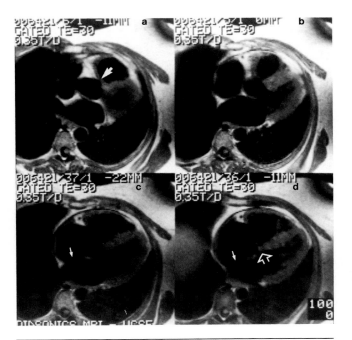

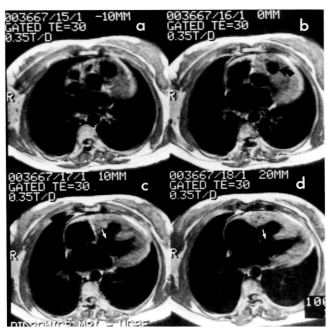

Figure 9-34. Series of transaxial images extending from cranial (*upper left panel*) demonstrate the various portions of the ventricular septum. The outlet septum (*arrow*) is shown in the upper left panel, separating the aorta from the right ventricular outflow region. The perimembranous portion of the VSD is demonstrated in the lower left panel as a thin region of the ventricular septum just beneath the aortic valve. The inlet ventricular septum is demonstrated in the lower right panel (*open arrow*) as the portion of ventricular septum separating the tricuspid and mitral valves. The trabecular septum is essentially the remainder of the ventricular septum, consisting entirely of muscle. A secundum ASD is indicated (*small arrows*). The defect is recognized on two adjacent transverse levels.

Figure 9-35. Multilevel spin-echo images extending from the base of the heart (*upper left panel*) to the middle of the right ventricle (*lower right panel*) in a patient with a perimembranous VSD that extends into and involves the inlet portion of the ventricular septum. In the lower panels the VSD is indicated (*small arrows*), involving the perimembranous portion of the ventricular septum and extending into the inlet ventricular septum, which separates the tricuspid and mitral valves. Note the substantial thickening of the right ventricular free wall, indicating right ventricular hypertrophy and suggesting the presence of pulmonary arterial hypertension as a consequence of the left-to-right shunt.

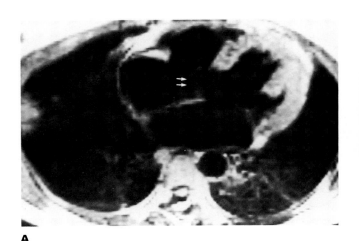

A

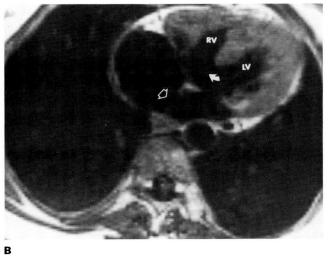

B

Figure 9-36. *A:* Transaxial image through the middle of the left ventricle demonstrates a perimembranous VSD with a ventricular septal aneurysm. Note the thin, low-signal-intensity, curvilinear structure at the region of the VSD (*small arrows*). This aneurysm bulges towards the right ventricle. This rupture represents an aneurysm of the ventricular septum. *B:* Transaxial image at the level of the atrioventricular valves demonstrates a VSD (*curved arrow*) involving the portion of the ventricular septum that normally separates the tricuspid and mitral valves (inlet septum). There is a substantial increase in the thickness of the right ventricle, indicating right ventricular hypertrophy. There is also an interatrial communication (*open arrow*).

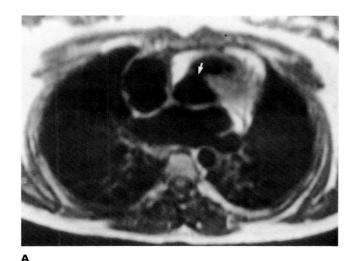

A

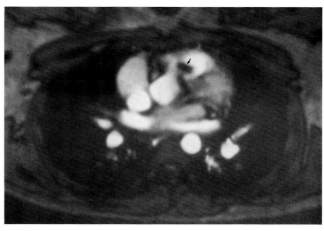

B

Figure 9-37. Transaxial spin-echo (*A*) and cine MR (*B*) images in a patient with supracristal VSD. The spin-echo image demonstrates a discontinuity in the portion of the septum separating the right ventricular outflow region and the base of the aortic valve (*arrow*). The cine MR image demonstrates a flow void projecting into the right ventricular outflow tract (*small arrow*). The signal void emanates from the region of the defect in the outlet portion of the ventricular septum. The flow void at this site represents the left-to-right shunting across the small supracristal VSD.

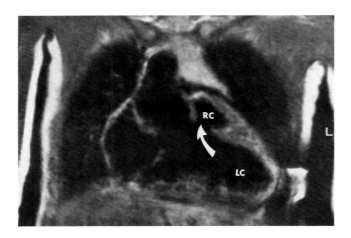

Figure 9-38. Coronal image in a patient with a single ventricle of the left ventricular type demonstrates the bulboventricular foramen (*curved arrow*) connecting the left ventricular chamber (LC) to the small right ventricular outlet chamber (RC). Visualization of the bulboventricular foramen as displayed in this image permits measurement of the diameter of this foramen. Determination of the diameter of the foramen in relation to the diameter of the annulus and valve of the outlet vessel is important in determining management of patients with single ventricle.

ventricle. The atrioventricular valves always reside in their appropriate ventricles. The tricuspid valve is part of the right ventricle and the mitral valve is part of the left ventricle under normal circumstances; the exception occurs in double-inlet (single) ventricle. A right ventricle contains the tricuspid valve, whether or not it occupies its normal position. The same holds for the left ventricle.

Although the atrioventricular valves cannot be distinguished from each other by their morphology on MRI, the recognition of the ventricular morphology indicates the nature of the valve within the ventricle.

Atrioventricular connections can be concordant or discordant (Fig. 9-39). Concordance is right atrium–left ventricular connection and left atrium–left ventricular connection. Discordance is right atrium–left ventricular and left atrium–right ventricular connection. An example of discordant atrioventricular connection is corrected transposition (situs solitus with L-ventricular loop).

Anomalies of atrioventricular connections include ventricular connections of the double-inlet type (both atrioventricular valves connect to one ventricle); straddling atrioventricular valve (one of the valves overlies both ventricles and empties blood into both ventricles), and atrioventricular valve atresia (one of the valves does not form or is not patent because of an imperforate membrane). These three groups of anomalies of connection are shown diagrammatically in Fig. 9-40. Univentricular atrioventricular connection is sometimes called single ventricle. Typically, a large ventricle with morphologic characteristics of a left ventricle receives both atrioventricular valves. The dominant ventricle is connected to a right ventricular outlet component through a bulboventricular foramen. Anomalies of arterioventricular connection commonly occur in association with abnormal atrioventricular connections. Consequently, these anomalies are extremely complex and must be analyzed precisely. The tomographic nature of MRI provides images that can be precisely examined and described using a segmental

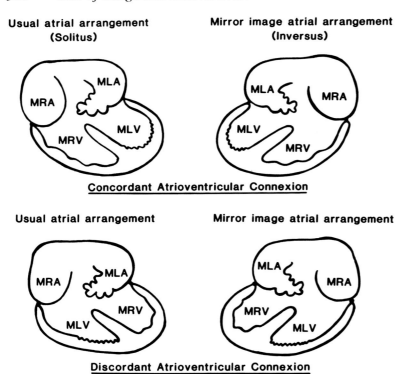

Usual atrial arrangement (Solitus)

Mirror image atrial arrangement (Inversus)

<u>Concordant Atrioventricular Connexion</u>

Usual atrial arrangement

Mirror image atrial arrangement

<u>Discordant Atrioventricular Connexion</u>

Figure 9-39. Diagram depicting the various types of atrioventricular connections (connexions). Concordant connection consists of a right atrium connected to a right ventricle and a left atrium connected to a left ventricle. Discordant connection is indicated by a morphologic right atrium connected to a morphologic left ventricle and a morphologic left atrium connected to a morphologic right ventricle. (MLA, morphologic left atrium; MLV, morphologic left ventricle; MRA, morphologic right atrium; MRV, morphologic right ventricle.) (Reproduced with permission from Anderson RH, Hoy SY. The tomographic anatomy of the normal and malformed heart. In: Tomographic imaging of congenital heart disease: echocardiography and magnetic resonance imaging. New York: Raven Press, 1990.)

approach. The segmental approach consists of five discrete steps:

1. Determination of situs (atrial position).
2. Determination of atrioventricular connections.
3. Determination of type of ventricular loop (D or L).
4. Determination of orientation of the great arteries to each other (*d* or *l*).
5. Determination of arterioventricular connections.

Coronal and transverse tomograms are generally used to assess complex cardiovascular anomalies and to diagnose possible abnormalities of atrioventricular connections. These images demonstrate both atrioventricular valves entering the dominant ventricle in univentricular atrioventricular connections of the double-inlet type, or connection of both valves to one ventricle with atresia of one of the atrioventricular valves (see Fig. 9-40A). Transverse images show a solid bar of muscle and fat between the right atrium and right ventricle in tricuspid atresia (Fig. 9-41). In tricuspid atresia, MRI can also be effective for showing the volume of the right ventricle and associated anomalies such as VSD, pulmonary stenosis or atresia, and arterioventricular abnormalities (Fig. 9-42). About 40% of patients with tricuspid atresia have transposition of the great arteries. Transverse MR images are also effective for determining the diameter of the atrial septal defect (ASD) or VSD in these patients. A restrictive VSD is one that is shown by MRI to have a max-

imum diameter less than the diameter of the pulmonary annulus for normally related great arteries or less than the diameter of the aortic annulus for transposition of the great arteries. For accurate measurement of the defect the imaging plane must be nearly perpendicular to the defect.

Complex Ventricular Abnormalities

The components of complex ventricular abnormalities may be difficult to unravel using any imaging technique. In these complex lesions, transverse MR images can clearly define the visceroatrial situs, the type of bulboventricular loop, the relationship of the great arteries, and the position of the cardiac apex.[18–20] Evaluation of these complex anomalies should be done by sequential analysis to formulate a complete description of the abnormal cardiovascular morphology. Abnormalities of arterioventricular connection, atrioventricular connection, and situs are frequently concomitant with complex ventricular anomalies. Abnormalities of arterioventricular connection include transposition and double-outlet ventricles. Abnormalities of atrioventricular connection include double-inlet ventricle, atresia of one of the atrioventricular valves, over-ride or straddling of one of the atrioventricular valves, criss-cross atrioventricular connections, and common atrioventricular valve.

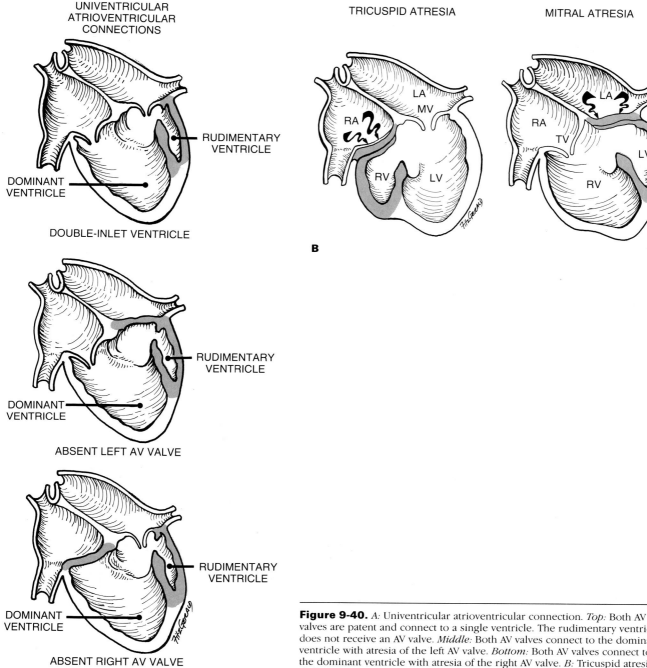

Figure 9-40. *A:* Univentricular atrioventricular connection. *Top:* Both AV valves are patent and connect to a single ventricle. The rudimentary ventricle does not receive an AV valve. *Middle:* Both AV valves connect to the dominant ventricle with atresia of the left AV valve. *Bottom:* Both AV valves connect to the dominant ventricle with atresia of the right AV valve. *B:* Tricuspid atresia (left) and mitral atresia (right). The right AV (tricuspid) valve connects to the right ventricle but is atretic. The left AV valve (mitral) connects to the left ventricle but is atretic.

It may not always be possible for angiography to differentiate among the various types of complex ventricular anomalies such as single ventricle (double-inlet ventricle), hypoplasia of one ventricle with atresia of its atrioventricular valve, common atrioventricular valve with asymmetric relationship of the valve to the ventricular system, and common ventricle (essentially absence of a ventricular septum, with each ventricle receiving an atrio-ventricular valve). In the analysis of these complex anomalies, MRI can define the presence and connections of the atrioventricular valves, the size of the VSD or bulboventricular foramen, the size of the two ventricles, the size of the ventricular septum, and the arterioventricular connections (Figs. 9-41 to 9-46).[18–20]

(*Text continues on page 311*)

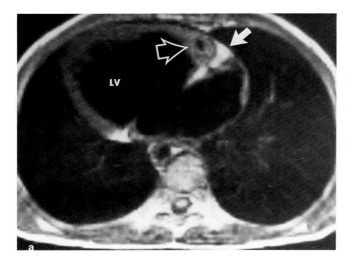

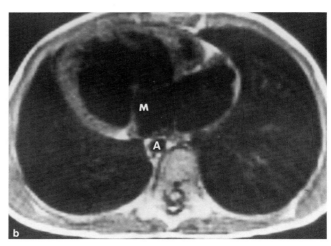

Figure 9-41. Transaxial images in a patient with tricuspid atresia, common atrium, and dextrocardia. *A* is located cranial to *B.* Note that the cardiac apex and the descending aorta (A) are located on the right side of the body. The right ventricle (*open arrow*) is hypoplastic and there is a solid bar of muscle and fat (*closed arrow*) that separates the hypoplastic right ventricle from the atrial chamber. This finding indicates the presence of tricuspid atresia. (LV, left ventricle; M, mitral valve.)

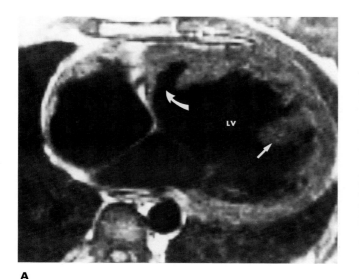

A

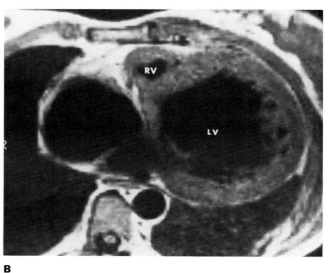

B

Figure 9-42. Transaxial images in a patient with tricuspid atresia and hypoplastic right ventricle. *A* is located cranial to *B.* Note the hypoplastic right ventricle, which is connected to the large left ventricle through a small VSD (*curved arrow*). There is a solid bar of muscle and fat that separates the right atrium from the hypoplastic right ventricle (RV). This indicates the presence of tricuspid atresia. There is a large papillary muscle (arrow) located in the middle of the left ventricle (LV).

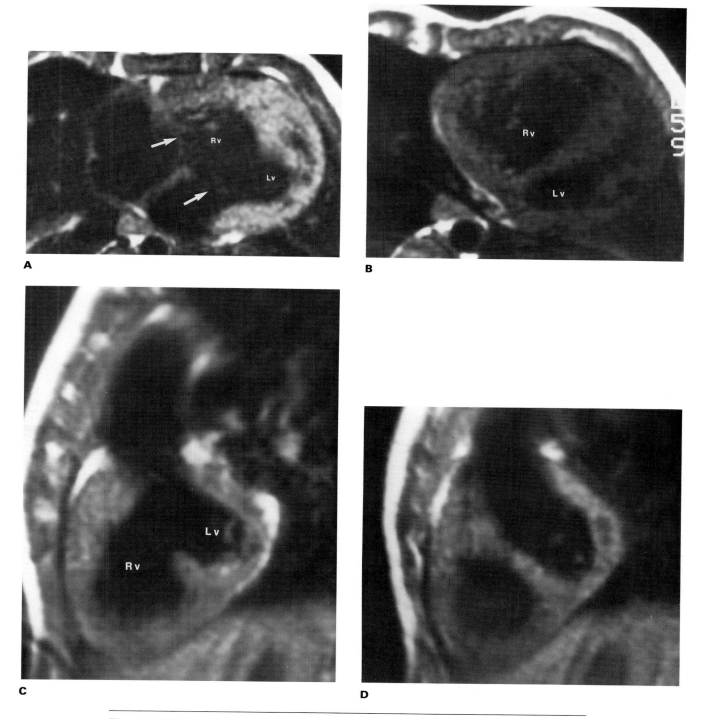

Figure 9-43. Transaxial (*A, B*) and sagittal (*C, D*) images in a patient with common ventricle. There is a large VSD (*arrow*) separating the morphologic right ventricle (Rv) from the morphologic left ventricle (Lv). Each of the ventricles receive an atrioventricular valve (*arrows*). This finding aids in the differentiation between a common ventricle, which is essentially a large VSD, from a single ventricle. Single ventricle is an anomaly in which one ventricle receives both atrioventricular valves; both valves may be patent or one might be atretic.

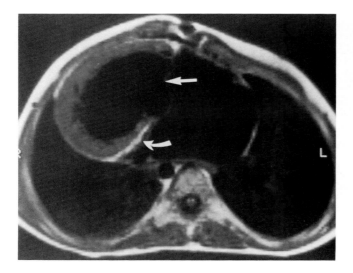

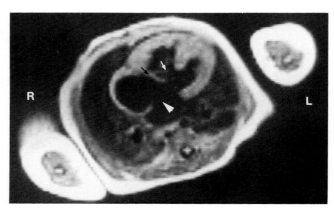

Figure 9-44. Transaxial image of the middle of the ventricle in a patient with mitral atresia. Note the large common atrium and the single ventricular chamber. This single ventricle receives the tricuspid valve, which is located anteriorly (*arrow*). In the posterior portion of the ventricle there is a solid bar of muscle (*curved arrow*) separating the ventricle from the atrium, which indicates the presence of mitral atresia.

Figure 9-45. Transaxial image at the middle of the ventricles in a patient with complete atrioventricular canal defect. This entity is also referred to as an atrioventricular septal defect. Note the large primum ASD (*arrowhead*) and large inlet VSD (*small arrow*). Portions of the right component of the single atrioventricular valve can be visualized (*closed small black arrow*). The atrioventricular valve spans the two ventricles.

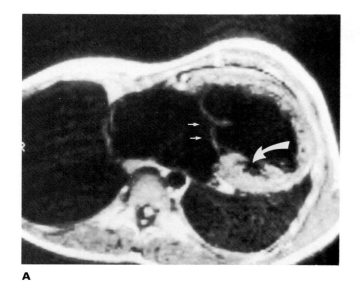

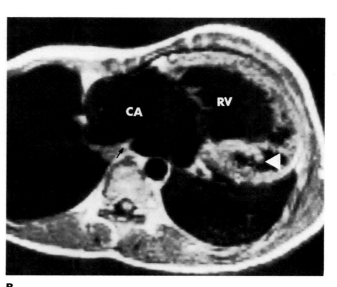

A   **B**

Figure 9-46. Transaxial images in a patient with single ventricle of the right ventricular type. *A* is located cranial to *B*. There is a large common atrium (CA). The common atrium connects to the predominant right ventricular chamber (RV). The predominant chamber is connected to a small posterior left ventricular chamber (*arrowhead*) through a small ventricular foramen (*curved arrow*).

In single ventricle, the MR images must be examined to determine the type of single ventricle. The major criterion when MRI is used to identify a chamber as a right or left morphologic ventricle is the presence of infundibulum as indicative of a right ventricle. When there is no detectable muscle separating either AV valve from the adjacent semilunar valve, the chamber is considered a left ventricle. In instances of single ventricle, both AV valves are attached to a dominant ventricle, and a rudimentary portion of the other ventricle is discernible (see Figs. 9-38 and 9-46). The position of the rudimentary right ventricle usually is anterior and superior to the dominant ventricle (see Fig. 9-38), whereas the rudimentary left ventricle usually is posterior and inferior to the dominant ventricle (see Fig. 9-46). This configuration is used as a secondary sign for deciding on the type of single ventricle. The trabecular pattern observed on transverse MR images is less useful for ventricular identification. Heavy trabeculation of the apical portion of the ventricular septum is characteristic for the right ventricle. Thus, MRI shows the following features for the various types of single ventricle. The left ventricular type is recognized by a morphologic left ventricle into which both AV valves are attached. This predominant chamber is connected to a right ventricular outflow chamber through a bulboventricular foramen (see Fig. 9-38). The right ventricular type is recognized by a predominant chamber characterized by a ventral position and an infundibulum; both AV valves enter this chamber if both are patent. The isolated remnant of the left ventricle is located posterior and connected to the dominant chamber by a VSD (see Fig. 9-46). A primitive type of single ventricle has morphologic features characteristic of neither right nor left ventricle. MRI has been effective for displaying great-vessel abnormalities that are frequently associated with single ventricle (see Fig. 9-38).

In common ventricle, both the right and left ventricular sides of the chamber receive AV valves (see Fig. 9-43). The morphologically distinct components are separated by a small ridge of muscle in the trabecular region of the ventricles.

Differentiation of tricuspid atresia or mitral atresia with a large VSD from single ventricle necessitates demonstration of the atretic valve region. Atresia of an AV valve has been shown on transverse MR images as a layer of muscle separating the atrium from the ventricle at the expected level of the valve (see Figs. 9-41, 9-42, and 9-44). MRI also displays the hypoplasia or absence of the inflow portion of the afflicted ventricle.

Complete AV canal defect with marked inequality in the size of the two ventricles occurs because a disproportionate portion of the common AV valve lies to either the right (right ventricular predominance) or left (left ventricular predominance) of the ventricular septum.

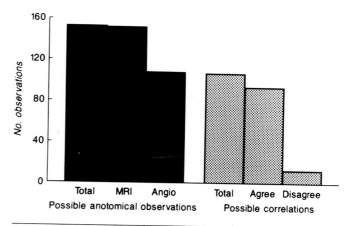

Figure 9-47. Block diagram demonstrating a comparison between MRI and angiography for recognizing the various segmental components of hearts with complex ventricular anomalies. In this series of 17 patients there were 9 critical anatomic observations which could potentially be reorganized in the imaging studies. Nearly all these observations could be attained from the MR images that encompassed the entire heart. Whereas the angiograms in these patients provided only partial assessment of these anatomic features. In instances where the evaluation was possible by both angiography and MRI, there was agreement in about 90% of instances and disagreement in 10%.

Figure 9-45 shows a transverse MR image from a patient with the left-predominant type in which there is commitment of more than 50% of the single AV valve to the left ventricular side of the septum. The opposite relationships have been noted on MR images in the right-predominant form.

Both our experience in complex ventricular abnormalities and the findings of others in patients with single ventricle show that MRI may be at least as accurate as angiography in defining all the components of these lesions (Fig. 9-47).[18–20] MRI has defined internal ventricular morphology, connections of the great vessels, and any associated atrioventricular abnormalities with an accuracy equivalent to angiography.

Displacement of the leaflets of the tricuspid valve, particularly the septal leaflet toward the apex, and atrialization of the inflow portion of the right ventricle have been defined on transverse and coronal images in patients with Ebstein's anomaly.[21] Transverse MR images have failed to demonstrate any abnormalities of the tricuspid valve in some patients with a mild form of this anomaly, however.

Atrial Abnormalities

Transverse or short-axis MR images clearly display the sinus venosus, secundum, and primum portions of the atrial septum (see Fig. 9-1).[22,23] The thinned region at the site of the fossa ovalis may produce little or no MR signal and can be misinterpreted as a secundum ASD. The septum gradually thins toward the site of signal absence in this circumstance, rather than the thickened edge of the septum adjacent to the true secundum defect. Cine MRI can be used to demonstrate that the septum is intact in the fossa ovalis region and to exclude a signal void at an atrial septal site, which could occur in the presence of a left-to-right shunt through a defect.

Spin-echo MRI has been found to be accurate for detection and determination of the site of ASDs. We have found greater than 90% sensitivity at the 90% specificity level for MRI in identifying defects at any level of the atrial septum.[22] Our criteria for stating the definite presence of an ASD is to visualize a defect at two adjacent levels on multislice transverse images (Figs. 9-34 and 9-48) or to visualize the defect at multiple phases of the cardiac cycle at the same anatomic level. Dinsmore et al. used images in the short-axis plane to estimate the size of the defect; MRI measurements correlated well with measurements made at operation.[23] Another report indicated only moderate sensitivity and specificity of gated MRI for detecting ASDs, however.[24]

MRI displays a defect in the portion of atrial septum between the superior vena cava and the left atrium and the sinus venosus defect (Fig. 9-49), as well as the anom-

alous connection of the right upper pulmonary vein. The defect is shown in the middle of the atrial septum in secundum ASD (see Figs. 9-34 and 9-48). The atrial septum usually shows increased thickness at the margin of the defect. Transverse images have also displayed a very thin layer of tissue bulging toward the right atrium in patients with aneurysm of the atrial septum.

Defects in the lower portion of the atrial septum adjacent to the AV valves have been shown in patients with primum ASDs (Figs. 9-45, 9-50, and 9-51). This type of ASD is observed on the transverse images that include the AV valves. Associated signs of ASD (atrioventricular canal or endocardial cushion defects) have also been demonstrated, such as a truncated inlet ventricular septum with both AV valves located at the same dorsoventral level because of the abnormal mitral valve orientation and attachments (Fig. 9-50). Left ventricular outflow tract elongation has also been seen on coronal scans. Conversely, the mitral valve cleft has not been imaged. In the complete form of this anomaly, leaflets of the single AV valve are observed spanning the two ventricles and there is an inflow VSD (Figs. 9-45, 9-51, and 9-52). Jacobstein et al. reported similar features in all of nine patients with endocardial cushion defect.[17] These characteristic findings were deficiency of the primum atrial and inlet ventricular septa, a common AV valve ring, and absence of

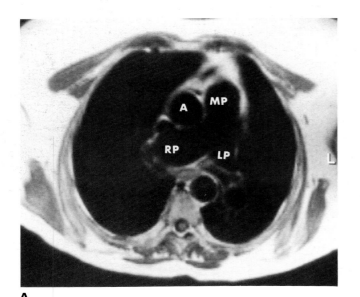

A

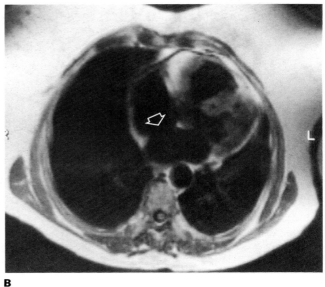

B

Figure 9-48. Transaxial images at the level of the pulmonary arteries (*A*) and middle of the atria (*B*) in a patient with the secundum type of ASD. There is enlargement of the pulmonary arteries. The ASD is relatively large and can be measured on the transaxial image through the middle of the defect (*open arrow*). (A, ascending aorta; LP, left pulmonary artery; MP, main pulmonary artery; RP, right pulmonary artery.)

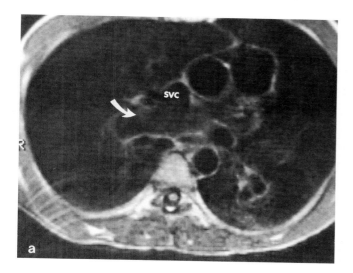

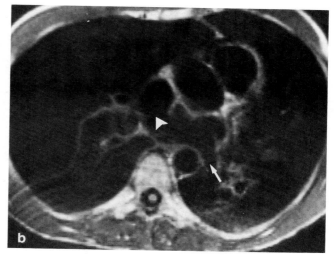

Figure 9-49. Transaxial images in a patient with sinus venosus type of ASD. *A* is located cranial to *B*. Note the connection of the right upper lobe pulmonary vein (*curved arrow*) to the lower portion of the superior vena cava (SVC). The left lower lobe pulmonary vein is indicated by the straight arrow. The sinus venosus VSD is shown by the *arrowhead*.

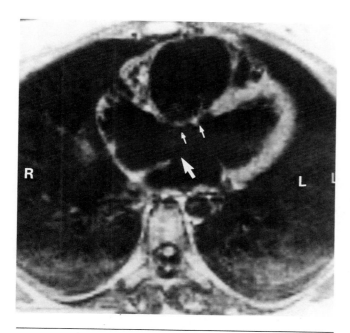

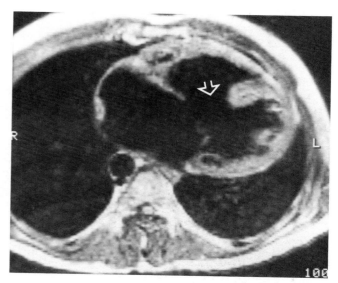

Figure 9-51. Transaxial image of the middle of the ventricle in a patient with a complete atrioventricular septal defect (atrioventricular canal defect). There is a large inlet VSD (*open arrow*). The single atrioventricular valve spans both ventricular chambers.

Figure 9-50. Transaxial image through the middle of the ventricles demonstrates an atrioventricular septal defect (atrioventricular canal defect). There is a primum ASD (*large arrow*). The atrioventricular valve (*small arrows*) is connected to the crest of the foreshortened inlet ventricular septum.

the cardiac crux. Patients with the incomplete form of the defect were found to have bridging tissue coursing from the AV septum to the crest of the truncated ventricular septum (see Fig. 9-50).

Complete absence of the primum and secundum portions of the septum is demonstrated in patients with common atrium (Figs. 9-52 and 9-53). A septum separating the junction of the superior vena cava from the left atrium (sinus venosus septum) is observed on MR images in these patients. Spin-echo MRI has been useful for assessing the size of the atrial septal defect after balloon septostomy or surgical excision. The diameter of the defect can be directly measured on transverse or short-axis MR images.[23]

Enlargement of the right-sided cardiac chamber, the pulmonary artery, and pulmonary veins is observed in patients with large left-to-right atrial shunts (see Fig. 9-48). Dilation of the left atrium and pulmonary veins has been demonstrated in patients with large left-to-right shunts below the atrial level. In patients with shunt lesions, dilation of the right atrium and reversed curvature of the ventricular septum (convexity toward the left ventricle) have been observed in the presence of severe pulmonary arterial hypertension.

Cine MRI demonstrates a signal void at the site of the shunt across the ASD. Cine MRI may be useful for documenting the presence and site of small interatrial communications.

Transverse MR images have been effective for demonstrating the membrane within the left atrial body in cor triatriatum (Figs. 9-54 and 9-55). The membrane lies between the pulmonary venous connection and the mitral valve. Demonstration of the membrane is provided by using thin section (3-mm) images (see Fig. 9-54).

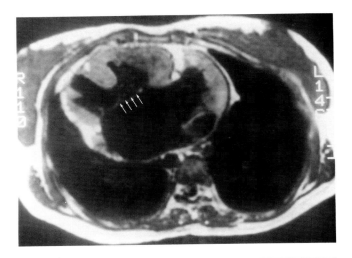

Figure 9-52. Transaxial image demonstrates dextrocardia, common atrium, and complete atrioventricular canal defect. Note the absence of a septum within the atrium. The atrioventricular valve spans the two ventricles. The small *arrows* indicate the common atrioventricular valve. The ventricular septum is defective in the inlet portion.

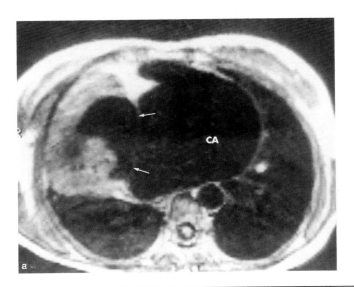
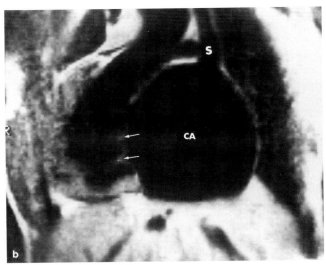

Figure 9-53. Transaxial (*A*) and coronal (*B*) images in a patient with common atrium (CA) and dextrocardia. The absence of an atrial septum is indicated both on the transaxial and coronal images. There is a single large atrioventricular valve (*arrows*) that connects the common atrium to the ventricular chamber. The superior vena cava enters the left side of the common atrium. (S, superior vena cava.)

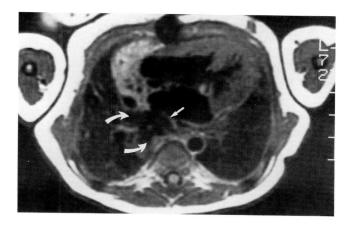

Figure 9-54. Transaxial image through the middle of the left atrium in a patient with cor triatriatum. The pulmonary veins (*curved arrows*) connect to a right posterior atrial chamber. The atrial portion of the atrial chamber containing the pulmonary veins is separated from the main atrial chamber by a membrane (*arrow*). Note the substantial increase in thickness of the right ventricular wall, indicating the presence of right ventricular hypertrophy as a consequence of pulmonary arterial hypertension.

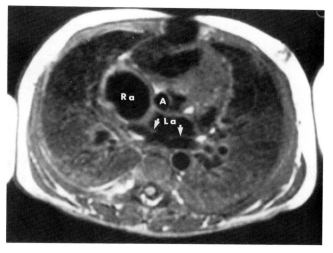

Figure 9-55. Transaxial image through the middle of the atria in a patient with cor triatriatum. The pulmonary veins enter the posterior portion of the left atrial chamber. The posterior portion of the atrial chamber is separated from the anterior portion by a membrane (*arrow*). There is a narrow ostium between the two portions of the atrial septum (curved arrow). Note the increased signal of the lungs caused by pulmonary edema. (A, aortic valve; La, left atrium; Ra, right atrium.)

Patent Ductus Arteriosus

The connection between the aorta and pulmonary artery can be discerned on MR images (Fig. 9-56). The ductus as an isolated anomaly courses from the proximal descending aorta to the left pulmonary artery just beyond the pulmonary arterial bifurcation. MRI can also reveal the focal dilation of the aorta at the site of ductal attachment (aortic spindle) and the large aortic arch, usually observed in association with patent ductus arteriosus. In our experience, however, a narrow patent ductus has not always been identified on MR tomograms with a thickness of 5 to 10 mm. It is also likely that the ductus could be missed in small infants even using 3- to 5-mm section thickness.

Pulmonary Venous Abnormalities

Partial anomalous pulmonary venous connection occurs in nearly all patients with sinus venosus defects and also occurs with an increased frequency in other types of ASD. Because MRI can clearly define the connection of the pulmonary veins to the left atrium, it is important to locate the connection of these veins in patients with ASD.[22,25] These connections are nearly always clearly defined on transverse images (Figs. 9-6, 9-57). Coronal images can also be used to demonstrate this anatomy (see Fig. 9-57).

Transverse images show the right upper pulmonary vein entering the superior vena cava (see Fig. 9-58) above

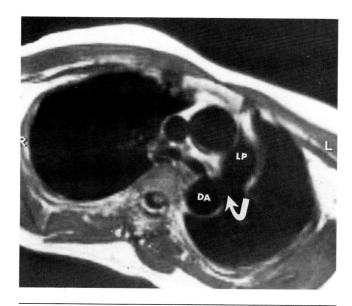

Figure 9-56. Transaxial image in a patient with patent ductus arteriosus. There is a discontinuity between the anterolateral wall of the descending aorta (DA) and the left pulmonary artery (LP). The *curved arrow* indicates the site of the patent ductus arteriosus.

its junction with the right atrium with partial anomalous connection. Transverse MR images display the coronary sinus; a dilated sinus may be a sign of anomalous connection to this structure. MR images in transverse, sagittal, and coronal planes have shown the connection of a com-

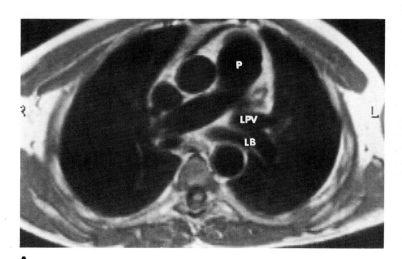

A

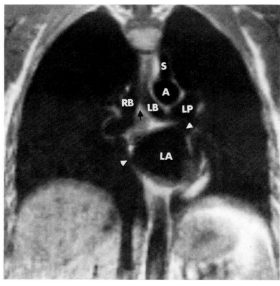

B

Figure 9-57. *A.* Transaxial image at the level of the left upper lobe pulmonary vein. The left upper lobe pulmonary vein is the one that is most difficult to follow into its connection with the left atrium. The left upper lobe pulmonary vein, when in a normal location, is located just ventral to the left bronchus. Recognition of the pulmonary vein of this site indicates normal pulmonary venous connection. (LB, left bronchus; LPV, left upper pulmonary vein; P, pulmonary artery.) *B:* Coronal image in the region of the connection of the left upper pulmonary vein to the left atrium. Note the entrance of the upper lobe pulmonary veins to the left atrium (*arrowheads*). (A, posterior aortic arch; LA, left atrium; LB, left bronchus; LP, left pulmonary artery; RB, right bronchus; S, left subclavian artery.)

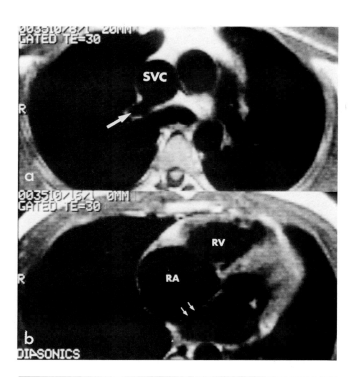

Figure 9-58. Transverse images through the lower portion of the superior vena cava (SVC) (*top*) and middle of the atria (*bottom*). The right upper lobe pulmonary vein enters the superior vena cava (*arrow*). A discontinuity in the atrial septum is also demonstrated (*small arrows*). (RA, right atrium; RV, right ventricle.)

mon right-sided pulmonary vein to the inferior vena cava in patients with scimitar syndrome.

Total anomalous pulmonary venous connection should be suspected when no pulmonary veins entering the left atrium can be identified. MRI can define the common pulmonary vein behind or above the left atrium (Fig. 9-59), a dilated left superior vena cava, or the dilated coronary sinus, thereby providing clues to the site of anomalous drainage. A recent study has indicated the capability of MRI for the diagnosis of partial and total anomalous pulmonary venous connections.[25]

Systemic Venous Abnormalities

Several anomalies of the systemic venous system have been depicted by MRI (Figs. 9-60 to 9-62).[26] Transverse images can reveal persistent left superior vena cava lying lateral to the main pulmonary artery (see Fig. 9-60 to 9-62). Transverse images can also show the enlarged vertical and horizontal limbs of the coronary sinus. The persistent left superior vena cava is variable in size; its diameter is reciprocal to the size of the right superior vena cava. In the rare instance of atretic right superior vena cava, the left cava and coronary sinus are markedly enlarged. Venous anomalies, including a left superior vena cava, may raise concern regarding a superior me-

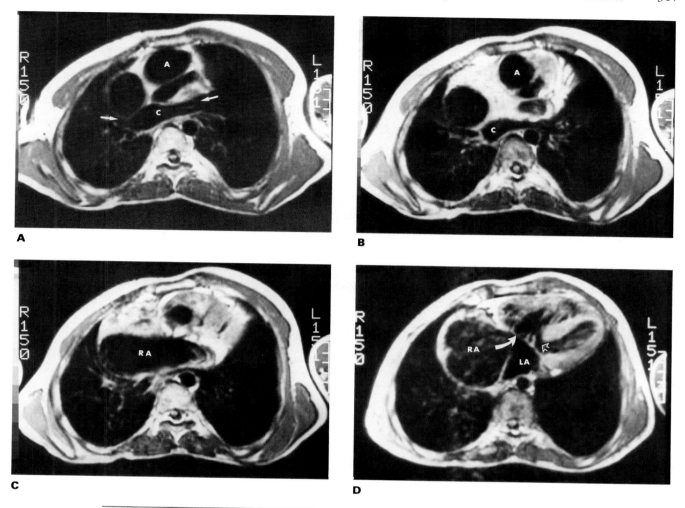

Figure 9-59. Series of transverse images (*A* to *D*) extending from cranial (*A*) to caudal (*D*) in a patient with total anomalous pulmonary venous connection, complete atrioventricular septal defect (atrioventricular canal), transposition of the great arteries, and pulmonary atresia. There is a confluence (C) of pulmonary veins (*arrows*) cranial to the right atrium (RA). The confluence of the pulmonary veins appear to enter the right atrium. Further caudally there is a small left atrium (LA). The common atrioventricular valve (*curved arrow*) spans both ventricles. There is a large inlet VSD (*open arrow*). (A, aorta.)

diastinal mass on chest x-ray. MRI provides a simple, noninvasive method for identifying this vascular anomaly and excluding a mediastinal mass. Transverse MR images have demonstrated the substantially enlarged coronary sinus into which the persistent left superior vena cava drains in most patients. Drainage of the left superior vena cava directly into the left side of the atrium has been observed in patients with asplenia syndrome (unroofed coronary sinus defect).

Interruption of the inferior vena cava (IIVC) with azygous continuation is clearly recognized on MR images (see Fig. 9-61). MRI has been used to diagnose this anomaly clearly when the enlarged azygous vein has suggested a posterior mediastinal mass on chest x-ray. Identification

of this anomaly before catheterization can also be useful in facilitating this procedure. The IIVC occurs as an isolated anomaly (see Fig. 9-61) and is associated with complex congenital heart disease (see Fig. 9-62). IIVC is a characteristic anomaly in the polysplenia syndrome (see Fig. 9-62); it occurs in most patients with polysplenia syndrome.

Quantification of Shunts

Shunts can be quantified by measurement of left and right ventricular volume from cine MR images or by simultaneous measurement of flow in the ascending aorta and main pulmonary artery using velocity-encoded cine MR (Table 9-1).[3,27,28] With the former technique, transverse cine MR images are acquired that encompass the entire right and left ventricle. The end-diastolic and end-systolic images are identified at each level; usually these are the first image obtained after the R wave (end diastole) and the smallest image (end systole). The area of the high signal-intensity blood pool is outlined and measured by planimetry on each image. Previous studies in healthy subjects demonstrated that right and left ventricular stroke volumes measured by cine MR images are equivalent.[29] The areas of the right and left ventricles are summed from the multiple images to calculate the volumes. The difference between right and left ventricular stroke volume is the net volume of atrial level shunts and patent ductus arteriosus.

Right ventricular stroke volume is greater than left ventricle stroke volume for ASD and partial anomalous pulmonary venous connection. Left ventricular stroke volume is greater than right ventricular stroke volume for patent ductus arteriosus. The volume of the shunt for VSD cannot be calculated using ventricular volumetrics. The opposite relationship exists for right-to-left shunt at the various levels. The calculations of the net shunt volume is complicated in the presence of valvular regurgitation since valvular regurgitation also causes a disparity between the ventricular stroke volumes.

The second method is to measure blood flow in the proximal aorta and pulmonary artery using a new flow quantification technique called velocity-encoded cine MRI.[22] This method uses the quantitative phase image in order to calculate instantaneous flow in the proximal aorta and main pulmonary artery. It is described in detail

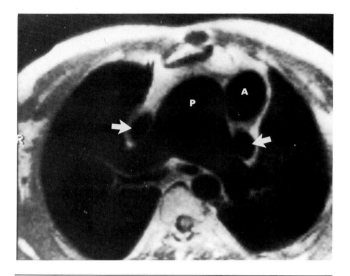

Figure 9-60. Transaxial image at the level of the pulmonary arterial bifurcation demonstrates bilateral superior vena cavae (*arrows*). The aorta is located anterior and to the left of the pulmonary artery, indicating the presence of an *l*-transposition of the great arteries.

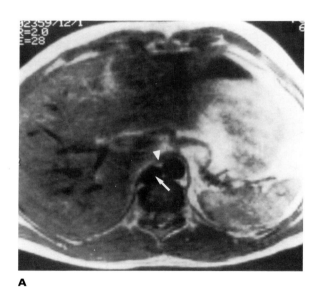

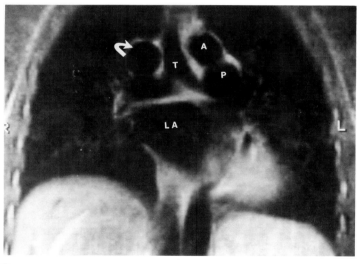

A   B

Figure 9-61. Transaxial (*A*) and coronal (*B*) images of a patient with intrahepatic interruption of the inferior vena cava. The transaxial image (*A*) demonstrates absence of the intrahepatic portion of the inferior vena cava and a markedly enlarged azygous vein (*arrow*). Note that the azygous vein is located posterior to the diaphragm (*arrowhead*). The coronal image (*B*) demonstrates the markedly enlarged arch of the azygous vein (*curved arrow*) located above the right bronchus. Note that the arch of the azygous is as large as the posterior portion of the left-sided aortic arch. (A, aortic arch; LA, left atrium; P, left pulmonary artery; T, trachea.)

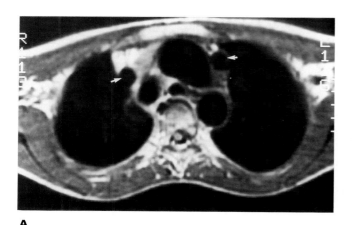

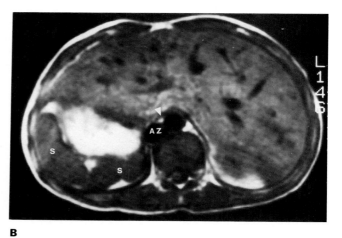

A **B**

Figure 9-62. Transaxial images at the level of the aortic arch (*A*) and liver (*B*) in a patient with bilateral superior vena cavae and interruption of the aortic arch. Note the bilateral superior vena cavae (*arrows*). There is absence of the intrahepatic portion of the inferior vena cava. Note that dorsal to the diaphragm (*arrowheads*) there is a markedly enlarged azygous vein (*AZ*). Note also the multiple spleens (*S*) in this patient with abdominal situs inversus. The liver is located on the left side and the stomach on the right side.

Table 9-1

Calculation of Left-to-Right Shunts by Cine MRI Techniques

	Cine MRI Volumetrics	*Velocity-encoded Cine MRI*
ASD PAPVC	Shunt = RVSV − LVSV	Shunt = RVSV − LVSV
VSD	LVSV = RVSV*	Shunt = RVSV − LVSV
PDA	Shunt = LVSV − RVSV	Shunt = LVSV − RVSV

ASD, atrial septal defect; LV, left ventricle; PAPVC, partial anomalous pulmonary venous connection; RV, right ventricle; SV, stroke volume; VSD, ventricular septal defect.
*Quantification of the shunt for a VSD is not possible using ventricular volumetrics.

later in this chapter. In healthy people volume flow in the aorta and pulmonary artery are nearly equivalent. The small volume of systolic coronary flow that is not interrogated apparently does not importantly influence this relationship; most of coronary blood flow occurs during diastole. Thus, flow measurements in the aorta during systole include most of the coronary flow in the stroke volume measurement. The difference in mean blood flow per heart beat (stroke volume) for the aorta compared with the pulmonary artery can be used as a measure of the shunt flow per beat.

In ASD, partial anomalous pulmonary venous connection, and VSD, the pulmonary blood flow is greater than aortic flow by a value equal to the left-to-right shunt. In patent ductus arteriosus the flow is greater in the aorta than in the pulmonary artery by a value equal to the left-

to-right shunt. The opposite relationship exists for right-to-left shunts.

Thoracic Aortic Anomalies

MRI is effective for the definitive diagnosis of a number of thoracic aortic abnormalities.[30–34] MRI should be considered the preferable imaging technique for thoracic aortic abnormalities and can usually be substituted for angiography. For most abnormalities it provides diagnostic information at least equivalent to that obtained with angiography.

Arch Anomalies

MRI has demonstrated aortic arch anomalies, including double aortic arch and right aortic arch with retroesophageal left subclavian artery.[32,33] MRI displays both the vascular anomaly and the compression of the airway. Compression of the airway is displayed optimally on the sagittal images (Figs. 9-63 and 9-64). In right aortic arch, transverse MR images show the arch lying to the right of the trachea and the proximal descending aorta on the right aspect of the vertebral bodies (see Figs. 9-63 and 9-64). Usually, the right arch crosses to the left of the spine in the upper thoracic region; however, this crossing site is variable and is readily defined by MRI. Transverse images readily show the diameter of the right and left arches in double aortic arch (see Figs. 9-63 and 9-64).

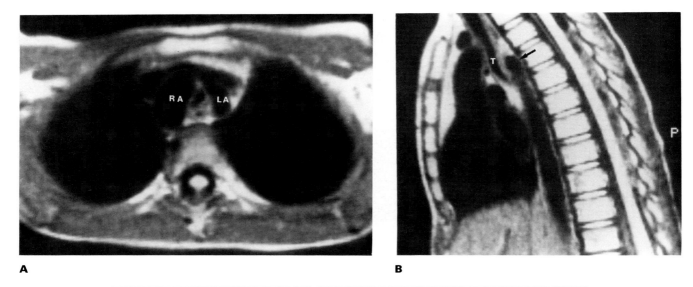

Figure 9-63. Transaxial (*A*) and sagittal (*B*) images in a patient with double aortic arch. The sagittal image demonstrates a vascular structure (*arrow*) posterior to the esophagus and trachea (T). The transaxial images demonstrate a large right arch (RA) and a smaller left arch (LA).

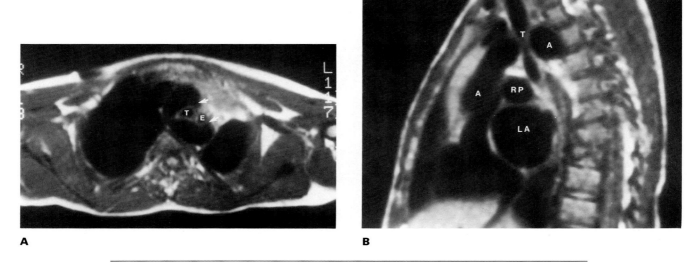

Figure 9-64. Transaxial (*A*) and sagittal (*B*) images in a patient with a double aortic arch. The sagittal image demonstrates compression of the trachea (T) by the double aortic arch. The transaxial image demonstrates the large right aortic arch and the anterior and posterior component of the smaller left aortic arch (*arrows*). (A, aorta; E, esophagus; LA, left atrium; RP, right pulmonary artery.)

Transverse images also reveal the diameter of the retro-esophageal subclavian artery (Fig. 9-65). Usually, right retroesophagal subclavian artery (with left arch) has a normal diameter, whereas left retroesophageal subclavian artery (with right arch) has a focal dilation at the site of origin from the descending aorta and consequently narrows the trachea and esophagus.

Aortic Coarctation

The most frequently encountered congenital anomaly of the thoracic aorta is coarctation. MRI has been found to be effective for evaluating coarctation before and after treatment.[30,31] For evaluation of coarctation and other thoracic aortic anomalies, gated images are obtained in

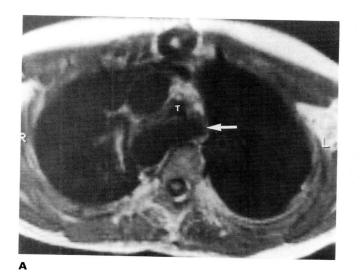

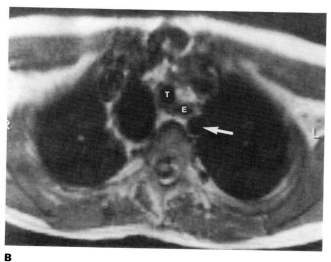

A **B**

Figure 9-65. Transaxial images in a patient with right aortic arch and retroesophageal left subclavian artery. *A* is located approximately 1 cm cranial to *B*. Note that the retroesophageal left subclavian artery (*arrow*) is located posterior to the trachea (T). At a more cranial level the top of the aortic arch is identified and the left subclavian artery is situated in the posterior portion of the mediastinum (*arrow*). It is located posterior to the trachea and esophagus (E).

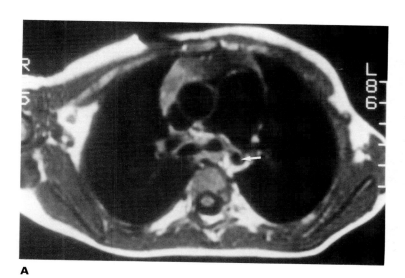

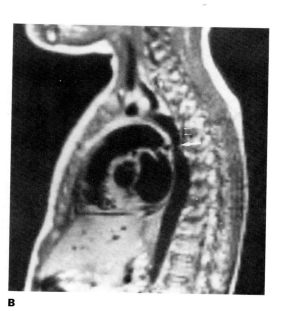

A **B**

Figure 9-66. Transaxial (*A*) and sagittal (*B*) MR images in a patient with coarctation of the aorta. The marked narrowing of the proximal portion of the descending thoracic aorta (*arrow*) is demonstrated. There is also a prominent collateral artery (*small arrows*).

planes perpendicular to each other. The imaging planes used when this diagnosis is suspected are the transverse and the sagittal (Figs. 9-66 and 9-67), or a plane reproducing the LAO view (Fig. 9-68). The latter view is obtained by elevating the right shoulder 30° and imaging in the sagittal plane or angulating the slice-selective gradient so that it cuts through the middle of the arch. Iden-

tification of the stenotic segment is sometimes easier in the sagittal or LAO-equivalent plane than in the transaxial planes because these planes are perpendicular to the coarctation and thereby the narrowing is less obscured by partial-volume effects (Figs. 9-66 to 9-69). These partial-volume effects encountered in the transverse plane may lead to underestimation or overestimation of the se-

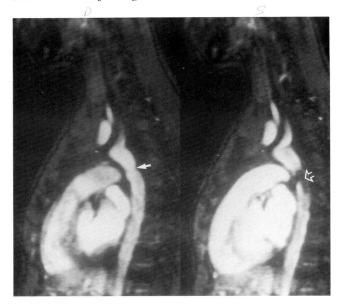

Figure 9-67. Cine MR images in a patient with coarctation of the aorta. The image on the left was obtained during diastole. The image on the right was obtained during systole. A transverse lucency across the descending thoracic aorta is recognized in diastole (*small arrow*). At the site of the coarctation a flow void (*open arrow*) is recognized, due to high-velocity turbulent flow across the coarctation site.

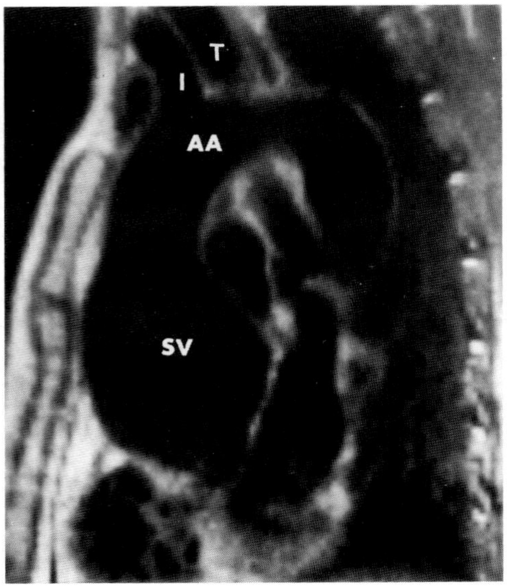

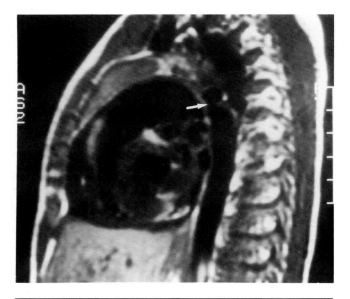

Figure 9-68. Oblique sagittal view of the thoracic aorta. The oblique sagittal view demonstrates the ascending aorta, aortic arch, and proximal portion of the descending aorta on a single tomogram. Note the aneurysmal dilation of the proximal ascending aorta; this pear-shaped configuration is called "marfanoid aorta." (AA, ascending aorta; I, innominate artery; SV, sinus of Valsalva; T, trachea.)

verity of coarctation. A 3-mm thick sagittal image centered in the middle of the coarctation should be used to measure the luminal diameter of the coarctation site (see Figs. 9-66 and 9-69).

A report of results of MRI in 15 patients with coarctation of the thoracic aorta showed that this modality identified all but one coarctation and also showed the site, extent, and involvement of the arch vessels by the coarctation.[30] In addition, MRI was able to visualize post-stenotic dilation and dilated collaterals. Cine MR images can demonstrate the abnormal flow pattern caused by the aortic coarctation; a signal void originates from the site of the coarctation (see Fig. 9-67). A recent study has shown the capability of a velocity-sensitive cine MRI technique for estimating the gradient across the coarctation.[31]

MRI can be used to distinguish between discrete coarctation or isthmus hypoplasia. The sagittal and LAO-equivalent views usually display the long-segment coarctation. MRI can also define abnormalities associated with coarctation of the aorta, such as dilation of the left subclavian artery and stenosis of the left subclavian artery.

After treatment, MRI can be used to demonstrate the diameter at the site of repair (Figs. 9-69 and 9-70), aortic arch bypass grafts in patients with long-segment coarctation, postoperative mediastinal hematoma, and false aneurysms developing at the site of patch angio-

Figure 9-69. Sagittal image in a patient after repair of coarctation of the aorta. There is a discrete coarctation (*arrow*) in the proximal portion of the descending aorta.

plasty (Fig. 9-71) or caused by balloon angioplasty. Coarctation may be associated with obstruction at other sites, such as the aortic valve and above and below the aortic valve. Although valvular aortic stenosis is not well de-

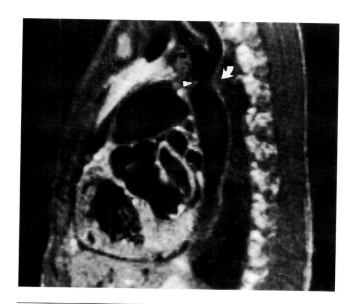

Figure 9-70. Sagittal image in a patient with recurrent coarctation after previous operative repair. Note the ledge (*arrowhead*) of fibrous tissue projecting from the ventral wall into the aortic lumen. There is also a dorsal indentation (*arrow*) of the aorta, which accentuates the coarctation.

fined by MRI, supravalvular (Fig. 9-72) and subvalvular narrowing can be reliably assessed by MRI. The LAO-equivalent view is especially useful for evaluating supravalvular and subvalvular of aortic stenosis. MRI can also show the severity of left ventricular hypertrophy.

Postoperative Evaluation

The various types of cardiovascular operations and the abnormalities in which they are used are described in Table 9-2. A recent study indicated the value of MRI compared with angiography for the evaluation of complex surgical procedures for cyanotic CHD.[15]

MRI has applications for the monitoring of patients after operations for congenital heart disease. These include the attractiveness of performing repeated studies with a technique free of the concerns of radiation exposure or contrast media; the capability for displaying extracardiac anatomy as well as intracardiac anatomy, and the capability of unequivocally demonstrating patency of

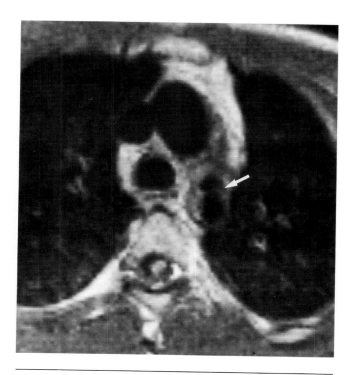

Figure 9-71. Transaxial image through the aorta in a patient with a pseudoaneurysm at the site of the coarctation repair. Note the small ostium (*arrow*) connecting the descending aorta to the pseudoaneurysm.

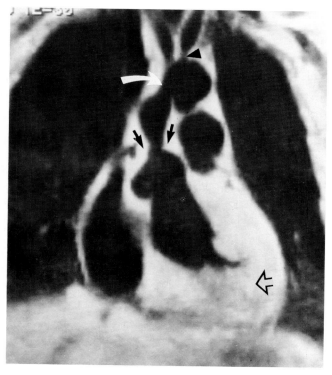

Figure 9-72. Coronal image in a patient with supravalvular aortic stenosis. There is severe stenosis (*arrow*) at the sinotubular junction of the ascending aorta, and in the distal ascending aorta (*curved arrow*). There is also a stenosis at the origin of the left carotid artery (*arrowhead*). There is severe left ventricular hypertrophy (*open arrow*).

Table 9-2

Cardiovascular Surgical Procedures

Name of Procedure	Structural Alterations	Indications
Mustard Senning	Atrial rerouting of venous blood flow	Transposition
Rastelli	Conduit from right ventricle to pulmonary artery(ies)	Pulmonary atresia Severe infundibular stenosis Transposition with pulmonary stenosis
Fontan	Anastomosis of right atrium to pulmonary artery or conduit between the two	Tricuspid atresia Severe tricuspid stenosis Hypoplastic right ventricle, single ventricle
Jatene	Switch in position of great arteries and reanastomosis of coronary arteries	Transposition
Damus	End-to-side anastomosis of proximal main pulmonary artery to the ascending aorta with shunt from aorta to disconnected distal pulmonary artery	Single ventricle of the left ventricular type with transposition and subaortic stenosis. Other complex CHD with subaortic stenosis
Norwood	First stage: end-to-side anastomosis of main pulmonary artery to the ascending aorta; gusset enlargement of aortic arch; graft from aorta to distal pulmonary artery. Second stage: anastomosis of superior vena cava to right pulmonary artery. Third stage: conduit from inferior vena cava to pulmonary artery. Alternative: Fontan procedure instead of second and third stages	Hypoplastic left heart syndrome
Blalock-Taussig shunt	Subclavian to pulmonary artery anastomosis, either directly or by interposition of a tube graft.	Obstruction to pulmonary blood flow; i.e., tetralogy, pulmonary atresia, tricuspid atresia
Waterston (Cooley)	Ascending aorta to right pulmonary artery anastomosis	Obstruction to pulmonary blood flow; i.e., tetralogy, pulmonary atresia, tricuspid atresia
Potts	Descending aorta to left pulmonary artery anastomosis	Obstruction to pulmonary blood flow; i.e., tetralogy, pulmonary atresia, tricuspid atresia
Central shunt	Graft from aorta to pulmonary artery	Obstruction to pulmonary blood flow; i.e., tetralogy, pulmonary atresia, tricuspid atresia
Glenn	Superior vena caval to right pulmonary artery anastomosis. Bidirectional type provides flow to both pulmonary arterial branches	Tricuspid atresia; hypoplastic right ventricle; pulmonary atresia with intact ventricular septum; single ventricle

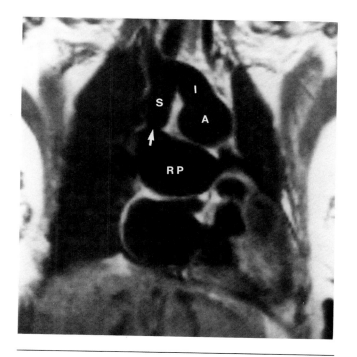

Figure 9-73. Coronal image in a patient with a right subclavian-to-right pulmonary artery anastomosis (*arrow*). Note the aneurysmal dilatation of the right pulmonary artery (RP). (A, aortic arch; I, innominate artery; S, right subclavian artery.)

shunts and the blood flow rate in systemic pulmonary shunts and conduits. The availability of echocardiography and MRI should substantially decrease the use of angiography for the postoperative evaluation of congenital heart disease. The potential advantage of MRI compared with echocardiography in this evaluation is the reliable and nearly unequivocal demonstration of conduits and anastomoses at the level of the great vessel and the quantitative assessment of the dimensions of the central and hilar pulmonary arterial segments.

MRI has been shown to be effective for demonstrating patency of systemic-to-pulmonary shunts (Figs. 9-73 and 9-74).[35] In general these shunts are depicted optimally on transverse images. In some cases a long segment of a graft may be depicted well on the coronal images (Figs. 9-73 and 9-74). The major complications are occlusion, stenosis, pseudoaneurysm of an anastomosis, lymphocele, seroma or chyloma surrounding a graft (see Fig. 9-74), and distortion of the pulmonary artery at the anastomotic site or proximal to it (see Fig. 9-32).

Operations involving supracardiac anastomoses are demonstrated well by MRI (Figs. 9-75 to 9-79).[15,16] The surgical procedures in which MRI has been found to be useful are the Rastelli (see Figs. 9-22 and 9-77) Fontan (see Fig. 9-78), Damus (see Fig. 9-75), Jatene (Fig. 9-79), and Norwood (see Fig. 9-76) procedures. Each of these operations involves grafts or anastomoses performed above the level of the cardiac chambers; consequently MRI is particularly useful. MRI has also been used to as-

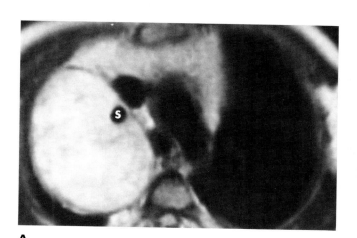

A

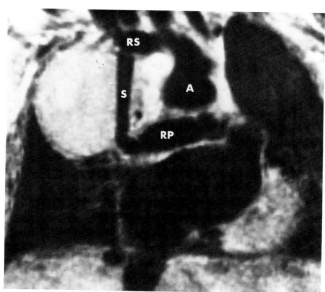

B

Figure 9-74. T$_2$-weighted transaxial (*A*) and coronal (*B*) MR images in a patient with a localized chyloma formed around a right subclavian-to-pulmonary artery shunt. The graft shunt (S) is placed between the right subclavian (RS) and the right pulmonary artery (RP). The localized chyloma has a bright signal intensity on the T$_2$-weighted sequence. (A, ascending aorta.)

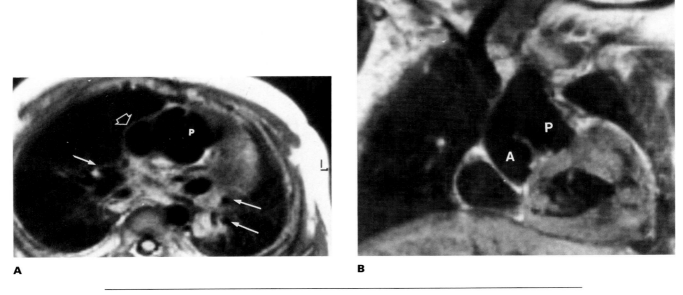

Figure 9-75. Transaxial (*A*) and coronal (*B*) MR images in a patient after the Damus procedure. The anastomosis between the main pulmonary artery and the ascending aorta is demonstrated. (A, ascending aorta; P, pulmonary artery; open arrow, superior vena cava; closed arrows, segmental pulmonary arteries.)

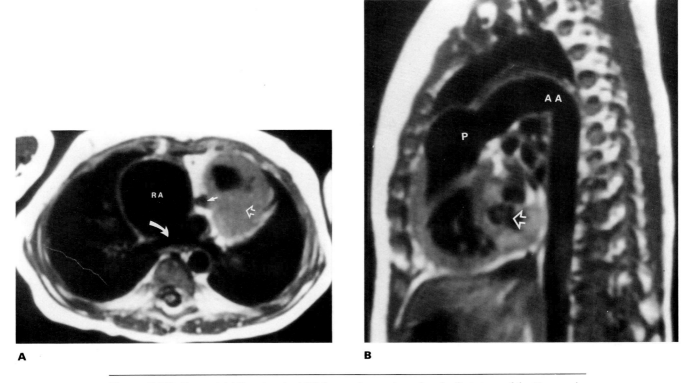

Figure 9-76. Transaxial (*A*) and sagittal (*B*) images in a patient after the first stage of the Norwood procedure for palliation of hypoplastic left heart syndrome. The sagittal image demonstrates the connection of the main pulmonary artery to the aortic arch and continuing into the descending aorta. The transaxial view demonstrates the large interatrial communication (*curved arrow*) connecting the large right atrium to the small left atrium. The left ventricular cavity is nearly completely obliterated by muscle (*open arrow*). The base of the ascending aorta is severely hypoplastic (*small arrow*). (AA, aortic arch; P, pulmonary artery; RA, right atrium.)

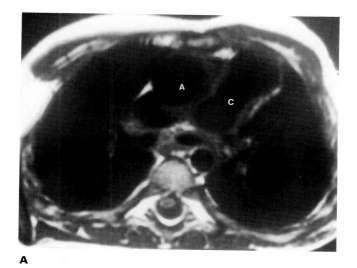

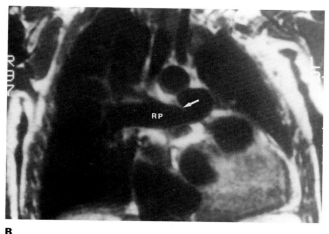

Figure 9-77. Transaxial (*A*) and coronal (*B*) images in a patient with conduit from the right ventricle to the pulmonary artery. Note the focal stenosis within the right pulmonary artery (*arrow*) beyond the anastomosis with the conduit. (A, ascending aorta; C, conduit, RP, right pulmonary artery.)

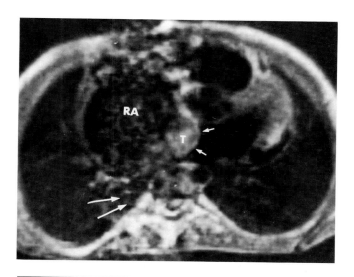

Figure 9-78. Transaxial image in a patient after the Fontan procedure. Note the marked enlargement of the right atrium (RA) and thrombus (T) along the wall of the atrial septum. The atrial septum (*small arrows*) is bowed towards the left atrium, indicating right atrial hypertension. There is compression of the right lower lobe pulmonary vein (*arrows*).

sess intracardiac reconstructions such as the Mustard and Senning procedures, repairs of the right ventricular outflow tract in tetralogy of Fallot, and intraventricular baffles used in the repair of double-outlet ventricles.

In the Rastelli and Fontan procedures, MRI demonstrates the size of the conduit or anastamosis and the size and interval growth of the central pulmonary arteries (Figs. 9-22 and 9-77).[15,16] The Rastelli conduit can be dis-

played along most of its length on sagittal images (see Fig. 9-22). MRI has also displayed the effect of right atrial hypertension in some patients after the Fontan procedure; the right atrium is severely dilated, and the atrial septum markedly bowed into the left atrium, and this bowing sometimes causes obstruction at the entrance of the right pulmonary vein with the left atrium (see Fig. 9-78). In the Norwood and Damus procedures, MRI clearly demonstrates the end-to-side anastomosis between the proximal main pulmonary artery to the ascending aorta and the patency and size of the shunt from the aortic arch or subclavian artery to the distal main pulmonary artery (see Figs. 9-75 and 9-76). The coronal and sagittal imaging planes are usually effective for demonstrating the pulmonary–aortic anastomoses (see Figs. 9-75 and 9-76). The sagittal image is preferred for this purpose and is generally acquired as the initial sequence in the evaluation of patients after the Rastelli, Jatene, and Norwood procedures.

When evaluating the Jatene (arterial switch) procedure, MRI in the transverse and sagittal plane is performed.[15] In these planes there is good visualization of the anastomosis of the aorta with the sinus portion of the pulmonary artery and the anastamosis of the pulmonary artery to the sinus portion of the aorta (see Fig. 9-79). The usual sites of stenoses are at the latter anastomosis or in the right ventricular outflow tract. Transverse MR images have been more effective than echocardiography for demonstrating obstruction of the proximal portion of the right and left pulmonary arteries. The pulmonary arteries are sometimes stretched and compressed as they pass around the proximal ascending aorta after performance of the Jatene procedure (see Fig. 9-79).

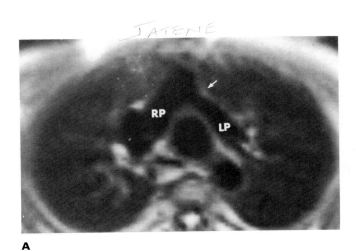

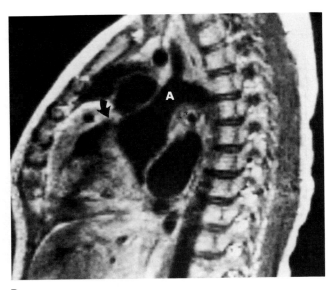

A

B

Figure 9-79. Transaxial (*A*) and sagittal (*B*) images in a patient after the Jatene procedure for correction of transposition of the great arteries. The transaxial images show the right (RP) and left (LP) pulmonary arteries coursing around the ascending aorta. There is a mild stenosis in the proximal portion of the left pulmonary artery (*small arrow*). Sagittal view demonstrates the ascending aorta (A) with a normal caliber and narrowing of the right ventricular outflow region (*black arrow*).

Functional Evaluation in CHD

Quantification of central cardiovascular function is a necessary step in the complete evaluation of CHD. Recent advances have made MRI a comprehensive technique for depicting morphology and measuring ventricular dimensions, mass, and function. Moreover, velocity-sensitive imaging sequences provide measurement of flow velocity and flow volume in the vena cavae, pulmonary veins, pulmonary artery, and aorta.[27,28] Abnormal flow velocities and profiles can be identified using cine MRI; recognition of disturbed flow patterns facilitates the diagnosis of valvular stenosis and regurgitation and the site of cardiovascular shunts (see Figs. 9-2, 9-3, 9-38, 9-67, and 9-80).[2,3,36]

Cine MRI permits the segmentation of the cardiac cycle into multiple time-resolved images. To isolate images corresponding to end diastole and end systole, gradient-echo pulses are performed at a rate that produces 15 to 30 images per cardiac cycle. When such sequences are repeated so that they encompass both ventricles, it is possible to measure the area of the blood volume of the right and left ventricles. Measurements done on the stack of tomograms acquired at end diastole and end systole provide end-diastolic (EDV) and end-systolic (ESV) volumes, stroke volume (SV = EDV − ESV), and ejection fraction (SV/EDV) for both the right and left ventricles.

Studies have indicated that the stroke volumes are equivalent for the right and left ventricles in healthy subjects.[29] SV is greater for one of the ventricles in circumstances of volume overload lesions of a ventricle, such as valvular regurgitation and atrial and arterial level shunts.[3,37] The SV of the left ventricle exceeds that of the right ventricle in aortic and mitral regurgitation; the total regurgitant volume of the left ventricle is the difference in SV of the two ventricles. In tricuspid or pulmonic regurgitation, the SV of the right ventricle exceeds that of the left ventricle in the same manner.

Using volume quantification of the stack of cine MR images it is possible to estimate the volume of some shunt lesions.[3] For VSD and patent ductus arteriosus, the left ventricular SV exceeds the right ventricular SV by an amount equal to the net left-to-right shunt. The right ventricular SV exceeds the left ventricular SV by an amount equal to a left-to-right shunt at the atrial level. The opposite relationship holds for net right-to-left shunts at the various levels. The left ventricular SV equals the right ventricular SV for ventricular septal defects; consequently, this shunt cannot be measured using cine MR volumetrics.

Parameters of global systolic function of the two ventricles are readily derived from the stack of cine MR images. The most useful parameter of global function of

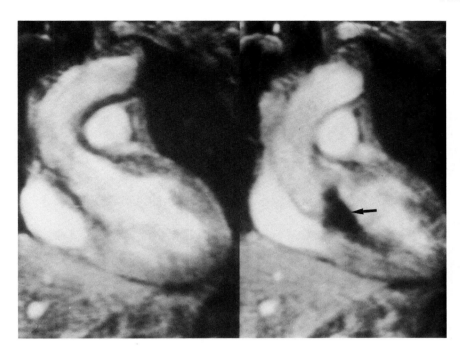

Figure 9-80. Cine MR images in a patient with aortic regurgitation. Image on the left is obtained during systole and the image on the right during diastole. During diastole there is a signal void (arrow) originating at the closed aortic valve and projecting into the left ventricular chamber. The signal void represents the aortic regurgitation.

the ventricle is ejection fraction. Ejection fractions for each ventricle using cine MRI have been established.[29] A study has also shown the reproducibility of volume and functional measurements of the ventricles between sequential studies in patients with normal, hypertrophied, and dilated ventricles.[38,39]

The velocity-encoded cine MRI technique can be used to measure blood flow in the central circulation.[27,28] This technique depends on the phenomenon of a change in the phase of a spin in proportion to its velocity as it moves along (parallel to) a magnetic field gradient. With this technique, magnitude and velocity images are produced for each sequence (see Fig. 9-81). Two imaging sequences are done for each line of the image; the difference in phase of the spins from one sequence to the second sequence is the change in phase angle. This change in phase angle is displayed as a gray scale value on the phase image and also exists as a computer value. Velocity can be calculated using this measured value and other known values, such as the strength of the magnetic gradient. Velocity values for each voxel of the image and a mean instantaneous velocity value for the entire cross-section of the vessel can be measured. Since this is done for each image acquired during the cardiac cycle (usually 16 to 30 images per cycle), it is then possible to integrate these sequential values and provide a measure of mean blood flow velocity per heart beat (Fig. 9-82). The cross-sectional area of the vessel of interest can be measured from the transverse image, and mean blood flow calculated by the formula: mean blood flow = mean velocity × cross-sectional area. These calculations are

optimal when the vessel of interest is interrogated perpendicular to the axis of blood flow.

The phase (velocity) image can discriminate between forward and retrograde blood flow. Regurgitant flow in the pulmonary artery and aorta can be recognized and appropriate accommodation made for it in the volume flow calculation in the great arteries. Left and right ventricular SVs can be measured by integrating the flow values from the multiple images acquired during the cardiac cycle from regions of interest encompassing the proximal aorta and main pulmonary artery.[27] This technique measures the effective forward flow from each ventricle if the aortic or pulmonary values are competent. In the absence of aortic or pulmonary regurgitation, this technique can also be used to measure the volume of shunts. For instance, calculated left ventricular SV exceeds right ventricular SV by a volume equal to the net left-to-right shunt of a patent ductus arteriosus. Conversely, calculated right ventricular SV exceeds left ventricular SV by a volume equal to the net left-to-right shunt of ASD, partial anomalous pulmonary venous connection, and VSD. It should be noted that the volumetric calculations of the ventricles obtained by planimetry of the stack of cine MR images measures the volume of blood pumped by each ventricle (total stroke volume), whereas the velocity-encoded cine MRI technique measures the volume of blood ejected from the ventricles into the great arteries (effective stroke volume). Consequently, the formulas used to calculate the shunts at various sites are different for the two techniques (Table 9-2).

With velocity-encoded cine MRI, blood flow can be

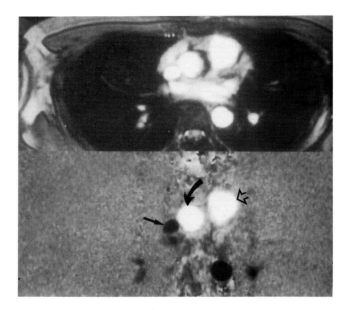

Figure 9-81. Magnitude (*upper panel*) and phase (*lower panel*) images through the region of the great vessels. The phase image indicates that only regions within the image with blood flow are visible. Each pixel within the blood vessel provides a measurement of velocity at that site. Note that the direction of blood flow is indicated by the reverse polarity in the superior vena cava (*arrow*) and descending aorta compared with the ascending aorta (*curved arrow*) and pulmonary artery (*open arrow*).

measured in the right or left pulmonary artery as well as the main pulmonary artery. Thus, this technique serves as one of the only techniques to quantitate flow separately in the right and left pulmonary arteries. A study in healthy volunteers has verified that the sum of the flow measured in the right and left pulmonary arteries is equal to the flow measured in the main pulmonary artery (Fig. 9-83).[40] The application of flow measurements in CHD are many. For instance, this technique can estimate the gradient across stenotic valves and correction by measuring the peak velocity of the stenotic jet flow. Future work will probably indicate numerous uses of this technique for the comprehensive evaluation of CHD.

Acknowledgment. Portions of the text in this chapter and many of the illustrations have been used with permission from *Magnetic Resonance Imaging of the Body,* 2nd edition, Higgins CB, Hricak H, eds., published by Raven Press, Ltd., New York, 1991.

References

1. Didier D, Higgins CB, Fisher M, Osaki L, Silverman N, Cheitlin M. Congenital heart disease: gated MR imaging in 72 patients. Radiology 1986;158:227.
2. Sechtem U, Pflugfelder PW, White RD, et al. Cine MRI: potential for the evaluation of cardiovascular function. AJR 1987;148:239.

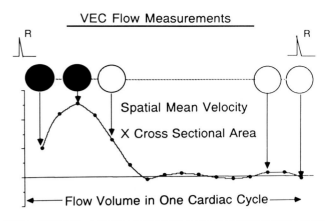

Figure 9-82. Diagram demonstrating a velocity-versus-time curve for blood flow within the pulmonary artery. The diagram demonstrates the images of the blood vessel (*arrow*) at each of the phases during the cardiac cycle, extending from one R wave to another. Each point on the curve represents the mean blood flow within the artery at a phase of the cardiac cycle. Each value is derived from a separate velocity-encoded cine MR image. The blood flow is a product of the spatial mean velocity times the cross-sectional area of the vessel.

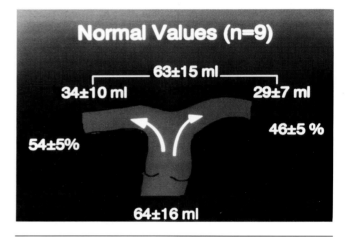

Figure 9-83. Diagram demonstrating the values for right and left pulmonary blood flow as well as total blood flow in the main pulmonary artery as measured by the velocity-encoded cine MR technique. These values were obtained from nine healthy volunteers. Notice that the sum of blood flow in the right and left pulmonary arteries equals 63 ml and compares closely with the 64 ml measured in the main pulmonary artery. The blood flow in the right pulmonary artery is slightly higher than that in the left pulmonary artery.

3. Sechtem U, Pflugfelder P, Cassidy MC, Holt W, Wolfe C, Higgins CB. Ventricular septal defect: visualization of shunt flow and determination of shunt size by cine magnetic resonance imaging. AJR 1987;149:689.
4. Anderson RH, Ho SY. The tomographic anatomy of the normal and malformed heart. In: Tomographic imaging of congenital heart disease: echocardiography and magnetic resonance imaging, 1st ed. New York: Raven Press, 1990, ch. 1.
5. Didier D, Higgins CB. Identification and localization of ventric-

ular septal defects by gated magnetic resonance imaging. Am J Cardiol 1986;57:1363.

6. Higgins CB, Silverman N, Kersting–Sommerhoff B, Schmidt K. Congenital heart disease: echocardiography and MRI. New York: Raven Press, 1990.

7. Kersting–Sommerhoff BA, Diethelm L, Teitel DF, et al. Magnetic resonance imaging of congenital heart disease: sensitivity and specificity using receiver operating characteristic curve analysis. Am Heart J 1989;118:155.

8. Higgins CB, Byrd BF III, Farmer D, Silverman N, Cheitlin M. Magnetic resonance imaging in patients with congenital heart disease. Circulation 1984;70:851.

9. Guit GL, Bluemm R, Rohmer J, et al. Levotransposition of the aorta: identification of segmental cardiac anatomy using MR imaging. Radiology 1986;161:673.

10. Mayo JR, Roberson D, Sommerhoff B, Higgins CB. MRI of double outlet right ventricle. J Comput Assist Tomogr 1990;14:336.

11. Mirowitz SA, Gutierrez FR, Canter CE, Vannier MW. Tetralogy of Fallot: MR findings. Radiology 1989;171:207.

12. Kersting–Sommerhoff BA, Sechtem U, Higgins CB. Evaluation of pulmonary blood supply by nuclear magnetic resonance imaging in patients with pulmonary atresia. J Am Coll Cardiol 1988; 11:166.

13. Gomes AS, Lois JF, Williams RG. Pulmonary arteries: MR imaging in patients with congenital obstruction of the right ventricular outflow tract. Radiology 1990;174:51.

14. Chung KJ, Simpson IA, Glass RF, Sahn DJ, Hesselink JR. Cine magnetic resonance imaging after surgical repair in patients with transposition of the great arteries. Circulation 1988;77: 104.

15. Kersting–Sommerhoff BA, Seelos KC, Hardy C, Kondo C, Higgins SS, Higgins CB. Evaluation of surgical procedures for cyanotic congenital heart disease using MR imaging. AJR 1990;155:259.

16. Julsrud PR, Ehman RL, Hagler DJ, Ilstrup DM. Extracardiac vasculature in candidates for Fontan surgery: MR imaging. Radiology 1989;173:503.

17. Jacobstein MD, Fletcher BD, Goldstein S, Riemenschneider TA. Evaluation of atrioventricular septal defect by magnetic resonance imaging. Am J Cardiol 1985;55:1158.

18. Kersting–Sommerhoff BA, Diethelm L, Stanger P, et al. Evaluation of complex congenital ventricular anomalies with magnetic resonance imaging. Am Heart J 1990.

19. Peshock RM, Parrish M, Fixler D, Parkey RW. Magnetic resonance imaging of single ventricle. Circulation (Suppl III)1985;72:III29.

20. Jacobstein MD, Portman MA, Fletcher BD. Magnetic resonance imaging in univentricular atrioventricular connection. Am J Cardiac Imaging 1987;1:221.

21. Link KM, Herrera MA, D'Souza VJ, Formanek AG. MR imaging of Ebstein anomaly: results in four cases. AJR 1988;150:363.

22. Diethelm L, Dery R, Lipton MJ, Higgins CB. Atrial level shunts: sensitivity and specificity of MR in diagnosis. Radiology 1987; 162:181.

23. Dinsmore RE, Wismer GL, Guyer D, et al. Magnetic resonance imaging of the interatrial septum and atrial septal defects. AJR 1985;145:697.

24. Lowell DG, Turner DA, Smith SM, et al. The detection of atrial and ventricular septal defects by gated MRI. Circulation 1986; 73:89.

25. Seelos KC, Masui T, Kersting–Sommerhoff BA, Higgins CB. Depiction of anomalies of the pulmonary venous return by means of MR imaging, angiography, and echocardiography. Radiology 1990;177P:99.

26. Fisher MR, Hricak H, Higgins CB. Magnetic resonance imaging of developmental venous anomalies. AJR 1985;145:705.

27. Kondo C, Caputo GR, Semelka R, Foster E, Shimakawa S, Higgins CB. Right and left ventricular stroke volume measurements with velocity encoded cine NMR imaging: in vitro and in vivo validation. AJR 1991 (in press).

28. Nayler GL, Fermin DN, Congmore DB. Blood flow imaging by cine MR. J Comput Assist Tomogr 1986;10:715.

29. Sechtem U, Pflugfelder PW, Gould RG, Cassidy MM, Higgins CB. Measurement of right and left ventricular volumes in healthy individuals with cine MR imaging. Radiology 1987;163:697.

30. von Schulthess GK, Higashino SM, Higgins SS, Didier D, Fisher MR, Higgins CB. Coarctation of the aorta: MR imaging. Radiology 1986;158:469.

31. Rees S, Somerville J, Warad C, et al. Coarctation of the aorta: MR imaging in late postoperative assessment. Radiology 1989; 173:499.

32. Bisset GS III, Strife JL, Kirks DR, Bailey WW. Vascular rings: MR imaging. AJR 1987;149:251.

33. Kersting–Sommerhoff BA, Sechtem UP, Fisher MR, Higgins CB. MR imaging of congenital anomalies of the aortic arch. AJR 1987;149:9.

34. Sommerhoff BA, Sechtem UP, Schiller NB, Lipton MJ, Higgins CB. MRI of the thoracic aorta in Marfan patients. J Comput Assist Tomogr 1987;11:633.

35. Jacobstein MD, Fletcher BD, Nelson AD, et al. Magnetic resonance imaging: evaluation of palliative systemic-pulmonary artery shunts. Circulation 1984;70:650.

36. Wagner S, Auffermann W, Buser P, et al. Diagnostic accuracy and estimation of the severity of valvular regurgitation from the signal void on cine MR. Am Heart J 1989;118:760.

37. Sechtem U, Pflugfelder PW, Cassidy MM, et al. Mitral or aortic regurgitation: quantification of regurgitant volumes with cine MR imaging. Radiology 1988;167:425.

38. Semelka RC, Tomei E, Wagner S, et al. Normal left ventricular dimensions and function: interstudy reproducibility of measurements with cine MR imaging. Radiology 1990;174:763.

39. Semelka RC, Tomei E, Wagner S, et al. Interstudy reproducibility of dimensional and functional measurements between cine magnetic resonance studies in the morphologically abnormal left ventricle. Am Heart J 1990;119:1367.

40. Caputo GR, Kondo C, Masui T, et al. Determination of right and left lung perfusion with oblique angle velocity encoded cine MR imaging: in vitro and in vivo validation. Radiology 1991 (in press).

Chapter 10

Nuclear Imaging of Acquired Heart Disease

Elias H. Botvinick

Michael W. Dae

J. William O'Connell

Douglas A. Ortendahl

Robert S. Hattner

The last 15 years have seen a revolution in noninvasive cardiac imaging techniques. Scintigraphic methods have been applied widely, impacting on the diagnosis and care of all forms of cardiac illness.[1–4] They are safe, have been adopted by the cardiologist, and integrated into the cardiac evaluation. An appreciation of the technical and physical aspects of the method is critical if it is to be employed appropriately and to the best advantage of the patient, however.[1–8]

Scintigraphy is a tracer technique. A radioactive substance, a radionuclide, physically unstable as it emits an energetic particle, is used to label a pharmaceutical or is itself administered intravenously and detected within the patient. Localization within the subject depends on the physiologic characteristics of the radiopharmaceutical. The pharmaceutical is nonallergenic, and it is given in small tracer amounts that have no effect on the process it seeks to characterize. The label allows the body and organ pharmaceutical distribution to be determined using a radioactivity detector, generally a component of the scintillation camera. Cardiac scinitgraphy is successful because of the ability of modern cameras to map tracer distribution accurately and computers to analyze this distribution.

The Method and Its Technology

The Radionuclide

The choice of radionuclide is based on a consideration of the particle emitted; its energy level; its half-life, both physical and biologic; and its labeling and localizing properties (Table 10-1). For imaging applications, gamma rays or x-rays in the energy range 70 to 250 keV are preferred. Lower energies are easily attenuated and have difficulty penetrating human tissue, whereas higher energies may be too penetrant to permit proper registration and can be accommodated only with reduced image quality. Gamma rays and x-rays are forms of electromagnetic radiation or photons. The former are the result of a nuclear interaction; the latter are due to atomic interactions. Other emissions, particularly charged particles, have reduced penetration and often deliver prohibitive radiation doses. Characteristic whole-body doses for clinical tests range from 100 to 300 mrad, roughly equivalent to two sets of posteroanterior and lateral chest x-ray films, or to a flat and upright x-ray film of the abdomen. Best not performed during pregnancy and with reduced pediatric dosage, the application should be based on the

Table 10-1

Physical Properties of Radionuclides Commonly Used in Cardiac Evaluation

Radionuclide	Physical Half-Life	Principal Photon(s)
^{11}C	20.5 min	511
^{127}Cs	6.2 hr	125,411
^{129}Cs	32 hr	375,411
^{18}F	110 min	511
^{67}Ga	3.3 days	93,185,300
^{111}In	2.8 days	172,247
^{43}K	22.2 hr	373,618
^{81m}Kr	13 sec	190
^{15}O	2 min	511
^{13}N	10 min	511
^{82}Rb	75 sec	511
^{99}Tc	6 hr	140
^{127}Xe	36 days	172,203,375
^{133}Xe	5.3 days	81
^{201}Tl	73 hr	69,083,167

Absorbed Total Body Radiation Dose for Commonly Used Radiopharmaceuticals

Radiopharmaceutical	rad/mCi
^{99m}Tc pyrophosphate	0.013
^{99m}Tc-labeled red cells	0.017
^{99m}Tc DTPA	0.016
^{99m}Tc pertechnetate	0.014
Tc-MAA	0.015
^{201}Tl	0.24
^{133}Xe	0.0009–0.0018 (single breath)
	0.0011 (5 min. rebreathing)

Data from Freeman LM, ed. Freeman and Johnson's clinical radionuclide imaging. 3rd ed. Orlando, FL, Grune & Stratton, 1984.

overall clinical cost-to-benefit ratio. Technetium 99m, the most commonly used isotope, emits a gamma ray at 140 keV, near optimal for imaging purposes, while thallium (Tl) 201, used for cardiac perfusion studies, decays by electron capture to mercury (Hg) 201, which emits x-rays in the range of 80 keV used for imaging. ^{201}Tl is cyclotron produced, has a long, 73-hour physical half-life and a significantly longer biologic half-life, whereas the short, 6-hour physical half-life of ^{99m}Tc better suits patient evaluation and is conveniently eluted from a molybdenum-99 generator, which can be replaced weekly. Although not optimal for first-pass applications, this duration does permit more prolonged imaging studies. Most other imaging radionuclides, including many of those used for positron emission tomography, are short-lived and cyclotron-produced.

The Imaging Device

Although a variety of radioisotope detectors have been used, the material of choice remains sodium iodide.[1,5] The interaction of a high-energy particle, such as x-rays or gamma rays, with the sodium iodide crystal, a scintil-lator, causes the emission of light, which is detected and amplified by a photomultiplier tube. The magnitude of the photomultiplier signal depends on the amount of energy deposited in the scintillator and is proportional to the number and energy of incident photons. Relative signal strength and location of each tube determine the energy and spatial coordinates of the incident photon.

Scintillation Camera. Valuable information regarding regional ventricular function requires an imaging detector such as the scintillation, Anger, or gamma camera. It consists of a larger sodium iodide crystal, at least 25 cm in diameter and 6 to 9 mm thick, and a bank of closely arrayed photomultiplier tubes. Sophisticated electronic circuitry senses the signal at each tube and assigns a position on the face of the crystal, localizing the point of gamma-crystal interaction. The scintillation camera analyzes a random serial sample of target radioactivity and can be set to sample regional radioactivity in brief temporal intervals. This permits the analysis and display of dynamic events. To ensure the relationship between the origin of the emitting isotope within the patient and the perceived location on the camera face, the direction of the gamma ray, constrained by means of the collimator, must be known.

Camera Collimation. The simplest design is the pinhole collimator, which spreads emissions from a small aperture over the camera face. For small, superficial organs, such as the thyroid, this is advantageous, magnifying the image and improving its spatial resolution. Sensitivity varies with depth, however, creating problems when evaluating the large, deep heart, where it has been applied to perfusion scintigraphy in adults. Pinhole and converging collimators are useful for cardiac imaging in the small pediatric patient.

The parallel hole collimator is most commonly used for cardiac applications. It constrains detected photons to travel down the length of holes that are spread uniformly over the camera face. The longer the holes and the smaller their diameter, the better will be the resultant spatial resolution. The high-resolution collimator, often used for equilibrium blood pool studies and now recommended for imaging ^{99m}Tc sestaMIBI, presents the most extreme example of collimator selectivity. Since this configuration rejects more photons, sensitivity is reduced, increasing the time of image acquisition. The high sensitivity is the least selective parallel hole collimator. It has advantages for use with temporally dependent studies such as first-pass blood pool and planar perfusion imaging, increasing photon acceptance and reducing imaging time. A price is paid in reduced spatial resolution, however. Because of its rapid myocardial clearance, the high sensitivity collimator may be required to image ^{99m}Tc teboroxime, another new myocardial perfusion agent.

The optimal trade-off between resolution and sensitivity will depend on the particular application. For many cardiac applications, the low-energy, all-purpose (LEAP) collimator is used. Alternatively, the parallel slant-hole collimator can be used with intermediate sensitivity and spatial resolution.

Tomography

Single Photon Tomographic Methods

Limited Angle Techniques. Important information may be obscured by superimposed activity using planar imaging. This may be ameliorated in part with the acquisition of multiple projections. Spatial integration may be computerized if the relationships between projections are known, yielding tomographic images. The seven-pinhole method projects seven images of the heart onto a large-field camera face through seven holes drilled centrally into a pinhole collimator.[6] Each aperture is separated by a lead septum to prevent image overlap. The rotating slant-hole method employs a slant-hole collimator with holes tilted at 20° or 30° from the normal.[7] By rotating the collimator 60° between acquisitions, six distinct images are obtained in a given projection. In both cases, multiple projections taken at different well-defined angles with respect to the target are processed using an algebraic reconstruction technique, yielding tomographic sections at different depths. Owing to their limited angular sampling, however, such reconstructions are susceptible to artifacts and do not reliably permit quantitative measurement. Although there is sufficient sampling for gross tomographic evaluation, sampling is insufficient to provide a mathematically closed solution.

Single Photon Emission Computed Tomography. Single photon emission computed tomography (SPECT) employs a camera rotating on a gantry to solve these problems.[8] Data acquired over 180° or 360° are reconstructed using standard algorithms developed for x-ray computed tomography.[9,10] One unique problem of the scintigraphic method that must be addressed is that of attenuation, producing undersampling of deep organs. Algorithms to deal with this problem are not completely satisfactory. Emission computed tomography of ^{201}Tl perfusion images applies only 180° rotation, since the posterior projections show severe attenuation of the 70 keV photons.

With cardiac scintigraphy, SPECT has been most widely applied to perfusion imaging with ^{201}Tl. Although quality control of planar perfusion scintigraphy is important, these factors become absolutely critical in relation to computer-enhanced images as SPECT studies. Issues related to image acquisition, processing, and display are

all important. Field homogeneity, center of rotation, the applied smoothing algorithm, and frequency cutoff must be carefully scrutinized. Furthermore, identical angulation and appropriate comparison of postintervention and delayed images, as well as careful avoidance or recognition of movement artifact with appropriate methods of intensity setting and display, must be provided to avoid major pitfalls in image interpretation and take full advantage of the SPECT method.[11-13] Issues of soft tissue attenuation, prominent with thallium imaging, especially in women, are somewhat improved but continue to be a source of concern in SPECT imaging. Also, diaphragmatic attenuation has been a problem in some cases, which may be aided by prone rather than supine imaging.[14]

A radionuclide body surface marker, imaged with the heart during SPECT acquisition, serves as an excellent method to detect patient motion; however, such detection does not generally permit reprocessing with removal of resultant image artifacts. The best way to deal with motion is to avoid it and if a patient cannot or will not lie still for the required 20 to 30 minute imaging period, planar images should be acquired. One or two planar images directly preceding SPECT acquisition provide important data regarding lung uptake, cavitary dilation, and basal uptake. They also demonstrate the distribution of soft tissue attenuation, provide information regarding inferior wall uptake, and present gross corroboration of defects seen in SPECT but may be artifactual in origin. Scrupulous attention to the 32 planar projection images applied to SPECT reconstruction provides another tool to assess findings in the final SPECT product.

Unlike other tomographic imaging methods as echocardiography, computed tomography, or magnetic resonance imaging, SPECT presents image sections in relation to the cardiac, not the body, axis. Generally, oblique or short-axis images, orthogonal to the left-axis sections, are produced from the data set and presented. The volume of data calls for an organized presentation and experience in image orientation. Methods of three-dimension reconstruction and display are now under investigation to condense the data and potentially optimize image assessment.

Beyond planar methods, SPECT permits recognition and assessment of regional perfusion without contamination of overlying structures. The anterior and posterior septum are well separated and, with proper attention to technical factors and interpretive pitfalls, image interpretation is more easily and more accurately learned. This is true in spite of comparative studies in the literature, demonstrating only an increased sensitivity of SPECT diagnosis for circumflex lesions involving the lateral left ventricular wall.[15,16] Although perfusion imaging can certainly be performed by planar methods, SPECT is optimal. The new technetium-based agent sestaMIBI will possibly require SPECT imaging to avoid obscuring defects by the more penetrant photons of the higher energy radionuclide in the opposite wall.[17] Although gated SPECT imaging of blood pool studies presents potential advantages for ventricular function analysis, it has been lightly applied because of the duration of acquisition and processing. Gated SPECT imaging of technetium-based perfusion agents with a long myocardial residence time promise to provide in a single imaging study objective, quantitative, and reproducible evaluation of regional myocardial perfusion *and* function, however.[18,19] Triple-headed rotating cameras have been developed to speed SPECT acquisition.

Positron Emission Tomography. Positron emission tomography (PET) is another tomographic scintigraphic modality.[10,20-21] The positron emitted in positron decay interacts with an electron, quickly annihilating both particles to produce two 511 keV photons, which travel at 180° to one another. By detecting each of these photons, the event is constrained to lie on the line between the two points. The reconstruction, determining the depth of origin, can then be performed using algorithms similar to those used in emission computed tomography or computed tomography, yielding highly resolved transaxial images of the target organ. PET requires completely new hardware compared with other scintigraphic studies. The high-energy 511 keV photons require a 2.5 cm crystal thickness and make the standard scintillation camera unsuitable for use because of its poor detection efficiency. The latter is an important issue in PET because both photons must be detected, making sensitivity proportional to the square of detection efficiency. Conversely, each of the detectors will see a large number of noncoincident events that can be automatically discounted, a kind of internal collimation. PET imaging strategy uses multiple individual detectors arranged in a ring about the patient, where components link detectors on opposite sides. This instrument provides a single cross-section or slice. If additional simultaneous sections are desired, then additional rings must be added, increasing the cost. Increased efficiency is obtained with a high-density detector such as bismuth germanate.[20] Another detection strategy employs time of flight information to improve spatial resolution.[21] Since annihilation photons are emitted simultaneously, the time to each detector could localize the event along the line. Currently fast scintillators, such as cesium fluoride, give timing resolution of 600 picoseconds and can localize the event to within 9 mm. In combination with the reconstruction algorithm, this constraint on position can lead to even better resolution, approaching 9 mm in some new devices. These faster detectors have poorer detection efficiency, however, and again, one must sacrifice total counts for better localizing information. It is not clear at this point which technology will prevail. PET imaging attracts special in-

terest owing to the biologically active nature of many of the positron-emitting radionuclides. They are generally cyclotron produced, however, their short half-life acts as both an advantage and a detriment, and they require, as shown, new expensive technology.

Computers in Cardiac Scintigraphy

Commercial equipment is widely available with much prepackaged software; however, the proper application and further development of these methods depend on an understanding of computer operations by physicians both generating and applying study results.

Computer applications represent a great advantage of the scintigraphic method, permitting objective, quantitative calculation of parameters measured only with difficulty by other methods or in no other way. The computer has several functions involved in the collection and storage of the study, requiring an interface to the camera and considerable mass storage. The analog data of the imaging device are easily digitized, making processing possible by microcomputers or minicomputers. The operating system provides overall control of acquisition, analysis, and display functions. Acquisition software should be adaptable, permitting the selective choice of study parameters. Analysis should be performed by programs designed to generate specific required data. Display software selects the display matrix dimension and makes the data accessible to video monitors as well as hard copy. Programs to enhance contrast and perform quantitative analysis of images should be available.[22-24] SPECT camera and software are important and the full range of computer capabilities to acquire, process, and display blood pool and other functional and dynamic data is necessary for full capability.

Myocardial Perfusion Scintigraphy

Myocardial perfusion scintigraphy seeks to characterize relative myocardial perfusion noninvasively.[25-27] It is among the most widely used and clinically valuable cardiac scintigraphic studies.

The Radionuclide

Previously, potassium (K) 43 or rubidium (Rb) 81 were used.[26,27] The current methodology employs thallium-201. Each of these is an intracellular cation that is extracted rapidly after its intravenous administration, distributing intracellularly in proportion to relative myocardial perfusion.[28,29] Behaving and localizing like native body potassium, their proper intracellular localization serves also as a strong indicator of myocardial viability (Table 10-2).[3,28] These agents are not myocardial specific, but localize, according to similar kinetics, in cells of all parenchymal tissues.[27,30,31]

Except for the small radiation dose, ^{201}Tl is entirely innocuous in the imaging dose administered. It is superior to other agents in some respects, owing to its longer half-life and the lower energy of emission; but it is imperfect, as the former is too long and the latter is too low for optimal image applications. Because of its rapid blood clearance, approximately 80% on the first pass, and the finite period of its intracellular localization, ^{201}Tl can be administered during a short-lived intervention and imaged shortly thereafter to reflect the distribution of perfusion at the time of administration.[30–32]

Except in the presence of severe obstruction, compensatory coronary arteriolar dilation or collateral perfusion permits relatively normal flow at rest through even significantly stenotic vessels. Most patients with coronary disease are asymptomatic at rest. As coronary flow demands increase with stress, however, compensation is insufficient and supply is limited. The inability to provide the full flow demands of stress represents insufficient flow reserve and is itself the pathophysiologic definition of a significant coronary stenosis. However, beds supplied by nonstenotic or minimally stenotic vessels augment regional perfusion in relation to demands (Fig. 10-1).[33] If ^{201}Tl is administered during such stress-induced regional heterogeneity, it will distribute in this heterogeneous pattern. Recognition of regions of reduced relative perfusion indicates an abnormality in the related coronary supply.

Thallium appears to gain cellular entry as does potassium, via membrane Na[+]/K[+] ATPase.[34] Yt is seems relatively stable once inside. Subsequent to its localization, regional intracellular ^{201}Tl follows its gradient with the blood. Those areas with most radioactivity lose thallium most rapidly. Reappearance in the blood is followed by cellular uptake in the resting distribution. In this way, myocardial regions slowly come to equilibrium with attainment of the baseline perfusion pattern.[35,36] The regional ratio, initial radioactivity-delayed radioactivity/initial radioactivity, background and time corrected, comprises the parameter of percent washout, an established objective measure of regional perfusion (Fig 10-2).[3,24,37] Relatively underperfused regions seen on immediate poststress imaging, which become less apparent or "fill in," are viable and indicate stress-induced regional myocardial ischemia. If defects remain "fixed" on delayed imaging, they are, in most cases, related to irreversible infarction and scar.[36] Partial redistribution with a mixture of fixed and improving abnormalities indicates elements of both ischemia and infarction, a common clinical substrate.

Table 10-2

Scintigraphic Methods

For Assessment of Myocardial Viability and Functional Reversibility

1. Reversible perfusion abnormalities using [201]T1 or other indicator
2. Delayed redistribution on [201]T1 perfusion imaging
3. Normal wall motion in the presence of apparently fixed perfusion defect
4. Abnormal wall motion in the presence of apparently normal perfusion
5. Normalized or improved wall motion after nitroglycerin

For Identification of Significant Myocardium at Ischemic Risk and Poor Prognosis

1. Impressive reversible perfusion defect
2. Relatively mild perfusion defect at a low level of stress or in the presence of extensive fixed defects
3. In patients with prior infarction-perfusion defect in the distribution of a noninfarcted vessel (outside the infarct zone)
4. In the presence of ischemic heart disease—stress-induced lung uptake, "cavitary dilation," basal uptake on [201]T1 imaging
5. In the presence of stress-induced heart rate over 85% predicted for age—extensive washout abnormalities
6. Heterogeneity of washout in association with low achieved double product or dipyridamole infusion
7. Extensive washout in association with minor reversible perfusion defects at a low double product*
8. Preserved LVEF at rest in a patient with a history of recurrent pulmonary edema
9. Extensive stress-induced wall motion abnormalities
10. Extensive stress-induced reduction in LVEF

Possible but not yet firmly established.

The Method

Dynamic Stress Perfusion Scintigraphy. In practice, the study is performed in association with a standard stress test, generally performed on a treadmill.[38] Patients are studied in the fasting state. The stress test is conducted according to the standard method with the placement of an intravenous line to ensure accessibility during peak exercise. Symptoms, signs, blood pressure, and electrocardiogram are monitored as testing proceeds to the clinically indicated end point. The patient informs the physician of any symptoms, especially those that may limit testing. Thirty seconds to 1 minute before the symptom, sign, or heart rate limited stress end point, 2 mCi of ^{201}Tl is injected through the intravenous line. A saline flush is used to clear the line as stress continues for another minute. The line is preferably placed away from joints, and the agent is administered quickly, but gently, during tension-free full arm extension to avoid back pressure and potential extravasation with infiltration or area contamination.

Full monitoring is again performed in recovery, as the scintigraphic information serves to complement the

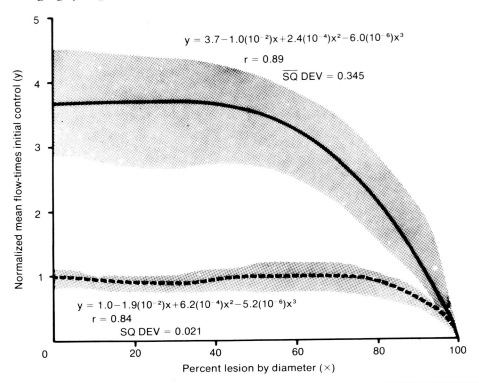

$$y = 3.7 - 1.0(10^{-2})x + 2.4(10^{-4})x^2 - 6.0(10^{-6})x^3$$

$$r = 0.89$$

$$\overline{SQ}\ DEV = 0.345$$

$$y = 1.0 - 1.9(10^{-2})x + 6.2(10^{-4})x^2 - 5.2(10^{-6})x^3$$

$$r = 0.84$$

$$SQ\ DEV = 0.021$$

Figure 10-1. Coronary flow at rest and at stress. Coronary flow is measured at rest (*dotted line*) and at stress (*solid line*). Normal flow is maintained by coronary dilation at rest up to subtotal stenosis. With stress, here provided by the dilation related to intracoronary contrast infusion, flow augmentation is submaximal in relation to coronary stenosis of about 70%, defining a critical coronary lesion. Such a loss of coronary flow reserve results in regional flow heterogeneity. When ^{201}Tl is administered under such circumstances, heterogeneity of radionuclide distribution produces "cold" areas and permits regional noninvasive definition of perfusion abnormalities. (Reproduced with permission from Gould KL, Lipscomb K, Hamilton GW. Physiologic basis for assessing critical coronary stenosis: instantaneous flow response and regional distribution during coronary hyperemia as measures of coronary flow reserve. Am J Cardiol 1974;33:87.)

results of stress testing, not replace it. Monitoring during imaging is generally impractical. Since image data are temporally dependent, imaging is begun as soon as possible. Thus, recovery is monitored for 7 minutes to capture pertinent ST or arrhythmic abnormalities not seen during stress.[39] Imaging in multiple planar projections or using tomographic methods begins immediately on termination of monitoring, within 10 minutes of radionuclide administration, barring serious arrhythmias, hypotension, or other problems.[38,40] ST changes are not a reason to delay imaging but rather may, in fact, indicate its need. If necessary, an electrocardiogram is performed after imaging, which can confirm return to baseline. Antianginal medications can be administered after ^{201}Tl localization without influencing its distribution or test results.[3] Imaging is repeated after "redistribution," approximately 4 hours later.

Reinjection Technique. Numerous studies of thallium perfusion scintigraphy have documented an overestimation of irreversible infarction in myocardial re-

gions proven to be viable by related function, serially improving function, or perfusion.[41] A better estimation of the full extent and distribution of viable myocardium was demonstrated possible with delayed, 24-hour thallium imaging.[42] This difficulty in the identification of viable myocardium by conventional scintigraphic methods has demonstrated superiority over even 24-hour imaging.

Budinger and coworkers have demonstrated that an obvious reason for the lack of redistribution in viable myocardium relates to the unavailability of the agent in the perfusing blood. This adverse effect is enhanced by eating soon before imaging, even 24-hour imaging. Recent work by Dilsiziam and associates and Bonow and coworkers demonstrated the value of a second administered thallium dose before delayed 4-hour imaging.[44,45] This *reinjection* method has demonstrated an enhanced ability to identify viable myocardium, essentially equivalent to PET metabolic image evaluation.[46]

Image Acquisition. Both planar and tomographic methods are acceptable.[24,38,40] For the former, a state-of-

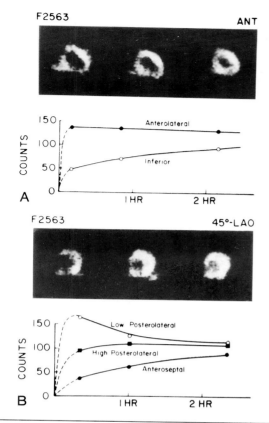

Figure 10-2. Myocardial washout of ²⁰¹Tl. Shown are perfusion images acquired serially over the course of 2 hours after stress administration of ²⁰¹Tl in anterior (*A*) and left anterior oblique (*B*) projections. Normal regions lose radioactivity rapidly, while visually abnormal regions show flat or upsloping curves of serial regional radioactivity. Other regions, as the high posterolateral wall in the LAO projection, may appear visually normal, yet their true relation to abnormal perfusion is exposed by the generation of an abnormal (flat) washout curve. (Reproduced by permission of the Society of Nuclear Medicine from Campbell NP, et al. Spatial and temporal quantitation of planar thallium myocardial images. J Nucl Med 1981;22:577.)

coronal, or horizontal, and a sagittal or vertical long-axis projection.

Image Processing. Visual recognition on analog images requires gross regional perfusion differences,[4,5] whereas computer enhancement increases defect recognition and test sensitivity.[48,49] Computer enhancement to "correct" for background is necessary for planar image interpretation. Tomographic images are less influenced by background and, by nature, are computer processed. The method is not immune to artifacts, however, and may not be performed in large or uncooperative patients. Processing enhances image heterogeneity and makes subtle image perfusion defects more obvious.[3,24,37,47,50] This may also result in reduced specificity,[49,51] and does not resolve problems related to soft tissue attenuation, most commonly the female breast, probably the most common cause of false positive readings.[51] Although tomography helps resolve this difficulty, reduced radioactivity is even seen in tomographic slices underlying the breast.[51,52]

Reduced radioactivity in the normal image relates to the ventricular base, the valve planes, membranous septum and apex, and myocardial regions with reduced mass.[29,50,51] Cardiac rotation adds to the variability (Fig. 10-3). To objectify image interpretation, circumferential profiles of the distribution of peak counts along multiple radii subtended from background subtracted poststress images have been made in populations of healthy patients.[24] Normalized to peak counts and plotted graphically in each projection, these normal values are best calculated for images rotated to a similar angulation relative to their long axis.

Similar count profiles in redistribution images, expressed in absolute counts, are compared with absolute peak radial values in each projection of the immediate

the-art scintillation camera should acquire at least anterior and two left anterior oblique projections. The initial poststress projection is acquired to optimal counts, and other poststress and redistribution images are obtained to isotime at fixed intensity to permit assessment of changes in regional radioactivity over time. A LEAP collimator is most often employed because a high-resolution device adds to acquisition time. A high-sensitivity collimator decreases imaging time, permitting rapid acquisition at a small cost to resolution, and permits acquisition of additional images.[3,24,35,38] Alternatively, tomographic methods may be employed.[40,47] The multiple pinhole method, successfully used by some investigators, yields suboptimal reconstruction and is technically difficult. Currently, SPECT methods with an orbiting camera are optimal and are generally reconstructed in cardiac short-axis projections, as well as two long-axis projections, a

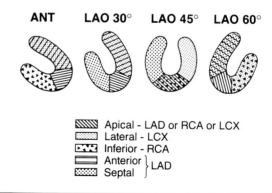

Figure 10-3. Illustrated is the relationship between perfusion image and cardiac anatomy. The base can be seen to rotate from left in anterior to right in left lateral projections. The indicated relationship between anatomy and coronary distribution is approximate and varies with specific coronary size, dominance, collateralization, and cardiac rotation. Some regions are projected and may relate to any of the perfused vascular regions.

poststress images. The difference in these profiles, compared to the initial radioactivity level, yields a plot of radial "washout," which appears to be an absolute perfusion indicator (Fig. 10-4).[3,24,37,47] Since the parameter depends on established myocardial/blood gradients, it is significantly affected by the achieved stress level and related double product. Washout levels below normal can be given little significance when associated with suboptimal stress.[53] An apparent perfusion defect seen best on the redistribution image has been termed *reverse redistribution.* Although originally thought to be related to widespread ischemia in other regions, the phenomenon is most frequently related to differential but normal global washout or a limited region of infarction. Because of the improved contrast resolution of SPECT images, washout analysis may not be of added value.

Planar color functional images of regional myocardial washout have been generated that can be related to normal values.[43] Functional images of uptake, redistribution, and washout can be generated from compressed tomographic slices presented in a "bull's eye" configuration.[47] Alternatively, superimposition of stress and redistribution SPECT slices can be processed, yielding functional SPECT washout slices.[54] Both methods permit a graphic, anatomic, and visual assessment of perfusion.

Some claim that the improved anatomic definition and increased sensitivity of SPECT imaging make washout unnecessary; however, computer methods have been developed to superimpose individual SPECT slices and analyze regional tomographic washout. These washout images appear to add to diagnostic sensitivity of regional ischemia, maximizing assessment of coronary involvement. Most valuable is the application of washout analysis to assess regional perfusion and exclude global ischemia in the setting of a normal scintigram related to a high coronary likelihood. Such normal images also appear unlikely with SPECT application. Dependent as they are on the effects of exercise on thallium distribution, washout methods have not demonstrated efficacy in relation to pharmacologic intervention, where generally reduced levels are seen. Of course, addition of a second, reinjection thallium dose obscures evaluation of the kinetics of the initial injected dose. Washout must be performed before reinjection if it is to be used.

Planar Image Interpretation. Regardless of the variety of sophisticated computer enhancement and processing methods employed, or possibly because of them, strict attention must be given to the assessment of the analog image pattern. Processed curves and images will only be as reliable as the original data set. Without an appreciation of the baseline distribution pattern, artifacts will not be recognized. The blind acceptance of such data is fraught with danger.[48,49,54,55]

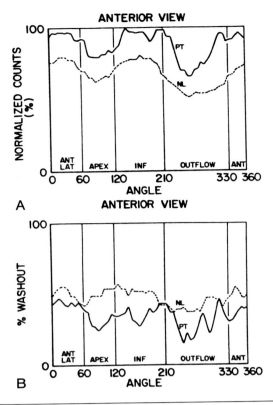

Figure 10-4. Advantages of washout analysis. Radial distribution of counts (*A*) in the anterior projection is normal. However, radial washout (*B*) analysis is abnormal in all segments, indicative of global ischemia in the presence of what might appear to be a normal perfusion image. (Reproduced by permission of the American Heart Association, Inc., from Abdulla A, Maddahi J, Garcia E, et al. Slow regional washout of myocardial thallium-201 in the absence of perfusion defects: contribution to detection of individual coronary artery stenosis and mechanisms for occurrence. Circulation 1985;71:72.)

The anterior and lateral projections present as a horseshoe configuration (see Fig. 10-4). Since the left ventricle has several times the muscle mass of the right, the myocardial perfusion image is composed primarily of the left ventricular contour. The right ventricle is often well seen only in the immediate poststress image. Prominent right ventricular visualization, especially in a rest or redistribution image, often relates to the presence of right ventricular hypertrophy.[56] The identification of right ventricular perfusion defects is tenuous.

Left anterior oblique projections present as a "doughnut" configuration in horizontal hearts or as a "horseshoe" with the base oriented superiorly in vertical hearts. The septal and lateral walls have varying radioactivity depending on rotation, with the greatest intensity in walls viewed in tangent. Multiple left anterior oblique projections help visual assessment by presenting rotational progression of regional radioactivity. Both visual and circumferential profile interpretations of the perfusion scintigram are made in regions viewed in tangent.

Conventional planar image evaluation permits assessment only of the walls seen in tangent. The myocardium seen *en face* is thinner, has less radioactivity, and permits the apparent imaging of the radionuclide-poor cavity. Only planar color washout images or tomographic evaluation permits assessment of the full extent of projected myocardium (see Fig. 10-4).[40,50]

Perfusion image interpretation requires significant experience and insight into factors related to radionuclide distribution. An evaluation of the cause of false positive perfusion images revealed that most of these occurred in women, and frequently these images revealed evidence of soft tissue breast attenuation, extending into the noncardiac soft tissues. This artifact often presents as an anterior defect, confused with pathology in the left anterior descending coronary artery distribution. Although generally fixed, some of these apparent lesions seemed reversible, but they frequently spared the apex, which was generally involved in anterior descending coronary disease.[51]

Pathologic lung uptake is related to a prolonged pulmonary transit time of any cause with increased ^{201}Tl extraction and may be seen with congestive cardiomyopathy, mitral disease, or extensive myocardial ischemia.[51,54] It must be differentiated from normal chest radioactivity seen at a low level of stress. Although nonspecific in the presence of limited but apparent perfusion abnormalities, lung uptake suggests extensive myocardium at ischemic risk.[54] It is one of three supplementary indices for image evaluation of myocardial perfusion defects in the assessment of the extent of ischemia (Fig. 10-5).[58] Another, basal uptake, reflects a general reduction of distal radioactivity in the distribution of all coronary vessels. The third, apparent cavitary dilation, is rarely related to actual stress-induced chamber enlargement, but is probably most often due to relative underperfusion of the wall overlying the cavity.[50]

The localization of defects is broadly related to the expected distribution of coronary arteries where the septum and anterior wall relate to the left anterior descending coronary artery, the lateral wall to the circumflex, and the inferior wall to the right coronary artery (see Fig. 10-3).[28,38,51,60] This correlation will vary with the specific coronary distribution, collateralization, and the effects of revascularization procedures (Fig. 10-6). The absence of an apparent left ventricular cavity suggests left ventricular hypertrophy, whereas reduced regional cavitary radioactivity suggests overlying scar (Fig. 10-7).[61] Cavitary size should be assessed cautiously, owing to the ungated nature of the study. The presence of defects should be expressed as well in terms of the extent and density of myocardium affected, since both these parameters as well as the extent of coronary involvement are important indicators of coronary risk.[62,63] Defects must also be defined as fixed or reversible, infarcted or ischemic (Fig. 10-8).

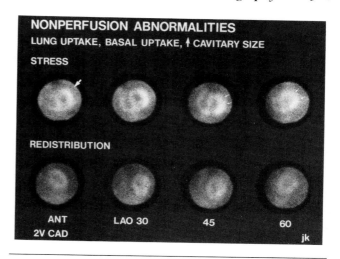

Figure 10-5. Example of supplementary indicators. Stress and redistribution images illustrating nonperfusion or supplementary indicators of ischemia are shown. Here, lung uptake (*arrow, upper left*), basal uptake (*arrows, upper right*), and cavitary dilatation are each evident. When seen in perfusion changes, especially in association with perfusion abnormalities, they indicate extensive myocardium at ischemic risk. (Reproduced with permission from Canhasi B, Dae M, Botvinick E, et al. The interaction of "supplementary" scintigraphic indicators and stress electrocardiography in the diagnosis of multivessel coronary disease. J Am Coll Cardiol 1985;6:581.)

Myocardial regions perfused by tight coronary lesions may not redistribute in 4 hours, however, but will show normalization on delayed imaging performed as long as 24 hours after radionuclide administration (Fig. 10-9).[64] It may be clinically important to differentiate such delayed redistribution patterns in viable myocardial regions from those of fixed scar. Functional reversibility may be expected in dyssynergic myocardial segments related to normal perfusion or reversible stress-induced abnormalities after coronary revascularization (Fig. 10-10 and Table 10-2).[41,65,66] Recently it has been shown that even some myocardial regions with fixed patterns at 4 and even at 24 hours may be viable. These generally relate to less dense defects. Reinjection of a small thallium dose or metabolic assessment with PET scanning may aid in identification of viable tissue.

Similarly, defects seen on a rest image are generally related to infarction. Although perfusion defects are extremely sensitive indicators by which to diagnose acute infarction, especially early after the event (Fig. 10-11), they are nonspecific and may relate to prior infarction or to noncoronary pathology.[61,67-71] Nevertheless, a negative study has been said to be a cost-effective measure for screening admissions to the coronary care unit.[72] Primary cardiomyopathy may present with widespread and mul-

(*Text continues on page 344*)

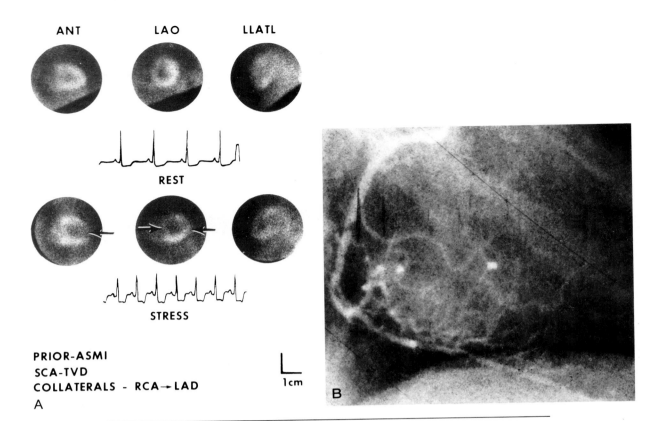

ANT   LAO   LLATL

REST

STRESS

PRIOR-ASMI
SCA-TVD
COLLATERALS - RCA→LAD

A

B

|___
| 1cm

Figure 10-6. High-risk pattern. *A:* Shown are stress and rest ^{201}Tl perfusion images in a patient with triple vessel disease (TVD) on angiography (SCA). A prior anteroseptal infarction (ASMI) is evident in the rest images. Extensive defects in the stress image indicate ischemia in the distribution of multiple vessels and extensive myocardium at risk. The inferior wall looked "normal," although the right coronary artery (RCA) was also stenotic. This demonstrates the relative nature of the study or relates to the fact that the RCA ischemic threshold was not reached. The RCA territory was, in fact, likely the best perfused, as the vessel served as collaterals to the left anterior descending (LAD) coronary artery, as shown in *B.* (Reproduced by permission of the American Heart Association, Inc., from Dash H, Massie B, Botvinick E, et al. The noninvasive identification of left main and three vessel coronary artery disease by myocardial stress perfusion scintigraphy and treadmill electrocardiography. Circulation 1979;60:276.)

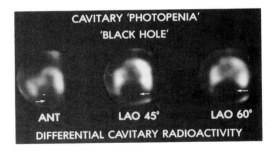

CAVITARY 'PHOTOPENIA'
'BLACK HOLE'

ANT   LAO 45°   LAO 60°
DIFFERENTIAL CAVITARY RADIOACTIVITY

Figure 10-7. Cavitary photopenia. Shown in anterior (ANT) and 45° and 60° left anterior oblique (LAO) projections are perfusion scintigrams in a patient with a large apical aneurysm. Note the area of reduced radioactivity, an apparent "black hole" in the apical wall and appearing to extend into the region of the "cavity." The latter most likely relates to reduced radioactivity in the overlying myocardial wall. (Reproduced with permission from Canhasi B, Dae M, Botvinick E, et al. The interaction of "supplementary" scintigraphic indicators and stress electrocardiography in the diagnosis of multivessel coronary artery disease. J Am Coll Cardiol 1985;6:581.)

Tl-201 Image Interpretation

Stress	*Rest/Redist.	Interpretation
Normal	Normal	No infarction No "ischemia"
Abnormal	Normal	Stress induced "ischemia"
Abnormal	Abnormal—less than stress	"Ischemia" and infarction
Abnormal	Abnormal—no change	†Infarction without apparent "ischemia"

*Rest and delayed redistribution images may not be the same in the setting of ongoing ischemia.

†Some of these segments may be viable and can possibly be identified only by PET metabolic evaluation.

Figure 10-8. Perfusion image interpretation. Shown is the general pattern for interpretation of perfusion scintigrams. Subtitles reviewed in the text provide qualification of this outline.

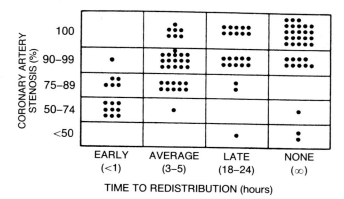

TIME TO REDISTRIBUTION (hours)

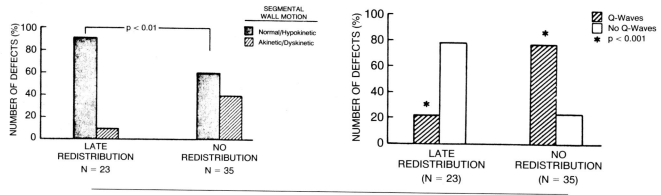

Figure 10-9. Delayed redistribution. Shown above is the relationship between the time to full perfusion image redistribution and the degree of coronary stenosis. The time to redistribution is directly related to the degree of narrowing. Late distributing segments, unlike those not redistributing, are viable and generally demonstrate preserved regional wall motion and no specific electrocardiographic evidence of infarction. Important clinical errors may be committed and viable segments interpreted as infarcted if delayed redistribution is not sought in select situations. (Reproduced with permission from Gorman J, Berman D, Freeman M. Time to completed redistribution of ²⁰¹Tl in exercise myocardial scintigraphy: relationship to the degree of coronary artery stenosis. Am Heart J 1983;106:989.)

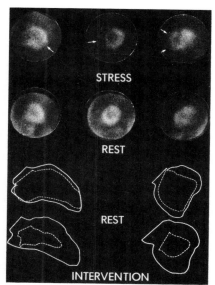

Figure 10-10. Functional reversibility. Large reversible abnormalities (*arrows*) are noted in the perfusion images above. Below, end-diastolic (*solid lines*) and end-systolic (*dotted lines*) outlines from the left ventriculogram of the same patient obtained at rest and postventricular ectopy indicate reversibility of wall motion abnormalities. Normal resting perfusion indicates viability and reversibility of functional abnormalities with a ventricular premature contraction (VPC), after nitroglycerin, or after successful revascularization. (Reproduced with permission from Brundage BH, Massie BM, Botvinick EH, et al. Improved regional ventricular function after successful surgical revascularization. J Am Coll Cardiol 1984;3:902.)

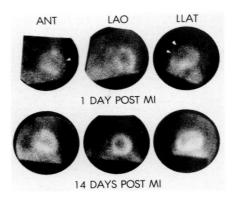

ANT   LAO   LLAT

1 DAY POST MI

14 DAYS POST MI

Figure 10-11. Serial perfusion images. Serial rest ^{201}Tl perfusion images obtained 1 day and 14 days after an acute anterior infarction demonstrate reduction of defect size. This may be due to resolution of ischemia. (Reproduced with permission from Botvinick E, Shames D. Nuclear cardiology: clinical applications, p. 5. © 1979, the Williams & Wilkins Co., Baltimore.)

tiple abnormalities, but may be difficult to differentiate from segmental ischemic abnormalities.[69]

The distribution of the radionuclide administered at rest need not be the same as that seen on delayed redistribution imaging.[73,74] Imaging after injection at rest, like that performed immediately poststress, reflects the relative distribution of perfusion at the time of administration. The delayed pattern rather relates to the distribution of the potassium, or viable intracellular space. Thus, if reversible ischemia exists at the time of imaging after rest injection, defects may redistribute on later image. This is an appropriate method to assess the nature of resting symptoms and the extent of related ischemia. Since some new technetium-based perfusion agents redistribute little, they may not be ideal for the evaluation of resting ischemia.

Similar considerations apply to SPECT image interpretation. Limited planar images should precede SPECT acquisition to aid identification of lung uptake, cavitary dilation, and soft tissue attenuation.

Accuracy of Dynamic Stress Perfusion Scintigraphy. Although the method is imperfect, diagnostic accuracy of dynamic stress perfusion scintigraphy compared with coronary angiography is high.[3,24,36,38,40,75–77] Defining a significant stenosis as 50% to 70% or more area narrowing, planar methods with computer enhancement but without the application of washout techniques achieve diagnostic sensitivity in the range of 80% to 95%. Of course, when exercise is conducted to suboptimal levels, when the radionuclide is administered prematurely, or when imaging is delayed, sensitivity is reduced. Similarly, the full extent of coronary involvement is less likely to be identified in the presence of collaterals.[49,78,79] This may relate to the lack of ischemia in the region of collateral supply (see Fig. 10-6). Tomographic methods appear

to have added diagnostic security in image interpretation and, in some studies, have added to diagnostic sensitivity.[40,47,80] Washout methods appear to aid the more complete identification of involved coronary vessels and the full amount of myocardium at ischemic risk.[3,24,47,50,80–83] Some studies have demonstrated the ability of the method to identify almost 70% of all involved vessels.[16,24,84,85] Rarely, washout evaluation will identify extensive perfusion abnormalities where none are visible, apparently due to balanced ischemia.[85]

This, along with lung uptake and other indicators of widespread ischemia, has added to the ability of the method to identify patients at high coronary risk, and has helped to establish the prognostic value of the test. Also, normal washout aids the identification of a normal study and makes coronary disease unlikely, even in the presence of induced ST depression.[86–88]

It is important to consider the difference between the pathophysiologic nature of the scintigraphic method and the anatomic nature of the angiographic technique. Although angiographic method is the standard for diagnostic assessment, interpretation of the degree and significance of coronary lesions is extremely variable.[89]

Pharmacologic "Stress" Perfusion Scintigraphy

A large percentage of patients who need evaluation for coronary disease are ill, debilitated, or even timid or anxious and cannot or should not undergo dynamic exercise stress. Nevertheless, their symptoms, when recognized, are often atypical, and the diagnosis and related risk remain in doubt. This group comprises as many as one third of all patients requiring evaluation for known or suspected coronary disease. Compounding the problem is the fact that these patients often face a significant intervention. Patients with peripheral vascular disease claudicate, and limited activities prevent the early appearance of cardiac symptoms. Yet their major morbidity and mortality relate to associated, frequently occult, coronary disease.[90]

Dipyridamole inhibits circulating red cell-bound adenosine deaminase,[91] resulting in reduced degradation and increased levels of adenosine, a potent arteriolar dilator. Administered intravenously, the dipyridamole has significant delayed effects on the coronary resistance vessels, resulting in a three- to fivefold coronary flow augmentation in normal vessels.[92] Alternatively, however, adenosine can be infused directly. This flow augmentation is limited by a fixed stenosis. Applying this differential response, Gould demonstrated a high sensitivity for coronary disease diagnosis with a relatively unimpressive peripheral hemodynamic effect in dogs.[93] Animal experiments indicate differential augmentation of coronary perfusion in both normal and stenotic vessels,[94,95] but ischemia has rarely been documented, possibly due to a "steal" effect or to an actual reduction in coronary flow.[96] Here, in the presence of collateral coronary perfusion, reduced resistance in the normal bed beyond that in the diseased bed results in reduced or absent collateral flow. Alternatively, reduced perfusion pressure in the presence of a fixed coronary stenosis and limited coronary flow reserve can also produce coronary underperfusion and ischemia.

An intravenous saline solution of 0.57 mg/kg of body weight is infused over 4 minutes, with full hemodynamic and symptomatic monitoring.[97] Ingestion of a dipyridamole slurry has also been found effective, but vagaries related to the absorbed dose make this route suboptimal.[98] Thallium is administered at the seventh minute and images acquired shortly thereafter and 4 hours later at redistribution, or with reinjection technique. Uniform flow augmentation, in the absence of significant coronary lesions, leads to a homogeneous ^{201}Tl distribution and a normal image. The presence of significant coronary lesions causes heterogeneous flow augmentation and perfusion image defects (Fig. 10-12). Washout values are lower in patients who are pharmacologically stressed where normal values have not been clearly established and where the effects of the intervention cannot be clearly quantitated.[99]

The effects of the drug are generally benign, producing a mild hypotensive response and a mild increase in heart rate.[97] Test sensitivity seems to increase with increasing peripheral hemodynamic response.[100]

Many now recommend the intravenous administration of 100 to 200 mg of aminophylline, 3 to 4 minutes after thallium administration, to end the test and avoid side effects or complications which might otherwise occur during imaging or later. Side effects are generally mild and relate to vascular dilation with headache, flushing, and nausea.[97] Although ischemic indicators are uncommon, an occasional dramatic ischemic response may be seen and rare fatalities have been reported. The method has proven safe in the elderly and may be of value for the assessment of myocardium at ischemic risk in specific cases of unstable angina.[101]

Drug-induced chest pain is nonspecific. Recently adenosine has been presented as an agent to directly stimulate pain neurons and may be the cause of nonspecific pain symptoms, both during dipyridamole and with adenosine infusion.[102]

Drug effects can be immediately reversed by the intravenous administration of aminophylline, which specifically blocks the adenosine receptors.[104] Although the functional correlate of such induced ischemia may be qualitatively assessed in some cases with echocardiography, that method will fail to identify the much more frequently induced malperfusion not associated with ischemia.[103] Most studies applying echocardiography to the

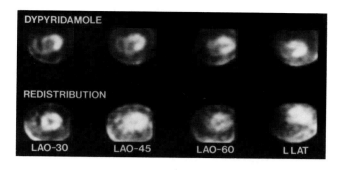

Figure 10-12. Abnormal dipyridamole image. The induced reversible anterior apical defect relates to left anterior descending coronary disease.

demonstration of dipyridamole-induced ischemia, assessed particularly high risk populations and infused dipyridamole at higher rates. Still, such methods will succeed only with induced ischemia and requires the proper anatomy.

Another potentially serious side effect of dipyridamole infusion is bronchospasm. Theophylline-like drugs to treat bronchospasm must optimally be discontinued for 2 days before dipyridamole testing, but the patient can be supported with adrenergic inhalants which do not interfere with the study. Although unlikely because of their half-lives and the protocol sequence, diminished aminophylline levels could again unmask dipyridamole effects, still circulating until its blood levels decay.

The diagnostic sensitivity of the imaging method approaches that related to dynamic stress imaging, in the range of 80% to 90%. Specificity is also high.[77,105–107] The test has proven extremely useful and has been noted to influence diagnosis and management in almost 80% of patients evaluated.[108] Additionally, the method, like dynamic perfusion evaluation, appears to have prognostic value.[109,110]

Unlike exercise-related defects, however, dipyridamole-induced regional abnormalities do not relate clearly to levels of related double product or exercise level. Dipyridamole-induced defects should not necessarily indicate the risk of events or correlate with predictable risk unless test results aid identification of symptoms seen in daily life or unless the patient faces a potential high stress, high risk procedure, as surgery.

For prognostic purposes, such pharmacologic "stress" testing seems of greatest value in assessing risk in patients facing an active cardiovascular stressful intervention, and who cannot provoke a sufficient coronary stress at dynamic exercise testing to challenge their coronary flow reserve. The classic patient group in this category is comprised of those with peripheral vascular disease who will be coming to surgical revascularization. In this group cardiovascular, and specifically coronary, complications are the greatest risk and cause of greatest surgical morbidity and mortality.[111,112]

In a group of patients studied before peripheral vascular surgery, perioperative coronary events were noted only in those with reversible scintigraphic defects. Although dipyridamole initially appeared to be of great prognostic value in all patients who were to undergo peripheral vascular surgery, recent studies suggest its greatest effectiveness is in high-risk subgroups.[113,114] Further, patients with reversible perfusion abnormalities were those developing coronary events after subendocardial infarction. Wolfe and coworkers demonstrated that prognostic value of dipyridamole perfusion scintigraphy in patients after relatively uncomplicated myocardial infarction.[115]

Most antianginal drugs effect the heart rate and blood pressure response to dynamic exercise, and indirectly reduce coronary flow demands. They do not affect dipyridamole function or adenosine coronary dilation, and so do not influence the dipyridamole-related test of coronary flow reserve. Thus, scintigraphic findings after dipyridamole "stress" should be little affected by antianginal therapy.[116] Since these drugs limit exercise response, however, which limits the exercise-related test of coronary flow reserve, antianginal drugs can reduce the extent of the exercise-related scintigraphic defect and that of the related ischemic region. Thus, dynamic exercise testing while on antianginal drugs will demonstrate the related myocardium at treatment; however, it will not reveal the full extent of scintigraphy performed off medication, or dipyridamole scintigraphy performed on or off most antianginal medications.

While all suggest the value of the method in patients who cannot achieve adequate exercise testing. Recently, some have suggested the diagnostic and prognostic value of dipyridamole pharmacologic "stress" testing in patients who "should not" have dynamic exercise testing. The method has been shown to be relatively safe and useful in patients soon after acute infarction, and in those with known or suspected unstable angina.[110,117,118] It is already a much sought-after and seemingly clinically important method. Because of the value of exercise-related data and the superiority of stress-related images, however, it is not recommended as a replacement for dynamic stress perfusion imaging.

Although the method seems to aid identification of coronary disease and related myocardium, the study gives no assessment of exercise tolerance and fails to relate involved myocardial regions to an ischemic threshold. This is not a replacement for a submaximal test after infarction and has not been proven superior to submaximal dynamic exercise evaluation; however, the pharmacologic "stress" may well prove superior if it identifies greater elements of myocardium at ischemic risk. A recent study has demonstrated that pharmacologic "stress"

testing provides similar prognostic value postinfarction.[119]

Recently, the direct intravenous infusion of adenosine has been applied as an alternative pharmacologic "stress."[120] The appeal of this approach relates to the direct delivery of the agent with definite establishment of blood levels as opposed to the indirect and indefinite nature of dipyridamole adenosine delivery. The 10-second adenosine half-life necessitates a constant infusion for maintenance of effects and permits rapid resolution of side effects with infusion termination. However, adenosine is a potent blocker of arteriovenous conduction and its brief infusion is now approved for termination of supraventricular tachycardia. Although infused at a lower rate, early results indicate a 1% incidence of heart block when infused in association with scintigraphy. Diagnostic accuracy appears similar to dipyridamole infusion but has not been compared directly. Its acceptance will depend on its patient tolerance and relative accuracy, safety, and cost. In the presence of coronary collateral perfusion, reduced resistance in the collateral source vessel beyond that in the diseased collateralized vessel results in reduced or reversed collateral flow.

Echocardiography has also been applied to identify adenosine-induced ischemia, which also seems relatively infrequent compared with that of exercise testing or that of adenosine-induced perfusion defects.[121-123] Although central effects may exceed those of dipyridamole, peripheral effects and side effects also appear more dramatic and there is no current evidence of adenosine superiority for diagnostic or prognostic purposes. Yet, its activity and brief half-life make the agent appealing for this purpose. Direct adenosine infusion is believed to be a more potent stimulus to the coronary circulation. Some investigators have applied a higher than standard dipyridamole dose, yet the standard dipyridamole infusion rate as employed in the standard dipyridamole protocol employs an administered dosage found to approach the optimal test of coronary flow reserve in both animal and patient studies.

Recent work has focused on the not infrequent occurrence of pain-free or "silent" myocardial ischemia.[124-126] Initially confirmed by the related findings of induced scintigraphic defects, it is now commonly sought with electrocardiographic ambulatory (Holter) monitoring.[127] It has been found that most ischemic episodes incurred during the daily activities of the coronary patient are silent.[128,129] Early investigators noted the occurrence of silent ischemia and ST depression in the absence of increased heart rate, suggesting a dissociation from factors of increased coronary flow demands and suggesting coronary vasospasm as a common cause.[130] More recent work indicates a relationship between silent ST depression and increased ambulatory blood pressure, confirming a relationship with myocardial determinants of coronary flow demand and fixed coronary lesions.[131] Regardless of their etiology, silent ischemic episodes appear as lethal, with as great a relationship to clinical outcome as the "audible" variety.[132,133] Detection of silent ischemia is a critical clinical concern. Many scintigraphic studies that demonstrate reversible ischemic defects of function or perfusion are unrelated to ischemic symptoms, and often, to definitive electrocardiographic evidence of ischemia. Scintigraphy is a critical method for detection of silent as well as symptomatic ischemic events and endpoints.[125,131] Further, recent work has demonstrated that Holter recordings rarely demonstrate evidence of ischemic episodes in the presence of negative exercise or pharmacologic "stress" scintigraphic studies.[125] In fact, it is those scintigraphic studies that demonstrate the most extensive evidence of myocardium at ischemic risk that are related to the highest and most frequent yield of ischemic and silent ischemic episodes on ambulatory electrocardiographic monitoring.[125] These same scintigraphic defects have been shown in other studies to relate to the greatest degree of coronary risk.[123,128,131] Thus, although ambulatory recording is of value for detection of ischemic episodes during the patient's daily activities, the greater test of coronary flow reserve provided by "stress" scintigraphic study provides an excellent method for identification of patients at greatest coronary risk and greatest yield on Holter recording.[131]

Clinical Utility

Thallium scintigraphy evaluates the primary pathophysiologic ischemic abnormality, insufficient myocardial perfusion. Blood pool scintigraphy and other modalities evaluate the secondary functional response. Additional ischemic responses include chest pain, a subjective and relatively insensitive measure; electrocardiographic ST changes, often a nonspecific finding; and myocardial lactate production, an insensitive invasive parameter.

Diagnostic Application. Many patients can be successfully evaluated for ischemic disease by exercise testing alone (Table 10-3). A high-level stress test in the absence of pain or electrocardiographic changes may be all that is required to practically exclude the diagnosis. In evaluating test utility in any patient, however, the pretest likelihood and Bayes theorem must be considered.[134–137] The posttest likelihood of disease is a function of test accuracy and the pretest likelihood. The latter is a function of the patient population assessed and can be estimated.[138] Thus, if the patient is a 35-year-old man with nonanginal chest pain, representing a population with a low pretest probability, the probability after a negative stress test is low enough to exclude coronary disease. If the patient is a 45-year-old man with atypical pain, however, representing a population with a 50% pretest prob-

Table 10-3

Clinical Applications of Stress Perfusion or Blood Pool Scintigraphy

Diagnosis of Coronary Disease
1. Where the stress test is equivocal in the presence of resting baseline electrocardiographic abnormalities
2. When the diagnosis is ambiguous and disease likelihood is indeterminant on where the stress electrocardiogram is abnormal in a patient with a low disease likelihood or the converse
3. When the stress electrocardiogram is negative at a low achieved double product*
4. To establish the pathophysiologic significance of coronary lesions of questionable significance

Evaluation of Coronary Disease Treatment
1. Localizes ischemia to specific vessels aiding the administration of revascularization procedures
2. Aids prediction of response to angioplasty or bypass surgery
3. Determines the effectiveness of collaterals
4. Determines myocardial viability, differentiating ischemia from infarction
5. Determines effectiveness of revascularization and thrombolytic therapy
6. Aids assessment of bypass graft patency

Evaluation of Coronary Disease Risk and Prognosis
1. Aids identification of main left and triple-vessel disease
2. Provides a measure of the extent of myocardium at ischemic risk, presenting an accurate independent prognostic measure
3. Assists in the selection of patients for revascularization procedures
4. Assists the evelation and management of patients after uncomplicated infarction

Possible but not yet firmly established.

ability, the probability of disease after a negative stress test would still be in the range of 20%. Here a negative perfusion scintigram reduces disease likelihood to approximately 3%, not significantly different from disease incidence in an asymptomatic population of the same age and sex (Fig. 10-13). Although it does not eliminate the diagnosis entirely, it reduces (or increases) disease likelihood to levels of diagnostic security where appropriate clinical management can be delivered.[136,137]

Scintigraphy is probably most valuable in patients presenting diagnostic difficulty (Fig. 10-14). Prominent among these are patients presenting with stress electrocardiograms that are uninterpretable for ischemia owing to the presence of left ventricular hypertrophy, digitalis use, electrolyte abnormalities, or other causes for resting ST abnormalities.[38,139] Recently, the value of the study in patients with left bundle branch block has been questioned. Experience here varies and many consider the study valuable even in the setting where pharmacologic stress may be advantageous.

Not infrequently, patients are sent to scintigraphic study after coronary angiography. In some cases, patients are returned for noninvasive pathophysiologic assess-

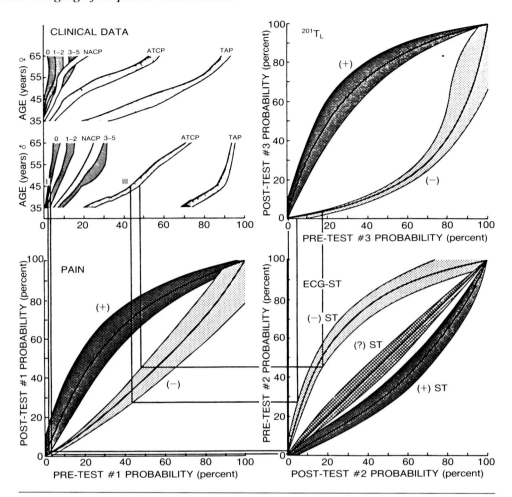

Figure 10-13. Diagnosis of coronary artery disease. Illustrated is the interaction of clinical data (*upper left*) and noninvasive stress-induced pain (*lower left*), ischemic electrocardiogram (*lower right*), and scintigraphic perfusion changes (*upper right*) in formulating the likelihood of coronary disease. The type of presenting pain, nonanginal (NACP), atypical (ATCP), or typical angina (TAP), in addition to patient age and sex present an initial estimate of disease likelihood according to the data of Diamond and Forrester.[138] Thereafter, the results of noninvasive stress testing influence likelihood assessment. Charted diagrammatically are examples presenting clinical data related to low and intermediate coronary likelihood. The effects of negative noninvasive results are traced and have little impact on the patient with initial low disease likelihood. However, a patient presenting with initial, intermediate, 40% to 50% likelihood relates to a 2% to 3% likelihood of coronary disease after negative noninvasive tests. This incidence is not significantly different from a similar asymptomatic population. (Reproduced with permission from Patterson RE, Eng C, Horowitz SF, et al. Practical diagnosis of coronary artery disease: a Bayes theorem nomogram to correlate clinical data with noninvasive exercise tests. Am J Cardiol 1984;53:252.)

ment when lesions are of uncertain significance or when their relation to ischemia and salvageable myocardium is questioned.

Prognostic Utility. Even in the clear presence of ischemic coronary disease patients are often sent for scintigraphy to determine the significance of lesions and the presence and extent of myocardium at ischemic risk (Fig. 10-15).[88,140] This measurement now more than ever appears most closely related to prognosis, an important parameter guiding management.[38,59,139,140] Further, such re-

gions are by definition viable and present an important opportunity for aggressive treatment. Especially important is the evaluation of risk postinfarction, where both the quantitative assessment of resting ventricular function and stress-induced perfusion abnormalities have been shown to augment identification of high-risk patients.[141–143] PET metabolic assessment may add significantly to viability and prognosis evaluation.[144,145]

Evaluation of Treatment. Most valuable is the application of scintigraphic ischemic indicators to the as-

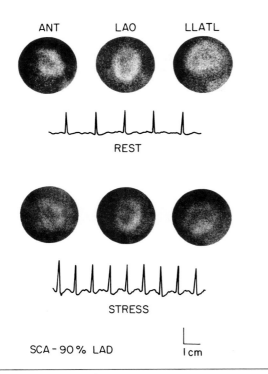

Figure 10-14. False negative stress electrocardiogram. Shown is scintigraphic evidence of stress-induced septal ischemia in a patient with a 90% left anterior descending stenosis. The stress electrocardiogram was normal. (Reproduced with permission from Botvinick EH, Taradash MR, Shames DM, et al. Thallium-201 myocardial perfusion scintigraphy for the clinical clarification of normal, abnormal and equivocal electrocardiographic stress tests. Am J Cardiol 1978;41:43.)

sessment of the results of angioplasty and bypass surgery (see Fig. 10-16).[59,62,142,146–150] Objective, pathophysiologic evauation of perfusion and viability is especially important in the setting of postintervention symptoms, where a comparison baseline study is valuable. Serial studies must be evaluated in terms of related stress level, however. Persistent abnormalities of diminished size, often related to a more advanced stress level, are not unusual after successful surgery. Perfusion imaging presents pathophysiologic advantages over the anatomic evaluation of graft patency by computed tomography (Fig. 10-17).[15] Yet in many cases the two studies may be complementary. Similarly, the method has been useful in determining the effects on perfusion and viability of streptokinase-induced postinfarction reperfusion.[152] The new technetium-based perfusion agents may be most valuable in this acute setting.[153]

Effects of Drugs on Study Interpretation

Although digitalis preparations affect membrane function, no cardiac drugs are known to interfere with the localization and dynamics of ^{201}Tl, and the method is effectively applied in patients on digitalis. Beta blockers, which reduce the achieved double product, may influence stress duration or delay the level of stress at which ischemia appears or even prevent its appearance. Most antianginal drugs affect coronary flow demands rather than the supply, which is affected by revascularization procedures. For this reason, in studies performed in patients on antianginal drugs, defects may appear unchanged but associated with higher induced stress levels. Unlike blood pool imaging, perfusion imaging may find difficulty identifying the stress level at which ischemia initially appears (Table 10-4). Although scintigraphic study while the subject is on medications is nevertheless useful for the assessment of treatment, coronary risk is best evaluated while the subject is off drugs. An exception may relate to pharmacologic "stress" testing.[115]

Perfusion and Blood Pool Scintigraphy

Although blood pool scintigraphy appears accurate for the assessment of stress-induced ischemia, the response is less specific.[154–156] Practitioners have varying preferences for the scintigraphic study of choice for the diagnosis of ischemia. Individual experience, skills, equipment, and personnel also influence the choice. Rarely, both studies may be useful. Stress blood pool evaluation is recommended when presented with a functional equivalent of angina or in evaluation of function in the setting of noncoronary heart disease.[157,158]

The Prospect of New Imaging Agents

Two new technetium-based radiopharmaceuticals have been recently approved for perfusion imaging. Like ^{201}Tl, they distribute rapidly intracellularly in relation to relative myocardial perfusion but present the inherent imaging advantages of [99m]Tc. Because of its ready availability and physical characteristics, a ^{99m}Tc label is extremely desirable. The isonitriles and neutral lipophilic complexes of boronic acid present members which can be tagged with ^{99m}Tc and distribute in proportion to myocardial perfusion.[153,159,160] Specifically, ^{99m}Tc methoxyisobutyl isonitrile or sestaMIBI, and ^{99m}Tc teboroxime, are now available for use as myocardial perfusion imaging agents.[161,162] Each bears the advantage of the technetium label, but each is different in physical characteristics, resulting in totally different imaging protocols and, likely, varying utility. Although both sestaMIBI and teboroxime distribute in relation to regional myocardial perfusion, teboroxime is more avidly extracted. When used with exercise or pharmacologic intervention, sestaMIBI will likely require a longer period after injection before terminating or abort-

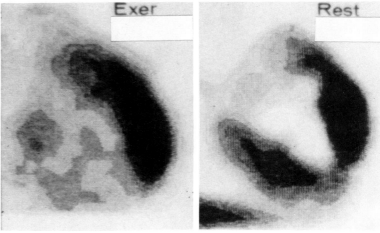

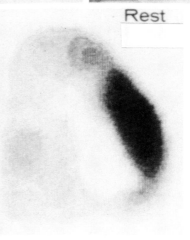

Figure 10-15. Myocardium at ischemic risk. Shown above are stress (*left*) and rest (*right*) myocardial perfusion scintigrams in a patient with right coronary stenosis estimated to be 40%. The scintigram clearly reveals evidence of reversible inferior ischemia. Subsequently, the patient went on to have a spontaneous infarction of the same region as shown on the rest image illustrated below. This study illustrates the difference between angiographic anatomy and scintigraphic pathophysiology while providing one form of evidence for the ability of scintigraphy to identify myocardium at ischemic risk. (Courtesy of Dr. M. Goris, Stanford University, Stanford, California.)

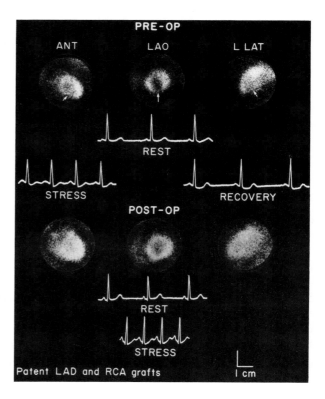

Figure 10-16. Effects of coronary bypass. Shown are serial perfusion studies performed before (*above*) and after (*below*) coronary artery bypass graft surgery. The induced inferior wall defect was no longer present postoperatively at a higher related double product. (Reproduced with permission from Greenberg BH, Hart R, Botvinick EH, et al. Thallium-201 myocardial perfusion scintigraphy to evaluate patients after coronary bypass surgery. Am J Cardiol 1978;42:167.)

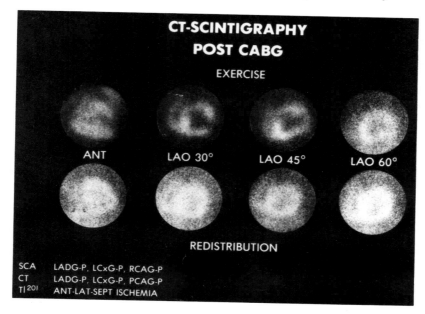

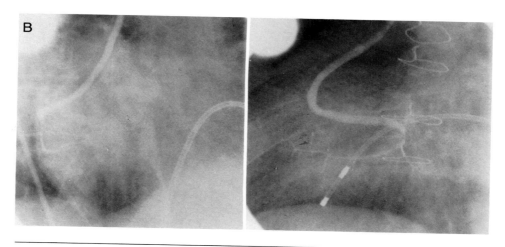

Figure 10-17. Computed tomography (CT) and perfusion scintigraphy. Rest CT examination of this patient with chest pain late after bypass surgery revealed flow through the left anterior descending and circumflex (LC$_x$) grafts, and reported them both patent. *A:* Scintigraphy reveals stress-induced ischemic changes in anterior, septal, and lateral regions (ANT-LAT-SEPT), the distribution of both vessels. *B:* Angiography revealed stenosis at the insertion sites of both vessels. The scintigram provides pathophysiologic information, often clarifying anatomical information. (Reproduced with permission from Englestad B, Wagner S, Herfkens R, et al. Evaluation of the post coronary bypass patient by myocardial perfusion scintigraphy and computed tomography. AJR 1983;141:507. © American Roentgen Ray Society.)

ing the "stress." This raises a minor concern regarding the myocardial distribution of sestaMIBI.

Both agents present significant hepatobiliary uptake, requiring specific, though minor, patient preparation and presenting a potential imaging difficulty. Myocardial transit of teboroxime is extremely rapid, necessitating rapid imaging, beginning within 1 to 2 minutes and completed within 10 to 15 minutes. Even with this restriction, SPECT may be done rapidly using a continuous, rather than a stop and shoot mode of acquisition. Multiheaded cameras may also increase the speed of ac-

quisition and could provide a more efficient imaging tool specifically matched for the kinetics of teboroxime. The agent also promises a more rapid laboratory throughput, with rapid rest study acquisition, soon after myocardial clearance of the agent. At this time, no relationship has been drawn between myocardial perfusion and teboroxime myocardial clearance rate. Conversely, sestaMIBI presents significant imaging advantages as well. Heralded as a nonselective, noninvasive microsphere, the agent has a prolonged myocardial dwell time and redistributes little if at all, presenting the freedom to delay imaging for an

Table 10-4

*Comparison of Perfusion and Blood Pool Scintigraphy**

	Perfusion Imaging	Blood Pool Imaging
Images perfusion	+	−
Evaluates function	−	+
Assessment made at peak stress	+	−
Assessment averaged over last minutes of stress	−	+
Assessment made serially during stress	−	+
Multiple projections convenient	+	−
Tomography routinely possible	+	−
Cost	+	+
Technically difficult	−	+
Computer intensive	+	+
Requires most camera/computer time	−	+
Volume assessment	−	+
Test sensitivity	+	+
Test specificity	+	−
Permits objective identification of extent of myocardium at ischemic risk	+	−
Prognostic assessment	+	+
Identification of functional reversibility	+	+

Tabulated is a comparison of perfusion and blood pool imaging. A + indicates an advantage in the category noted and + in both columns indicates equal capabilities in the designated category.

hour or 2 after injection.[159] This allows enhanced hepatic clearance and, in the acute setting, permits time for physicians to treat a patient, institute thrombolytic therapy, or perform angiography before imaging. The generator produced nature of the technetium-based radiopharmaceutical provides, as it does for teboroxime, 24-hour availability. Application to acute cardiac patients will be limited to sestaMIBI, however, owing to its kinetics, which alone permit delayed image acquisition. Here a preintervention injection will be made with imaging after intervention, permitting assessment of regional perfusion at presentation. A subsequent same- or next-day study will demonstrate intervention-related changes and salvaged myocardium after acute thrombolysis. Preliminary studies indicate a relationship of sestaMIBI distribution to myocardial viability as well as to regional perfusion, thus providing hope that this agent will be of value for assessment of infarction, normal myocardium, and myocardium at ischemic risk after infarction.[159]

Same-day or next-day imaging protocols have been devised where the initial study would use approximately 50% of the agent dose of the subsequent study. When performed in relation to dynamic exercise or pharmacologic "stress," it appears as though rest should precede stress evaluation.[163] A number of computer programs are being developed to compare the serial studies, which ap-

pear as accurate as thallium perfusion scintigraphy for the diagnosis of coronary lesions.[164] Although washout analysis will not be possible, objective assessment can be made of serial variation in regional radionuclide distribution.

The lack of redistribution may present clinical disadvantages. Patients with ongoing ischemia may continue to demonstrate perfusion defects in spite of, or possibly because of, thallium reinjection, the currently favored injection method.[46] This relates to the fact that the initial thallium distribution reflects regional myocardial perfusion, and in the face of ongoing ischemia, perfusion abnormalities will be visualized and even enhanced with reinjection. Only delayed imaging with a redistribution interval will permit imaging of regional cell volume or potassium space, a marker of cell viability. If sestaMIBI relates to the distribution of perfusion rather than regional cell volume, imaging with this agent, requiring a "reinjection method," risks overlooking regions of ongoing ischemia at rest. In this case, only delayed thallium redistribution imaging will permit such identification. Future studies will determine the frequency and likelihood of this problem. Although preliminary studies indicate the overall similarity of reinjection, thallium imaging at 4 hours and subsequent 24-hour imaging, there are bothersome exceptions, suggesting an increased yield in occasional cases that seem to require a delay period for optimal redistribution between thallium reinjection and imaging. This and other factors may have a bearing on the eventual application of technetium-based perfusion agents and their potential replacement of currently employed [201]Tl.

Another advantage of the ^{99m}Tc based perfusion agents relates to the high injected dose made possible due to the agent's shorter 6 hour half-life and reduced radiation exposure per administered milliCurie compared with that of ^{201}Tl, with its 73-hour half-life.

Left ventricular function can be assessed with these agents while still in the blood pool during exercise. This requires a special multicrystal camera to optimize first pass acquisition (see section on Blood Pool Imaging) and needs to overcome the difficulties of patient motion artifact.[12] However, exercise-related function will then be apparent. Alternatively, assessment of function at rest may be performed with gated SPECT images of the localized perfusion agent, and the assessment of wall motion, thickening, and even left ventricular ejection fraction. Additionally, a direct comparison with regional perfusion could permit identification of "stunned," perfused but dysfunctional, and "hibernating" myocardium (see section on Assessment of Myocardial Viability). This latter application will only be possible with the longer myocardial persistence of the sestaMIBI agents.

Regardless of the method employed, these new agents promise to provide the first practical noninvasive method to acquire accurate information regarding both perfusion and function in the same study. Both agents will provide the 24-hour availability of the generator-produced agent, influencing cost and clinical use. The short, 6-hour half-life and larger permitted injected dose yields improved photon flux and improved image resolution. Of course the increased energy of emission will reduce problems related to soft tissue attenuation. The dose presented will also permit the practical acquisition of gated SPECT studies to provide a rigorous functional assessment based on and absolutely correlated with the localization of the perfusion imaging agent.[165,166]

These agents have been successfully imaged by planar methods. However, some studies suggest their optimal imaging with SPECT technique. This relates to the potential image distortion due to "radioactivity shine-through" because of the higher energy of emission and increased penetrance of the technetium agents. Thus, a well-labeled myocardial wall could obscure perfusion of defects located between it and the detector. Of course, such defects would be obvious on SPECT reconstruction.[164] A practical necessity then, would be the placement of SPECT imaging capability in acute cardiac care units to employ these agents in acute situations, as with acute infarction and thrombolytic therapy. This would appear to be a leading potential application of such agents. The short teboroxime transit time makes SPECT imaging difficult, however. Although possible, it will take a concerted effort and organized approach with methodologic adaptation to apply this agent in this way. Gated SPECT studies with teboroxime present similar difficulties.

Blood Pool Scintigraphy

There are two scintigraphic methods for evaluating right and left ventricular size and function: the first-pass and equilibrium techniques.[167–170] In addition to their noninvasive nature, they provide quantitative, reproducible, pathophysiologic evaluation and permit computer analysis with derivation of a variety of useful measurements. Both methods permit accurate serial volume and function measurements, as well as regional and global evaluation of ventricular function.

First-Pass Methodology

This technique generates data during the first transit of a radionuclide bolus through the central circulation. Using a low radiopharmaceutical dose, only the time-versus-radioactivity curve can be analyzed.[171,172] With a high dose, associated images can be generated.[169,173,174] First-pass evaluation can be performed with virtually any pharmaceutical passing through the central circulation.

Short-lived, rapidly excreted ^{99m}Tc diethylenetriamine pentaacetic acid (DTPA) is commonly used. For quantitative volume assessment or equilibrium evaluation, however, a long-lived blood pool marker, such as labeled red cells, should be used.[140] First-pass quantitation of ventricular size and function depends on principles of the indicator dilution technique, requiring a compact bolus injection proximal to the mixing chamber and homogeneous mixing of the blood pool indicator.[176]

A sensitive camera or probe over the central circulation, generally in the 30° right anterior oblique projection, follows the bolus through the heart.[7,169,171,174,176] Its arrival and departure in each chamber produce a low-frequency radioactivity peak. The sequential variations of the cardiac cycle superimpose high-frequency spikes and valleys, proportional to end-diastolic (ED) and end-systolic (ES) volumes, respectively, on the time versus radioactivity curve (Fig. 10-18). These values will yield accurate right and left ventricular ejection fractions.[167,169,173,177,178] The difference in ED and ES counts (C) is proportional to stroke volume (SV), which, divided by background-corrected EDC, yields the EF, or

$$EF = EDC - ESC/EDC - background$$

With proper choice of background, these values have been well correlated with invasive methods.[169,174,178]

The background-subtracted area under the low-frequency ventricular component of the time versus radioactivity curve is related to cardiac output and can be readily quantitated,[179] like indicator concentration, as

$$F = R/-C(t) \, dt$$

where F is flow or cardiac output, R is the amount of radionuclide injected in counts per minute, and the denominator is the area under the time versus radioactivity curve extrapolated to correct for recirculation. As de-

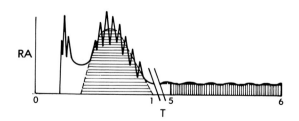

Figure 10-18. First-pass analysis. In this dramatic sketch of a first-pass curve, the area under the left ventricular component (*horizontal lines*) is proportional to cardiac output. It is calibrated for volume by dividing it into the integrated area under 1 minute of the equilibrium time versus radioactivity curve (*vertical lines*). Alternatively, volumes may be calculated from ventricular outlines using geometric considerations. (Reproduced with permission from Botvinick EH, Glazer H, Shosa D. What is the reliability and the utility of scintigraphic methods for the assessment of ventricular function? In: Rahimtoola S, ed. Controversies in coronary artery disease. Philadelphia: FA Davis, 1981:65.)

scribed by Holman,[180] the total amount of radionuclide injected (R) also equals the equilibrium radionuclide concentration (Ceq) in counts per minute per millimeter times the blood volume (BV) in milliliters or

$$R = Ceq \times BV$$

and the indicator dilution equation becomes

$$F = \frac{Ceq \times BV}{\int_0^x C(t)\, dt}$$

There is no need, however, to sample this data from the total circulation. In first-pass scintigraphy, counts information is evaluated over the central circulation and over the left ventricle. The imaging device samples the same area during passage of the bolus and at equilibrium, and the fraction of the blood volume sampled need not appear in the flow equation.

In practice, measurements are made of the area under the first-pass curve and the equilibrium concentration of radionuclide is measured after a 5-minute delay. A blood sample at this time is related to the injected dose to yield the absolute blood volume in milliliters. The area under a 1-minute segment of the equilibrium curve is divided by the area under the first-pass curve to yield left ventricular (cardiac) output in volumes per minute (see Fig. 10-18). This can easily be converted to liters per minute. With the cardiac output, heart rate, and ejection fraction, the stroke volume, either right ventricular or left ventricular end-diastolic and end-systolic volumes, can be accurately calculated.[180] In addition, pulmonary transit time, left ventricular ejection rate, and fractional emptying measures may be generated.[181] The dose (as low as 2 mCi) and related exposure (less than 50 mrad) permit frequent repetitive studies, and the brief acquisition time makes the study applicable, even in uncooperative patients. Nonimaging probes with high sensitivity and temporal resolution detect beat-to-beat left ventricular variations.[72,182]

To permit ventricular visualization and the assessment of ventricular shape and wall motion by first-pass techniques, a higher dose (10 to 20 mCi) is employed. Acquired on a high-sensitivity camera and processed on a minicomputer with high count rate acceptability, the study may be displayed to reveal the anatomical features of a right-sided angiogram with subsequent levophase.[174,183] This flow study can be useful in the evaluation of congenital cardiac abnormalities and may demonstrate the presence and quantitate the size of central left-to-right or right-to-left shunts.[184] Subsequent temporal separation permits dynamic evaluation of ventricular wall motion, cardiac output, and ventricular volumes by the classic method noted above or employing a geometric method (Fig. 10-19).[168]

High-dose first-pass data in the temporal window of the respective ventricle can be spatially isolated and

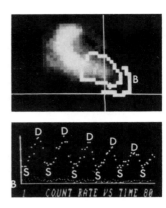

Figure 10-19. First-pass levophase analysis. Shown above is the levophase of a first-pass radioangiogram. A region of interest has localized the left ventricle. High-frequency analysis of the time versus radioactivity data in this region yields the curve below. Correcting for background, the peaks and valleys may be compared to calculate left ventricular ejection fraction. (Reproduced with permission from Botvinick EH, Glazer H, Shosa D. What is the reliability and the utility of scintigraphic methods for the assessment of ventricular function? In: Rahimtoola S, ed. Controversies in coronary artery disease. Philadelphia: FA Davis, 1981:65.)

formulated using postprocessing or gated to the R wave of the electrocardiogram, yielding alternating end-diastolic and end-systolic images, or framed to provide a cyclic display of ventricular contraction. First-pass methodology requires specialized equipment for optimal performance to avoid statistical difficulties at low count rates. Multicrystal cameras allow count rates up to 450,000/second without significant deterioration, but their resolution is suboptimal for other techniques.

In gaining the imaging advantage, the high-dose first-pass method becomes less suitable for study repeatability. Nonetheless, such methods have been applied to the evaluation of changes in ventricular function with dynamic stress, pharmacologic intervention, and in a variety of clinical situations.[185–189]

It would take a count rate five times that available on first-pass analysis to reduce the statistical error to that generally obtained with equilibrium blood pool studies.[190] Nevertheless, the high-dose first-pass technique compares favorably for ejection fraction determination with equilibrium and selective ventriculographic methods, with an extremely low level of intraobserver and interobserver variability.[191] This method may be applied to gain functional data from technetium-based perfusion agents.

Equilibrium Methodology

Equilibrium multiple gated blood pool scintigraphy is the most widely employed scintigraphic method for the evaluation of both right and left ventricular size and function.[192-196] Imaging is performed in synchrony with or gated to the surface electrocardiogram, at equilibrium, at least 5 minutes after intravenous administration, with complete mixing of the stable ^{99m}Tc blood pool label. At this time, each volume of blood contains the same amount of radioactivity. There are several methods to label the red cells. Although simply performed in vivo, greater labeling efficiency and stability are offered by the convenient modified in vitro method.[197] From 20 to 25 mCi of ^{99m}Tc pertechnetate (O_4^-) is combined with 10 mL of the patient's blood, previously combined with stannous ions. The labeled cells are then readministered and imaged. In vitro labeling adds efficiency and stability, sometimes necessary in the presence of multiple medication.[198] Radionuclide stability permits repeated imaging in multiple projections without temporal constraints, yet lacks the speed and temporal and spatial selectivity of first-pass methods. Resolution of anatomy and wall motion is optimized by acquisition in three projections, anterior, 70° left anterior oblique, to view the inferior wall,[199] and the "best septal" left anterior oblique projection. The best septal separates the two ventricles and is often obtained with a caudal tilt to reduce left atrial overlap. A high-resolution, single-crystal camera and a high-resolution or slant-hole collimator should optimally be used in adults.

Since equilibrium studies depend on image analysis of a composite sum of serial cardiac cycles, they are always computer acquired and triggered by or "gated" to the R wave. The mean length of the R–R interval is established before acquisition. Frame mode acquisition serially images a predetermined fraction (40 msec or less) of the mean cardiac cycle, and is best employed with regular rhythms. In each temporal interval, or frame, image data are combined to yield a summed picture over 200 to 600 cycles (Fig. 10-20). The study is terminated when each monitored frame contains sufficient data to permit

the generation of images with adequate spatial resolution of chamber anatomy and to provide adequate statistical counts analysis (Figs. 10-21 and 10-22).

List mode acquisition employs an expanded computer memory to individually identify each scintillation temporally, in relation to the R wave, and spatially. Subsequently, an R–R histogram plotting beat length versus frequency can be generated and the data framed for the cycle length desired. List mode acquisition is of particular value in the presence of a variable heart rate, or in the compilation of specific parameters referable to end-diastole, the region of the cycle most affected by heart rate variability. Again, sequential frames, regardless of the method of their derivation, can be displayed as a cyclic, endless loop movie or, alternatively, end-diastolic and end-systolic images may be extracted and viewed to evaluate wall motion.[200]

It is possible to accurately assess wall motion and calculate ejection fraction using certain classic geometric assumptions.[201] The great advantage of the scintigraphic method lies in the fact that counts within the ventricular region of interest are proportional to volume, however. Thus, in the best septal left anterior oblique projection, background-corrected ESC may be subtracted from EDC and divided by EDC to yield an ejection fraction independent of geometry (Fig. 10-23).[167,170,193,196,202] Ejection fraction, as calculated by this method, demonstrates an extremely low intraobserver and interobserver variability; however, background correction is critical.[203] Multiple gated acquisition provides a simple, reproducible, and accurate serial assessment of ventricular size and function at rest after infarction[194,204-208] and during pharmacologic interventions[209,210] or exercise,[155,156,203,205-219] which affect heart rate and the relative duration of systole (Fig. 10-24). Equilibrium time versus radioactivity curves can be employed as well to measure mean and peak ejection and filling rates[220,221] and a variety of other functional

R WAVE SYNCHRONIZED BLOOD POOL IMAGING

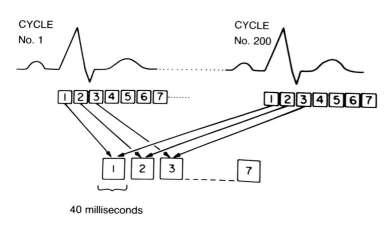

40 milliseconds

Figure 10-20. ECG gating of the blood pool images. With frame mode acquisition, image data representing preset fractions of the R–R interval, generally measuring 40 msec or less, are collected during each cardiac cycle. These individual frames are pooled with the same frame of subsequent beats until, after several hundred beats, summed frames (*below*) containing the sum of data representing all image intervals are displayed as an endless loop movie and analyzed for parameters of ventricular size and function. (Reproduced with permission from Strauss HW, Zaret BL, Hurley PJ, et al. A scintographic method for measuring left ventricular ejection fraction in man without cardiac catheterization. Am J Cardiol 1971;28:575.)

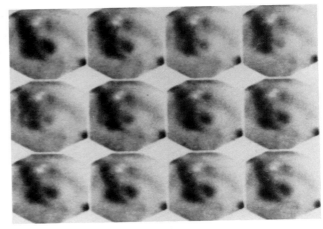

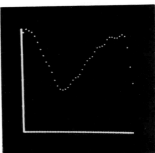

Figure 10-21. Multiple gated image. Shown in the "best septal" projection are 12 frames from a multiple gated equilibrium study. Contraction progresses left to right, top to bottom. End-diastole is in upper left and end-systole is immediately below it. A clear halo around left ventricular images indicates hypertrophy. At the bottom is a time versus radioactivity curve derived from left ventricular counts in this study, where peak counts are proportional to end-diastolic left ventricular volume and lowest counts are proportional to end-systolic volume. Curve count fall-off relates to irregular R–R intervals over the period of acquisition, where short cycles do not augment terminal frames. (Reproduced by permission of the Society of Nuclear Medicine from Green MV, Ostrow HG, Douglas MA, et al. High temporal resolution ECG gated scintigraphic angiocardiography. J Nucl Med 1975;16:95.)

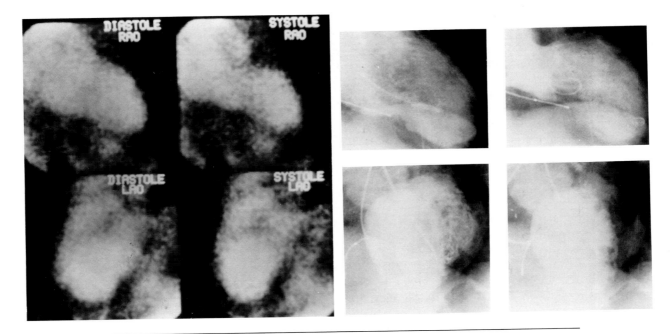

Figure 10-22. Blood pool/ventriculography comparison. Shown are diastolic (*left*) and systolic (*right*) frames from the rest blood pool scintigram of a patient with a left ventricular aneurysm in anterior (*above*) and "best septal" left anterior oblique projection. Similar images are shown by the same format from the selective ventriculogram in the same patient. Note both studies reveal best contraction in the postero-lateral base in the left anterior oblique projection. Scintigraphic anatomic information regarding regional wall motion is available and accurate and is further enhanced by functional image display. (Reproduced with permission from Botvinick EH, Glazer H, Shosa D. What is the reliability and the utility of scintigraphic methods for the assessment of ventricular function? In: Rahimtoola S, ed. Controversies in coronary artery disease. Philadelphia: FA Davis, 1981:65.)

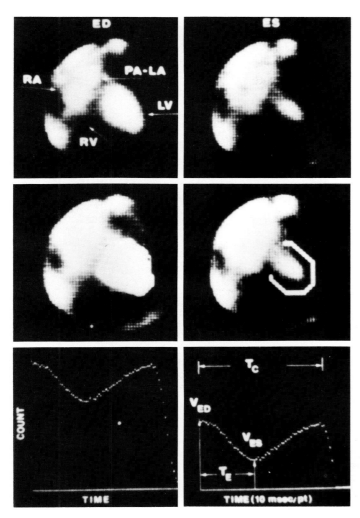

Figure 10-23. Equilibrium blood pool ejection fraction calculation. End diastolic (ED) and end systolic (ES) frames of a blood pool study are shown in the "best septal" projection (*above*). The region of the left ventricle is defined in the "best septal" projection (*middle left*) and a background region is selected adjacent to the end-systolic left ventricle (*middle right*). Applying this background value to the raw time versus radioactivity curve (*bottom left*) generates the corrected curve (*bottom right*). Since in this equilibrium method counts are proportional to volume, the curve peak is proportional to end-diastolic volume (V_{ED}), while the lowest curve value is proportional to the end-systolic volume (V_{ES}). This permits an accurate, reproducible method of ejection fraction calculation. (ED, end-diastolic frame; ES, end-systolic frame; LA, left atrium; LV, left ventricle; PA, pulmonary artery; RA, right atrium; RV, right ventricle; T_c, cycle duration; T_E, ejection time) (Reproduced by permission of the American Heart Association, Inc., from Green M, Ostrow HG, Douglas MA, et al. High temporal resolution ECG-gated scintigraphic angiocardiography. Circulation 1977;56:1024.)

parameters (Fig. 10-25).[222,223] In addition, curves can be assessed serially for relative volume changes or standardized for absolute volume.[224,225] A number of ventricular edge-detection methods are available to objectify these measurements, but all require occasional observer interventions.[226]

As for all methods, interobserver variability for the equilibrium scintigraphic calculation of right ventricular ejection fraction is greater than for left ventricular ejection fraction.[183,203] Yet, both scintigraphic methods are accurate and reproducible and have been useful for the single and serial evaluation of right ventricular ejection fraction and right ventricular wall motion in the assessment of right ventricular disease (Fig. 10-26).[183,192,219,222] and in the diagnosis of right ventricular infarction.[228,229] Both calculated right ventricular and left ventricular ejection fractions correlate well with hemodynamic parameters. Serial reproducibility of functional measurements of both ventricles may be altered by changes in blood pressure and ventricular compliance, food intake, and variations in blood volume.[230–233]

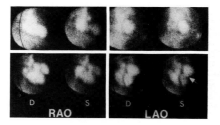

Figure 10-24. False left ventricular aneurysm. Above, in right anterior oblique (RAO) and left anterior oblique (LAO) projections, are end-diastolic (D) and end-systolic (S) images from the equilibrium blood pool study in a patient with a true aneurysm. Below, in the same projections and in the same format, are images from a patient with false left ventricular aneurysm. Unlike the former, the latter is not stabilized by myocardium and is actually formed by a contained myocardial rupture. The false aneurysm cavity is separated from the ventricle by a thin neck (*arrow*). (Reproduced with permission from Botvinick E, Shames D, Hutchinson J, et al. The noninvasive diagnosis of a false left ventricular aneurysm by gated blood pool imaging. Am J Cardiol 1976;37:1089.)

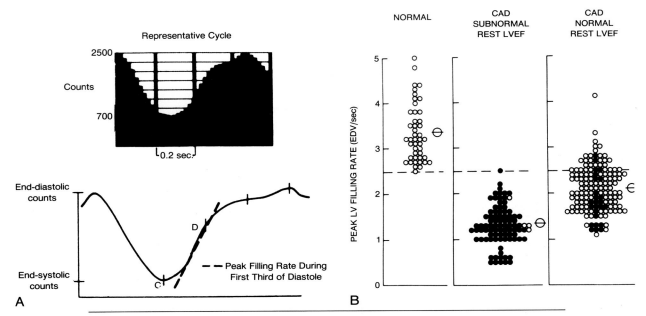

Figure 10-25. Evaluation and importance of diastolic filling measurements. *A:* Using first-pass data as shown here, or using equilibrium data (*B*), accurate noninvasive measurement of ventricular filling rate can be performed and applied to evaluation of a variety of problems. *B:* Bonow and coworkers found the scintigraphic peak left ventricular filling rate, expressed in end-diastolic volumes (EDV)/sec, to be lower than normal in most patients with coronary disease (CAD), studied at rest, regardless of the level or resting systolic function (LVEF). While this presents the promise of noninvasive coronary artery disease diagnosis without stress, filling rates may be nonspecific and depressed in a variety of conditions other than coronary disease. (*A,* reproduced with permission from Reduto LA, Wickemyer WJ, Yank JB, et al. Left ventricular diastolic performance at rest and during exercise in patients with coronary artery disease: assessment with first-pass radionuclide angiography. Circulation 1981;63:1228. *B,* reproduced with permission from Bonow RO, Bacharach SL, Green MV, et al. Impaired left ventricular diastolic filling in patients with coronary artery disease: assessment with radionuclide angiography. Circulation 1981;64:315. *A* and *B* reproduced by permission of the American Heart Association, Inc.)

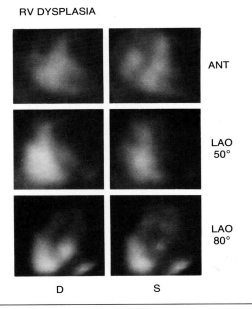

Figure 10-26. Right ventricular dysfunction. Shown are end-diastolic (D) and end-systolic (S) images in anterior (ANT) and 50° and 80° left anterior oblique (LAO) projections in a patient with right ventricular (RV) dysplasia. Note the large, poorly contracting right ventricle, which lifts the diminutive, vigorously contracting left ventricle.

A small, hand-guided, nonimaging probe has been developed that can perform first-pass and equilibrium studies.[182] However, in many cases problems of positioning could lead to gross inaccuracies in patients with segmental contraction abnormalities.[172] The technique has been applied to evaluate such serial changes after ergonovine administration in patients with variant angina[234] and during anesthesia administration in surgical patients with known or suspected heart disease,[235] and appears to be useful for measurement of emptying and filling phase indices. An extension of this approach is a miniature semiconductor detector, which, when mounted as a vest on a patient, can monitor ejection fraction continuously for hours in ambulatory subjects.[236]

Absolute Volume Calculation. At equilibrium, counts are proportional to volume. Relative volumes may be converted to absolute volumes by a number of methods. The proportionality factor is related to the duration of imaging, a product of the frame duration and the number of cycles imaged, the injected dose, and the mixing volume, and is affected by the attenuation of radioactivity imaged at depth. All methods seek to normalize acquired background-corrected counts within the left ventricular

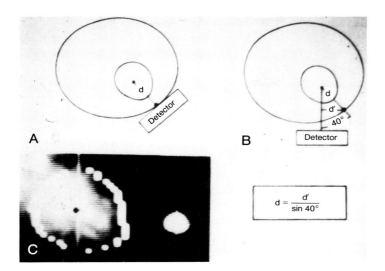

Figure 10-27. Attenuation correction. Shown is the mathematical basis for the measurement of an attenuation distance required to apply an attenuation correction, converting counts within the left ventricular region of interest to absolute volumes. The attenuation distance illustrated at the lower left is estimated from the measured distance from the center of the left ventricle to the chest wall marker overlying the center of the "best septal" projection, measured in the anterior projection (d'). If the "best septal" projection is the 40° left anterior oblique, the attenuation distance is given by d'/sin 40°. (Reproduced by permission of the American Heart Association, Inc., from Links JM, Becker LC, Schindledecker JG, et al. Measurements of absolute left ventricular volume from gated blood pool studies. Circulation 1982;65:82.)

region of interest for frame duration and time of acquisition, and use a blood sample to correct for the injected dose and blood volume. Links and coworkers placed a radioactive marker on the left chest wall over the center of the left ventricular region of interest in the best septal left anterior oblique projection.[225] The measured distance between the center of the left ventricle and the marker, as seen in the anterior projection, corrected for angulation, was taken as the attenuation distance of the left ventricle from the collimator face (Fig. 10-27). A number of recent studies have used phantoms or theoretical models to demonstrate the importance of attenuation and present various methods of correcting for this factor in the calculation of left ventricular volume.[237-239] Similar methods have been applied to right ventricular volume calculation. Bourguignon and coworkers measured the radioactivity in a volume of the cylindrical ascending aorta and used this value to correct left ventricular counts internally and thereby derive absolute volume.[240] Application of SPECT to the calculation of absolute ventricular volume requires extensive computer memory and software, but has obvious advantages related to spatial resolution.[241] Although some investigators have demonstrated accuracy and reproducibility for calculation of both right ventricular and left ventricular volumes in the absence of attenuation correction, the physical facts make attenuation hard to ignore.[224] Attenuation distances from 6 to 12 cm are common, which, when employing the attenuation coefficient of water, $\mu = 0.16$/cm, relates to an attenuation correction of roughly two to six times the measured radioactivity in the image region of interest. Practical and technical issues have led us to establish in our laboratory the relatively straightforward method of Links and coworkers.[225] The formula employed to calculate ventricular volume relates measured background-corrected left ventricular or right ventricular counts to the factors influencing its proportionality to volume:

$$\frac{\text{left ventricular counts*/time per frame} \times \text{cardiac cycles}}{\dfrac{(e^{-\mu d})\dagger}{(\text{venous blood counts/cc/sec})\ddagger}}$$

where μ = attenuation coefficient of water and d = left ventricular depth. Practically speaking, these values are available from a combination of computer-acquired measurements and from counting a blood specimen drawn at the time of imaging. With the proper software, decay correction is automatically performed, and calculations of end-diastolic volume, end-systolic volume, stroke volume, ejection fraction, and cardiac output follow quickly. Such quantitative assessment of ventricular size and function requires careful quality control but offers important advantages in the evaluation of blood pool images. The extreme amenability of equilibrium methods to computer manipulation would then make available a variety of absolute volumetric markers related to emptying and filling phases, as well as absolute values for regional parameters of ventricular function. Additionally, computer analysis permits the generation of a variety of functional data and images that are of great potential clinical value and that, in many cases, cannot be practically obtained by other methods.[158,188,211,222,223,242,247]

Quantitation is an extremely important aspect of clinical cardiology. Whereas qualitative methods may be satisfactory for diagnostic purposes, quantitation is required for accurate serial study, the evaluation of therapeutic effects,[157,248] and prognosis.[205,206,218,220] Specifically, quantitative estimates of ventricular volumes may be quite useful for evaluating the course of illness over time,[204,217,249] the effects of exercise,[216,218] the results of pharmacologic and surgical interventions[158,250,251] the ef-

*Background-corrected end-diastolic and end-systolic counts
†Correction factor for depth and attenuation
‡Correction for dose, blood volume, dilution

fects of potentially cardiotoxic drugs,[37,157,248] and the functional response to conduction sequence altered by pacemakers.[252]

Other Capabilities of the Method. Blood pool scintigraphy has been reported to demonstrate intracavitary masses and atrial myxomas,[253] identify the presence of ventricular hypertrophy,[254,255] differentiate pericardial effusion,[254] approximate pulmonary circuit hemodynamics from right ventricular ejection fraction,[228,229,256] and even estimate left atrial volumes.[258] Although such visual findings should be reported and such calculated measurements show promise, echocardiography appears to be the definitive and appropriately more widely used technique for the evaluation of such abnormalities. An exception in the evaluation of pericardial effusion relates to the scintigraphic ability to identify and quantitate the volume of bloody pericardial effusion, a useful aid after coronary bypass graft surgery (Fig. 10-28).[258] The scintigraphic method, however, remains the simplest and the most reproducible method for the quantitative assessment of parameters of left ventricular and right ventricular size and function after infarction, with various interventions, and during serial follow-up.[259,260]

Scintigraphic techniques afford the opportunity to quantitate left-sided or right-sided regurgitation fraction or intracardiac shunts, employing xenon washout techniques,[262] computer analysis of left-sided time versus radioactivity curves,[158,262] or the comparison of equilibrium stroke volume ratios or their equivalent (Fig. 10-29).[188,263] The latter calculation equals the left ventricular stroke volume expressed in counts divided by the counts equivalent of the right ventricular stroke volume. This regurgitant index (RI) should equal unity in healthy patients, increase in the setting of left-sided regurgitant lesions and left-to-right shunts distal to the atrial level, and decrease in the setting of right-sided regurgitant lesions or right-to-left shunts. For practical purposes, the regurgitant fraction, the fraction of the total stroke volume passing retrograde through the insufficient valve, equals (RI − 1)/RI. A number of investigators have reported an excellent association between scintigraphic and angiographic measurements of regurgitant fraction in patients with mitral and aortic insufficiency. Although useful for assessing the major hemodynamic lesion, quantitative assessment of a regurgitant or shunt lesion by this method can only optimally be done when that lesion is strongly dominant or isolated. In the presence of mixed lesions, the scintigraphic method accurately portrays their sum. The application of mathematical assumptions and new scintigraphic methods promises to overcome difficulties related to geometry and overlap in the physiologic assessment of regurgitant lesions.[263,264]

Regional counts and their serial alterations can be compared to yield information relating to regional stroke volume, ejection fraction, and regional and global ventricular emptying and filling rates.[188,211,222] Such derived stroke volume can be compared to yield accurate, reproducible regurgitant fractions.[158,265] Additionally, parameters relating to the degree and sequence of regional ventricular or atrial emptying can be derived and displayed.

Functional or Parametric Imaging. One of the great advantages of the equilibrium scintigraphic method is its ability to generate parametric or functional images.[265] Each functional image represents the distribution of some parameter related to or derived from the time versus radioactivity curve (Fig. 10-30).

The stroke volume image is generated by a pixel-by-pixel computer subtraction of background-corrected

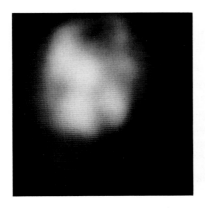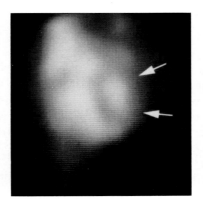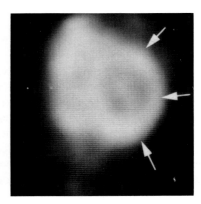

Figure 10-28. Bloody pericardial effusion. The arrows indicate the serial accumulation of a blood pericardial effusion over the course of 1 hour in these blood pool images after coronary bypass surgery. (Reproduced with permission from Viquerat CE, Hansen R, Botvinick EH, et al. Undrained bloody pericardial effusion in the early postoperative period after coronary bypass surgery: a prospective blood pool study. Am Heart J 1985;110:335.)

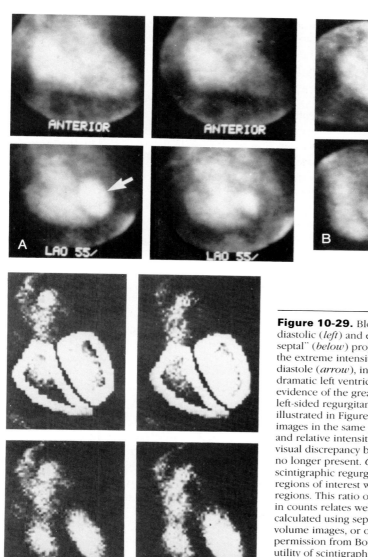

Figure 10-29. Blood pool imaging in mitral regurgitation. *A:* Shown are end-diastolic (*left*) and end-systolic (*right*) images in the anterior (*above*) and "best septal" (*below*) projections in a patient with significant mitral regurgitation. Note the extreme intensity of the left ventricle compared to the right ventricle in diastole (*arrow*), indicative of the large left ventricular volume. This, with the dramatic left ventricular ejection compared to the right ventricular, gives visual evidence of the greater left ventricular stroke volume, indicative of a significant left-sided regurgitant lesion, which was related to a regurgitant index of 2.7 illustrated in Figure 10-38A. *B:* Shown in the same format are the blood pool images in the same patient studied soon after mitral valve replacement. The size and relative intensity of the diastolic left ventricle are much diminished and the visual discrepancy between left ventricular and right ventricular stroke volumes is no longer present. *C:* Regurgitant index. In this initial calculation of the scintigraphic regurgitant index, the same left ventricular and right ventricular regions of interest were used in systole and diastole with efforts to exclude atrial regions. This ratio of left ventricular and right ventricular stroke volume expressed in counts relates well to the extent of valvular regurgitation but is more accurately calculated using separate end-diastolic and end-systolic regions of interest, stroke volume images, or other functional images illustrated below. (*B,* reproduced with permission from Botvinick EH, Glazer H, Shosa D. What is the reliability and the utility of scintigraphic methods for the assessment of ventricular function? In: Rahimtoola S, ed. Controversies in coronary artery disease. Philadelphia: FA Davis, 1981:65. *C,* reproduced by permission of the American Heart Association, Inc., from Rigo P, Alderson PO, Robertson RM, et al. Measurement of aortic and mitral regurgitation by gated cardiac blood pool scans. Circulation 1979;60:306.)

end-systolic from end-diastolic frames. Similarly, the ejection fraction image further divides these values by regional end-diastolic counts. In each case, regional stroke volume or ejection fraction is gray scale or color-coded for its local value.[222] These images are derived from global left ventricular end-diastolic and end-systolic frames and so are temporally dependent. That is, in the case of incoordinate contraction or conduction abnormalities, stroke volume or ejection fraction may not be accurate in image regions not sharing the systolic and diastolic timing of the global left ventricle. Regional stroke volume and ejection fraction images have been extremely useful for the assessment of changes after therapeutic interventions and after myocardial infarction[266,267] and are valuable for objectifying the response to stress or pharmacologic intervention.[188,210,211]

The phase image is a parametric image derived by fitting the time versus radioactivity curve to a cosine function of the following form on a pixel-by-pixel basis:

$$F_1(t) = A_0 + A_1 \cos(\theta_1 + W_0 t)$$

This is the first harmonic of the Fourier series, in which the frequency of the function is equal to the heart rate. For each pixel, A_1 (amplitude) is a measure of the excursion of the cosine curve approximating one-half the stroke counts. A_0 represents the mean amplitude; θ_1 is the phase angle, a measure of curve symmetry that describes the relative position of the curve peak in the acquisition

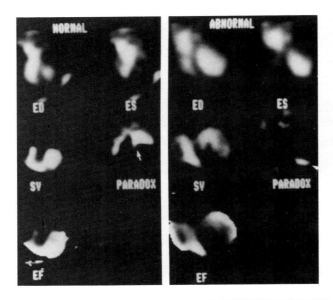

Figure 10-30. Functional images. Shown are end-diastolic (ED) and end-systolic (ES), stroke volume (SV), paradox, and ejection fraction (EF) images in a normal patient (*left panel*) and in a patient with a left ventricular aneurysm (*right panel*). The stroke volume image intensity codes regional, "positive" stroke volume, whereas the paradox image, made by subtracting end-diastolic from end-systolic data, reveals atrial and paradoxical ventricular segments (*arrows*). (Reproduced with permission from Botvinick E, Dae M, Schechtmann N. The current status of cardiovascular nuclear medicine: selected topics. In: Margulis A, Goodman C, eds. Diagnostic radiology. St. Louis: CV Mosby, 1985:513.)

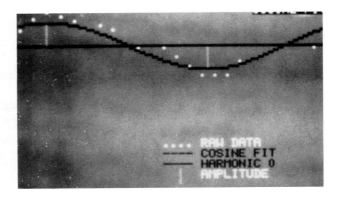

Figure 10-31. Cosine curve fit. Shown are the raw time versus radioactivity curve (*dots*) and first harmonic curve fit. The fitted curve peak defines the phase angle, measured from 0° to 360°, while the amplitude parallels the stroke volume and represents one-half the depth of the curve excursion. (Reproduced with permission from Frais M, Botvinick E, Shosa D, et al. Phase image characterization of ventricular contraction in left and right bundle block. Am J Cardiol 1982;50:95.)

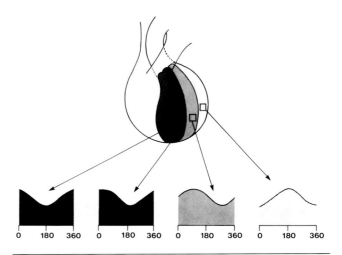

Figure 10-32. Phase analysis. The diagram presents a ventricle that is gray scale coded for increasing delay in contraction sequence, from septum to lateral wall. Resultant cosine curves fitted to the regional time versus radioactivity curves are shown below. The septum and its corresponding curve begin contraction at the R wave. The region has a phase angle of 0° and is coded dark gray. The lateral wall and its related curve fill when the ventricle should empty. This wall would demonstrate paradoxical motion and the curve would have a phase angle of 180°. (Reproduced with permission from Frais M, Botvinick E, Shosa D, et al. Phase image characterization of ventricular contraction in left and right bundle branch block. Am J Cardiol 1982;50:95.)

interval, the R–R interval; W_0 represents a parameter that converts time to degrees as the phase angle is expressed from 0°, the onset of the R wave gating trigger, to 360°, the onset of the subsequent cycle (Fig. 10-31). Values of amplitude A_1, and phase angle, θ_1, are extracted for each pixel and are gray scale or color-coded to provide amplitude and phase "maps" (Figs. 10-32 and 10-33). The evaluation of fitted data is employed, rather than sampling the raw data in each pixel in order to enhance sampling statistics.[223]

Unlike the stroke volume image, the amplitude image is not temporally dependent and does reflect the maximum excursion, proportional to stroke volume, regardless of where in the cardiac cycle this occurs. Although related to both systolic and diastolic curve features and influenced strongly by curve symmetry, the phase function has been related to the sequential pattern and extent of ventricular contraction and may be of value for identification of stress-induced ischemia[246] and assessment of serial function changes, as well as the extent of left ventricular aneurysm (Fig. 10-34).[244] The parameter has been applied to the assessment of the serial pattern of electrical excitation, has identified sites of ventricular impulse formation and the origin of sites of preexcitation (Fig. 10-35), has demonstrated characteristic patterns in

complete bundle-branch block[242,245,247] and left anterior hemiblock,[269] and has been shown to be accurate for the identification of the focus in patients studied during ventricular tachycardia.[248] Parametric images permit evaluation of measurements of ventricular function and structure that are not available with other methods.

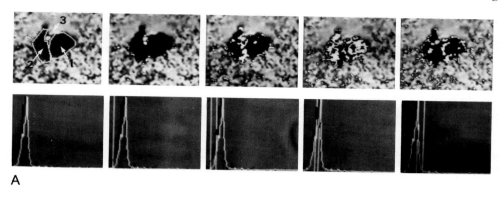

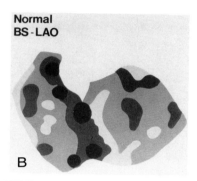

Figure 10-33. Normal phase analysis. *A:* Shown, above left, is the phase image in a patient with normal conduction and contraction. Early, homogeneous phase angle is evident from the dark gray shade of the left ventricle (*first arrow*) and right ventricle (*second arrow*) region of interest. The more proximal atrial regions are out of phase with the ventricles and have light gray shade and delayed phase angle in this "best septal" projection. The movement of background structures, bearing no relationship to cardiac contraction, is a random salt-and-pepper distribution of gray shades. Below are the left ventricular (*white*) and right ventricular (*black*) phase histograms generated from the respective regions above and plotting phase angle on the abscissa versus its frequency on the ordinate. Phase histograms are early, virtually superimposed and narrow based, indicating early, coordinate, and rapid onset of contraction through both ventricles. The pattern of phase progression, taken to roughly parallel the sequence of contraction, can be assessed by sequentially sampling the histograms via a set window of phase angles, vertical bars with corresponding whitening of the related pixels in the respective regions of interest. The site of earliest phase angle is seen in the proximal septum (*third arrow*), with subsequent homogeneous spread. *B:* Shown diagrammatically is the phase image of the same patient illustrated in part *A* of this figure. The site of earliest phase angle, in darkest gray, is again seen to occur in the septal region with subsequent symmetrical delay. (Reproduced with permission from Botvinick E, Frais M, O'Connell W, et al. Phase image evaluation of patients with ventricular pre-excitation syndrome. J Am Coll Cardiol 1984;3:799.)

The parametric stroke volume image and the amplitude image have been employed to derive the ratio of ventricular stroke volumes or their equivalent, the regurgitant ratio. Right atrial overlap tends to blunt the assessment of right ventricular stroke volume, however, falsely elevating the ratio. Using a simple correction that combines geometric considerations to correct for overlap and a regional phase evaluation to correct for incoordinate contraction, these effects can be largely eliminated (Fig. 10-36).[243]

Stress Evaluation. The reproducibility of blood pool measurements makes them eminently suitable for the assessment of quantitative serial changes with dynamic exercise.[93,202,203,269] These measurements have been applied to the detection of myocardial ischemia and to the evaluation of ventricular function in patients with valvular disease,[194] where it serves as a measure of valve disease severity and an indicator for surgical intervention.[270] Stress measurements have been used as well to assess the effects of chemotherapy. Although the latter can probably be effectively assessed at rest,[157,251] exercise blood pool imaging appears to have diagnostic accuracy for ischemia similar to exercise perfusion scintigraphy with ^{201}Tl (Fig. 10-37).[156,185,213,214,271] Generally, no change or a reduced ejection fraction with stress represents a pathologic response. Yet the response to stress varies with resting ejection fraction, age,[272] and stress end point. The complete

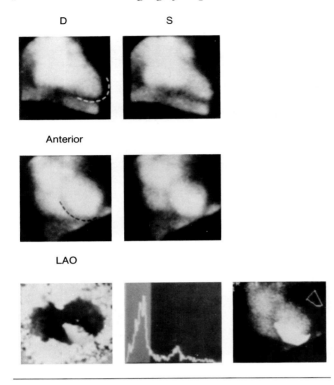

D   S

Anterior

LAO

Figure 10-34. Phase aneurysm evaluation. Shown in anterior and "best septal" projections are diastolic (D) and systolic (S) frames of a study in a patient with large left ventricular aneurysm. The akinetic segment has been outlined. Below, the left anterior oblique (LAO) phase image and histogram are shown. Pixels corresponding to an abnormal phase angle (*dark gray accentuation*) are highlighted on the phase image. The related area correlates with the percent akinetic segment and can be used to estimate the extent of aneurysm involvement. (Reproduced with permission from Frais M, Botvinick E, Shosa D, et al. Phase image characterization of localized and generalized left ventricular contraction abnormalities. J Am Coll Cardiol 1984;4:987.)

stress evaluation should include quantitation of volumes and their alteration, since a stress-induced increase in end-systolic volume has been shown to be a sensitive indicator of the ischemic response.[185] Similarly, filling rate may also prove sensitive to the identification of ischemia.[221,273] The "ischemic" response is not entirely specific, however, and can be encountered in hypertensive patients,[220,231] or in any condition with exercise-induced ventricular dysfunction. Nonetheless, the scintigraphic evaluation of the functional response to stress appears to relate to the extent of myocardium at ischemic risk, and eventual prognosis,[205,206,211,214–216] as well as to the potential for functional benefit related to invasive treatment of coronary disease.[249,261]

Pitfalls in Blood Pool Imaging. Errors in background selection are the most common type influencing blood pool results. A poor blood pool label may result in incomplete or erroneous image evaluation. Omission of the priming dose, drug interference, administration

through 5% dextrose in water, or label decomposition may be the cause. Errors in gating are also important and must be recognized, although soft tissue attenuation, though less common than that seen with ^{201}Tl, must still be considered. In addition to background errors, the faulty measurement of any involved parameter will lead to error in ventricular volume calculation. Most common are errors in the attenuation distance, where an underestimation will lead to a reduced volume. Particularly troublesome is the withdrawal of the blood sample from an intravenous line, where any dilution will lead to an overestimation of ventricular volume (Table 10-5).[274]

Comparison of Scintigraphic Methods

Each scintigraphic method provides some advantages that may make it more suitable for the performance of a given task. The methodologic differences should be seriously considered to determine the most appropriate scintigraphic method (Table 10-6). Both equilibrium and first-pass methods require a computer for full analysis. In spite of their differences, both techniques are capable of providing accurate, reproducible, and quantitative data regarding both right and left ventricular size and function.[167,181,183,192,193,207] Moreover, both techniques can be employed as complementary methods in the same patient.[192–194,200,275]

Schen and Jennings described calcium accumulation in myocardial cells early after the occurrence of necrosis.[276] Bonte and coworkers demonstrated the localization of ^{99m}Tc stannous pyrophosphate (TcPYP), already a common bone-imaging agent, in acute infarcts in dogs.[277] Similar to its localization in bone, myocardial localization appears to occur in regions of hydroxyapatite deposition in mitochondria and other subcellular fractions.[278,279] Intramyocardial TcPYP localization does not depend on the presence of calcium or leukocytic infiltration and has been documented to be confined to regions of irreversible damage.[280–282] Recently, other phosphate compounds, particularly ^{99m}Tc imidodiphosphonate (TcIDP), have been shown to have superior infarct affinity and accelerated blood clearance, providing advantages for infarct imaging.[283]

Relationship to Blood Flow

At higher levels of blood flow, TcPYP uptake appears to parallel the density of myocardial necrosis. However, TcPYP uptake falls precipitously below flow levels 30% to 40% of normal, regardless of the extent of cellular damage (Fig. 10-38).[279] It appears that TcPYP gains access into acutely infarcted myocardium, in relation to a total arte-

(*Text continues on page 368*)

WPW-Left Bypass
BS-LAO

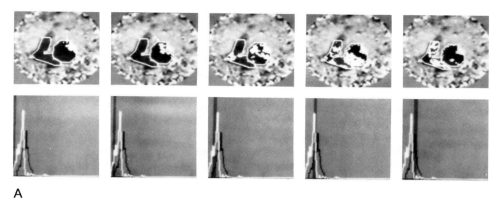

A

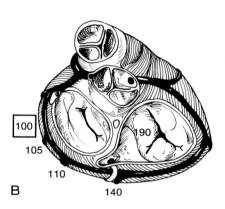

B

WPW-Right Bypass
BS-LAO

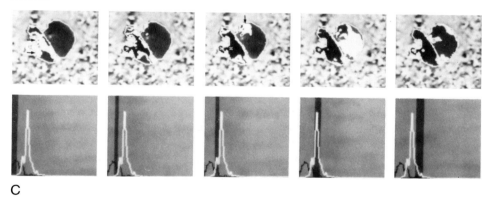

C

Figure 10-35. Phase analysis of atrioventricular connections. *A:* Shown, according to the same format as in the preceding figure, are phase images and histograms from a patient with Wolff–Parkinson–White syndrome studied during preexcitation in the "best septal" (BS-LAO) projection. Note the image site of earliest phase angle in the lateral left ventricular wall (*white arrow, above*), with parallel delay in the right ventricle phase histogram. *B:* Illustrated is the electrophysiologic map performed in the same patient as in *A* during preexcitation. The shortest interval of retrograde atrioventricular conduction, 100 msec, also occurred in the lateral left ventricular wall. *C:* Shown, according to the same format as shown in *B,* are phase images and histograms from a patient with preexcitation via a right-sided pathway. The sight of earliest phase angle appears in the lateral aspect of the right ventricle (*arrow, upper left*) with delayed phase angle in the left ventricle base (*arrow above, center panel*) and corresponding delay in the left ventricle (*white*) histogram. (Reproduced with permission from Botvinick E, Frais M, O'Connell W, et al. Phase image evaluation of patients with ventricular pre-excitation syndrome. J Am Coll Cardiol 1984;3:799.)

PHASE
REGURGITANT FRACTION

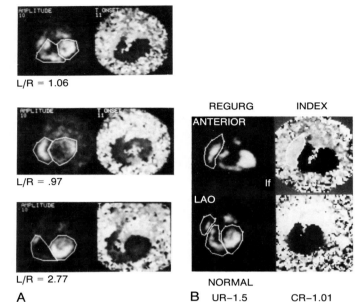

Figure 10-36. Atrial correction for regurgitation index. *A:* Shown are amplitude (*left*) and phase (*right*) images in the "best septal" left anterior oblique projections in a normal subject (*above*), a patient with cardiomyopathy without regurgitation (*middle*), and in the patient with mitral regurgitation illustrated in Figure 10-32. The ratio of left ventricular to right ventricular amplitude in outlined regions of interest yields a regurgitant index. Although accurate and reproducible, this index tends to overestimate the amount of regurgitation owing to a blunting of the apparent right ventricular amplitude due to right atrial overlap. *B:* Shown are phase (*right*) and amplitude (*left*) images in a patient without valvular regurgitation in anterior (*above*) and "best septal" (*below*) projections. The ratio of left ventricular to right ventricular amplitude in the regions outlined in the lower amplitude image again yields an uncorrected regurgitant index. The difference between the full projected and the atrial area evident in the LAO image represents an estimate of the right ventricular region obscured by the atrium. The right ventricular amplitude is then augmented by the mean right ventricular amplitude, multiplied over the area affected. In this example, the index falls from 1.5 uncorrected to 1.0 in this patient without valvular insufficiency.

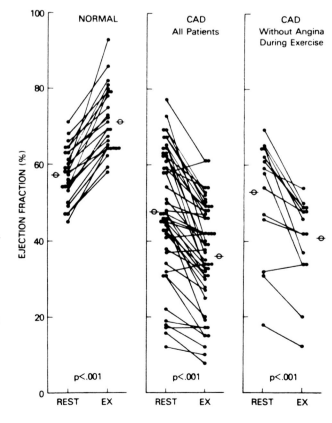

Figure 10-37. Stress blood pool evaluation. Shown from the initial study is the effect of dynamic stress on left ventricular ejection fraction. Left ventricular ejection fraction increases significantly in normals but shows little change or falls in patients with coronary disease, regardless of symptoms development. Subsequent studies revealed the response to be less specific and less sensitive with a normal ejection fraction response often seen in patients with coronary disease exercised to a nonischemic endpoint. (Reprinted by permission of the New England Journal of Medicine, from Borer J, Bacharach S, Green M, et al. Real time radionuclide cineangiography in the noninvasive evaluation of global and regional left ventricular function at rest and during exercise in patients with coronary artery disease. N Engl J Med 1977;296:839.)

Table 10-5

Pitfalls of Equilibrium Blood Pool Imaging

Poor red cell label
 Stannous ions omitted
 Drug interference
 Radionuclide decomposition
 Injection in 5% dextrose in water
 ^{99m}Tc administration—milking an old generator
Soft tissue attenuation
 Makes variations in right and left ventricular counts and
  inaccuracies in calculation of regurgitant index
Erroneous gating
 Bad beat acceptance
 Rhythm irregularity
Erroneous choice of left ventricular region of interest
Poor choice of background

Pitfalls of Equilibrium Blood Pool Volume Distribution

Erroneous entry of acquisition parameters
 Time of day
 Acquisition time
 Blood sample counts
 Sample volume
Blood drawn from IV infusion—diluted specimen
Blood drawn from IV radionuclide injection site—overestimate
 blood counts
Error in estimate of attenuation distance
Error in delineation of left ventricular region of interest
Erroneous background correction

Table 10-6

*Relative Advantages of Blood Pool Imaging Methods**

	First Pass		Equilibrium
	Low Dose	High Dose	
Technique	−	−	+
Quality control	−	−	+
Computer required	+ +	+	+ +
Acquisition time	+	+	−
Processing time	−	−	+
Radiopharmaceutical	+	+	−
Dose (radiation exposure)	+	−	−
Repeatability	+ +	−	+
Reproducibility	+	+	+
Image quality	−	+	+ +
Segmental wall motion	−	+	+ +
Left ventricular ejection fraction	+	+	+
Left ventricular volumes	+	+	+
Right ventricular ejection fraction	+ +	+ +	+
Functional parameters and images	−	−	+
Use with interventions	+	+	+ +

*Advantages of the method in the respective category are noted in
increasing order from − to + to + +.*

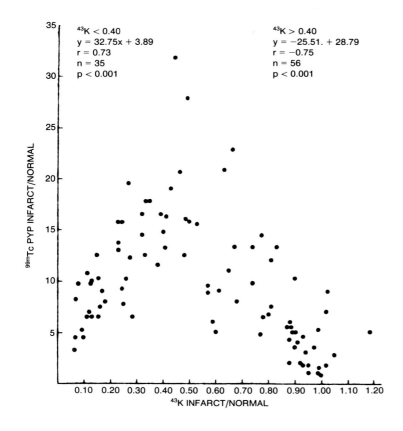

Figure, $^{43}K < 0.40$
$y = 32.75x + 3.89$
$r = 0.73$
$n = 35$
$p < 0.001$

$^{43}K > 0.40$
$y = -25.51. + 28.79$
$r = -0.75$
$n = 56$
$p < 0.001$

Axes: ^{99m}Tc PYP INFARCT/NORMAL (vertical); ^{43}K INFARCT/NORMAL (horizontal)

Figure 10-38. Relationship of ^{99m}Tc to perfusion. Shown is the relationship between ^{99m}Tc pyrophosphate and ^{43}K infarcted and normal tissue. Although perfusion relates inversely to ^{99m}Tc pyrophosphate and apparent infarct density at high flow levels, at low flow levels, ^{99m}Tc pyrophosphate density also falls. (Reproduced by permission of the American Heart Association, Inc., from Zaret BL, DiCola UC, Donbedial RK, et al. Dual radionuclide study of myocardial infarction. Circulation 1976;53:422.)

rial occlusion, via residual and collateral flow to the region. The "doughnut pattern" of TcPYP uptake, seen in association with proximal occlusion of the left anterior descending coronary artery in animals and humans, has been related to a poor prognosis (Fig. 10-39).[284] Some ascribe the central clear area to reduced radionuclide localization in a region of ischemic infarction. However, the origin of the pattern may relate to projectional factors.

Image Dynamics, Methods, and Interpretation

After infarction, the radionuclide depends for its localization on access to the involved area and maturation of a

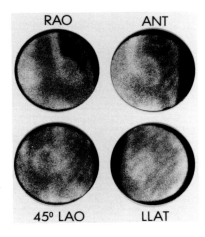

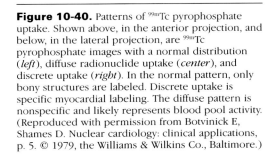

Figure 10-39. Doughnut configuration. Shown are [99mTc] pyrophosphate images in multiple projections in a patient with a recent anterior lateral infarction. The doughnut configuration has been associated with a large infarct area and a poor prognosis, and may relate to poor central infarct perfusion. (Reproduced with permission from Botvinick E, Shames D. Nuclear cardiology: clinical applications, p. 5. © 1979 the Williams & Wilkins Co., Baltimore.)

biochemical process. Although increased radioactivity is present in involved tissue as early as 4 to 6 hours after infarction, these cellular processes do not generally result in positive TcPYP images until at least 12 hours after the onset of necrosis. This may relate, in part, to progressive increase in collateral supply to the infarct zone. In most patients with infarction, cardiac radioactivity is maximum at 48 to 72 hours, becomes less intense by 6 to 7 days, and is usually absent by 10 to 14 days after the event.[280–282] Reduced radionuclide avidity relates to progressive replacement of necrotic myocardium by granulation tissue and scar.

Distribution of "cardiac" radioactivity has been interpreted as localized and discrete, or diffuse (Fig. 10-40).[285] The former is specific for myocardial damage, whereas the latter, originally thought to be related to subendocardial infarction, is most frequently related to blood pool radioactivity.[286] Further, diagnostic security increases with the intensity of uptake, graded 1+ to 4+. "Diffuse" should not be confused with "generalized" myocardial uptake. The latter is occasionally localized to widespread subendocardial, "shell" infarction, but projected, in these ungated images, throughout the left ventricular myocardium (Fig. 10-41). Combined blood pool and infarct imaging with computer comparison or computer subtraction of background has been suggested as a method to distinguish myocardial from cavitary radioactivity.[287] The interpretation of multiple projections, radiopharmaceutical choice and care in preparation, and imaging are more practical approaches, however. Rotating slant-hole tomography at the bedside or rotating camera ECT has recently been shown to aid diagnostic accuracy (Fig. 10-42).[288]

Figure 10-40. Patterns of [99mTc] pyrophosphate uptake. Shown above, in the anterior projection, and below, in the lateral projection, are [99mTc] pyrophosphate images with a normal distribution (*left*), diffuse radionuclide uptake (*center*), and discrete uptake (*right*). In the normal pattern, only bony structures are labeled. Discrete uptake is specific myocardial labeling. The diffuse pattern is nonspecific and likely represents blood pool activity. (Reproduced with permission from Botvinick E, Shames D. Nuclear cardiology: clinical applications, p. 5. © 1979, the Williams & Wilkins Co., Baltimore.)

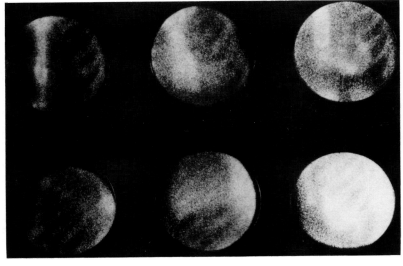

bo

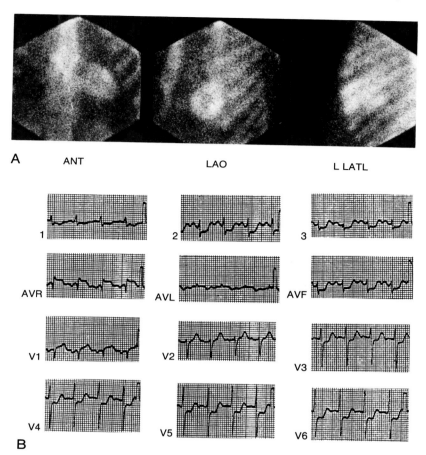

A   ANT   LAO   L LATL

B

Figure 10-41. Extensive ^{99m}Tc pryophosphate (TcPYP) uptake. *A:* The extensive pattern of TcPYP uptake illustrated in multiple projections is related to a poor prognosis. In surviving patients, it indicates a widespread subendocardial or shell infarction. *B:* The related electrocardiogram shows widespread ST segment depression without Q waves. (Reproduced by permission of the American Heart Association, Inc., from Botvinick E, Shames D, et al. Acute myocardial infarction: clinical application of technetium 99m stannous pyrophosphate infarct scintigraphy. Circulation 1979;59:257.)

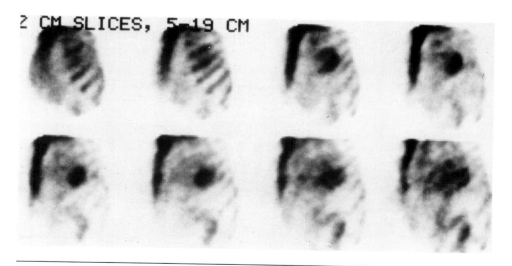

Figure 10-42. Rotating slant-hole tomographic ^{99m}Tc pyrophosphate imaging. Six planar images acquired at 60° angles in the 45° left anterior oblique projection were employed to reconstruct the normal tomographic images shown in the bottom row. Beginning with the first tomographic image in the top row, and proceeding left to right in this and the following row, the sternum and aspects of the ribs can be seen to come into and out of focus as slices are reconstructed from 5- to 19-cm depths at 2.0-cm intervals. The patient illustrated has an obvious apicolateral infarction.

Diagnostic Accuracy

Early animal studies revealed the ability of the method to detect regional transmural infarction as small as 3 g.[289] Parkey and coworkers demonstrated positive discrete uptake in all 23 patients admitted with transmural infarction.[285] Massie and coworkers revealed a direct relationship between image visualization and enzymatic infarct size.[290] They also demonstrated reduced sensitivity in subendocardial infarction, while others suggested a "diffuse" pattern of radionuclide distribution in subendocardial infarction. Soon a variety of investigators reported false positive TcPYP scintigrams in association with valvular disease,[291] unstable angina, stable angina pectoris,[292] heart failure,[293] after cardiopulmonary bypass,[294] and at a time remote from past infarction.[295,296] Although an occasional patient in these series revealed discrete uptake associated with a punctate area of valvular calcification, in association with unstable angina and enzyme release in relation to postinfarction pericarditis, most of these reported "false positives" were of the relatively low intensity, nonspecific "diffuse" pattern. Others, with discrete uptake, could largely be explained in reference to actual associated myocardial necrosis. Subsequent studies strongly suggested a relationship of diffuse uptake with blood pool labeling. Lyons and coworkers have reported decreased specificity of TcPYP for acute infarction due to a significant number of positive images weeks and months after the event.[295] However, a study of TcPYP scintigrams performed in 55 patients 9 days to 10 years after a documented transmural infarction revealed only two with discrete uptake. Both had extensive prior infarction and aneurysm.[296] Pathologic studies revealed evidence of ongoing necrosis in patients with remote infarction and scintigraphic myocardial uptake before demise in the absence of an acute coronary event.[297] Accepting the 2+ intensity classification as only equivocal, Berman and coworkers demonstrated a dramatic improvement in test specificity with only 3% false positives.[287]

Discrete uptake appears specific for acute infarction and correlates with electrocardiographic and pathologic infarct localization. Numerous studies suggest a diagnostic sensitivity to transmural infarction of 85% to 90%

probably best in relation to anterior infarction.[298] However, small transmural and subendocardial infarctions are less easily resolved and the study has a sensitivity to subendocardial infarction of 60% to 70%.[290,299] Although discrete uptake is more common in transmural and dense infarction, its presence cannot itself differentiate transmural from subendocardial infarction. Further, discrete uptake may be seen as well in relation to penetrating chest trauma, tumor invasion, or other conditions related to actual myocardial necrosis but bearing no relationship to an acute ischemic event.

"Primary" cardiac amyloidosis provides an exception to this analysis (Fig. 10-43).[300] Here, the infiltrative process is frequently associated with dense accumulation of the radiotracer. Although this may relate, in part, to an associated element of necrosis, there also appears to be a relationship with the amyloid deposit itself. Images in such cases may be impressive and, as in all circumstances, care must be taken to relate image findings to the clinical presentation.

Relation to Other Diagnostic Methods. Although sensitive to the presence of acute infarction, infarct avid scintigraphy is less sensitive than serial electrocardiographic changes, induced contraction abnormalities, serum enzyme release, and the presence of perfusion scintigraphic defects (Table 10-7). Neither wall motion nor perfusion scintigraphic abnormalities are specific for acute infarction, however, and electrocardiographic changes may also be nonspecific or concealed, or mimicked by a multitude of conduction abnormalities, drug or electrolyte effects, pericarditis, or other concomitant conditions. "Hot spot" infarct imaging maintains its specificity.

The presence of cellular damage and pathophysiologic evidence of necrosis does not itself determine clinical management. Infarction with extensive necrosis would precipitate a conservative approach. Prolonged or recurrent episodes of chest pain with evidence of only minimal necrosis, in the setting of unstable angina and evidence of enzyme release, would encourage an aggressive approach. Acute myocardial infarction scintigraphy adds to the specificity of infarction diagnosis and pro-

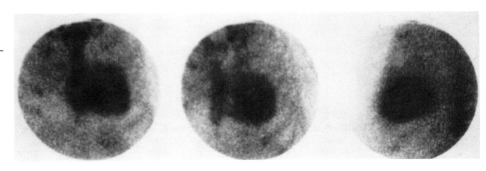

Figure 10-43. [99m]Tc pyrophosphate in amyloidosis. Shown are markedly abnormal ^{99m}Tc pyrophosphate images in (*left to right*) anterior, left anterior oblique, and left lateral projections acquired in a patient with primary amyloidosis. (Courtesy of Dr. R. Lull, Letterman Army Hospital, San Francisco, California.)

Table 10-7

Relative Accuracy of Infarct Diagnostic Methods

Sensitivity
Serial electrocardiogram changes
Wall motion abnormalities
Enzyme (CK-MB) abnormalities
Perfusion image abnormalities
Focal ^{99m}Tc pyrophosphate abnormalities

Specificity
Enzyme (CK-MB) abnormalities
Focal ^{99m}Tc pyrophosphate abnormalities
Serial electrocardiogram changes
Perfusion image abnormalities
Wall motion abnormalities

vides information relating to infarct size, localization, and prognosis. The method often provides better understanding of the clinical presentation and a more rational approach to patient management. Infarct scintigraphy appears to be of greatest value for infarct diagnosis in patients where acute electrocardiographic and enzymatic findings are nonspecific or unavailable.

Diagnosis of Postoperative Infarction. The diagnosis of perioperative infarction can be difficult, especially after coronary bypass graft surgery. Although the appearance of new Q waves after bypass surgery seems significant, the diagnosis may still remain in doubt. The presence of previous infarction, conduction abnormalities, nonspecific ST-T abnormalities, and pericarditis-related repolarization changes frequently make electrocardiographic findings nonspecific.[301] In this setting, even the MB-CK fraction may not be a useful clinical indicator of significant myocardial necrosis after coronary bypass surgery.[294,301,302] Several studies have demonstrated infarct scintigraphy to be a useful adjunct for the diagnosis of perioperative infarction after revascularization.[298,303] Preoperative images may be of added utility in gauging the extent of perioperative necrosis, especially in the presence of a known or potential and relatively recent preoperative event. In this case, the high specificity but limited sensitivity of the method work to clinical advantage. Patients with negative images generally bear an excellent prognosis and a benign postoperative course, regardless of associated electrocardiographic or enzymatic findings, whereas positive images generally relate to new contraction abnormalities and reduced ejection fraction and, occasionally, clarify the cause of new symptoms after surgery.

Evaluation Postcardioversion. Another important diagnostic subgroup is composed of patients in whom cardioversion or defibrillation has been carried out. Frequently comprised of patients suffering unex-

pected hemodynamic collapse or survivors of out-of-hospital sudden death, confirmation or exclusion of acute infarction is of considerable importance for both acute and chronic management. Classification in this population may be difficult where persistent enzyme and electrocardiographic abnormalities may relate to the trauma of resuscitation or prior unrelated infarction or conduction abnormalities. Although false positive studies have been reported with cardioversion,[303] the method appears to maintain its specificity postcoronary bypass graft surgery, even after direct electrical defibrillation,[304] and in the setting of catheter ablation of ectopic electrical foci or pathways. Care must be taken to avoid confusion with chest wall uptake, however, and, in turn, paddles must be placed judiciously to permit visualization of myocardial uptake.

Infarct Localization. The imaging method permits accurate infarct localization. Although of some importance for prognostic value, this also facilitates the differentiation of current from prior infarction. With serial study, infarct imaging may permit the identification of infarct extension and its differentiation from other postinfarction pain syndromes.

A number of studies have demonstrated the relationship between right ventricular TcPYP uptake, right ventricular wall motion abnormalities, and inappropriate elevation of right-sided pressures (Fig. 10-44).[229] Such scintigraphic findings parallel pathologic findings and are seen in roughly one third of all acute inferior infarctions. TcPYP imaging is the only specific direct, noninvasive method of diagnosing right ventricular infarction, which is of considerable clinical importance. To derive the full value of the method, technical errors must be avoided (Table 10-8).

Prognostic Value. Several reports have documented the relationship of infarct size to the development of power failure and an inverse relationship between estimates of infarct size and subsequent survival.[305] Imaging methods have been assessed for their ability to evaluate infarct size and assess methods to limit its extent and related prognosis. Although some workers have shown a correlation between CK enzyme infarct size and projected image infarct area, it is not surprising, owing to differences in their mechanisms, to note disagreement in the relationship between the amount of enzyme release and the magnitude of image infarct size.[298] TcPYP image infarct size correlated well with the weight and projected area of infarction in living dogs.[289,307,308] In patients, the infarct area correlated inversely with the stroke work index and with morbidity and mortality postinfarction (Fig. 10-45).[306] Although it was possible to differentiate infarct survivors from nonsurvivors by infarct image area, it

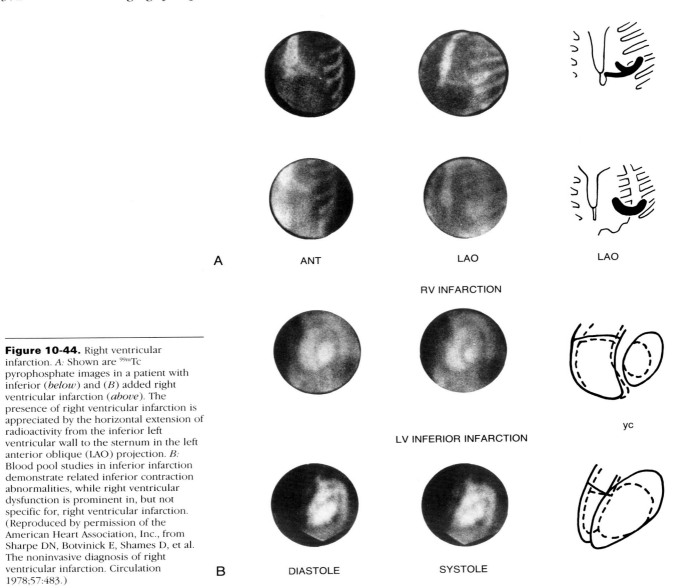

Figure 10-44. Right ventricular infarction. *A:* Shown are ^{99m}Tc pyrophosphate images in a patient with inferior (*below*) and (*B*) added right ventricular infarction (*above*). The presence of right ventricular infarction is appreciated by the horizontal extension of radioactivity from the inferior left ventricular wall to the sternum in the left anterior oblique (LAO) projection. *B:* Blood pool studies in inferior infarction demonstrate related inferior contraction abnormalities, while right ventricular dysfunction is prominent in, but not specific for, right ventricular infarction. (Reproduced by permission of the American Heart Association, Inc., from Sharpe DN, Botvinick E, Shames D, et al. The noninvasive diagnosis of right ventricular infarction. Circulation 1978;57:483.)

could not be used to prognosticate subgroups among survivors, as could the size of perfusion scintigraphic abnormalities and left ventricular ejection fraction (Fig. 10-46).[147,307]

New Agent

Recently, interest has focused on the ^{111}In-labeled FAB fragment of antimyosin antibody to label acute infarction.[309,310] The agent appears specific for acute infarction. However, it requires 24 to 48 hours for clearance of background and deposits significant radioactivity in the liver, possibly interfering with visualization of inferior infarction. Animal and patient studies thus far conducted indi-

Table 10-8

Pitfalls of "Hot Spot" Infarct-Avid Scintigraphy

Uptake in bony structures: ribs, cartilage, spine
Blood pool radioactivity
Poor label—free pertechnetate
Early imaging—before radionuclide localization or infarct maturation
Late imaging
Superficial uptake

cate excellent diagnostic accuracy and acceptable imaging characteristics. Most enticing is the independence of agent localization from regional flow. This could make localization a more direct function of infarct density and presents an excellent prospect for accurate infarct sizing.

Scintigraphic Evaluation of High-Risk Coronary Artery Disease

A great deal of interest has been directed at the identification of coronary patients at greatest risk. This is appropriate in light of the extreme morbidity, mortality, tragedy, and suffering caused by coronary disease, as well as its cost. The importance of this effort increases along with our ability to modify that risk.

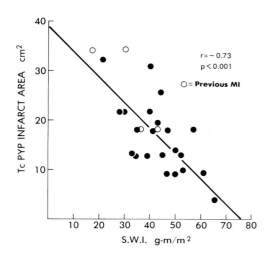

Figure 10-45. Functional infarct size. Shown is the relationship between "hot" spot, 99mTc pyrophosphate (TcPYP) image infarct size and stroke work index (S.W.I.), an index of ventricular function that correlates closely with patient prognosis. (Reproduced by permission of the American Heart Association, Inc., from Sharpe DN, Botvinick EH, Shames DM, et al. The clinical estimation of acute myocardial infarct size with Tc-99m pyrophosphate scintigraphy. Circulation 1978;57:307.)

Clinical Measures of High Risk

A variety of clinical parameters, including historical factors, behavioral characteristics, and hemodynamic and anatomic variables, are known to affect the overall risk and prognosis of patients with coronary disease. Risk is certainly related to the amount of scarred myocardium.[305,311] Most important among prognostic indicators are those related to the total amount of myocardium permanently lost or at reversible ischemic risk.

The Importance of Anatomy

Early natural history studies documented the reduced survival of patients with left main and multivessel coronary disease.[62] The presence of ventricular dysfunction reduced the survival in every anatomic subgroup.

The Contribution and Problem of Surgical Studies

Even if anatomy were the single determinant of coronary risk, it would be difficult to identify patients on this basis at presentation.[312] Further, the incidence of such high-risk anatomy varies widely in different coronary syndromes.[208,313] A number of controlled studies have demonstrated a limited but significant benefit of surgical intervention in the presence of triple-vessel disease, especially when related to reduced left ventricular function, and a greater benefit in the setting of left main coronary artery disease. Not all patients in the groups at risk benefit from the intervention, and surgery must be performed on many patients to provide a benefit to a few.[316,317]

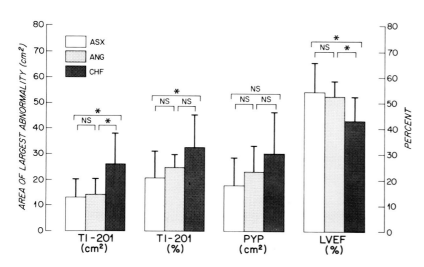

Figure 10-46. Scintigraphic prognosis. Perfusion defect size (Tl-201 cm²) and left ventricular ejection fraction (LVEF) were the best discriminators of asymptomatic patients (ASX) from those who suffered recurrent angina (ANG) or heart failure (CHF) postinfarction. (PYP, Tc pyrophosphate image infarct size) (Reproduced by permission of the American Heart Association, Inc., from Perez-Gonzales J, Botvinick E, Dunn R, et al. The late prognostic value of acute scintigraphic measurements of myocardial infarction size. Circulation 1982;66:960.)

Further, these studies often eliminated from analysis large numbers of patients with severe ischemic symptoms,[318] employed gross clinical markers and end points, and failed to use established pathophysiologic indicators of ischemia or recently developed image indicators of ischemia and infarction.[57,58] They also failed to consider the difference between coronary pathophysiology and anatomy, a factor of increased importance given the documented inaccuracy and variability of the visual evaluation of coronary stenosis.

None of these studies could document either an improvement in resting left ventricular function or reduction in subsequent infarction rate. Numerous population studies have identified those with greatest likelihood of postsurgical functional improvement, however, and scintigraphic studies have identified myocardial segments at greatest risk and likelihood for improvement after revascularization.[41,66,189] Would study results differ if patient populations were expanded and more selectively classified?

The Real Culprit: Salvageable Myocardium at Ischemic Risk

Since surgery and angioplasty offer nothing to infarcted, scarred segments, the full and specific component of patients at greatest risk who have the greatest possibility of benefit are those with a large or significant component of salvageable myocardium at ischemic risk.[318] This group includes postinfarction patients with preserved left ventricular ejection fraction after an episode of pulmonary edema,[319] a subgroup of those previously noted by Schuster and Bulkley to have "ischemia at a distance."[320] These and other studies suggest that the patient at greatest risk of death from coronary disease is that person who will have extensive nonfunctioning myocardium after the next event.[59,321]

Identification of Myocardium at Ischemic Risk

The extent of myocardium at ischemic risk can best be currently identified by a variety of noninvasive pathophysiologic electrocardiographic and scintigraphic markers for ischemia. Reduced exercise duration,[322] a low achieved double product,[323] the presence of stress-induced symptomatology and hypotension,[324] as well as deep ST segment depressions, particularly down-sloping and early in exercise,[325] and multiple extensive perfusion abnormalities have been highly correlated with the presence of main left or triple-vessel coronary disease.[326] Although scintigraphy seems to complement electrocar-

diography,[16,59,83,84,142] Canhasi and coworkers found that many more patients with "high-risk" anatomy could be identified by the presence of lung uptake or other supplementary scintigraphic indicators.[58]

Grouping Populations According to Coronary Risk

A recent thrust in cardiology research seeks to subgroup apparently high-risk populations in an effort to identify specific individuals at risk and estimate the presence and extent of reversible ischemia.[59,139,319] Such added prognostic discrimination permits the proper diagnostic and therapeutic focus to target invasive study and aggressive treatment at those who would most likely benefit, while excluding from such consideration patients not benefiting from it. Recent evaluation has demonstrated added advantages of surgery compared to medical treatment of coronary disease when pathophysiologic indicators of ischemia were considered.

Advantages of Scintigraphic Evaluation

Although able to separate patients into differing prognostic subgroups, stress tests continue to remain relatively nonspecific and insensitive, lack localizing information, and find particular difficulty in the presence of resting baseline abnormalities.[319,327] Reports document the value of both perfusion and blood pool scintigraphy in interpreting the significance of electrocardiographic changes in the setting of baseline abnormalities,[38] and the importance of "reciprocal" ST depressions outside an infarct zone,[328] of ST elevations within it,[329] and of T wave normalization. Multiple perfusion scintigraphic abnormalities identified patients who became hypotensive during stress on an ischemic basis,[330] better even than did extensive coronary involvement. Although the relative regional sensitivity of perfusion scintigraphy varies,[16,79] visual scintigraphic patterns specific for left main or triple-vessel disease have been identified.[83] Although relatively insensitive, scintigraphic and electrocardiographic findings were complementary in identifying "high-risk" coronary lesions.[83,328] Jones and coworkers demonstrated a direct relationship between the extent of decremental ejection fraction response and the extent of coronary involvement.[185] Within each coronary subgroup, however, there were wide variations, possibly related to pathophysiologic but real variation in stress response in patients with otherwise similar anatomy. Could scintigraphic variability better reflect the underlying risk than even the anatomy? The results of stress perfusion and blood pool study can be critical in determining relative coronary risk.[59,331,334]

Quantitative Computer Analysis

Attention to supplementary perfusion indicators and the objective, quantitative application of computer methods, including tomographic displays and "washout" analysis, promise to add to our sensitivity for the identification of extensive myocardial ischemia.[16,24,40,47,50] With this should come a further increase in our ability to assess risk and related prognosis. As important as the identification of those at greatest risk could be the elimination from consideration of those with little risk.[86,87,335]

High-Risk Patients Postinfarction

In the setting of acute infarction, the quantitative scintigraphic assessment of resting left ventricular ejection fraction and the extent of regional akinesis have been well correlated with survival.[206,306,312,336,337] Serial measures of left ventricular ejection fraction early and late after infarction have been identified as prognostic measures.[204] Further, the effect of nitroglycerin on regional ejection fraction and the findings on perfusion scintigraphy may predict those with associated viable but ischemic and nonfunctioning myocardium after the event.[41,65,66,189,190] Brown and coworkers determined that left ventricular ejection fraction was the leading independent indicator of risk after infarction, but in the absence of infarction it was the extent and distribution of scintigraphic perfusion abnormalities.[141] Gibson and coworkers have shown that multiple perfusion abnormalities predicted a high complication rate in patients with inferior infarction compared with the low rate seen in patients having isolated inferior defects, however.[329]

"Hot Spot" Imaging. These agents have been shown to correlate well with pathologic measures of acute infarction size in animals and in patients.[289,338] Image infarct size related inversely to left ventricular stroke work index and directly with prognosis in patients with crescendo angina,[339] negative images related to a benign prognosis. Poor prognosis was associated with a doughnut configuration,[284] persistent image positivity,[295] and large scintigraphic abnormalities.[340,341] Infarct images were prognostic but less discriminating than the scintigraphic evaluation of function or perfusion postinfarction. This probably relates to the fact that infarct imaging cannot offer the full identification of myocardium at reversible ischemic risk (see Fig. 10-46),[142,143] including regions of prior infarction and ongoing ischemia. Differences in size of abnormalities on perfusion or blood pool and infarct images may give clues to the extent and nature of myocardium at risk and related prognosis.

Perfusion Scintigraphy Postinfarction. Wackers and coworkers have documented the extreme diagnostic sensitivity of myocardial perfusion scintigrams during the early hours to days after acute infarction.[67,68] A postmortem study by Bulkley and coworkers identified a subgroup of patients demonstrating large perfusion scintigraphic abnormalities premortem but relatively smaller areas of pathologic scar, likely owing to the prior presence of significant ischemic myocardium.[342] Becker and coworkers documented the extreme complementary prognostic value of combined scintigraphic evaluation of perfusion defect size and left ventricular ejection fraction (Fig. 10-47).[142]

Gibson and coworkers have documented the value of predischarge perfusion scintigraphy for the identification of postinfarction patients at greatest risk for future cardiac events (Fig. 10-48).[59] Most revealing was the finding that the number and extent of perfusion abnormalities were the most important predictors of a subsequent event, more predictive than stress-induced ST depression or the documented presence of multivessel coronary disease. Further, neither did the presence of multivessel disease ensure a poor prognosis, nor did its absence

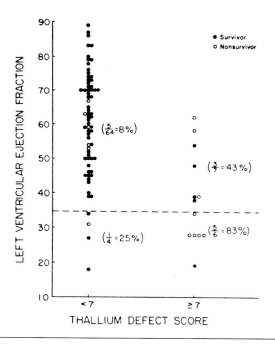

Figure 10-47. Prognosis postinfarction. In this study, the scintigraphic evaluation of left ventricular ejection fraction and the extent of the perfusion abnormality best subgrouped patients into risk subgroups. (Reproduced by permission of the American Heart Association, Inc., from Becker LC, Silverman KJ, Bulkley BH, et al. Comparison of early thallium-201 scintigraphy and gated blood pool imaging for predicting mortality in patients with acute myocardial infarction. Circulation 1983;67:1272.)

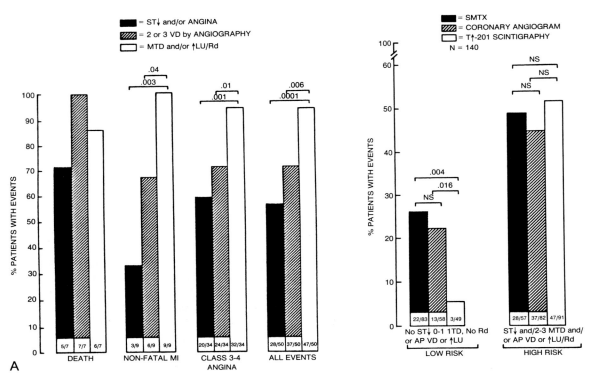

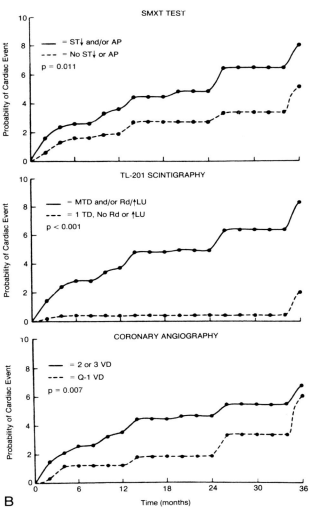

Figure 10-48. Prognosis of perfusion scintigraphy. *A:* Shown at the left is the incidence of positive stress test ischemic ST depression or angina, two or three vessel coronary disease (VD), or positive scintigrams (multiple perfusion defects or lung uptake with evidence of redistribution) among patients who experienced death, nonfatal infarction (MI), severe angina, and all events. At the right is the frequency of events among patients not demonstrating these stress-induced, anatomical or scintigraphic abnormalities compared to those that did. Scintigraphic findings were best both for identifying patients with highest risk of postinfarction events and separating high-risk from low-risk subgroups. Patients could not be subgrouped by any other parameter. *B:* Plotted for this same patient population is the probability over time, of cardiac events in the presence or absence of multivessel coronary disease, scintigraphic or stress test (SMXT) abnormalities (from below upward). Scintigraphy provided a significantly better separation of high-risk and low-risk subgroups than parameters noted or any other considered. (Reproduced by permission of the American Heart Association, Inc., from Gibson RS, Watson DD, Craddock GB, et al. Prediction of cardiac events after uncomplicated myocardial infarction: a prospective study comparing predischarge exercise thallium-201 scintigraphy and coronary angiography. Circulation 1983;68:321.)

ensure a benign prognosis. Hung and Corbett and coworkers[205,334] have each documented a strong independent relationship between the response on stress blood pool scintigraphy and the occurrence of subsequent events in the postinfarction period.

Dipyridamole Perfusion Scintigraphy

Perfusion scintigraphy during infusion of dipyridamole appears able to identify coronary disease and ischemic myocardium.[97] It is most valuable in patients unable to undergo dynamic stress, a group often at greatest coronary risk. The method appears to have prognostic value in important patient subgroups.[109,110]

The Clinical Approach to the High-Risk Patient

Several publications have sought to integrate the results of this body of literature in the evaluation and treatment of patients with known or suspected coronary disease. Silverman and Grossman[343] mention scintigraphic evaluation of ischemia prominently in their evaluation of risk and determination of treatment of coronary patients (Fig. 10-49). DeBusk and coworkers[344] recently noted that quantitative blood pool evaluation of resting function and stress scintigraphic identification of reversible ischemia complement standard stress testing in the identification of approximately 30% of the population at high coronary risk who would not otherwise be recognized. Such analysis appreciates the relative imperfection and complementary nature of all noninvasive methods. Accepting the numerous indicators of extensive coronary disease and, more specifically, of coronary events and risk, the modern, aggressive cardiologist applies historic, physical, electrocardiographic, and scintigraphic findings to selected patients for invasive study and revascularization. Even after catheterization, proper treatment can often be designed only after the appropriate evaluation of both physiologic and anatomic assessment. Depending on the combined evaluation and the personnel and skills available, the proper course of treatment can be chosen.

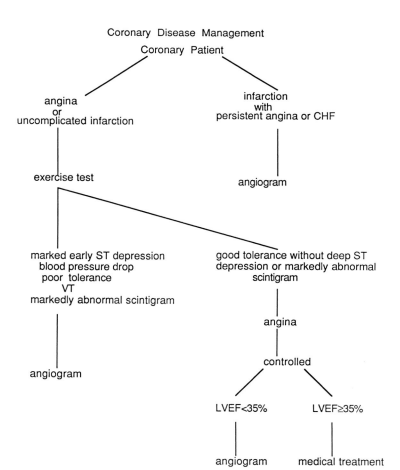

Figure 10-49. Coronary disease management. Shown is the relationship of scintigraphic studies with symptomatology and other test results in the determination of patient management. Left ventricular ejection fraction can be quantitatively and reproducibly calculated *only by blood pool scintigraphy.* (Adapted by permission of the New England Journal of Medicine, from Silverman KJ, Grossman W. Angina pectoris: natural history and strategies for evaluation and management. N Engl J Med 1986;314:161.)

A Consideration of Scintigraphic Cost-Effectiveness in Coronary Disease Evaluation

There are a host of studies that can be performed in the evaluation of patients with known or suspected ischemic heart disease. The characteristics of the ideal imaging method can be summarized by a number of parameters related to safety, cost, and clinical effectiveness. Bell assessed clinical efficacy or utility to be of three varieties: diagnostic efficacy, confirmed by comparison with the standard; management efficacy, considering how a test influences management; and outcome efficacy, gauging the ability of the test to prognosticate the clinical outcome.[345] Scintigraphic study has been assessed from each of these perspectives.

One certain observation relates to the fact that if a test is not useful in a specific clinical situation, any advantage the test may have in other circumstances is lost. Although pericardial effusion[255] and sometimes an intracavitary mass[254] can be seen on blood pool scintigraphy, or hypertrophy on perfusion scintigraphy,[69] the echocardiogram is the imaging test of choice for these abnormalities.[346,347] Conversely, exercise echocardiography is qualitative and here scintigraphy appears to be the study of choice for the evaluation of ventricular function with stress or other intervention.[167,344,348] Cost-effectiveness is clear in such situations: where the tests are of similar clinical value, the less expensive test is the clinically preferred; when the specific question clearly demands a given application, that test is to be applied. Neither do considerations related to ionizing radiation generally alter a scintigraphic preference if its advantages are otherwise apparent, since the exposure is small. Similar considerations must be made when seeking to noninvasively quantitate shunts,[184] the extent of valvular regurgitation,[303,322] or determine the location of a preexcitation pathway.[217] For these studies, there is no substitution and the choice simply relates to the clinical contribution of the data presented. Similarly, cost-effectiveness of infarct-avid imaging is related to the need and ability to make the diagnosis and localize and quantitate the event without the study.[291,294,298,301,302]

Cost-effectiveness is often difficult to assess objectively, especially in relation to coronary disease, where the choices are numerous and varied. In considering cost effectiveness, a variety of situations and parameters must be considered. Obviously, the cost, advantages, and disadvantages of the test, the specific clinical question, and the patient population are important. Specifically, test predictive value will vary with the pretest disease likelihood, regardless of test accuracy. Any test will be somewhat less cost-effective in a population with a relatively low prevalence.[349–351]

The ability of cardiac scintigraphy or any test to influence the pretest probability and come to a different posttest probability is greatest where the pretest probability is in an indeterminate range, that is, where the diagnosis is insecure.[134] Unlike the situation with populations at very low or very high levels of the scale, where test results do not strongly influence pretest probability, patients with an intermediate probability have the greatest realization of cost effectiveness.

Patterson and coworkers[136] evaluated the effects of perfusion scintigraphy on pretest probability calculated by the method of Diamond and Forrester.[138] The study illustrates test effectiveness in the diagnosis and exclusion of disease to be greatest when diagnosis is in doubt and the pretest probability is intermediate. They have also illustrated that test results in parallel (e.g., an abnormal scintigram supporting an abnormal stress electrocardiogram) add a degree of diagnostic security. There is a certain potential benefit in using combined test diagnostic or predictive power. Conversely, since errors related to two tests are additive, such assessment must be carefully applied.[352]

Another study by Patterson and coworkers[135] evaluated cost-effectiveness in terms of dollars and cents. Here, a theoretical population of 1000 men aged 45 was used as a model of test effectiveness for the assessment of asymptomatic coronary disease. Although costs have increased since the study publication, relative values and study conclusions still appear valid. By this analysis, were catheterization performed on patients who have both positive stress electrocardiogram and scintigram, rather than on all patients with a positive stress electrocardiogram alone, costs would be halved while still identifying 85% of those patients with significant coronary lesions. This excludes any benefits of eliminating the risk and discomfort of needless angiography and does not consider anatomic–pathophysiologic differences, which would add to the scintigraphic advantage.

In yet another analysis, these same investigators sought to assess coronary disease diagnosis and cost effectiveness in terms of years of life preserved in relation to four testing approaches.[135] The authors assessed costs in relation to disease prevalence as well. The lowest cost was seen in relation to the performance of angiography only if both stress test and scintigram were positive. Conversely, when prevalence is plotted versus mortality, it is clear that this approach pays the greatest penalty for patient misdiagnosis in terms of mortality when both tests are required to be positive. Again, mortality was relatively low and stable at all prevalence rates, when angiography was done on all patients. The same data were assessed taking into account all possible factors and the cost per patient diagnosed was calculated. This parameter, most closely related to what we could call cost-effectiveness, was lowest for the approach calling for angiography but only after positive scintigraphy. The difference was most significant at low disease prevalence, yet persisted to rates well over 50%. When test effectiveness was assessed in terms of survival, this approach again yielded the lowest cost per year of quality life preserved. This analysis is strictly based on diagnostic costs and fails to consider advantages related to less tangible values, which also must be factored into the cost-effectiveness equation.

This group also presented a cost-effectiveness analysis for coronary disease diagnosis in a population of 96 patients who had symptoms of unknown cause.[88] If stress testing, scintigraphy, and angiography were done on all patients, no patients with disease would be missed, but the cost per patient diagnosed would be high. If angiography is omitted when both stress electrocardiogram and scintigraphy are negative, or when the history is diagnostic, again no patients are missed, but the costs dramatically fall (Table 10-9). In addition to demonstrating cost-effectiveness, this analysis also demonstrates the value of the scintigraphic method in excluding coronary disease. Although these analyses demonstrate the interaction of tests in affecting costs, cost-effectiveness must be assessed as well in terms of the diagnostic sacrifices we find acceptable. These considerations are as much ethical as clinical.

Patterson and coworkers performed a more complicated analysis in seeking to estimate the cost-effectiveness of screening postinfarction patients for left main and triple-vessel disease.[81] Most cost-effective was the performance of angiography on those patients with stress scintigraphic perfusion abnormalities outside the infarct zone or in those with other clinical or stress test indicators of extensive ischemia, and few patients were missed. Here, the use of all diagnostic and clinical parameters resulted in both high diagnostic and, if we recognize the poor prognosis related to the anatomy identified, outcome efficacy.

Dipyridamole perfusion scintigrams are performed in patients who cannot or should not undergo dynamic stress testing. These patients often have rest pain and, if this is ischemic in origin, it is related to severe coronary disease. Frequently they are to undergo noncardiac surgery and are placed at significant coronary risk without any reasonable method of evaluation. Performing angiography in all of these patients is certainly ill advised, as abnormalities would be found. But could their related risk be evaluated or the anatomic information applied to properly determine the course of management?

In the initial population of 61 patients assessed with dipyridamole perfusion scintigraphy, we sought to evaluate test effects on clinical management.[108] We calculated pretest disease probability[137] and determined test influence on patient management by set criteria. These included patients with a low pretest probability and revers-

Table 10-9

Estimated Cost-Effectiveness of Exercise Tests to Evaluate Patients With Chest Pain

Cost × Patients (n)	Total (Dollars)	Patients with CAD Who Would Be Missed (% of All CAD Patients)
All Tests in Every Patient		
Angiography $3000 × 96	$288,000	
Exercise tests $300 × 96	$ 28,800	
Total	$316,800	0%
Angiography Only		
Angiography $3000 × 96	$288,000	
Exercise tests $300 × None	$ 0	
Total	$288,000	0%
Avoid Angiography if Exercise Tests Are Both Negative		
Angiography $3000 × 79	$237,000	
Exercise tests $300 × 96	$ 28,800	
Total	$265,800	6%
Avoid Angiography if Exercise Tests Are Both Negative and Avoid Exercise Tests if History Reflects Typical Angina in a Patient over 40 Years of Age		
Angiography $3000 × 82	$246,000	
Exercise tests $300 × 43	$ 12,900	
Total	$258,900	0%

Reprinted with permission from Patterson RE, Horowitz SF, Eng C, et al. Can exercise electrocardiography and thallium-201 myocardial imaging exclude the diagnosis of coronary artery disease? Am J Cardiol 1982;49:1127.

ible image abnormalities who went on to catheterization or an aggressive medical management; patients with a high pretest probability and a benign image who were discharged or managed conservatively; and patients with an intermediate pretest probability or known coronary disease who were sent to image evaluation with ambiguous coronary anatomy and who demonstrated image findings consistent with subsequent management. The preliminary results were impressive, since dipyridamole scintigraphy influenced management in almost 80% of this initial group of patients with known or suspected coronary disease who could not undergo dynamic stress testing. Further, since scintigraphic and angiographic findings were generally consistent, such influence was apparently appropriate. The rate of such test influence is extremely high and relates to the diagnostic difficulty presented by these patients, the lack of acceptable diagnostic alternatives, and the need and willingness, more so in these patients, to let image results guide management decisions. This test then is an excellent example of high management efficacy as well as cost-effectiveness. Studies have already been noted that demonstrate the potential outcome efficacy of the method.[109,110] Because of such results and the findings of Gibson and other workers[59] documenting the value of the scintigraphic method in identifying coronary patients at greatest risk,[1-4,142,206,306,340,341] a number of recent publications indicate the importance of the role of stress scintigraphic study in the evaluation of patients with known or suspected coronary disease.[342-344]

The cost-effectiveness of other diagnostic and therapeutic procedures is also of interest. In a study by Moorman and coworkers,[353] the value of 1410 rest electrocardiograms was assessed. The diagnostic yield was extremely small. Even regarding the rest electrocardiogram, the most benign test imaginable, there is still a question of cost effectiveness. Among those 775 done for screening, the electrocardiogram aided assessment in only 1% of patients, a calculated cost of $24,000 per life saved. The authors observed that much of the increased costs of current medical care is contributed by the widespread repeated use of individual inexpensive tests. Thus, just because a test is inexpensive, benign, and safe does not mean it is cost-effective.

Evaluating coronary bypass surgery, one of the most expensive interventions, the net cost per quality-adjusted year of life gained ranges from $3800 for left main to $30,000 for single-vessel disease.[354] Again, cost-effectiveness varies with the patient population as well as the anatomic and pathophysiologic nature of disease.

Today no methodology should be immune to extensive evaluation and review of cost-effectiveness. The new high-tech modalities such as cine computed tomography, as well as more established methods such as echocardiography and angiography, must be evaluated as conventional scintigraphy has been. The more expensive the

modality, the greater must be its demonstrated clinical advantage in order to justify its application. In the context of these new, expensive modalities, conventional scintigraphic methods must be seen as relatively inexpensive. The clinical value and expense of these tests should be evaluated in reference to the patient population and the specific clinical question being considered. Then, when the situation arises, the response will be appropriate and cost-effective.

Myocardial Viability: Its Assessment and Clinical Importance

Overview

In many clinical situations, the clinical objective is to identify ischemic myocardium and differentiate it from normally perfused myocardium. Here the diagnosis of coronary disease is often in doubt and the study is performed for both diagnostic and prognostic indications. In other situations, the diagnosis of coronary disease may be known or is easily established from clinical and scintigraphic cues. Yet regions of myocardium are dysfunctional at rest or present clinically as irreversibly infarcted tissue. Years ago there seemed to be little difficulty in differentiating ischemic from infarcted myocardium. Now it is clear that many "indicators" of infarction may be, in fact, nonspecific. These include pain, evidence of reduced perfusion, reduced function, acidosis, ATP or creatine phosphate depletion, and arrhythmias. Even enzyme release and electrocardiographic changes may be nonspecific or misleading in certain clinical settings and do not give specific regional information. Only altered metabolism, altered staining characteristics, and pathology can provide specific indication of viability or necrosis. Obviously these may be hard to apply at the bedside.

The designation of myocardial viability is a critically important clinical need. Recognition of ischemic myocardium and its differentiation from infarct may be difficult since it may be both underperfused and dysfunctional. The differentiation of severe ischemia from infarction is important if not possible on clinical grounds, however, and can be aided by scintigraphic indicators. Even if infarction is evident clinically, the regional assessment of viable myocardium may be clinically crucial and often needs scintigraphic evaluation. The issue is important, since the risk of intervention rises with the extent of irreversible dysfunctional infarction, whereas benefit relates to the extent of reversibly ischemic myocardium, the extent of myocardium at ischemic risk, and our ability to preserve and protect it. Mistaking intarction for ischemia can expose patients to needless risk, pain, and expense, whereas the converse can deprive patients of the potential benefits of intervention. The objective of the scintigraphic effort is to identify, aiding salvation of ischemic myocardium. The search for ischemic myocardium is motivated by the clinical need to preserve and restore ventricular function in these territories.

In the presence of demonstrated stress-induced ischemia, an increasing margin of benefit results from revascularization in relation to less extensive coronary disease. With the exception of left main coronary lesions, early studies revealed no survival benefit from surgical revascularization in the presence of normal left ventricular function, regardless of the extent of coronary disease.[315,316,318,355,356] Similar anatomy revealed a survival advantage with surgery compared with medical treatment, when associated with significantly depressed left ventricular function.[317,357,358] One reason for this difference relates to the use of survival as the measured endpoint, a hard and reliable indicator, but one insensitive to less final, nonetheless critical, intermediate events. Another reason relates to the severe degree of diminution of ventricular functional reserve, where further functional deterioration and loss is intolerable and more likely prevented by surgical rather than medical management.

Currently we seek to intervene earlier, in part because of the increased safety of reperfusion intervention, and to preserve the function of myocardium at ischemic risk, even, or especially, in the presence of preserved left ventricular function. In this way, we seek to delay the time when function will deteriorate to the edge of survival. This approach is supported by numerous studies relating electrocardiographic and scintigraphic ischemic indicators to increased risk.[59,109,110,141,142,319,320] Recent analysis has confirmed an expanded population with improved survival after coronary bypass surgery compared with medical management, when coronary anatomy is associated with evidence of induced ischemia.[317,357,358] This provides further validity to the current approach and makes even more critical the differentiation of viable ischemic or postischemic myocardium from irreversibly infarcted myocardium.

Myocardial Survival. The survival of myocardium after an ischemic insult depends on the depth and duration of ischemia. Myocardium ischemic for 3 hours or more is not likely to recover function even weeks after the event. The extent of necrosis increases rapidly after 15 minutes of ischemia and exceeds 70% after 45 minutes.[358–361]

In patients, cell death is more variable and less predictable because of the variability of flow reduction, the chronicity of coronary disease, the effects of functional compensation, the presence of collaterals,[362] and the protective effects of drugs. These latter factors can prolong cell life and preserve myocardial function. The delay in cell death permits increased time for revascularization.

Survival in coronary disease relates to myocardial preservation and with it, preservation of function. Recognition of viable ischemic myocardium permits attempts at its preservation. Not infrequently, severe ischemia may correspond to dysfunction at rest in the absence of scar.[363] This is supported by pathologic studies. Such segments most likely fall into the category of stunned or hibernating myocardium.[364,365]

Recognition of Ischemia. Recognition of ischemic myocardium may then be difficult, since ischemic myocardium may be both underperfused and dysfunctional and may look similar to infarction. The differentiation of severe ischemia from infarction is critical, however, and if not possible on clinical grounds can be aided by scintigraphic indicators. The differentiation is important, since the risk of intervention rises with increasing extent of irreversible dysfunction, infarction, whereas benefit relates to the extent of reversibly ischemic myocardium. Mistaking infarction for ischemia can expose patients to needless risk, pain, and expense. The converse can deprive patients of the benefits of intervention. The objective of the clinical effort is to identify and salvage ischemic myocardium. The search for ischemic myocardium is one of preserving and restoring ventricular function through restoration of perfusion.

Infarct-Specific Imaging. Twenty years ago we had no trouble differentiating ischemic from infarcted myocardium. Now we know that many indicators of infarction are nonspecific. Some indicators are thought to be more specific, however, and include enzyme release, electrocardiographic changes, altered metabolism, altered pathologic staining characteristics, and pathology.[366–369]

A long-standing application of the scintigraphic method has been the application of "hot spot" radiotracers that localize specifically in acutely infarcted myocardium.[369–371] Recent tracer studies[309,310] have led to the development and imminent introduction of radiolabeled antimyosin antibody. This is a fully specific agent for the imaging of necrotic myocardium, shown to be unrelated in its distribution to regional blood flow and thus not dependent for its localization on reperfusion and infarction. A disadvantage of all infarct imaging methods is their failure to identify regions of prior infarction and myocardium at ischemic risk. In this omission, which is of course critical to their success, they provide only a single component of coronary risk. Nonetheless, although an indicator of viability, such agents have a limited role to play in providing a piece of the "ischemic" puzzle.

Viability and Ventricular Function. Resting left ventricular function remains an important prognostic indicator and regional ventricular function provides important yet at times circumstantial evidence of myocardial viability, a critically important parameter in clinical decision making related to the coronary patient. Although a moving wall no doubt indicates an element of viable and therefore salvageable myocardium, an immobile region may relate to irreversible infarction or reversibly "stunned" or "hibernating" myocardium.

Evidence that dysfunctional myocardium at rest can be viable and recover with reperfusion includes:

1. 5% to 50% of akinetic and dyskinetic segments have normal myocardium on autopsy.[364]
2. Akinetic and dyskinetic segments can recover with time after infarction,[337] with thrombolytic therapy, as well as after PTCA or CABG, and these can be predicted by PESP/NTG response[336,372–379] and PET metabolic evaluation.
3. Most reversible and some fixed perfusion defects related to abnormal wall motion, normalize function after thrombolysis, PTCA or CABG.[41,380–383]

Stunned myocardium is dysfunctional after reperfusion and may be well identified by conventional scintigraphic perfusion imaging, demonstrating perfused but dysfunctional myocardium. Hibernating myocardium is both underperfused and dysfunctional at rest. It, as well as some areas of stunned myocardium, will require metabolic evaluation as well, to demonstrate active metabolism in dysfunctional, underperfused segments. This evaluation may represent an important potential application of PET, the success of which will depend on the frequency of such conditions, their clinical importance, the unique nature of PET to gain their identification, and our willingness and ability to pay for this information.

Perfusion Scintigraphy for the Identification of Myocardial Viability: Difficulties and Implications.

The scintigraphic evaluation of myocardial perfusion with ²⁰¹Tl is probably most important for the clinical evaluation of the patient assessed for the presence of viable myocardium at ischemic risk, either in an acute or more chronic clinical situation. The method presents a pathophysiologic indicator of coronary flow reserve and appears even better to relate to coronary risk then does the standard evaluation of coronary anatomy.[48,384]

In patients hospitalized with acute pain syndromes, the extent of infarction, recent and remote, as well as the extent of ischemia, can often be identified with the serial imaging of a rest-administered injection of the radiotracer. Recently, dipyridamole infusion has been applied as a successful alternative to dynamic stress in patients unable to exercise to a clinically meaningful endpoint. Both methods have proven to be both diagnostic and prognostic beyond other parameters in patients evaluated for known suspected coronary disease.[97,109,114]

It has been shown that ²⁰¹Tl distributes to viable myocardium in relation to its relative perfusion and, if administered during intervention as exercise, "redistributes" with time after the intervention to reflect the basal pattern of perfusion.[31,32]

Conventional wisdom suggests that perfused myocardial regions on delayed or rest imaging are viable, and underperfused or nonperfused regions are not viable. Prior studies indicated that fixed defects generally relate to scar. In prior studies there was a high correlation between fixed defects and the presence of severe wall motion abnormalities, whereas reversible defects seemed to correlate with improved regional perfusion and function post-PTCA or CABG. Normal or reversible segments related to normal wall motion or improved motion after a PVC or nitroglycerin, standard methods used to indicate viability and to predict functional improvement after revascularization. In fact, some studies revealed that among segments moving abnormally before bypass graft surgery, most of those with related redistribution abnormalities improved postoperatively, whereas those showing no redistribution at 4 hours postinjection generally showed no functional improvement.[66,385] Also, fixed defects generally related to a benign prognosis, whereas reversible defects relate to increased risk and a poor prognosis.[109,114] Owing to acutely changing parameters, the method presents some special considerations when applied to assess viability after thrombolytic therapy.[386] It has been found that 24-hour delayed imaging better estimates reversibly ischemic myocardium than 4-hour study, which may overestimate fixed defects or infarction.[41,387–390]

Positron Emission Tomography

Compared to conventional single photon scintigraphy, PET is intrinsically tomographic and provides uniform high-efficiency event detection over an extensive field of view.[10] It provides high spatial resolution, inversely related to detector size and approaching 5 mm.[5,391] Resolution is independent of depth and preserved over a wide range of the solid angle of detection.[392,393] As detectcor size is reduced, however, sensitivity falls and instrument complexity and cost increase.[392,393] The high energy of the annihilation photon greatly reduces difficulties related to tissue attenuation so common with low-energy emittors such as ²⁰¹Tl. This high energy necessitates increased crystal thickness, however.[392,393] Further, technical correction for photon attenuation and characteristics of the method permit quantitation of tissue tracers.[392–394] Many positron emittors are short-lived, permitting repeated study with low radiation exposure but requiring rapid use (see Table 10-1).[110,392,393] Most important, the biologic nature of many such radionuclides, ¹¹C, ¹⁵O, and ¹³N, permits the formulation of radiopharmaceuticals, which can partici pate as substrates in metabolic processes.[392,395-398] This allows their application in the evaluation of myocardial metabolism; however, their generally brief half-life and mode of production make an on-site cyclotron necessary for application of many of these agents.[10,393]

A number of studies have demonstrated reduced regional uptake of both metabolic, ^{11}C palmitate, and perfusion markers, [82]Rb and ^{13}N ammonia, respectively, in myocardial infarction.[398,399] Positron imaging has demonstrated augmented perfusion in the hypertrophied septum of asymmetric septal hypertrophy.[400] The method has defined a specific pattern with reduced posterior wall perfusion and augmented glucose metabolism, in association with the cardiomyopathy of Duchenne's muscular dystrophy,[401] and metabolic analysis promises differentiation among other probable heterogeneous members of the currently ill-defined group of dilated cardiomyopathies.[402]

The metabolic consequences of ischemia have been imaged and applied to its diagnosis. A significant decline in the myocardial turnover rate of ^{11}C acetic acid, detected noninvasively with PET during exercise in patients with coronary disease, implies reduced activity of the citric acid cycle in ischemia.[399,403] Augmented myocardial ^{11}C palmitate uptake was noted after release of a short-duration coronary occlusion in dogs, whereas reduced [13]NH₃ uptake was detected distal to a coronary stenosis of even 47% after dipyridamole administration.[397] During fasting, the substrate of myocardial metabolism shifts from glucose to fatty acids. Persistent myocardial glucose use during fasting in regions of reduced perfusion monitored by fluorine 18 deoxyglucose (FDG) serves as the marker for ischemic myocardium and has been induced with rapid pacing (Fig. 10-50). FDG 6-

phosphate provides ample stability for imaging and is preferable to the more transient ^{11}C-labeled glucose. Visualization of such alterations with persistent image evidence of glucose metabolism in areas of apparent prior infarction appears to attest to regional tissue viability in an animal model. Recently, myocardial regions of continued glucose use associated with abnormally perfused and contracting myocardial segments indicated viability in patient studies and served as a specific marker, superior to conventional perfusion scintigraphy, for functional improvement after revascularization.[404]

Both [13]NH₃ and [82]Rb distribute according to regional myocardial perfusion after their intravenous administration.[398,404-407] Unlike most other positron emitters, however, [82]Rb is generator produced,[407] making it potentially available as a positron perfusion agent without the need for an on-site cyclotron. Administered as a continuous infusion, its brief, 75-second half-life could permit performance of intervention evaluation in association with dipyridamole administration and baseline rest study even minutes apart. This would permit the efficient assessment of ischemia without the need for redistribution imaging, potentially increasing throughput with increased patient convenience and reduced radiation exposure compared to current methods employing [201]Tl.

Although gating and crude ventricular function evaluation is possible,[408] the major application of the method lies in the assessment of perfusion and metabolism. The method may provide insight into the underlying cause and earliest metabolic impairment of disease. With this comes the possibility of discriminating between currently indistinguishable conditions with individualization of therapy and of earlier disease recognition with the promise of more effective intervention. The work al-

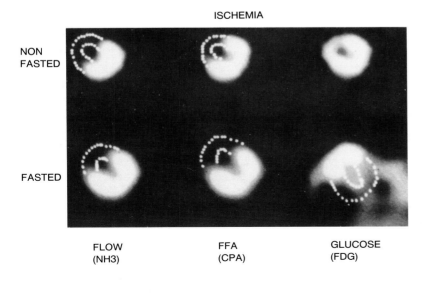

Figure 10-50. Metabolic PET imaging. Shown are myocardial PET images of perfusion using ^{15}N-labeled ammonia (NH₃), free fatty acid metabolism using ^{11}C-labeled palmitate (CPA), and glucose utilization using [11]F fluorodeoxglycose (FDG) acquired in fasted and nonfasted states. Fasting FDG uptake, glucose use in a region with reduced perfusion, indicates viable but ischemic myocardium (Reproduced with permission from Schelbert HR. The heart. In: Ell PJ, Holman BL, eds. Computed emission tomography. Oxford: Oxford University Press, 1982:91.)

ready done, the potential presented, and the more widespread commercial availability of perfusion and metabolically active positron imaging agents and imaging devices could make PET the next important clinical breakthrough in noninvasive cardiac imaging. Of course, the expense of method implementation and the success of current techniques make mandatory the careful evaluation of its relative diagnostic accuracy, clinical efficacy, and cost-effectiveness before its conversion from its present research application to that of a widely applied clinical tool.

The Promise of Cardiac PET

PET is a form of nuclear imaging or scintigraphy. PET images the distribution of radionuclides that decay by emission of positrons. Positrons are high energy photons that undergo annihilation with the release of two high-energy, 511 keV photons. The PET instrument is specially designed with detectors, generally placed in an orbital array, to register the annihilation events. Since the latter are of high energy and are released simultaneously and at 180° from each other, appropriate electronics can locate the origin of the event providing intrinsic tomographic capability without troublesome artifacts of tissue attenuation. PET radionuclides are often biologically reactive, providing a unique opportunity to apply radiotracer techniques to the evaluation of common, important, and otherwise obscure biologic processes, such as myocardial metabolism.

The agent fluoro-18-deoxyglucose (F-18 DOG) is used in PET imaging to assess glycolytic metabolism of the myocardium. The retention of F-18 DOG by the heart is the result of metabolic trapping, since it is a good substrate for the enzyme hexokinase but a poor substrate for subsequent metabolic steps of the glycolytic pathway. It is an excellent marker for the increase of glucose uptake and consumption accompanying the increased rate of anaerobic glycolysis in ischemia.[410] Myocardial glucose uptake and use are regulated by the dual determinants of fatty-acid levels and oxygen availability.[411]

In the fasting state, myocardial glucose uptake is suppressed when serum fatty acid levels are high. In the presence of ischemia, however, glucose uptake is not suppressed as myocardial metabolism shifts to anaerobic glycolysis. For metabolic assessment of myocardial ischemia by PET, we therefore image with F-18 DOG in the fasting state, when viable ischemic myocardium traps the agent, not normal or necrotic myocardium. To assess myocardial viability, we image FDG localization after a glucose load, when both normal and ischemic myocardium take up the agent but infarcted regions do not.

Some recent evidence indicates that there is no specific indicator, including EKG and functional measures, which would make late redistribution (and viability) more or less likely and that only PET could identify viable myocardium. PET seemed to be able to differentiate viable from infarcted myocardium, even among segments demonstrating persistent scintigraphic perfusion defects after 4 and 24 hours.[412] On the basis of data relating to active metabolism presented by PET, abnormal contraction before CABG could be predicted to be reversible or irreversible after CABG.[342,413,414] PET also appeared able to resolve an increased number of viable segments among those not reversible even after 24 hours.[51]

Much work suggests that PET metabolic assessment may be critically important and necessary to the assessment of myocardial viability, especially in the presence of fixed perfusion defects. Prior work, however, reviewed above, demonstrated the value of conventional thallium imaging to identify viable myocardium. Recently, Dilsiziam and coworkers have presented an exciting series of studies employing a reinjection technique to increase our ability to detect viable segments.[44] In this first effort they demonstrated that resolution of a scintigraphic defect after thallium reinjection at 4 hours correlated with preservation, or return of, wall motion after revascularization.[44] In other words, improved reinjection of thallium (as previously demonstrated with regard to redistribution defects[40]) seemed to identify underperfused and dysfunctional but viable segments—hibernating myocardium.[366] Subsequently, a segment-by-segment comparison demonstrated over 90% agreement with regard to segment viability when reinjection thallium technique was compared with PET metabolic evaluation.[45,46] Again, the question of the need for metabolic assessment and PET use for viability assessment is revitalized. It appears as though some cases cannot be resolved without PET. Can we identify them by conventional methods? How much are we willing to spend to get the ultimate assessment of tissue viability in all cases? These questions are now being investigated.

In the setting of new and developing treatment methods that can, by a number of techniques, reperfuse the myocardium, the identification of patients and specifically segments that may benefit from such reperfusion is critically important. The effort to fully develop diagnostic methods must continue in an effort to maximize the clinical benefit of therapeutic inverventions.

References

1. Freeman LM, ed. Freeman and Johnson's clinical radionuclide imaging. Orlando: Grune & Stratton, 1984.
2. Freeman LM, Blaufox MD, eds. Cardiovascular nuclear medicine I–III: seminars in nuclear medicine. Orlando: Grune & Stratton, 1979.
3. Beller G. Nuclear cardiology: current indications and clinical usefulness. Curr Probl Cardiol 1985;10:3.

4. Cardiac Imaging Symposium I–VI. Prog Cardiovasc Dis 1985; 28:85, 1986;29:434.

5. Sorenson JA, Phelps ME, eds. Physics in nuclear medicine. Orlando: Grune & Stratton, 1986.

6. Vogel R, Kirsch D, LeFree M, et al. Thallium-201 myocardial perfusion scintigraphy: results of standard and multi-pinhole tomographic techniques. Am J Cardiol 1979;43:787.

7. Herfkens R, Shosa D, Hattner R, et al. Clinical applications of rotating slanthole tomography to cardiovascular nuclear medicine. J Nucl Med 1980;21:70.

8. Holman B, Hill T, Wynne J, et al. Single photon transaxial emission computed tomography of the heart in normal subjects and in patients with infarctions. J Nucl Med 1979;20:736.

9. Tamaki N, Mukai T, Ishii Y, et al. Comparative study of thallium emission myocardial tomography with 180° and 360° data collection. J Nucl Med 1982;23:661.

10. Ell PJ, Holman BL, eds. Computed emission tomography. New York: Oxford University Press, 1982.

11. Eisner R, Churchwell A, Nowak D, et al. Quantitative analysis of the tomographic thallium-201 myocardial bullseye display: critical role of correcting for patient motion. J Nucl Med 1988;29:91.

12. Zhu YY, Botvinick EH, O'Connell JW, et al. Tolerance of SPECT perfusion imaging to patient motion. J Nucl Med 1990;31:841.

13. Croft BY. Single photon emission computed tomography. Chicago: Year Book Medical Publishers, 1990.

14. Esquerre JP, Coca FJ, Martinez SJ, et al. Prone decubitus: a solution to inferior wall attenuation in thallium-201 myocardial tomography. J Nucl Med 1989;30:398.

15. DePasquale EE, Nody AC, DePuey EG, et al. Quantitative rotational thallium-201 tomography for identifying and localizing coronary artery disease. Circulation 1988;77:316.

16. Maddahi J, VanTrain KF, Prigent F, et al. Quantitation of Tl-201 myocardial single photon emission computerized rotational tomography: development, validation and prospective evaluation of an optimized computerized method. J Nucl Med 1986;27:899.

17. Maddahi J, Kiat H, VanTrain KF, et al. Myocardial perfusion imaging with technetium-99m sestaMIBI SPECT in the evaluation of coronary artery disease. Am J Cardiol 1990;66:55E.

18. Jones RH, Borges-Neto S, Potts JM. Simultaneous measurements of myocardial perfusion and ventricular function during exercise from a single injection of technetium-99m sestaMIBI in coronary artery disease. Am J Cardiol 1990;66:68E.

19. Ziffer J, LaPidus A, Alazraki N, et al. Predictive value of systolic wall thickening for myocardial viability assessed by Tc-99m sestaMIBI using a count based algorithm. J Am Coll Cardiol 1991;17:251A.

20. Hoffman EJ, Ricci AR, Van der Stoe LM, Phelps ME. ECAT III—basic design considerations. IEEE Trans Nucl Sci 1983;NS-30:729.

21. Mullani NA, Gaeta J, Yerian W. Dynamic imaging with high resolution time-of flight PET camera—TOFPET I. IEEE Trans Nucl Sci 1984;NS-31:609.

22. Goris ML, Daspit SG, McLaughlin P, et al. Interpolative background image components. J Nucl Med 1977;18:781.

23. Ortendahl DA, Shosa DW, Kaufman L. Resolution and contrast recovery at depth in planar nuclear images. Phys Med Biol 1982;27:257.

24. Maddahi J, Garcia EV, Berman DS, et al. Improved noninvasive assessment of coronary artery disease: quantitative analysis of regional stress myocardial distribution and washout of thallium-201. Circulation 1981;64:924.

25. Strauss HW, Harrison BS, et al. Thallium 201: noninvasive determination of regional distribution of cardiac output. J Nucl Med 1977;18:1167.

26. Zaret BL, Strauss HW, Martin ND, et al. Noninvasive regional myocardial perfusion with radioactive potassium: study of patients at exercise, rest and during angina pectoris. N Engl J Med 1973;288:809.

27. Botvinick EH, Shames DM, Gershengorn KM, et al. Myocardial stress perfusion scintigraphy with rubidium-81 versus electrocardiography. Am J Cardiol 1977;39:364.

28. Nielsen AT, Morris KG, Murdock R, et al. Linear relationship between the distribution of thallium-201 and blood flow in ischemic and non-ischemic myocardium during exercise. Circulation 1980;61:797.

29. Strauss HW, Harrison K, Langan JK, et al. Thallium-201 for myocardial imaging: relationship of thallium-201 to regional myocardial perfusion. Circulation 1975;51:641.

30. Beller GA, Watson DD, Pohost GM. Kinetics of thallium distribution and redistribution: clinical applications in sequential myocardial imaging. In: Strauss H, Pitt B, James AE, eds. Cardiovascular nuclear medicine. St. Louis: CV Mosby, 1979:225.

31. Beller GA, Watson DD, Ackell P, et al. Time course of thallium-201 redistribution after transient myocardial ischemia. Circulation 1980;61:791.

32. Grunwald AM, Watson DD, Holzgrefe HH Jr, et al. Myocardial thallium-201 kinetics in normal and ischemic myocardium. Circulation 1981;64:610.

33. Gould KL, Lipscomb K, Hamilton GW. Physiologic basis for assessing critical coronary stenosis: instantaneous flow response and regional distribution during coronary hyperemia as measures of coronary flow reserve. Am J Cardiol 1974;33:87.

34. Britten JS, Blank M. Thallium activation of the Na^+–K^+ activated ATPase of rabbit kidney. Biochim Biophys Acta 1968; 159:160.

35. Berger BB, Watson DD, Taylor GJ, et al. Quantitative thallium-201 exercise scintigraphy for the detection of coronary artery disease. J Nucl Med 1981;22:585.

36. Pohost GM, Zir LM, Moore RH, et al. Differentiation of transiently ischemic from infarcted myocardium by serial imaging after a single dose of thallium-201. Circulation 1977;55:294.

37. Garcia E, Maddahi J, Berman B, et al. Space/time quantitation of thallium-201 myocardial scintigraphy. J Nucl Med 1981; 22:309.

38. Botvinick EH, Taradash MR, Shames DM, et al. Thallium-201 myocardial perfusion scintigraphy for the clinical clarification of normal, abnormal and equivocal electrocardiographic stress tests. Am J Cardiol 1978;41:43.

39. Ellestad MH. Stress testing: principles and practice. 2nd ed. Philadelphia: FA Davis, 1980:178.

40. Nohara R, Kambara H, Suzuki Y, et al. Stress scintigraphy using single-photon emission computed tomography in the evaluation of coronary artery disease. Am J Cardiol 1984;53:1250.

41. Brundage BH, Massie BM, Botvinick EH, et al. Improved regional ventricular function after successful surgical revascularization. J Am Coll Cardiol 1984;3:902.

42. Kiat H, Berman D, Maddahi J, et al. Late reversibility of tomographic myocardial thallium defects—an accurate marker of myocardial viability. J Am Coll Cardiol 1988;12:1456.

43. Budinger TF, Knittel BL. Cardiac thallium redistribution and model. J Nucl Med 1977;28:588.

44. Dilsiziam V, Swain J, Dextras R, Almagor Y, Bonow R. Prediction of viable myocardium by thallium reinjection at rest after stress redistribution imaging: a pre- and post-revascularization study. Circulation (Suppl II)1989;80:II–366.

45. Bonow RO, Bacharach SL, Cuocolo A, Dilsiziam V. Myocardial viability in coronary artery disease and left ventricular dysfunction: thallium-201 reinjection vs. fluorodeoxyglucose. Circulation (Suppl II)1989;80:II–377.

46. Dilsiziam V, Rocco TP, Freedman NMT, et al. Enhanced detec-

tion of ischemic but viable myocardium by the reinjection of thallium after stress-redistribution imaging. N Engl J Med 1990;323:141.

47. Berger HJ. Nuclear medicine's revival: new drugs and cameras lead the way. Diagn Imaging 1985;5:68.

48. Massie B, Botvinick EH, Arnold S, et al. Effect of contrast enhancement on the sensitivity and specificity of Tl-201 scintigraphy. Am Heart J 1981;102:37.

49. Botvinick EH, Dunn R, Hattner R, et al. A consideration of factors affecting the diagnostic accuracy of thallium-201 myocardial perfusion scintigraphy in detecting coronary artery disease. Semin Nucl Med 1980;10:157.

50. Botvinick EH, O'Connell W, Hattner R, et al. The color perfusion washout image provides advantages and insight. Circulation (Suppl) 1985;72:III–424.

51. Dunn R, Wolff L, Wagner S, et al. The inconsistent pattern of thallium defects: a clue to the false positive perfusion scintigram. Am J Cardiol 1981;48:224.

52. VanTrain K, Maddahi J, Wong C, et al. Definition of normal limits in stress Tl-201 myocardial rotational tomography. J Nucl Med 1986;27:899.

53. Kaual S, Chesler DA, Pohost GM, et al. Influence of peak exercise heart rate on normal thallium-201 myocardial clearance. J Nucl Med 1986;27:26.

54. O'Connell W, Botvinick E, Dae M. Anatomic functional images quantify distribution and regional washout in SPECT perfusion studies. J Nucl Med 1990;31:872.

55. Friedman J, VanTrain K, Maddahi J, et al. "Upward creep" of the heart: a frequent source of false positive reversible defection thallium-201 stress redistribution SPECT. J Nucl Med 1986; 27:899.

56. Ohsuzu F, Handa S, Kondo M, et al. Thallium-201 myocardial imaging to evaluate right ventricular overloading. Circulation 1980;61:620.

57. Boucher CA, Zir LM, Beller GA, et al. Increased lung uptake of thallium-201 during exercise myocardial imaging: clinical hemodynamics and angiographic implications in patients with coronary artery disease. Am J Cardiol 1980;46:189.

58. Canhasi B, Dae M, Botvinick E, et al. The interaction of "supplementary" scintigraphic indicators and stress electrocardiography in the diagnosis of multivessel coronary disease. J Am Coll Cardiol 1985;6:581.

59. Gibson RS, Watson DD, Craddock GB, et al. Prediction of cardiac events after uncomplicated myocardial infarction: a prospective study comparing predischarge exercise thallium-201 scintigraphy and coronary angiography. Circulation 1983;68: 321.

60. Dunn RF, Freedman B, Bailey IK, et al. Localization of coronary artery disease in exercise electrocardiography: correlation with thallium-201 myocardial perfusion scanning. Am J Cardiol 1981;48:837.

61. Bulkley BH, Rouleau J, Strauss HW, et al. Idiopathic hypertrophic subaortic stenosis: detection by thallium-201 myocardial perfusion imaging. N Engl J Med 1979;293:1113.

62. Proudfit WL, Bruschke AVG, Jones FM. Natural history of obstructive coronary disease: ten year study of 601 nonsurgical cases. Prog Cardiovasc Dis 1978;21:53.

63. Hammermeister KE, DeRouen TA, Dodge HT. Variables predictive of survival in patients with coronary disease. Circulation 1979;59:421.

64. Bateman TM, Maddahi J, Gray RJ, et al. Diffuse slow washout of myocardial thallium-201: a new scintigraphic indicator of extensive coronary artery disease. J Am Coll Cardiol 1984;4:55.

65. Massie BM, Botvinick EH, Brundage BH, et al. Relationship of regional myocardial perfusion to segmental wall motion: a

physiologic basis for understanding the presence of reversible asynergy. Circulation 1978;58:1154.

66. Massie B, Botvinick E, Shames D, et al. A physiologic basis for understanding the presence and reversibility of asynergy. Circulation 1978;58:1154.

67. Wackers FJT, Becker AE, Samson G, et al. Location and size of acute transmural myocardial infarction estimated from thallium-201 scintiscans: a clinical pathological study. Circulation 1977;56:778.

68. Wackers FJT, Busemann-Sokole E, Samson G, et al. Value and limitations of thallium-201 scintigraphy in the acute phase of myocardial infarction. N Engl J Med 1976;295:1.

69. Bulkley BH, Hutchins GM, Bailey I, et al. Thallium-201 imaging and gated cardiac blood pool scans in patients with ischemic and idiopathic congestive cardiomyopathy: a clinical and pathologic study. Circulation 1977;55:753.

70. Makier PT, Lavine SJ, Denenberg BS, et al. Redistribution on the thallium scan in myocardial sarcoidosis: concise communications. J Nucl Med 1981;22:428.

71. Gaffney FA, Wohl AJ, Blomquist CQ, et al. Thallium-201 myocardial perfusion studies in patients with the mitral valve prolapse syndrome. Am J Med 1978;64:21.

72. Wackers FJT, Lie KI, Liem KL, et al. Potential value of thallium-201 scintigraphy as a means of selecting patients for the coronary care unit. Br Heart J 1979;41:111.

73. Brown KA, Okada RD, Boucher CA, et al. Serial thallium-201 imaging at rest in patients with stable and unstable angina pectoris: relationship of myocardial perfusion at rest to presenting clinical syndrome. Am Heart J 1983;106:70.

74. Iskandrian AS, Hakki AH, Kane SA, et al. Rest and redistribution thallium-201 myocardial scintigraphy to predict improvement of left ventricular function after coronary artery bypass grafting. Am J Cardiol 1983;51:1312.

75. Rigo P, Bailey IK, Griffith LSC, et al. Stress thallium-201 myocardial scintigraphy for the detection of individual coronary artery lesions in patients with and without previous myocardial infarction. Am J Cardiol 1981;48:209.

76. Ritchie JL, Zaret BL, Strauss HW, et al. Myocardial imaging with thallium-201: a multicenter study in patients with angina pectoris or acute myocardial infarction. Am J Cardiol 1978;42:345.

77. Gibson RS, Beller GA. Should exercise electrocardiography be replaced by radionuclide methods? In: Rahimtoola SH, Brest AN, eds. Controversies in coronary disease. Philadelphia: FA Davis, 1981:1.

78. Berger BC, Watson DD, Taylor GJ, et al. Assessment of the effect of coronary collaterals on regional myocardial perfusion using thallium-201 scintigraphy. Am J Cardiol 1980;46:365.

79. Massie B, Botvinick E, Brundage B. Correlation of thallium-201 scintigrams with coronary anatomy: factors affecting region by region sensitivity. Am J Cardiol 1979;44:616.

80. Kirsch CM, Doliwa R, Buell V, et al. Detection of severe coronary heart disease with thallium-201: comparison of resting single photon emission tomography with invasive arteriography. J Nucl Med 1983;24:761.

81. Patterson RE, Horowitz SF, Eng C, et al. Can noninvasive exercise test criteria identify patients with left main or three vessel coronary disease after a first myocardial infarction? Am J Cardiol 1983;51:361.

82. Rehn T, Briffith LSC, Achuff SC, et al. Exercise thallium-201 myocardial imaging and left main coronary artery disease: sensitive but not specific. Am J Cardiol 1981;48:217.

83. Dash H, Massie BM, Botvinick EH, et al. The noninvasive identification of left main and three vessel coronary artery disease by myocardial stress perfusion scintigraphy and treadmill exercise electrocardiography. Circulation 1979;60:276.

84. Abdulla A, Maddahi J, Garcia E, et al. Slow regional clearance of myocardial thallium 201 in the absence of perfusion defects: contribution to detection of individual coronary stenoses and mechanism for occurrence. Circulation 1985;71:72.

85. Gerwitz H, Paladino W, Sullivan M, et al. Value and limitations of myocardial thallium washout rates in the noninvasive diagnosis of patients with triple vessel coronary artery disease. Am Heart J 1983;106:686.

86. Pamelia FX, Gibson RS, Watson DD, et al. Prognosis with chest pain and normal thallium-201 exercise scintigrams. Am J Cardiol 1985;55:920.

87. Uhl GS, Kay TN, Hickman JR Jr, et al. Computer enhanced thallium scintigrams in asymptomatic men with abnormal exercise tests. Am J Cardiol 1981;48:1037.

88. Patterson RE, Horowitz SF, Eng C, et al. Can exercise electrocardiography and thallium-201 myocardial imaging exclude the diagnosis of coronary artery disease? Am J Cardiol 1982;49:1127.

89. Zir LM, Miller SW, Dinsmore RE, et al. Interobserver variability in coronary angiography. Circulation 1976;53:627.

90. Cooperman M, Pflug B, Martin EW Jr, et al. Cardiovascular risk factors in patients with peripheral vascular disease. Surgery 1978;84:505.

91. Rall TW: Central nervous system stimulants. In: Gilman AB, Goodman LS, Gilman A, eds. The pharmacologic basis of therapeutics. New York: Macmillan, 1984:592.

92. Feldman RL, Nichols WW, Pepine CJ, et al. Acute effect of intravenous dipyridamole on regional coronary hemodynamics and metabolism. Circulation 1981;64:333.

93. Gould KL. Noninvasive assessment of coronary stenosis by myocardial imaging during pharmacologic coronary vasodilatation: physiologic basis and experimental vasodilation. Am J Cardiol 1978;41:267.

94. Okada RD, Leppo JA, Boucher CA, et al. Myocardial kinetics of thallium-201 after dipyridamole infusion in normal canine myocardium and in myocardium distal to a stenosis. J Clin Invest 1982;69:199.

95. Beller GA, Holzgrefe HH, Watson DD. Effects of dipyridamole induced vasodilation on myocardial uptake and clearance kinetics of thallium-201. Circulation 1983;68:1328.

96. Becker LC. Conditions for vasodilator induced coronary steal in experimental myocardial ischemia. Circulation 1978;57:1103.

97. Leppo J, Boucher CA, Okada RD, et al. Serial thallium-201 myocardial imaging after dipyridamole infusion: diagnostic utility in detecting coronary stenoses and relationship to regional wall motion. Circulation 1982;66:649.

98. Jakubowski AT, Huckell VF, Cooper JA, et al. Low dose oral dipyridamole produces coronary blood flow redistribution on thallium-201 myocardial imaging in patients with coronary artery disease. J Am Coll Cardiol 1986;7:215A.

99. O'Byrne GT, Maddahi J, VanTrain KF, et al. Myocardial washout rate of thallium-201: comparison between rest, dipyridamole with and without aminophylline, and exercise states. J Am Coll Cardiol 1986;7:175A.

100. Zhu YY, Lee W, Botvinick E, et al. The clinical and pathophysiologic implications of pain, ST abnormalities and scintigraphic changes during dipyridamole infusion: their relationship to the peripheral hemodynamic response. Am Heart J 1988;116:1071.

101. Lam YJT, Chaitman BR, Glaenzer M, et al. Safety and diagnostic accuracy of dipyridamole-thallium imaging in the elderly. J Am Coll Cardiol 1988;11:585.

102. Lagerquist B, Sylven C, Beerman B, et al. Intracoronary adenosine causes angina pectoris like pain—an inquiry into the nature of visceral pain. Cardiovasc Res 1990;24:609.

103. Indolfi C, Giustino G, Piscione F, et al. Intravenous dipyridamole in detecting coronary stenosis. Assessment by two-dimensional echocardiography and radionuclide angiography. J Am Coll Cardiol 1986;7:212A.

104. Alonso S. Inhibition of coronary vasodilating action of dipyridamole and adenosine by aminophylline in the dog. Circ Res 1970;26:743.

105. Ruddy TD, Dighero HR, Okada RD, et al. Detection and localization of coronary artery disease with quantitation of dipyridamole thallium images. J Nucl Med 1986;27:944.

106. Josephson MA, Brown BG, Hecht HS, et al. Noninvasive detection and localization of coronary stenosis in patients: comparison of resting dipyridamole and exercise thallium-201 myocardial perfusion imaging. Circulation 1982;66:649.

107. Albro PC, Gould KL, Wescott RJ, et al. Noninvasive assessment of coronary artery stenosis by myocardial imaging during pharmacologic coronary vasodilatation. III. Clinical trial. Am J Cardiol 1978;42:751.

108. Schectmann N, Dae M, Lanzer P, et al. The clinical impact of perfusion scintigraphy with dipyridamole. J Nucl Med 1984;25:86.

109. Boucher CA, Brewster DC, Darling RC, et al. Determination of cardiac risk by dipyridamole thallium imaging before peripheral vascular surgery. N Engl J Med 1985;312:389.

110. Leppo JA, O'Brien J, Rothendler J, et al. Dipyridamole thallium-201 scintigraphy in the prediction of future cardiac events after acute myocardial infarction. N Engl J Med 1984;310:1014.

111. Cooperman M, Pflug B, Martin EW Jr, et al. Cardiovascular risk factors in patients with peripheral vascular disease. Surgery 1978;84:505.

112. Hertzer NR, Beven EG, Young JR, et al. Coronary artery disease in peripheral vascular patients: a classification of 1000 coronary angiograms and results of surgical management. Ann Surg 1984;199:223.

113. Eagle KA, Coley CM, Newell JB, et al. Combining clinical and thallium data optimizes preoperative assessment of cardiac risk before major vascular surgery. Ann Intern Med 1989;110:859.

114. Eagle KA, Singer DE, Brewster DC, et al. Dipyridamole thallium scanning in patients undergoing vascular surgery: optimizing preoperative evaluation of cardiac risk. JAMA 1987;257:2185.

115. Wolfe C, Lee W, Botvinick EH, et al. The utility of dipyridamole thallium scintigraphy in predicting ischemic events after myocardial infarction. Circulation (Suppl II)1988;78:II–43.

116. Bonaduce D, Muto P, Morgano G, et al. Effect of beta-blockade on thallium-201 dipyridamole myocardial scintigraphy. Acta Cardiol 1984;39:399.

117. Zhu YY, Botvinick EH, Dae MW, et al. Dipyridamole perfusion scintigraphy: the experience with its application in 170 patients with known or suspected unstable angina. Am Heart J 1991;121:33.

118. O'Meara JR, Brown KA, Chambers CE. Intravenous dipyridamole-thallium-201 imaging very early post-MI is safe and predicts recurrent in-hospital ischemia. J Nucl Med 1988;29:781.

119. Gimple LW, Hutter AM, Buiney TE, et al. Prognostic utility of predischarge dipyridamole-thallium imaging compared to predischarge submaximal exercise electrocardiography and maximal thallium imaging after uncomplicated acute myocardial infarction. Am J Cardiol 1989;64:1243.

120. Verani MS, Mahmarian JJ, Hixson JB, et al. Diagnosis of coronary artery disease by controlled coronary vasodilation with

adenosine and thallium-201 scintigraphy in patients unable to exercise. Circulation 1990;82:80.

121. Landsberg J, Botvinick E, Schiller N, et al. Dipyridamole echocardiography reassessed. Clin Res 1987;35:109A.

122. Jain A, Suarez J, Marhmarian JJ, et al. Functional significance of myocardial perfusion defects inducted by dipyridamole using thallium-201 single photon emission computed tomography and two-dimensional echocardiography. Am J Cardiol 1990; 66:802.

123. Nguyen T, Heo J, Ogilby JD, et al. Single photon emission computed tomography with thallium-201 during adenosine-induced coronary hyperemia: correlation with coronary arteriography, exercise thallium imaging and two-dimensional echocardiography. J Am Coll Cardiol 1990;16:1375.

124. Deanfield JE, Maseri A, Selwyn AP, et al. Myocardial ischemia during daily life in patients with stable angina: its relation to symptoms and heart rate changes. Lancet 1983;2:753.

125. Selwyn AP, Fox K, Eves J, et al. Myocardial ischemia in patients with frequent angina pectoris. Br Med J 1978;2:1594.

126. Munoz del Romero L, Botvinick EH, Dae MW, et al. The relationship between ambulatory ST changes and perfusion imaging in association with dyanmic exercise and dipyridamole "stress." Clin Res 1980;37:99A.

127. Epstein S, Quyyumi A, Bonow R. Current concepts: myocardial ischemia—silent or symptomatic? N Engl J Med 1988;318:1038.

128. Fleg JL, Gerstenblith G, Zonderman AB, et al. Prevalence and prognostic significance of exercise-induced silent myocardial ischemia detected by thallium scintigraphy and electrocardiography in asymptomatic volunteers. Circulation 1990; 81:428.

129. Deanfield JE, Shea M, Ribiero P, et al. Transient ST segment depression as a marker of myocardial ischemia during daily life. Am J Cardiol 1984;54:1195.

130. Hirzel HO, Leutwyler R, Krayenbuehl HP. Silent myocardial ischemia: hemodynamic changes during dynamic exercise in patients with proven coronary artery disease despite absence of angina pectoris. J Am Coll Cardiol 1985;6:275.

131. Deedwania PC, Nelson JR. Pathophysiology of silent myocardial ischemia during daily life. Circulation 1990;82:1296.

132. Hecht HS, Shaw RE, Bruce T, et al. Silent ischemia: evaluation by exercise and redistribution tomographic thallium-201 myocardial imaging. J Am Coll Cardiol 1989;14:895.

133. Bonow RO, Bacharach SL, Green MV, et al. Prognostic implications for symptomatic versus asymptomatic (silent) myocardial ischemia induced by exercise in mildly symptomatic and in asymptomatic patients with angiographically documented coronary artery disease. Am J Cardiol 1987;60:778.

134. Hamilton GW, Trobaugh GB, Ritchie JL, et al. An analysis of clinical usefulness based on Bayes' theorem. Semin Nucl Med 1978;8:358.

135. Patterson RE, Eng C, Horowitz SF, et al. Bayesian comparison of cost effectiveness of different clinical approaches to diagnose coronary artery disease. J Am Coll Cardiol 1984;4:278.

136. Patterson RE, Eng C, Horowitz SF, et al. Practical diagnosis of coronary artery disease: a Bayes' theorem nomogram to correlate clinical data with noninvasive exercise tests. Am J Cardiol 1984;53:252.

137. Patterson RE, Eng C, Horowitz SF, et al. Bayesian anaysis of a nomogram of sequential tests for coronary disease: indicators for exercise ECG and thallium-201 imaging. Clin Res 1982; 30:212A.

138. Diamond GA, Forrester JS. Analysis of probability as an aid in the clinical diagnosis of coronary artery disease. N Engl J Med 1979;300:1350.

139. Iskandrian AS, Wasserman LA, Anderson GS, et al. Merits of

140. DePace NL, Iskandrian AS, Nadell R, et al. Variation in the size of jeopardized myocardium in patients with isolated left anterior descending coronary artery disease. Circulation 1983; 67:988.

141. Brown KA, Boucher CA, Okada RD, et al. Prognostic value of exercise thallium-201 imaging in patients presenting for evaluation of chest pain. J Am Coll Cardiol 1983;1:994.

142. Becker LC, Silverman KJ, Bulkley BH, et al. Comparison of early thallium-201 scintigraphy and gated blood pool imaging for predicting mortality in patients with acute myocardial infarction. Circulation 1983;67:1272.

143. Botvinick EH, Perez-Gonzalez JF, Dunn R, et al. Late prognostic value of scintigraphic parameters of acute myocardial infarction size in complicated myocardial infarction without heart failure. Am J Cardiol 1984;53:1244.

144. Marshall RC, Schelbert HR, Phelps ME, et al. Evaluation of infarcted and ischemic myocardium with 18-fluoro-deoxyglucose, $^{13}NH_3$, and positron computed tomography. Am J Cardiol 1981;47:481.

145. Schelbert HR, Phelps ME, Selin C, et al. Regional myocardial ischemia assessed by 18 fluoro-2-deoxyglucose and positron emission computed tomography. In: Kreuzer H, Parmley WW, Rentrop P, Heiss HW, eds. Advances in clinical cardiology. Vol. I. Quantification of myocardial ischemia. New York: Gehard Witzstrock, 1980.

146. Gibton RS, Watson DD, Taylor GJ, et al. Prospective assessment of regional myocardial perfusion before and after coronary revascularization surgery by quantitative thallium-201 scintigraphy. J Am Coll Cardiol 1983;1:804.

147. Greenberg BH, Hart R, Botvinick EH, et al. Thallium-201 myocardial perfusion scintigraphy to evaluate patients after coronary bypass surgery. Am J Cardiol 1978;42:167.

148. Hirzel HO, Nuesch K, Gruentzig AR, et al. Short and long term changes on myocardial perfusion after percutaneous transluminal coronary angioplasty assessed by thallium-201 exercise scintgraphy. Circulation 1981;63:1001.

149. Stuckey TD, Burwell LR, Nygaard TW, et al. Value of quantitative exercise thallium-201 scintigraphy for predicting angina recurrence after percutaneous transluminal coronary angioplasty. J Am Coll Cardiol 1985;5:531.

150. DePuey EG, Roubin GS, Cloninger KG, et al. Correlation of transmural coronary angioplasty parameters and quantitative thallium-201 tomography. J Nucl Med 1986;27:900.

151. Engelstad B, Wagner S, Herfkens R, et al. Evaluation of the postcoronary artery bypass patient by myocardial perfusion scintigraphy and computed tomography. AJR 1983;141:507.

152. Maddahi J, Ganz W, Ninomiya K, et al. Myocardial salvage by intracoronary thrombolysis in evolving acute myocardial infarction: evaluation using intracoronary injection of thallium-201. Am Heart J 1981;102:664.

153. Heo J, Hermann GA, Iskandrian AS, et al. New myocardial perfusion agents: description and applications. Am Heart J 1988;115:1111.

154. Osbakken MD, Okada RD, Boucher CA, et al. Comparison of exercise perfusion and ventricular function imaging: an analysis of factors affecting the diagnostic accuracy of each technique. J Am Coll Cardiol 1984;3:272.

155. Berger H, Goldman L, Reduto HL, et al. Global and regional left ventricular response to bicycle exercise in coronary artery disease: assessment by quantitative radionuclide angiography. Am J Med 1979;66:13.

156. Borer JS, Bacharach SL, Green MV, et al. Real time radionuclide

cineangiography in the noninvasive evaluation of global and regional left ventricular function at rest and during exercise in patients with coronary artery disease. N Engl J Med 1977; 296:839.

157. Alexander J, Dainiak N, Berger HF, et al. Serial assessment of doxorubicin cardiotoxicity with quantitative radionuclide angiography. N Engl J Med 1977;300:278.

158. Borer JS, Rosing DR, Kent KM, et al. Left ventricular function at rest and during exercise after aortic valve replacement in patients with aortic regurgitation. Am J Cardiol 1979;44:1297.

159. Beller GA, Sinusas AJ. Experimental studies of the physiologic properties of technetium-99m isonitriles. Am J Cardiol 1990; 66:5E.

160. Meerdink DJ, Leppo JA. Experimental studies of the physiologic properties of technetium-99m agents: myocardial transport of perfusion imaging agents. Am J Cardiol 1990;66:9E.

161. Maddahi J, Kiat H, VanTrain K, et al. Myocardial perfusion imaging with technetium-99m sestaMIBI SPECT in the evaluation of coronary artery disease. Am J Cardiol 1990;66:55E.

162. Johnson LL, Seldin DW. Clinical experience with technetium 99m teboroxime, a neutral, lipophilic myocardial perfusion imaging agent. Am J Cardiol 1990;66:63E.

163. Taillefer R. Technetium-99m sestaMIBI; myocardial imaging; same day rest-stress studies and dipyridamole. Am J Cardiol 1990;56:80E.

164. Garcia EV, Cooke CD, VanTrain KF, et al. Technical aspects of myocardial SPECT imaging with technetium-99m sestaMIBI. Am J Cardiol 1990;56:23E.

165. Jones RH, Borges-Neto S, Potts JM. Simultaneous measurement of myocardial perfusion and ventricular function during exercise from a single injection of technetium-99m sestaMIBI in coronary artery disease. Am J Cardiol 1990;66:68E.

166. Ziffer J, LaPidus A, Alarak N, et al. Predictive value of systolic wall thickening for myocardial viability assessed by Tc-99m sestaMIBI using a count based algorithm. J Am Coll Cardiol 1991;17:251A.

167. Botvinick EH, Glazer H, Shosa D. What is the reliability and utility of scintigraphic methods for the assessment of ventricular function? Cardiovasc Clin 1983;13(1):65.

168. Ashburn WL, Schelbert HR, Verba JW. A review of several radionuclide angiographic approaches using the scintillation camera. Prog Cardiovasc Dis 1978;20:267.

169. Schelbert HR, Verba JW, Johnson AD, et al. Nontraumatic determination of left ventricular ejection fraction by radionuclide angiocardiography. Circulation 1975;51:902.

170. Strauss HW, Zaret BL, Hurley PJ, et al. A scintiphotographic method for measuring left ventricular ejection fraction in man without cardiac catheterization. Am J Cardiol 1971;28: 575.

171. Steele PP, VanDyke D, Trow RW, et al. Simple and safe bedside method for serial measurement of left ventricular ejection fraction, cardiac output and pulmonary blood volume. Br Heart J 1974;136:122.

172. Zema MJ, Restwig B, Munsey D, et al. Potential pitfalls of the nuclear stethoscope. Clin Nucl Med 1980;5:504.

173. Zaret BL, Strauss HW, Hurley PJ, et al. A noninvasive scintigraphic method for detecting regional ventricular dysfunction in man. N Engl J Med 1971;284:1165.

174. Jengo JA, Mena I, Blaufuss A. Evaluation of left ventricular function, ejection fraction and segmental wall motion by single pass radioisotope angiography. Circulation 1978;57:326.

175. Pavel DG, Zimmer AM, Patterson VN. *In vivo* red blood cell labeling with ^{99m}Tc: a new approach to blood pool visualization. J Nucl Med 1977;18:1035.

176. Wagner HN Jr, Wake R, Nickoloff J, et al. The nuclear stethoscope: a simple device for generation of left ventricular volume curves. Am J Cardiol 1976;38:747.

177. Stewart GM. Researches on the circulation time and organs and on the influence which affect it. IV. The output of the heart. J Physiol 1897;22:159.

178. Marshall RC, Berger HJ, Cosbin JC, et al. Assessment of cardiac performance by quantitative radionuclide angiography: sequential left ventricular ejection rate and regional wall motion. Circulation 1977;56:820.

179. Harpen MD, Debulsson RL, Head B III, et al. Determination of left ventricular volume from first pass kinetics of labeled red blood cells. J Nucl Med 1983;24:98.

180. Holman L. Radioisotope examination of the cardiovascular system. In: Braunwald E, ed. Diseases of the heart. Philadelphia: WB Saunders, 1980:309.

181. Pierson RN Jr, VanDyke DC. Analysis of left ventricularl function. In: Pierson RN, Kriss JP, Jones RH, MacIntyre WJ, eds. New qualitative nuclear cardiology. New York: John Wiley & Sons, 1975.

182. Berger HJ, Davies RA, Batsford WP, et al. Beat to beat left ventricular performance assessed from the equilibrium cardiac blood pool using a computerized nuclear probe. Circulation 1981;63:133.

183. Berger HJ, Matthay RA, Loke J, et al. Assessment of cardiac performance with quantitative radionuclide angiocardiography: right ventricular ejection fraction with reference to findings in chronic obstructive pulmonary disease. Am J Cardiol 1978; 41:897.

184. Maltz OL, Treves S. Quantitative radionuclide angiocardiography: determination of Qp/Qs in children. Circulation 1973; 476:1049.

185. Jones RH, McEwan P, Newman GE. Accuracy of diagnosis of coronary disease by radionuclide measurement of left ventricular function during rest and exercise. Circulation 1981; 64:586.

186. Bodenheimer MM, Banka VS, Fooshee CM, et al. Comparison of wall motion and regional ejection fraction at rest and during isometric exercise. J Nucl Med 1979;20:724.

187. Poliner LR, Dehmer GJ, Lewis SE, et al. Left ventricular performance in normal subjects: a comparison of the responses to exercise in the upright and supine positions. Circulation 1980;62:528.

188. Marshall RC, Berger HJ, Reduto LA. Assessment of cardiac performance with quantitative radionuclide angiocardiography: effects of oral propranolol on global and regional left ventricular function in coronary artery disease. Circulation 1978; 58:808.

189. Salel N, Berman D, DeNardo F, et al. Radionuclide assessment of nitroglycerin influence on abnormal left ventricular segmental contraction in patients with coronary heart disease. Circulation 1976;53:975.

190. Williams DL, Hamilton GW. The effect of errors in determining left ventricular ejection fraction from radionuclide counting data. In: Sorenson JA, ed. Nuclear cardiology: selected computer aspects: symposium proceedings. New York: Society of Nuclear Medicine, 1978:375.

191. Burow R, Straus SH, Singleton R, et al. Analysis of left ventricular function from multiple gated acquisition cardiac blood pool imaging: comparison to contrast angiography. Circulation 1977;56:1024.

192. Maddahi J, Berman DS, Matsuoka DJ, et al. A new technique for assessing right ventricular ejection fraction using multiple gated equilibrium cardiac blood pool scintigraphy. Circulation 1979;60:581.

193. Wackers FJ, Berger H, Johnston DE, et al. Multiple gated cardiac

blood pool imaging for left ventricular ejection fraction: validation of the technique and assessment of variability. Am J Cardiol 1979;43:1159.

194. Borer J, Bacharach SL, Green MV. Exercise induced left ventricular dysfunction in symptomatic and asymptomatic patients with aortic regurgitation: assessment with radionuclide cineangiography. Am J Cardiol 1978;42:351.

195. Rigo P, Murray M, Strauss HW, et al. Left ventricular function in acute myocardial infarction evaluated by gated scintigraphy. Circulation 1974;50:678.

196. Dehmer GH, Lewis SE, Hillis LD, et al. Nongeometric determination of left ventricular volume from equilibrium blood pool scans. Am J Cardiol 1980;45:293.

197. Bunder RJ, Haluszcynski I, Langhammer H. *In vivo/in vitro* labeling of red blood cells with Tc^{99m}. Eur J Nucl Med 1983;8:218.

198. Hegge FN, Hamilton GW, Larson SM, et al. Cardiac chamber imaging: a comparison of red blood cells labeled with Tc-99m *in vitro* and *in vivo*. J Nucl Med 1978;19:129.

199. Freeman M, Berman D, Stanloff H, et al. Improved assessment of inferior segmental wall motion by the addition of 70-degree left anterior oblique view in multiple gated equilibrium scintigraphy. Am Heart J 1981;101:169.

200. Bacharach SL, Green MV, Borer JS. Instruments and data processing in cardiovascular nuclear medicine: evaluation of ventricular function. Semin Nucl Med 1979;9:257.

201. Greenberg B, Drew D, Botvinick E, et al. Evaluation of left ventricular volumes ejection fraction and segmental wall motion by gated radionuclide angiography. Clin Nucl Med 1980;5:245.

202. Green MV, Brody WR, Douglas MA, et al. Ejection fraction by count rate from gated images. J Nucl Med 1978;19:880.

203. Okada RD, Kirshenbaum HD, Kushner FG, et al. Observer variance in the qualitative evaluation of left ventricular wall motion and the quantification of left ventricular ejection fraction using rest and exercise multigated blood pool imaging. Circulation 1980;61:128.

204. Schelbert HR, Henning H, Ashburn WL, et al. Serial measurements of left ventricular ejection fraction by radionuclide angiography early and late after myocardial infarction. Am J Cardiol 1976;38:707.

205. Corbett JR, Dehmer GJ, Lewis SE, et al. The prognostic value of submaximal exercise testing with radionuclide ventriculography before hospital discharge in patients with recent myocardial infarction. Circulation 1981;64:535.

206. Nicod P, Corbett JR, Firth BG, et al. Prognostic value of resting and submaximal exercise radionuclide ventriculography after acute myocardial infarction in high risk patients with single and multivessel disease. Am J Cardiol 1983;52:32.

207. Botvinick EH, Shames D, Hutchinson J, et al. The noninvasive diagnosis of a false left ventricular aneurysm by gated blood pool imaging. Am J Cardiol 1976;37:1089.

208. Rapaport E, Remedio P. The high risk patients after recovery from myocardial infarctcion: recognition and management. J Am Coll Cardiol 1983;1:391.

209. Ritchie JL, Sorenson SG, Kennedy JW, et al. Radionuclide angiography: noninvasive assessment of hemodynamic changes after administration of nitroglycerine. Am J Cardiol 1979;43:278.

210. Marshall RC, Wisenberg G, Schelbert HR, et al. Effect of oral propranolol on rest, exercise and post-exercise left ventricular performance in normal subjects and patients with coronary artery disease. Circulation 1981;63:572.

211. Borer JS, Bacharach SL, Green MV, et al. Effect of nitroglycerin on exercise induced abnormalities of left ventricular regional function and ejection fraction in coronary artery disease. Circulation 1978;57:314.

212. Pfisterer ME, Ricci DR, Schuler G, et al. Validity of left ventricular ejection fractions measured at rest and peak exercise by equilibrium radionuclide angiography using short acquisition times. J Nucl Med 1979;20:484.

213. Gibbons RJ, Lee K, Cobb FR, et al. Ejection fraction response to exercise in patients with chest pain, coronary artery disease and normal ventricular function. Circulation 1982;66:643.

214. Iskandrian AS, Hakki AH, Marsch SK, et al. Prognostic implications of rest and exercise radionuclide ventriculography in patients with suspected or proven coronary heart disease. Am Heart J 1985;110:135.

215. Leong KH, Jones RH. Influence of the location of left anterior descending coronary artery stenosis on left ventricular function during exercise. Circulation 1982;65:109.

216. Bonow RO, Kent KM, Rosing DR, et al. Exercise induced ischemia in mildly symptomatic patients with coronary artery disease and preserved left ventricular function: identification of subgroups at risk of death during medical therapy. N Engl J Med 1984;311:1339.

217. Kent KM, Bonow RO, Rosing DR, et al. Improved myocardial function during exercise after successful percutaneous transluminal coronary angioplasty. N Engl J Med 1982;306:441.

218. Borer J, Kent K, Bacharach SL. Sensitivity specificity and predictive accuracy of radionuclide cineangiography during exercise in patients with coronary artery disease. Circulation 1979;60:572.

219. Maddahi J, Berman DS, Matsouka DT, et al. Right ventricular ejection fraction during exercise in normal subjects and in coronary artery disease patients: assessments by multi-gated equilibrium scintigraphy. Circulation 1980;62:133.

220. Bonow RO, Rosing DR, Bacharach SL, et al. Long-term effects of verapamil on left ventricular diastolic filling in patients with hypertrophic cardiomyopathy. Am J Cardiol 1981;47:409.

221. Bonow RO, Bacharach SL, Green MV, et al. Impaired left ventricular diastolic filling in patients with coronary artery disease: assessment with radionuclide angiography. Circulation 1981;64:315.

222. Maddox DE, Wynne J, Uren R, et al. Regional ejection fraction, a quantitative radionuclide index of regional left ventricular performance. Circulation 1979;59:1001.

223. Pavel D, Sweryn S, Lam W, et al. Ventricular phase analysis of radionuclide gated studies. Am J Cardiol 1980;45:398.

224. Slutsky R, Karliner J, Ricci D, et al. Response of left ventricular volume to exercise in man assessed by radionuclide equilibrium angiography. Circulation 1979;60:565.

225. Links MJ, Becker LC, Shindledecker JG, et al. Measurements of absolute left ventricular volume from gated blood pool studies. Circulation 1982;65:82.

226. Chang W, Henkin RE, Hals DJ, et al. Methods of detection of left ventricular edges. Semin Nucl Med 1980;10:39.

227. Matthey RA, Berger HJ, Loke J, et al. Right and left ventricular performance in ambulatory young patients with cystic fibrosis. Br Heart J 1980;43:474.

228. Rigo P, Murray M, Taylor DR, et al. Right ventricular dysfunction detected by gated scintiphotography in patients with acute inferior myocardial infarction. Circulation 1975;52:268.

229. Sharpe N, Botvinick E, Shames D, et al. The noninvasive diagnosis of right ventricular infarction. Circulation 1978;57:483.

230. Kolibash AJ, Leier CV, Bashore TM. Assessment of left ventricular pressure-volume relations using gated radionuclide angiography, echocardiography and micromanometer pressure recordings. Circulation 1983;67:844.

231. Wasserman AG, Katz RJ, Varghesi PJ, et al. Exercise radionuclide ventriculographic responses in hypertensive patients with chest pain. N Engl J Med 1984;311:1276.

232. Brown JM, White CJ, Sobol SM, et al. Increased left ventricular ejection fraction after a meal: potential source of error in performance of radionuclide angiography. Am J Cardiol 1983; 51:1709.

233. Sandler MP, Kronenberg MW, Formam MB, et al. Dynamic fluctuations in blood and spleen radioactivity: splenic contraction and relation to clinical radionuclide volume calculations. J Am Coll Cardiol 1984;3:1205.

234. Davies GJ, Chierchia S, Crea F, et al. The use of a scintillation probe to investigate ischemic heart disease. J Nucl Med 1981;22:23.

235. Giles RW, Berger JH, Barsh P, et al. Left ventricular dysfunction during anesthesia induction for coronary artery surgery assessed with the computerized nuclear probe. J Nucl Med 1981;22:17.

236. Berger HJ, Hoffer PB, Steidley J, et al. Serial assessments of left ventricular ejection fraction with the miniaturized Cadmium Telluride Detector Module: potential technique for continuous monitoring of ventricular function. J Nucl Med 1981;22:9.

237. Lerman B, Lamphan R, Walton J. Count based left ventricular volume determination utilizing a left posterior oblique view for attenuation, correction. Radiology 1984;150:831.

238. Petru MA, Sorensen SG, Chandhuri TK, et al. Attenuation correction of equilibrium radionuclide angiography: a noninvasive quantitation of cardiac output and ventricular volumes. Am Heart J 1984;107:1221.

239. Starling MR, Dell'Italia LI, Walsh RA, et al. Accurate estimates of absolute left ventricular volumes from equilibrium radionuclide angiographic counts data using a simple geometric attenuation correction. J Am Coll Cardiol 1984;3:789.

240. Bourguignon MH, Schindledecker JG, Caret GA, et al. Quantification of left ventricular volumes in gated equilibrium radioventriculography. Eur J Nucl Med 1981;6:349.

241. Bunker SR, Hartshorne MJ, Schmidt WP, et al. Left ventricular volume determination from single photon emission tomography. AJR 1985;144:295.

242. Swiryn S, Pavel D, Byrom E. Sequential regional phase mapping of radionuclide gated biventriculograms in patients with ventricular tachycardia: close correlation with electrophysiologic characteristics. Am Heart J 1982;103:319.

243. Dae MW, Botvinick EH, O'Connell W, et al. Atrial corrected Fourier amplitude ratios for the scintigraphic quantitation of valvar regurgitation. J Nucl Med 1984;25:36.

244. Frais M, Botvinick E, Shosa D, et al. Phase image characterization of localized and generalized left ventricular contraction abnormalities. J Am Coll Cardiol 1984;4:987.

245. Frais M, Botvinick E, Shosa D, et al. Phase image characterization of ventricular contraction in left and right bundle branch block. Am J Cardiol 1982;50:95.

246. Ratib O, Heinze E,. Schon H, et al. Phase analysis of radionuclide ventriculograms for the detection of coronary artery disease. Am Heart J 1982;104:1.

247. Botvinick EH, Frais M, O'Connell W, et al. Phase image evaluation of patients with ventricular pre-excitation syndromes. J Am Coll Cardiol 1984;3:799.

248. Colocci WS, Wynne J, Holman BL, et al. Long-term therapy of heart failure with prazosin: a randomized double blind trial. Am J Cardiol 1980;45:337.

249. Nichols AB, McKusick KA, Strauss HW, et al. Clinical utility of gated cardiac blood pool imaging in congestive heart failure. Am J Med 1978;65:785.

250. Kronenberg MW, Pederson RW, Harston WE, et al. Left ventricular performance after coronary artery bypass surgery: prediction of functional benefit. Ann Intern Med 1983;99:305.

251. Schwartz RG, Alexander J, McKenzie WB, et al. Adherence to radionuclide angiocardiographic guidelines reduces the incidence and severity of congestive heart failure in high risk patients: the Yale doxorubicin cardiotoxicity study. J Am Coll Cardiol 1986;7:24A.

252. Nitosh J, Seiderer M, Bull U, et al. Evaluation of left ventricular performance by radionuclide ventriculography in patients with atrioventricular vs. ventricular demand pacemakers. Am Heart J 1984;5:906.

253. Pohost GM, Pastore JO, McKusick KA, et al. Detection of left atrial myxoma by gated radionuclide cardiac imaging. Circulation 1977;55:88.

254. Berger HJ, Zaret BL. Radionuclide assessment of left ventricular performance. In: Freeman LM, ed. Clinical radionuclide imaging. New York: Grune & Stratton, 1984:386.

255. Bulkley BH, Hutchins GM, Bailey I, et al. Thallium-201 imaging and gated cardiac blood pool scans in patients with ischemic and idiopathic cardiomyopathy. Circulation 1977;55:753.

256. Korr KS, Gandsman EJ, Winkler ML, et al. Hemodynamic correlates of right ventricular ejection fraction measured with radionuclide angiography. Am J Cardiol 1982;49:71.

257. Bough EW, Gandsman E, Shulman R. Measurement of normal left atrial function with gated radionuclide angiography. Am J Cardiol 1981;48:473.

258. Viquerat CE, Hansen RM, Botvinick EH, et al. Undrained bloody pericardial effusion in the early postoperative period after coronary bypass surgery: a prospective blood pool study. Am Heart J 1985;110:335.

259. Ramanathan KB, Bodenheimer MM, Banka VS, et al. Severity of contraction abnormalities after acute myocardial infarction in man: response to nitroglycerin. Circulation 1979;60:1230.

260. Simoons ML, Wijns W, Balakumaran K, et al. The effect of intracoronary thrombolysis with streptokinase on myocardial thallium distribution and left ventricular function assessed by blood pool scintigraphy. Eur Heart J 1982;3:433.

261. Kirch D, Metz C, Steel P. Quantitation of valvular insufficiency by computerized radionuclide angiocardiogrphy. Am J Cardiol 1974;34:711.

262. Baugh E, Gandsman E, North D, et al. Gated radionuclide angiographic evaluation of valve regurgitation. Am J Cardiol 1980;46:423.

263. Sorensen SG, O'Rourke RA, Ghaudhur TK. Noninvasive quantitation of valvular regurgitation by gated equilibrium radionuclide angiography. Circulation 1980;62:1089.

264. Makler PJ Jr, McCarthy DM, Velchik MG, et al. Fourier amplitude ratio: a new way to assess valvular regurgitation. J Nucl Med 1983;24:204.

265. Goris ML. Functional and parametric images. J Nucl Med 1982;23:360.

266. Wynne J, Sayres M, Moaddox DE, et al. Regional left ventricular function in acute myocardial infarction: evaluation with quantitative radionuclide ventriculography. Am J Cardiol 1980; 45:203.

267. Wackers FJ, Berger HJ, Weinberg MA, et al. Spontaneous changes in left ventricular function over the first 24 hours of acute myocardial infarction: implications for evaluating early therapeutic interventions. Circulation 1982;66:748.

268. Dae M, Wen YM, Botvinick E, et al. Assessment of left anterior fascicular block by scintigraphic phase analysis. J Am Coll Cardiol 1984;3:591.

269. Upton MT, Rerych SK, Newman GE, et al. The reproducibility of radionuclide angiographic measurements of left ventricular function in normal subjects at rest and during exercise. Circulation 1980;62:126.

270. Boucher CA, Wilson RA, Kanarack DJ, et al. Exercise testing in asymptomatic or minimally symptomatic aortic regurgitation:

relationship of left ventricular ejection fraction to left ventricular filling pressure during exercise. Circulation 1983;67:1091.

271. Caldwell JH, Hamilton GW, Sorensen SG, et al. The detection of coronary artery disease with radionuclide techniques: a comparison of rest exercise thallium imaging and ejection fraction response. Circulation 1980;61:610.

272. Port S, Cobb FR, Coleman RE, et al. Effect of age on the response of the left ventricular ejection fraction to exercise. N Engl J Med 1980;303:1133.

273. Polak JF, Kemper AJ, Bianco JA, et al. Resting early peak diastolic filling rate: a sensitive index of myocardial dysfunction in patients with coronary artery disease. J Nucl Med 1982; 23:471.

274. Kaul S, Boucher CA, Okada RD, et al. Sources of variability in the radionuclide angiographic assessment of ejection fraction: a comparison of first pass and gated techniques. Am J Cardiol 1984;53:823.

275. Greenberg B, Drew D, Botvinick EH, et al. Evaluation of left ventricular volume, ejection fraction and segmental wall motion by gated radionuclide angiography. Clin Nuc Med 1980; 5:245.

276. Shen AC, Jennings RB. Myocardial calcium and magnesium in acute ischemic injury. Am J Pathol 1972;67:441.

277. Bonte FJ, Parkey RW, Graham KD, et al. A new method for radionuclide imaging of myocardial infarcts. Radiology 1973; 110:473.

278. Coleman RE, Klein MS, Ahmed SA, et al. Mechanisms contributing to myocardial accumulation of technetium-99m stannous pyrophosphate after coronary occlusion. Am J Cardiol 1977; 39:55.

279. Zaret BL, DiCola UC, Donbedial RK, et al. Dual radionuclide study of myocardial infarction. Circulation 1976;53:422.

280. Buja LM, Parkey RW, Dees JH, et al. Morphologic correlates of technetium-99m stannous pyrophosphate imaging of acute myocardial infarcts in dogs. Circulation 1975;52:596.

281. Buja LM, Tofe AJ, Kulkarni PV, et al. Sites and mechanisms of localization of technetium-99m phosphorous radiopharmaceuticals in acute myocardial infarcts and other tissues. J Clin Invest 1977;60:724.

282. Schelbert HR, Ingwall JS, Sybers HD, et al. Uptake of infarct imaging agents in reversibly and irreversibly injured myocardium in cultured fetal mouse heart. Circ Res 1976;39:860.

283. Joseph SP, Ell PJ, Ross P. ^{99m}Tc imidodiphosphonate: a superior radiopharmaceutical for in vivo positive myocarial infarct imaging. Br Heart J 1978;40:234.

284. Rude RE, Parkey RW, Bonte FJ, et al. Clinical implications of the technetium-99m stannous pyrophosphate myocardial scintigraphic "doughnut" pattern in patients with acute myocardial infarcts. Circulation 1979;50:540.

285. Parkey RW, Bonte FJ, Meyer SL, et al. A new method for radionuclide imaging of acute MI in humans. Circulation 1974; 50:540.

286. Prasquier R, Taradash MR, Botvinick EH, et al. The specificity of the diffuse pattern of cardiac uptake in myocardial infarction imaging with technetium-99m stannous pyrophosphate. Circulation 1977;55:61.

287. Berman DS, Amsterdam DS, Hines H, et al. New approach to interpretation of technetium-99m pyrophosphate scintigraphy in the detection of acute myocardial infarction. Am J Cardiol 1977;39:341.

288. Holman BL, Goldhaber SZ, Kirsch CM, et al. Measurement of infarct size using single photon emission computed tomography and ^{99m}Tc-pyrophosphate: a description of the method and a comparison with patient prognosis. Am J Cardiol 1982; 50:503.

289. Botvinick EH, Shames D, Lappin H, et al. Noninvasive quanti-

tation of myocardial infarction with technetium-99 pyrophosphate. Circulation 1975;52:909.

290. Massie BM, Botvinick EH, Werner JA, et al. Myocardial infarction scintigraphy with technetium 99m stannous pyrophosphate: an insensitive test for nontransmural myocardial infarction. Am J Cardiol 1979;43:186.

291. Righetti A, O'Rourke RA, Schelbert N, et al. Usefulness of preoperative and postoperative Tc-99m(SN) pyrophosphate scans in patients with ischemic and valvular heart disease. Am J Cardiol 1977;39:43.

292. Willerson JT, Parkey RW, Bonte FJ, et al. Technetium stannous pyrophosphate myocardial scintigrams in patients with chest pain of varying etiology. Circulation 1975;51:1046.

293. Ahmed M, Dubiel JP, Logan KW, et al. Limited clinical diagnostic specificity of technetium-99m stannous pyrophosphate myocardial imaging in acute myocardial infarction. Am J Cardiol 1977;39:50.

294. Klausner SC, Botvinick EH, Shames DM, et al. The application of radionuclide scintigraphy to diagnose perioperative myocardial infarction following revascularization. Circulation 1977; 56:173.

295. Lyons KP, Olson HG, Brown WT, et al. Persistence of an abnormal pattern on ^{99m}TC pyrophosphate myocardial scintigraphy following acute myocardial infarction. Clin Nucl Med 1976; 1:253.

296. Botvinick EH, Shames DM, Sharpe DN, et al. The specificity of technetium stannous pyrophosphate myocardial scintigrams in patients with prior myocardial infarction. J Nucl Med 1978; 19:1121.

297. Poliner LR, Buja LM, Parkey RW, et al. Clinicopathologic findings in 52 patients studied by technetium-99m stannous pyrophosphate myocardial scintigraphy. Circulation 1979;59:257.

298. Werner JA, Botvinick EH, Shames DM, et al. Acute myocardial infarction: clinical application of technetium 99m stannous pyrophosphate infarct scintigraphy. West J Med 1977;127:464.

299. Willerson JT, Parkey RW, Bonte FJ, et al. Acute subendocardial infarction in patients. Circulation 1975;51:436.

300. Braun SD, Lisbona R, Novales-Diaz JA, et al. Myocardial uptake of ^{99m}Tc-phosphate tracers in amyloidosis. Clin Nucl Med 1979;6:244.

301. Righetti A, Crawford MH, O'Rourke RA, et al. Detection of perioperative myocardial damage after coronary artery bypass graft surgery. Circulation 1977;5:173.

302. Coleman RE, Klein MS, Roberts R, et al. Improved detection of myocardial infarction with technetium-99m stannous pyrophosphate and serum MB creatine phosphokinase. Am J Cardiol 1976;37:732.

303. Pugh BR, Buja LM, Parkey RW, et al. Cardioversion and "false positive" technetium-99m stannous pyrophosphate myocardial scintigrams. Circulation 1976;54:399.

304. Werner JA, Botvinick EH, Shames DM, et al. Diagnosis of acute myocardial infarction following cardioversion: accurate detection with technetium-99m pyrophosphate scintigraphy. Circulation 1977;56:III-63.

305. Page DL, Caulfield JB, Kaster JA, et al. Myocardial changes associated with cardiogenic shock. N Engl J Med 1971;285:133.

306. Sharpe DN, Botvinick EH, Shames DM, et al. The clinical estimation of acute myocardial infarct size with 99m technetium pyrophosphate scintigraphy. Circulation 1978;57:307.

307. Holman BL, Chishold RJ, Braunwald E. The prognostic implications of acute myocardial infarct scintigraphy with ^{99m}Tc-pyrophosphate. Circulation 1978;57:320.

308. Stokeley EM, Buja LM, Lewis SE, et al. Measurement of acute myocardial infarcts in dogs with ^{99m}Tc-stannous pyrophosphate scintigrams. J Nucl Med 1976;17:1.

309. Khaw BA, Beller GA, Haber E. Experimental myocardial infarct

imaging following intravenous administration of iodine-131 labeled antibody (Fab')2 fragments specific for cardiac myosin. Circulation 1978;57:743.

310. Berger H, Alderson L, Becker L, et al. Multicenter trial of In-Ill antimyosin for infarct-avid imaging. J Nucl Med 1986;27:967.

311. Burggraf GW, Parker JO. Prognosis in coronary artery disease: angiographic, hemodynamic and clinical factors. Circulation 1975;51:146.

312. Block WJ Jr, Crumpacker EL, Dry TJ, et al. Prognosis of angina pectoris: observations in 6882 cases. JAMA 1952;150:259.

313. Bigger JT Jr, Heller CA, Wenger TL, et al. Risk stratification after acute myocardial infarction. Am J Cardiol 1981;42:202.

314. Forrestor JS, Diamond G, Swan HJC. Classification of clinical and hemodynamic function after acute myocardial infarction. Am J Cardiol 1977;39:137.

315. Harris PJ, Lee KL, Harrell FE Jr, et al. Outcome in medically treated coronary artery disease. Circulation 1980;62:718.

316. The Veterans Administration Coronary Artery Bypass Surgery Cooperative Study Group: Eleven year survival in the Veterans Administration randomized trial of coronary bypass surgery for stable angina. N Engl J Med 1984;311:1333.

317. Roberts WC, Manning MM. The coronary artery surgery study (CASS): do the results apply to your patient? Am J Cardiol 1984;54:440.

318. Frais M, Botvinick EH, Shosa D, et al. Are regions of ischemia detected on stress perfusion scintigraphy predictive of sites of subsequent myocardial infarction? Br Heart J 1982;47:357.

319. Warnowicz MA, Parker H, Cheitlin M. Prognosis of patients with acute pulmonary edema and normal ejection fraction after myocardial infarction. Circulation 1983;67:330.

320. Schuster EH, Bulkley BH. Early-post-infarction angina: ischemia at a distance and ischemia in the infarct zone. N Engl J Med 1981;305:1101.

321. Taylor GJ, Humphries JO, Mellitis ED, et al. Predictors of clinical course, coronary anatomy, and left ventricular function after recovery from acute myocardial infarction. Circulation 1980;62:960.

322. Bartel AG, Behar VS, Peter RH, et al. Graded exercise stress tests in documented coronary artery disease. Circulation 1974;49:348.

323. Ellstad MH, Wan MKC. Predictive implications of stress testing: follow-up of 2700 subjects after maximum treadmill stress testing. Circulation 1975;51:363.

324. Thompson P, Keleman M. Hypotension accompanying the onset of exertional angina: a sign of severe compromise of left ventricular ejection fraction. Circulation 1975;52:28.

325. Goldman S, Tselos S, Cohn K. Marked depth of ST segment depression during treadmill exercise testing: indicator of severe coronary artery disease. Chest 1975;69:729.

326. Dagenais GR, Rouleau JR, Christen A, et al. Survival of patients with a strongly positive exercise electrocardiogram. Circulation 1982;65:452.

327. Kattus AA. Exercise electrocardiography. In: Amsterdam EA, ed. Exercise in cardiovascular health and disease. New York: Yorke Medical Books, 1977:161.

328. Gibson RS, Crampton RS, Watson DD, et al. Precordial ST segment depression during acute inferior myocardial infarction: clinical scintigraphic and angiographic correlations. Circulation 1982;66:732.

329. Haines DE, Beller G, Cooper A, et al. Clinical, scintigraphic and angiographic correlates of exercise induced ST elevation, ten days after uncomplicated myocardial infarction. Circulation (Suppl)1985;72:III-462.

330. Hakki AH, Munley BM, Starvos H, et al. Physiologic and anatomic determinants of abnormal blood pressure response to exercise in patients with coronary artery disease. Circulation (Suppl)1985;72:III-104.

331. Chaitman BR, Brevers G, Dupras G, et al. Diagnostic impact of thallium scintigraphy and cardiac fluoroscopy when the exercise ECG is strongly positive. Am Heart J 1984;108:260.

332. Boucher CA, Leonard M, Beller G, et al. Increased lung uptake of thallium-201 during exercise myocardial imaging: clinical, hemodynamic correlates and their relationship to coronary artery disease. Am J Cardiol 1980;46:189.

333. Weld FM, King-Lee C, Bigger JT, et al. Risk stratification with low-level exercise testing 2 weeks after acute myocardial infarction. Circulation 1981;64:306.

334. Hung J, Goris M, Nash E, et al. Comparative value of maximal treadmill testing, exercise thallium myocardial perfusion scintigraphy and exercise radionuclide ventriculography for distinguishing high and low risk patients soon after acute myocardial infarction. Am J Cardiol 1983;51:361.

335. Wackers FJ, Russo DJ, Russo D, et al. Prognostic significance of normal quantitative planar thallium-201 stress scintigraphy in patients with chest pain. J Am Coll Cardiol 1985;6:27.

336. Dunn R, Botvinick EH, Benge W, et al. The significance of nitroglycerin-induced changes in ventricular function after myocardial infarction. Am J Cardiol 1982;95:590.

337. Misbach GA, Botvinick EH, Tyberg J, et al. The functional implications of scintigraphic measures of ischemia and infarction. Am Heart J 1983;106:996.

338. Buja LM, Parkey RW, Stokely EM, et al. Pathophysiology of technetium-99m stannous pyrophosphate and thallium-201 scintigraphy in acute anterior infarction in dogs. J Clin Invest 1976;57:1508.

339. Olson HG, Lyons KP, Aronow WS. The high risk angina patient: identification by clinical features, hospital course, electrocardiography, and technetium 99m stannous pyrophosphate scintigraphy. Circulation 1981;66:674.

340. Olson H, Lyons K, Aronow W, et al. Prognostic value of a persistently positive technetium-99m stannous pyrophosphate myocardial scintigram after myocardial infarction. Am J Cardiol 1979;43:889.

341. Holman LB, Chisolm RJ, Braunwald E, et al. The prognostic implications of acute myocardial infarction scintigraphy with 99m technetium pyrophosphate. Circulation 1978;57:326.

342. Bulkley BH, Silverman KJ, Weisfeldt ML, et al. Pathologic basis of thallium-201 scintigraphic defects in patients with fatal myocardial injury. Circulation 1979;60:785.

343. Silverman KJ, Grossman W. Angina pectoris: natural history and strategies for evaluation and management. N Engl J Med 1984;310:1712.

344. DeBusk RF, Blomquist CG, Kouchoukos NT, et al. Identification of low risk patients with acute myocardial infarction and coronary artery bypass surgery. N Engl J Med 1986;314:151.

345. Bell RS. Efficacy . . . What's that? Semin Nucl Med 1978;8:316.

346. Schiller NB, Botvinick EH. Noninvasive quantitation of the left heart by echocardiography and scintigraphy. Cardiology Clinics (in press).

347. Hatle L, Angelsen B. Doppler ultrasound in cardiology. In: Hatle L, Angelsen B, eds. Physical principles and clinical applications. Philadelphia: Lea & Febiger, 1982:221.

348. Botvinick EH, Engelstad BL, Glazer HB, et al. Blood pool scintigraphy of the heart: current status. In: Freeman LB, Wagner R, eds. Nuclear medicine annual. New York: Raven Press, 1982.

349. Lusted LB. Introduction to medical decision making. Springfield, IL: Charles C Thomas, 1968.

350. Weinstein MC, Fineberg HV, Elstein AS, et al. Clinical decision analysis. In: Lusted LB, ed. Clinical medicine. Philadelphia: WB Saunders, 1980.

351. Weinstein MC, Stason WB. Foundations of cost effectiveness

analysis for health and medical practices. N Engl J Med 1977;296:716.

352. Snedecor GW, Cochran WG. Statistical methods, 6th ed. Ames, Iowa: Iowa State University Press, 1967.

353. Moorman JR, Hlatky MA, Eddy DM, et al. The yield of the routine admission electrocardiogram. Ann Intern Med 1985; 103:590.

354. Weinstein MC, Stason WB. Cost-effectiveness of coronary artery bypass surgery. Circulation (Suppl 3)1982;66:56.

355. CASS/Principle Investigators and their associates: Coronary Artery Surgery Study (CASS). A randomized trial of coronary artery bypass surgery: survival data. Circulation 1983;68:939.

356. Weiner DA, Ryan TJ, McCabe CH, et al. The role of exercise testing in identifying patients with improved survival after coronary artery bypass surgery. J Am Coll Cardiol 1986;8:741.

357. Weiner DA, Ryan TJ, McCabe CH, et al. Value of exercise testing in determining the risk classification and the response to coronary artery bypass grafting in three vessel coronary artery disease: a report from the Coronary Artery Surgery Study (CASS) Registry. Am J Cardiol 1986;8:741.

358. Bush LR, Buja LM, Samowitz W, et al. Recovery of left ventricular segmental function after long term reperfusion following temporary coronary occlusion in conscious dogs. Comparison of 2 and 4 hour occlusions. Circ Res 1983;53:248.

359. Lavellee M, Cox D, Patrick TA, et al. Salvage of myocardial function by coronary artery reperfusion 1, 2, and 3 hours after occlusion in conscious dogs. Circ Res 1983;53:235.

360. Matzuzaki M, Gallagher KP, Kemper WS, et al. Sustained regional dysfunction produced by prolonged coronary stenosis: gradual recovery after reperfusion. Circulation 1983;68:170.

361. Reimer KA, Jennings RB. The "wavefront phenomenon" of myocardial ischemic cell death. Lab Invest 1979;40:633.

362. Piek JJ, Becker AE. Collateral blood supply to the myocardium at risk in human myocardial infarction: a quantitative postmortem assessment. J Am Coll Cardiol 1988;11:1290.

363. Stinson EB, Billingham ME. Correlative study of regional left ventricular histology and contractile function. Am J Cardiol 1978;39:378.

364. Braunwald E, Kloner RA. The stunned myocardium: prolonged postischemic ventricular dysfunction. Circulation 1982;66:1146.

365. Rahimtoola SH. The hibernating myocardium. Am Heart J 1989;117:211.

366. Nachlas MM, Shurtka TK. Macroscopic identification of early myocardial infarcts by alterations in dehydrogenase activity. Am J Pathol 1963;43:379.

367. Cox JL, McLaughlin VW, Flowers NC, et al. The ischemic zone surrounding acute myocardial infarction: its morphology as detected by dehydrogenase staining. Am Heart J 1968;76:650.

368. Schwaiger M, Neese RA, Araujo L, et al. Sustained nonoxidative glucose utilization and depletion of glycogen in reperfused canine myocardium. J Am Coll Cardiol 1989;13:745.

369. Buja M, Tofe AJ, Kulkarne PV, et al. Sites and mechanisms of localization of Tc-99m phosphorous radiopharmaceuticals in acute myocardial infarction. JCI 1977;60:724.

370. Poliner LR, Buja LM, Parkey RW, et al. Clinicopathologic findings in 32 patients studied by Tc-99m stannous pyrophosphate myocardial scintigraphy. Circulation 1979;59:527.

371. Long R, Symes J, Allard J, et al. Differentiation between reperfusion and occlusion myocardial necrosis with Tc-99m pyrophosphate sensitivity. Am J Cardol 1980;46:413.

372. Ramanathan K, Bodenheimer MM, Banka VS, et al. Natural history of contractile abnormalities after acute myocardial infarction in man: severity of response to NTG as a function of time. Circulation 1981;63:731.

373. Homans DC, Sublett E, Elsberger J, et al. Mechanism of remote myocardial dysfunction during coronary artery occlusion in the presence of multivessel disease. Circulation 1986;74:588.

374. Hood WB Jr. Experimental myocardial infarction III—recovery of left ventricular function in the healing phase: contribution of increased fiber shortening in noninfarcted myocardium. Am Heart J 1970;79:531.

375. Popio KA, Gorlin D, Bechtel D, et al. Postextrasystolic potentiation as a predictor of potential myocardial viability: preoperative analysis compared with studies after CABG. Am J Cardiol 1977;39:944.

376. Cohen M, Charney R, Hershman R, et al. Reversal of chronic myocardial ischemic dysfunction after transluminal coronary angioplasty. J Am Coll Cardiol 1988;12:1193.

377. Cornish AL, Hanley HG, O'Conner W, et al. Limitations of postextrasystolic potentiation in identifying ischemic myocardium. Am J Physiol 1981;241:H654.

378. McAnulty JH, Hattenaner MT, Rosch J, et al. Improvement in left ventricular wall motion following NTG. Circulation 1974; 51:140.

379. Helfant RH, Pine R, Meister SG, et al. Nitroglycerin to unmask reversible asynergy. Circulation 1974;50:108.

380. Schuler G, Schwartz F, Hofmann M, et al. Thrombolysis in acute myocardial infarction using intracoronary STK: assessment of Tl-201 scintigraphy. Circulation 1982;66:658.

381. Rankin JS, Newman GE, Muhlbaier LH, et al. The effects of coronary revascularization in left ventricular function in ischemic heart disease. Thor Cardiovasc Surg 1985;90:818.

382. Chatterjee K, Swan HJC, Parmley WW, et al. Depression of left ventricular function due to acute myocardial ischemia and its reversal after aortocoronary saphenous vein bypass. N Engl J Med 1972;286:1117.

383. Chatterjee K, Swan HJC, Parmley WW, et al. Influence of direct myocardial revascularization on left ventricular asynergy and function in patients with coronary heart disease. Circulation 1973;47:276.

384. Okada RD, Pohost GM. The use of preintervention and postintervention thallium imaging for assessing the early and late effects of experimental coronary arterial reperfusion in dogs. Circulation 1984;69:1153.

385. Rozanski A, Berman D, Gray R, et al. Use of Tl-201 redistribution scintigraphy in the preoperative differentiation of reversible and non-reversible myocardial asynergy. Circulation 1981;64:936.

386. Beller GA. Role of myocardial perfusion imaging in evaluating thrombolytic therapy for acute myocardial infarction. J Am Coll Cardiol 1987;9:661.

387. Budinger T, Knittel BL. Cardiac thallium redistribution and model. J Nucl Med 1987;28:588.

388. Yang LD, Berman D, Kiat H, et al. Frequency of late reversibility in SPECT Tl-201 stress studies: a prospective evaluation. J Nucl Med 1989;30:740.

389. Cloninger KG, DePuey EG, Garcia E, et al. Incomplete redistribution in delayed thallium-201 SPECT images: an overestimation of myocardial scarring. J Am Coll Cardiol 1988; 12:955.

390. Liu P, Kiess MC, Okada RD, et al. The persistent defect on exercise thallium imaging and its fate after myocardial revascularization: does it represent scar or ischemia? Am Heart J 1985;110:994.

391. Budinger TF, Rollo FD. Physics and instrumentation. In: Holman BL, Sonnenbleck EH, Lesch M, eds. Principles of cardiovascular nuclear medicine. New York: Grune & Stratton, 1979:170.

392. Goldstein RA, Mullani NA, Gould KL. Quantitative myocardial imaging with positron emitters. In: Goodwin JF, ed. Progess in cardiology. Philadelphia: Grune & Stratton, 1983:147.

393. Phelps ME. Emission computed tomography. Semin Nucl Med 1977;7:337.

394. Henze E, Huang SC, Plummer D, et al. Retrieval of quantitative information from positron emission computed tomographic images for cardiac studies with C-11 palmitate. J Nucl Med 1981;22:21.

395. Schelbert HR, Phelps ME, Hoffman EJ, et al. Regional myocardial perfusion assessed with N-13 labeled ammonia and positron emission computerized axial tomography. Am J Cardiol 1979;43:209.

396. Ter-Pogossian MN, Klein MS, Markham J, et al. Regional assessment of myocardial metabolic integrity in vivo by positron emission tomography with 11C labeled palmitate. Circulation 1980;61:242.

397. Gould KL, Schelbert HR, Phelps ME, et al. Noninvasive assessment of coronary stenoses with myocardial perfusion imaging during pharmacologic coronary vasodilatation. V. Detection of 47% diameter coronary stenosis with intravenous nitrogen-13 ammonia and emission computed transaxial tomography in intact dogs. Am J Cardiol 1979;46:200.

398. Selwyn AP, Allan RM, L'Abbate A, et al. Relation between regional myocardial uptake of rubidium-82 and perfusion: absolute reduction of cation uptake in ischemia. Am J Cardiol 1982;50:112.

399. Sobel BE, Weiss ES, Welch MJ, et al. Detection of remote myocardial infarction in patients with positron emission transaxial tomography and intravenous 11C-palmitate. Circulation 1977; 55:853.

400. McKenna WJ, Allan RM, Horlock P, et al. Hypertrophic cardiomyopathy: measurement of cation uptake. Am J Cardiol 1981;47:409.

401. Henze E, Perloff JK, Schelbert HR. Alterations of regional myocardial perfusion and metabolism in Duchenne's muscular dystrophy (DMD) detected by positron computed tomography (PCT). Circulation (Suppl)1981;64:IV-279.

402. Geltman EM, Smith JL, Beecher D, et al. Altered regional myocardial metabolism in congestive cardiomyopathy detected by positron tomography. Am J Med 1983;74:773.

403. Randle PJ, England PJ, Denton RM. Control of the tricarboxylic acid cycle and its interactions with glycolysis during acetate utilization in rat heart. Biochem J 1970;117:677.

404. Tillisch J, Brunken R, Marshall R, et al. Reversibility of cardiac wall motion abnormalities predicted by positron tomography. N Engl J Med 1986;314:884.

405. Schelbert HR, Wisenberg G, Phelps ME, et al. Noninvasive assessment of coronary stenoses by myocardial imaging during pharmacologic vasodilation. VI. Detection of coronary artery disease in man with intravenous N-13 ammonia positron computed tomography. Am J Cardiol 1982;49:1197.

406. Marshall RC, Tillisch JH, Phelps ME, et al. Identification and differentiation of resting myocardial ischemia and infarction in man with positron computed tomography, 18F-labeled fluorodeoxyglucose and N-13 ammonia. Circulation 1983;67:766.

407. Grant PM, Erdal BR, O'Brien HA. A 82Sr-82Rb isotope generator for use in nuclear medicine. J Nucl Med 1975;16:300.

408. Phelps ME, Schelbert HR, Hoffman EJ, et al. Physiologic tomography of myocardial glucose metabolism, perfusion and blood pools with multiple gated acquisition. In: Kreuzer H, Parmley WW, Rentrop P, Heiss HW, eds. Advances in clinical cardiology. New York: Gerhard Witzstrock, 1980.

409. Gallagher BM, Fowler JS, Gratterson NI, et al. Metabolic trapping as a powerful principle of radiopharmaceutical design: some factors responsible for the biodistribution of F-18-2Deoxy-Glucose. J Nucl Med 1978;19:1154.

410. Taegtmeyer H. Myocardial metabolism. In: Phelps M, Mazziotta J, Schelbert H, eds. Positron emission tomography and autoradiography: principles and applications for brain and heart. New York: Raven Press, 1986:149.

411. Schwaiger M, Schelbert HR, Ellison D, et al. Sustained regional abnormalities in cardiac metabolism after transient ischemia in the chronic dog model. J Am Coll Cardiol 1985;6:336.

412. Brunken R, Tillisch J, Schwaiger M, et al. Regional perfusion, glucose metabolism and wall motion in patients with chronic electrocardiographic Q wave infarctions: evidence for persistence of viable tissue in some infarct regions by positron emission tomography. Circulation 1986;73:951.

413. Brunken R, Schwaiger M, Grover-McKay M, et al. PET detects tissue metabolic activity in myocardial segments with persistent thallium perfusion defects. J Am Coll Cardiol 1987;10:557.

414. Brunken R, Mody FV, Hawkins RA, et al. Positron tomography detects glucose metabolism in segments with 24 hour tomographic thallium defects. Circulation 1988;78:II-91.

Chapter 11

Nuclear Imaging of Congenital Heart Disease

Michael W. Dae

Radionuclide imaging in congenital heart disease is used primarily for the assessment of cardiac physiology. The main techniques for the evaluation of congenital heart diseases are echocardiography and angiocardiography, which define morphology. The application of Doppler methodology to the echo has provided a powerful method for acquiring clinically useful information about hemodynamics as well. Even in this context, however, radionuclide methodology continues to offer useful and often unique information. Three major categories of studies are applicable to the assessment of congenital lesions: evaluation of shunts, accurate determination of right and left ventricular function, and assessment of myocardial perfusion. Currently, assessment of the presence and magnitude of left-to-right shunts is the most widely used radionuclide methodology in congenital heart disease.

Assessment of Shunts

Left-to-Right Shunts

The method of assessment involves the rapid injection of a bolus of a radionuclide (usually technetium diethylenetriamine pentaacetic acid [Tc-DTPA]) into the circulation while monitoring the transit through the heart and lungs with a gamma camera. For small infants (i.e., premature newborn infants) a butterfly needle can be used in a temporal scalp vein to deliver a compact bolus of activity to the central circulation. In older children and

adults either a butterfly needle or a small plastic catheter can be inserted into an external jugular vein. The delivery of a compact, nonfragmented bolus of activity is critical to allow accurate determination of the size of the shunt. With good technique, the success rate should be over 90%. It may be necessary to sedate infants and some children, since crying simulates a Valsalva maneuver, which can impede bolus entry into the thorax and lead to fragmentation of the bolus. Tc-DTPA is most commonly used for shunt studies. Doses are 200 μCi per kilogram of body weight, with a minimum dose of 2 mCi. The advantage of Tc-DTPA over other Tc-based agents is its fairly rapid renal excretion, which leads to prompt clearance of background activity. This becomes important if it is necessary to perform a second injection to improve the quality of the bolus. Generally no more than two sequential injections are done because of dosimetry concerns.

The study is done in the anterior projection using a converging collimator (which provides magnification) in infants, and ideally a high-sensitivity collimator (which maximizes count rate) in older children and adults. A dynamic acquisition with a framing rate of two to four frames per second should be adequate for evaluation of shunts. If ejection fraction measurements are to be made by the first pass method, a rate of at least 25 frames per second should be used. The sequential flow study is reviewed to provide useful information regarding chamber orientation and vascular connections. In the presence of normal anatomic relationships, right heart structures appear, followed by the main pulmonary artery, lungs, and subsequently, the left ventricle (levophase) and descend-

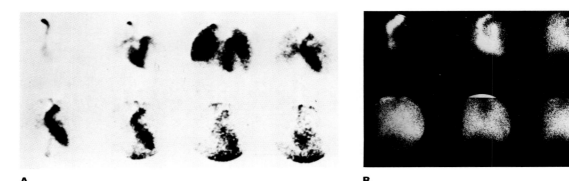

A   **B**

Figure 11-1. Radionuclide first-pass flow studies. Shown are radionuclide flow studies, progressing left to right in a patient without left-to-right shunt (*A*) and in a patient with left-to-right shunt (*B*). The absence of a levophase in the latter is consistent with a moderate to large shunt with a Qp/Qs over 1.5. (Reproduced by permission of the American Heart Association, Inc., from Botvinick E, Schiller N, Shames D. The role of echocardiography and scintigraphy in the evaluation of adults with suspected left-to-right shunts. Circulation 1980;62:1020.)

ing aorta. The absence of a good levophase is consistent with a moderate to large left-to-right shunt (Fig. 11-1). This appearance results from recirculation of activity from the heart back to the lungs and vice versa across the shunt. This appearance has been called the "smudge sign," and generally relates to a shunt of at least 1.6/1 (pulmonary to systemic flow [Qp/Qs]).

Time-versus-radioactivity curves are drawn from regions of interest over the superior vena cava to assess the quality of the bolus, and over the periphery of the right lung for shunt detection and quantitation (Fig. 11-2). A separate curve may be generated from a region over the left lung if differential shunting is expected (as may occur with a patent ductus arteriosus). The normal pulmonary arterial curve has an ascending limb, reflecting the arrival of tracer in the pulmonary circulation, and a descending limb, as the tracer leaves the lungs and enters the left side of the heart. A late peak appears, reflecting systemic recirculation. In the presence of a left-to-right shunt, a shoulder is present on the downslope, indicating recirculation of activity back to the lungs across the shunt. For shunt quantification, the shape of the pulmonary portion of the curve is approximated by an algebraic expression called a gamma variate function (Fig. 11-3).[1] In practice, the computer is given the coordinates of the upslope and initial downslope of the pulmonary curve and a curve is generated that approximates the shape of the pulmonary curve. The area under this curve is proportional to pulmonary flow (Qp). This fitted curve is then subtracted from the initial time-versus-radioactivity curve and another gamma variate fit is done on the remaining curve. The area under this second fitted curve is proportional to the shunt flow (Qsh). The difference between the two fitted curves is a measure of systemic flow (Qs). The re-

sulting calculation of pulmonary to systemic flow, Qp/Qs, is performed by the computer as:

$$Qp/Qs = \frac{Qp}{Qp - Qsh}$$

Ratios less than 1.2:1 are consistent with the absence of left-to-right shunts. The Qp/Qs calculation is quantitative over a clinically significant range of 1.2:1 to 3.0:1. The gamma variate method has shown excellent correlation with shunt size determined at cardiac catheterization.[1] This relationship remains valid even in the presence of pulmonary hypertension, tricuspid regurgitation, and heart failure.[1,2] In these conditions extensive dilution and slow flow lead to a slow downslope to the pulmonary curve. The upslope should be proportionately slowed, however, and the curve fit method should generally apply. Nevertheless, caution should be exercised in these cases. Since the method is dependent on the full passage of the administered radionuclide through the lungs, left-to-right shunts will be overestimated in the presence of right-to-left shunts. Shunts greater than 3.0:1 are difficult to fit by the gamma variate method because of distortions in curve shape as a result of the large and torrential shunt flow. This is not a practical limitation, however, because any shunt greater than 3.0:1 is considered large. In general, a shunt of 2.0 or greater is sufficient to warrant surgical correction.

Equilibrium Approach. It is possible to calculate the extent of left-to-right shunts using the equilibrium blood pool method. Stroke volume or amplitude images can be used to measure the difference in stroke volume

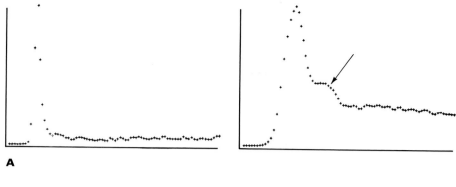

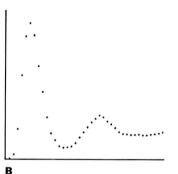
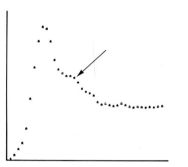

A

B

Figure 11-2. Time–activity curves at 2 frames/sec (2 fps). *A:* Time–activity histograms of the superior vena cava (*left*) and the right lung (*right*). The bolus of radiotracer is adequate because it produced a single peak. The lung curve is that of a left-to-right shunt showing premature recirculation of the tracer (*arrow*). *B:* Pulmonary time–activity curves. Normal (*left*). Left-to-right shunt (*right*). A shoulder on the downslope of the curve indicates a left-to-right shunt (*arrow*). (Reproduced with permission from Treves ST, et al. Pediatric nuclear medicine. New York: Springer–Verlag, 1985:248.)

between the ventricles, as is commonly performed for the evaluation of regurgitant lesions (Fig. 11-4).[3] For example, for a ventricular septal defect or a patent ductus arteriosus, the left ventricle handles the excess volume of the shunt flow. The left ventricular (LV) stroke volume is proportional to the pulmonary blood flow, and the right ventricular (RV) stroke volume is proportional to the systemic blood flow. The pulmonary-to-systemic flow ratio can be calculated as:

$$Qp/Qs = \text{LV stroke volume/RV stroke volume}$$

where LV stroke volume equals LV end-diastolic volume minus end-systolic volume, and RV stroke volume equals RV end-diastolic volume minus end-systolic volume.

For an atrial septal defect or anamolous pulmonary venous return, the right ventricle carries the excess shunt flow. The Qp/Qs can be calculated as:

$$Qp/Qs = \text{RV stroke volume/LV stroke volume}$$

A good correlation ($r = 0.79$) has been noted between the shunt Qp/Qs ratio calculated from stroke volume ratios and oximetry.[4] This approach may be particularly useful in situations where attempts at a good bolus injection were unsuccessful.

Clinical Applications. The radionuclide method is most often used to assess the size of left-to-right shunts in four major congenital lesions: atrial septal defect, ven-

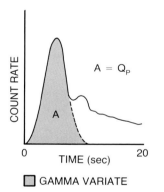
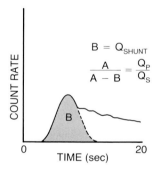

☐ GAMMA VARIATE

Figure 11-3. Calculation of pulmonary-to-systemic flow ratio (Qp/Qs) using pulmonary time–activity curves and the gamma variate model. *A:* Area under the first pass of tracer through the lungs as defined by a gamma variate extrapolation. (Qp, pulmonary flow.) *B:* Area under the portion of the curve corresponding to radiolabeled blood returning prematurely to the lung by the left-to-right shunt. (Q shunt, shunt flow. A − B = Qs = systemic flow.) (Reproduced with permission from Treves ST, et al. Pediatric nuclear medicine. New York: Springer–Verlag, 1985:252.)

tricular septal defect, patent ductus arteriosis, and partial anomalous pulmonary venous return. In each lesion, knowledge of the size of the shunt (Qp/Qs) is an essential component for decisions regarding corrective surgery. In fact, with the anatomic detail provided by echocardiography, the hemodynamic correlates from Doppler exam-

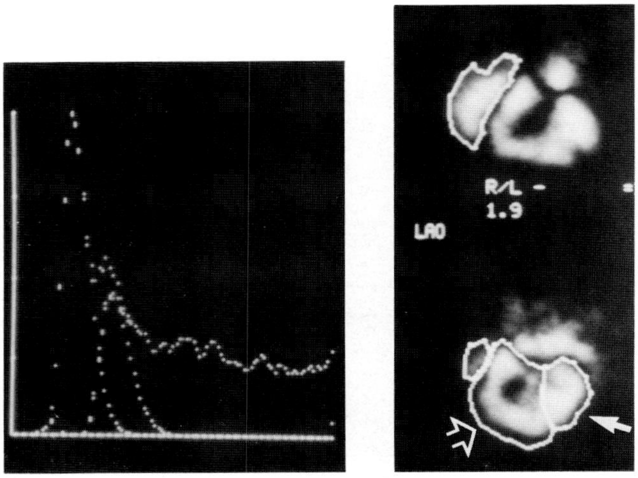

Figure 11-4. *A:* Fitted time-versus-radioactivity curves from a first-pass shunt study with a calculated Qp/Qs of 2.22 in a patient with an atrial septal defect. *B:* Amplitude functional images derived from a gated equilibrium study in the anterior (*upper*) and left anterior oblique (*lower*) projections in the same patient. Notice the increased amplitude of the right ventricle (*open arrow*) compared with the left ventricle (*solid arrow*), indicating a right-sided volume load in the presence of an atrial septal defect. The ratio of right ventricular amplitude-to-left ventricular amplitude is 1.9, similar in magnitude to the measured Qp/Qs from the first-pass study.

ination, and the precise quantitation available from a radionuclide shunt study, it is sometimes possible to proceed directly to surgery without the necessity of preoperative cardiac catheterization. This is particularly true with uncomplicated patent ductus and secundum atrial septal defect. In the situation of anomalous pulmonary venous return, the radionuclide determination of shunt size may be more accurate than that determined at catheterization by oximetric methods because of the inability to obtain a good mixed venous blood sample at catheterization.[5] The radionuclide method has also been used to measure changes in shunt magnitude in response to oxygen therapy to assess the reactivity of the pulmonary vascular bed in patients with large shunts and pulmonary hypertension.[6] This is an important consideration in determining operability in patients with moderate to large ventricular septal defects.

One of the leading indications for radionuclide shunt studies is the postoperative assessment of residual shunt size in patients with murmurs and echo Doppler evidence of persistent shunting after surgical correction of septal defects. Doppler quantification of shunt size is often unreliable after patch closure of defects because of the turbulence generated in the vicinity of the patch. In this situation, the radionuclide technique has been extremely helpful for assessing the need for repeat catheterization and possibly reoperation.

Right-to-Left Shunt Evaluation

Right-to-left shunts can be detected by inspection of the first-pass radionuclide angiogram, which reveals a premature appearance of radioactivity in the left-sided cham-

bers or aorta (Fig. 11-5). Time-versus-radioactivity curves generated from regions of interest over the carotid artery can be analyzed by curve-fitting methods to quantify shunt size.[7] Intravenous injections of an inert radioactive gas, such as ^{133}Xe or Krypton 81m, can also be used for detecting right-to-left shunts.[8] Significant systemic activity of these agents, which should be totally extracted by the lungs and exhaled in the alveolar gas, indicates shunting.

The easiest and most commonly used method is the intravenous injection of ^{99m}Tc-labeled macroaggregated albumin (MAA) particles, similar to those used for the assessment of pulmonary perfusion.[9] In the absence of right-to-left shunting all of the particles are trapped in the lungs. When right-to-left shunting occurs at any level, particles enter the systemic circulation in proportion to the shunt flow, lodging in the capillary and precapillary beds of systemic organs (Fig. 11-6). A series of whole-body images is taken to determine the percentage of right to left shunt as:

$$\frac{\text{Whole-body counts } - \text{ lung counts}}{\text{Whole-body counts}}$$

In spite of the general reluctance to administer particles to patients with known right-to-left shunts, the method has proven to be safe, accurate, and easy to perform.[9] The particle number should be kept below 50,000 in pediatric patients.

Assessment of Ventricular Function

Radionuclide methods are well suited for the assessment of ventricular size and function in congenital heart lesions. Both first-pass and gated equilibrium methods for

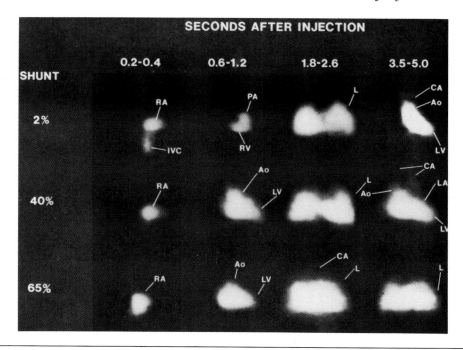

Figure 11-5. Scintigraphic flow studies in right-to-left shunts. The images depict tracer transit through the right side of the heart, lung (L), and the left side of the heart in small children, ages 9 months to 3 years, with a 2% right-to-left shunt through a ventricular septal defect (*top*), a 40% right-to-left shunt with tetralogy of Fallot (*middle*), and a 65% right-to-left shunt related to transposition of the great vessels. (Ao, aorta; CA, carotid artery; IVC, inferior vena cava; LA, left atrium; LV, left ventricle; PA, pulmonary artery; RA, right atrium.) (Reproduced by permission of the American Heart Association, Inc., from Peter C, Armstrong B, Jones R. Radionuclide quantitation of right-to-left shunts in children. Circulation 1981;64:572.)

the determination of ejection fraction have been validated in pediatric patients.[10,11] Quantitative assessment of absolute ventricular volumes and determination of regurgitant fraction have also been reported in children.[12-14] For infants, the imaging is optimized with the use of a converging collimator to improve spatial resolution and increase the sensitivity. It is feasible to measure ejection fraction in tiny premature infants with the use of the pinhole collimator.[15] Ventricular size and function evaluation is useful at rest and with dynamic stress in a variety of congenital lesions, both before and after surgical correction.[16,17] Residual structural and functional abnormalities are common and careful long-term follow-up is important.

Assessment of Myocardial Perfusion

In pediatric patients, perfusion imaging has been most widely used for the noninvasive identification of anomalous left coronary artery.[18,19] Generally, thallium 201 is injected intravenously at rest and images are acquired in multiplanar projections. The usual anatomy in this rather rare disease is for the left main coronary artery to arise

from the main pulmonary artery. This situation can lead to regional ischemia and infarction of the left ventricle due to low perfusion pressure from the pulmonary artery. Thallium scintigraphy typically reveals a segmental perfusion abnormality at rest (Fig. 11-7). This pattern is useful for identifying anomalous left coronary as opposed to myocarditis or cardiomyopathy as the cause of poor ventricular function in infants. The condition is often associated with Q waves on the electrocardiogram. Echocardiography is sometimes able to identify the aberrant origin of the left coronary artery, but catheterization is required for confirmation.

Another clinical condition for which perfusion scintigraphy is becoming increasingly important is Kawasaki disease, or the mucocutaneous lymph node syndrome.[20,21] This syndrome is initially associated with persistent fevers, rash, adenopathy, and mucous membrane abnormalities. Up to 20% of patients with the disorder develop aneurysms of the coronary arteries that may later thrombose and cause myocardial ischemia and infarction. Bypass surgery has been advocated for some patients with objective evidence of ischemia.[22] Perfusion abnormalities have also been induced by stress in adults with a variety of anomalous origins of the left coronary from

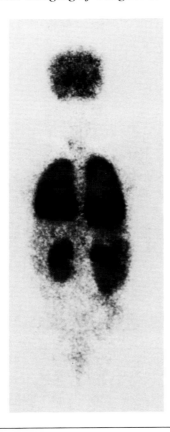

Figure 11-6. Posterior whole-body image. TC-labeled MAA particles were injected intravenously and show localization to lungs, kidneys, and brain, indicating a right-to-left shunt.

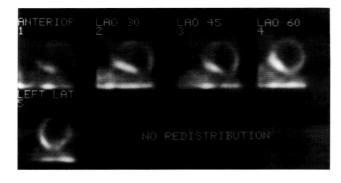

Figure 11-7. Thallium 201 images in the anterior, 30°, 45°, and 60° left anterior oblique and left lateral projections. The heart is dilated, and thallium uptake is heterogeneous with diminished intensity at the lateral wall, consistent with previous infarct to this area.

the right. Evaluation of the resting pattern of ventricular perfusion and function can help differentiate segmental pathology related to large-vessel coronary disease from other causes, including cardiomyopathy, myocarditis, and small-vessel embolization. The pattern of thallium uptake can also suggest right and left ventricular hypertrophy and help diagnose asymmetric septal hypertrophy.

References

1. Maltz OL, Treves S. Quantitative radionuclide angiocardiography. Determination of Qp/Qs in children. Circulation 1973; 47:1049.
2. Kuruc A, Treves S, Parker JA. Accuracy of deconvolution algorithms assessed by simulation studies. J Nucl Med 1983;24:258.
3. Dae M, Botvinick E, Schiller N, et al. Increased accuracy of valvar regurgitation using atrial corrected fourier amplitude ratios. J Noninvas Cardiol 1987;1:155.
4. Rigo P, Chevigne M. Measurement of left to right shunts by gated radionuclide angiography: concise communication. J Nucl Med 1982;23:1070.
5. Baker E, Ellam S, Lorber A, Jones O, Tynan M, Maisey M. Superiority of radionuclide over oximetric measurement of left to right shunts. Br Heart J 1985;53:535.
6. Fujii A, Rabinovitch M, Keane J, et al. Radionuclide angiographic assessment of pulmonary vascular reactivity in patients with left to right shunts and pulmonary hypertension. Am J Cardiol 1982;49:356.
7. Peter C, Armstrong B, Jones R. Radionuclide quantitation of right-to-left shunts in children. Circulation 1981;64:572.
8. Long R, Braunwald E, Morrow A. Intracardiac injection of radioactive krypton. Circulation 1960;21:1126.
9. Sty J, Starshak R, Miller J. Particle body imaging in cardiopulmonary disorders. In: Wagner HN, ed. Pediatric nuclear medicine. New York: Appleton-Century-Crofts, 1983:46.
10. Baker E, Ellam S, Tynan M, Maisey M. First-pass measurement of left ventricular function in infants and children. Eur J Nucl Med 1985;10:422.
11. Baker E, Ellam S, Maisey M, Tynan M. Radionuclide measurement of left ventricular ejection fraction in infants and children. Br Heart J 1984;51:275.
12. Parrish M, Graham T, Born M, et al. Radionuclide ventriculography for assessment of absolute right and left ventricular volumes in children. Circulation 1982;66:811.
13. Parrish M, Graham T, Born M, et al. Radionuclide stroke count ratios for assessment of right and left ventricular volume overload in children. Am J Cardiol 1983;51:261.
14. Hurwitz RA, Treves S, Freed M, Girod D, Caldwell R. Quantitation of aortic and mitral regurgitation in the pediatric population: evaluation by radionuclide angiocardiography. Am J Cardiol 1983;51:252.
15. Hannon D, Gelfand M, Bailey W, Hall J, Kaplan S. Pinhole radionuclide ventriculography in small infants. Am Heart J 1986; 111:316.
16. Reduto L, Berger H, Johnstone D, et al. Radionuclide assessment of right and left ventricular exercise reserve after total correction of tetralogy of Fallot. Am J Cardiol 1980;45:1013.
17. Hurwitz R, Papanicolaou N, Treves S, et al. Radionuclide angiography in evaluation of patients after surgical repair of transposition of the great arteries. Am J Cardiol 1982;49:761.
18. Findley J, Howman-Giles R, Gilday D, et al. Thallium-201 myo-

cardial imaging in anomalous left coronary artery arising from the pulmonary artery: applications before and after medical and surgical treatment. Am J Cardiol 1978;42:675.

19. Moodie D, Cook S, Gill C, et al. Thallium-201 myocardial imaging in young adults with anomalous left coronary artery arising from the pulmonary artery. J Nucl Med 1980;21:1076.

20. Spielmann R, Nienaber C, Hausdorf G, Montz R. Tomographic myocardial perfusion scintigraphy in children with Kawasaki disease. J Nucl Med 1987;28:1839.

21. Nakano J, Saito A, Ueda K, Nojima K. Clinical characteristics of myocardial infarction following Kawasaki disease. J Pediatr 1986; 108:198.

22. Suzuki A, Kamiya T, Ono Y, Takahashi N, Naito Y, Kou Y. Indication of aortocoronary by-pass for coronary arterial obstruction due to Kawasaki disease. Heart and Vessels 1985;1:94.

Chapter 12

Echocardiography in Acquired Heart Disease

Ronald B. Himelman

Since its evolution from M-mode echocardiography to two-dimensional, Doppler, color-flow, exercise, and transesophageal imaging, cardiac ultrasound has become the premier tool for the study of acquired cardiac pathology. This chapter provides a brief and simple overview of this rapidly growing field, including the physical principles of ultrasound; the basic echocardiographic examination; Doppler and hemodynamic evaluation; quantitative echocardiographic planimetry; abnormalities of left ventricular diastolic function; diseases of the coronary arteries, myocardium, pericardium, and valves; cardiac masses; and new developments in echocardiography.

Physical Principles and Instrumentation

Basic Principles

Ultrasound is the term applied to sound having a frequency greater than 20,000 cycles per second. The advantages of high-frequency sound for medical purposes are its abilities to be directed in a straight beam and be reflected by small objects.[1] Sound waves travel in a straight line through homogeneous human soft tissue at a velocity of 1540 meters per second. When an ultrasound beam encounters an interface between media of differing acoustic densities, part of the beam is reflected back toward the source and part is refracted. The more inhomogeneous the object of evaluation, the more acoustic interfaces encountered and the greater the attenuation of the beam. Ultrasound that has a very high frequency can reflect sound from small objects, thus improving resolu-

tion. Because of increased reflection and refraction off of these small objects, however, penetration into a medium decreases with increasing frequency. Thus, a complete sonographic evaluation of a large, inhomogeneous object may require a range of ultrasound frequencies.

Attenuation, or the loss of ultrasound as it travels through an object, is an important physical principle in echocardiography. At the same frequency, an ultrasound beam can travel easily through aqueous substances (such as water, blood, and soft tissue), but poorly through gaseous or solid materials (such as lung or bone, respectively). Thus, in ultrasound examination, the transducer (the source of ultrasound) must be placed in direct contact with the body at sites that avoid penetration through lung, ribs, and sternum. To accomplish this, cardiac views are usually obtained from the suprasternal notch, intercostal spaces at the left parasternal border and cardiac apex, and subcostal area. To promote airless contact between the transducer and the chest, ultrasound jelly is used liberally. Despite these strategies, when patients are very muscular, obese, or emphysematous, transmission of ultrasound may be impaired at all sites.

Properties of the Transducer

The primary component of an ultrasound transducer is the piezoelectric crystal, which rapidly expands and contracts under the influence of an electric current, thus emitting sound waves. The transducer is capable of both sending and receiving ultrasound signals. When a synchronized series of multiple small piezoelectric crystals is used, individual curved waves intersect to form a linear wave front moving away from the source (linear phased array). As this longitudinal wave front propagates, it remains parallel to the direction of propagation for a certain distance and then begins to diverge. The part of the beam close to the transducer is called the near field, whereas the diverging part of the beam is called the far field. In the near field, the beam is parallel and reflecting surfaces are more perpendicular to the transducer; thus, objects are imaged best when located in this part of the beam. The length of the near field can be extended by increasing the radius of the transducer or decreasing the wavelength. Increases in the radius of the transducer are limited by the size of the human intercostal space, however.

The beam can be focused acoustically (by placing a lens on the surface of the transducer) or electronically. When coupled with a system that focuses multiple small piezoelectric crystals in a controlled manner, electronic focusing allows for dynamic focusing of the beam. This system is known as a phased array transducer. When the phased array units are arranged in a circular pattern, the transducer is known as an annular phased array. Advantages of the annular phased array transducer include improved signal-to-noise ratio and greater penetration.

Receiver gain settings also influence beam width. When gain settings are high (often necessary in portable studies or in obese or mechanically ventilated patients), beam widths are larger and the potential for echocardiographic artifacts increases.

The transmitter of the echocardiograph machine controls the transmission of the ultrasound beam in the transducer by timing the duration and rapidity of ultrasound pulses. Reflected echoes return to the transducer, which converts sound waves to electrical impulses that are then directed to the receiver and signal amplifier, processed, and displayed on the oscilloscope.

M-Mode and Two-Dimensional Imaging

Using information on the velocity of sound traveling through a medium and the time for sound to leave the transducer, reflect off an interface, and return to the transducer, the distance from the transducer to the interface can be computed and displayed on the screen. Moving interfaces have changing echographs depending on the variation in the distance to the transducer. M-mode echocardiography provides a one-dimensional or "ice-pick" view of the heart that can be viewed on a screen or recorded on paper. Cardiac motion is displayed as a change in this one-dimensional recording over time (i.e., over the course of the cardiac cycle). Two-dimensional echocardiography involves rapid movement of a one-dimensional ultrasonic beam across the heart to provide real-time cross-sectional images. In current transducers,

the rapid movement of the ultrasound beam is accomplished mechanically or electrically. Since modern two-dimensional echocardiographs use scan converters and digital manipulation of the images, individual ultrasonic lines ("raster lines") are eliminated and the observer does not see the sweeping process occur.

Doppler Echocardiography

Doppler ultrasound is a relatively new addition to echocardiography. It allows for interrogation of the direction, velocity, and intensity or cardiac and extracardiac blood flow. Ultrasound is directed at moving red blood cells, which cause sound to reflect back toward the receiver. When the red blood cells are moving toward the source, the reflected frequency is greater than the transmitted frequency. When the red blood cells are moving away from the source, the reflected frequency is less than the transmitted frequency. The Doppler shift or Doppler frequency equals the difference between the reflected and transmitted frequencies, and is proportional to the product of the velocity of the blood flow and the cosine of the angle between the direction of blood flow and the ultrasound beam. For angles up to 20° the cosine function remains close to unity, so that the most accurate peak blood flow velocities are obtained when the ultrasound beam is directed close to parallel to the direction of blood flow.

Doppler echocardiography has been developed in two modes: continuous-wave and pulsed-wave. Continuous-wave Doppler involves the transmission and reception of a constant ultrasound beam that interrogates all moving targets along the beam. Although this mode is invaluable for the accurate measurement of high velocity flows, it cannot precisely localize the site of the flow along the beam. Continuous-wave Doppler has found wide application in the study of cardiac valvular pathology and the quantitation of stenotic and regurgitant flows. Fortunately, there are only four cardiac valves and these have disparate methods of Doppler interrogation; thus, confusion as to the location of continuous-wave Doppler signals within the heart can be minimized.

Pulsed-wave Doppler was developed as a complementary system to continuous-wave Doppler. Pulsed-wave Doppler mode sends and receives repetitive short bursts of ultrasound and permits precise spatial localization of flows based on the timing of reflected pulsed signals ("range-gating"). Although the pulsed-wave Doppler cursor can be superimposed on an M-mode or two-dimensional image to obtain a flow signal from any area of the heart or vasculature, pulsed Doppler is limited in its ability to measure high-velocity flow by its pulse repetition frequency (PRF, the rate of repetitive emission of bursts of ultrasound). When blood flow under study is

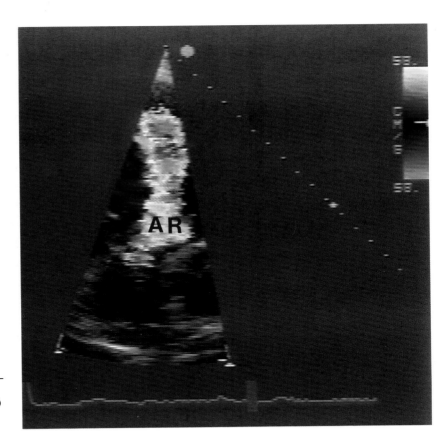

Plate 4. Apical four-chamber view with color Doppler; a turbulent aortic regurgitation jet (AR) originates in the aortic valve and penetrates all the way into the apex of the left ventricle.

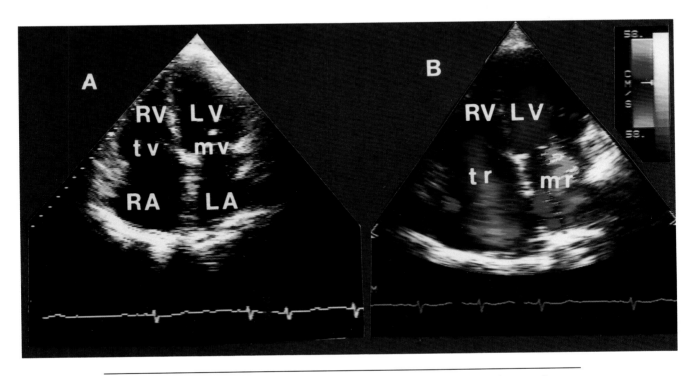

Plate 5. Apical four-chamber view displaying blue color-flow jets of mitral (mr) and tricuspid regurgitation (tr) emanating from the mitral (mv) and tricuspid (tv) valves, respectively. (LA, left atrium; LV, left ventricle; RA, right atrium; RV, right ventricle.)

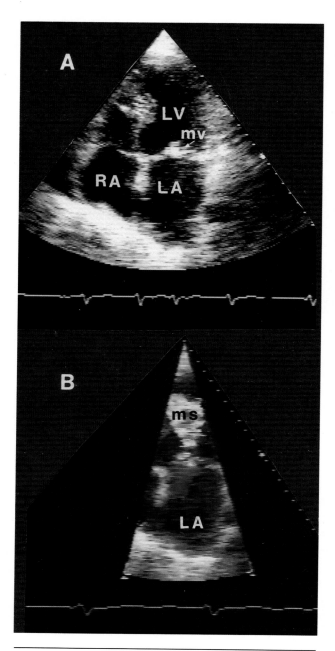

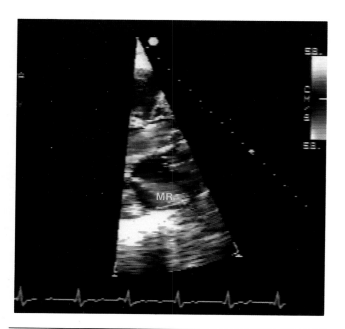

Plate 2. Parasternal long-axis view of the mitral valve and left atrium showing a blue mitral regurgitation jet (MR) that penetrates a relatively small percentage of the left atrium, correlating with mild mitral regurgitation.

Plate 1. *A:* Apical four-chamber view showing mitral valve (mv) thickening and calcification. (LA, left atrium; LV, left ventricle; RA, right atrium.) *B:* Same view with color flow turned on; a turbulent mitral stenotic jet (ms) emanates from the left atrium.

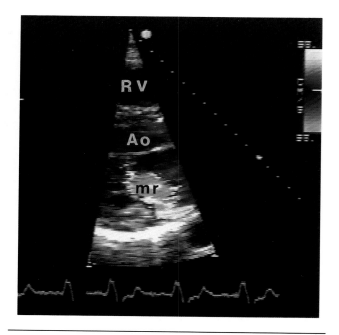

Plate 3. Parasternal long-axis view of moderate mitral regurgitation (mr). The turbulent blue jet occupies a greater area of the left atrium than in the patient in Plate 2, and the convergence of the jet as it forms on the atrial side of the valve is wider. (Ao, aortic valve; RV, right ventricle.)

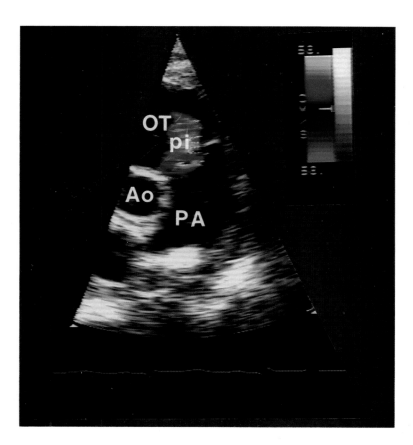

Plate 6. Pulmonary insufficiency (pi) by color-flow Doppler imaging appears in the parasternal short-axis view as a red jet moving retrograde from the pulmonary valve into the right ventricular outflow tract (OT). (Ao, aortic valve; PA, pulmonary artery.)

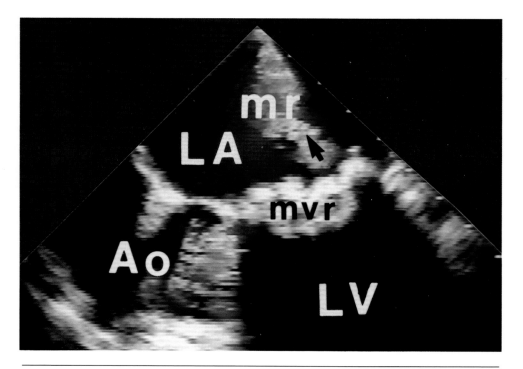

Plate 7. Transesophageal echocardiogram demonstrating paravalvular mitral regurgitation (mr, *arrow*) emanating from the sewing ring of a tilting-disc prosthesis (mvr). (Ao, aortic valve; LA, left atrium; LV, left ventricle.)

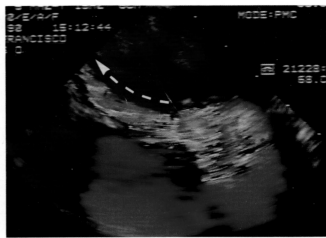

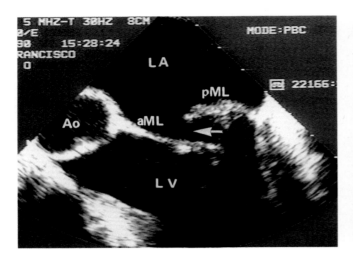

Plate 8. Transesophageal echocardiogram clearly delineates the abnormal coaptation of the mitral leaflets (*left*) and the eccentrically directed mitral regurgitation color-flow jet (*right,* arrow). (Ao, aortic valve; aML, anterior mitral leaflet; LA, left atrium; LV, left ventricle; pML, posterior mitral leaflet.)

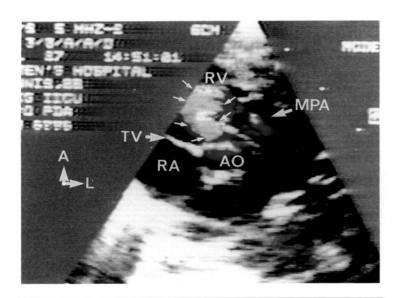

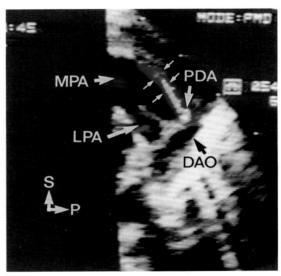

Plate 9. Parasternal short-axis view of a conoventricular septal defect with color flow Doppler. (RV, right ventricle; TV, tricuspid valve; RA, right atrium; MPA, main pulmonary artery; AO, aorta; A, anterior; L, left; *arrows,* left to right shunt.)

Plate 10. Patent ductus arteriosus (PDA) view using color flow Doppler. (MPA, main pulmonary artery; LPA, left pulmonary artery; DAO, descending aorta; S, superior; P, posterior; *arrows,* left to right flow.)

too rapid for a pulsed-wave Doppler system to measure its velocity, the "aliasing" phenomenon occurs, where flows appear to "wrap around" and are inscribed in opposite directions simultaneously. To successfully localize and quantitate all cardiac flows, clinical Doppler echocardiographic studies usually require the combination of continuous and pulsed-wave technology.

Although the original cardiac Doppler investigators worked with audible signals only, graphic displays have recently been developed. Most commercial systems now employ a fast Fourier transform approach of displaying Doppler signals that are measured in velocity units. Flows moving toward the transducer are displayed as positive (above the baseline), whereas flows moving away from the transducer are displayed as negative (below the baseline). Flows moving perpendicular to the transducer are not recorded. In general, using a gray scale, the intensity of a signal is indicative of the volume of flow. Thus low volume flows involving a small number of moving red blood cells reflect less ultrasound, and are inscribed as faint or light gray signals. High-volume flows involving a large number of cells are depicted as dark or black signals.

In general, peak forward flow velocities across normal cardiac valves are less than or equal to about 1.0 m/sec. Flow velocities are slightly higher for aortic and mitral valves than for pulmonary and tricuspid valves. In patients with high cardiac output states, such as those with anemia or fever, or those with valvular sclerosis or regurgitation, peak aortic forward flow velocity may increase up to 2.0 m/sec. Usually, peak aortic forward flow velocities exceeding 2.0 m/sec correlate with some degree of anatomic stenosis. Although pulsed-wave Doppler can be used to interrogate forward cardiac flows in normal valves, continuous-wave Doppler is often necessary to measure peak velocities in stenotic valves.

High-velocity valvular regurgitant flow also requires continuous-wave Doppler for assessment of peak velocity. In healthy subjects, Doppler evidence of trivial or mild tricuspid or pulmonary regurgitation may be present in up to 90% and mitral regurgitation in up to 50% of subjects. These faint regurgitant signals do not imply valvular disease, but may be caused by the retrograde movement of red blood cells during normal valve leaflet closure. The presence of aortic regurgitation is considered abnormal, however, and usually correlates with pathology in the aortic valve or root. In the absence of pulmonary hypertension, peak velocity of tricuspid and pulmonary insufficiency flow is in the range of 2.0 to 2.5 m/sec; however, mitral and aortic regurgitation usually demonstrate peak velocities greater than 4.0 m/sec.

Although Doppler signals are measured in velocity units, the modified Bernoulli formula permits a simple method to convert velocity of flow to pressure gradient. This formula of flow dynamics states that the pressure drop across a stenotic orifice equals the sum of the convective acceleration, flow acceleration, and viscous friction across the stenosis. In the human heart, the latter two terms are negligible, and the formula simplifies to the following:

$$P = 4V^2$$

where P indicates the peak pressure gradient in mm Hg, and V indicates the peak flow velocity by Doppler.

Thus if the peak velocity across a stenotic aortic valve is 4.0 m/sec, then the peak pressure gradient is 64 mm Hg. This noninvasive hemodynamic information is invaluable for the assessment of pressure gradients, valve areas, and pulmonary artery systolic pressure.

Color Flow Doppler Imaging

Color flow Doppler is a recent valuable advance in echocardiography that superimposes a color-coded, real-time display of blood flow velocity and direction on a two-dimensional cardiac image. The color flow map represents an extension of pulsed-wave Doppler technology, in that each pixel in the cardiac image is range-gated to provide selective pulsed-wave Doppler data. Usually about 120 sample volumes of about 0.4 mm each are placed in series along lines within the scan plane. Most systems image 90° of tissue and 30° to 45° of flow within the sector; narrowing the flow sector allows for a higher frame rate. Color sampling is slow because each sample volume of color flow information must be sampled at least 8 times more than each sample of two-dimensional echocardiographic data. The primary colors of red, green, and blue are used singly or in combination to express direction, mean velocity, aliasing, variance, and turbulence of blood flow. According to convention, red is assigned to represent flow toward the transducer and blue to represent flow away from the transducer. In addition, color brightness is proportional to mean velocity up to the Nyquist limit. When velocity is greater than these limits, the aliasing phenomenon occurs and the opposite color is assigned. Another option, the "power mode," displays the power of the Doppler shift, which is proportional to the number of red blood cells moving toward and away from the transducer. Although some systems claim to image "turbulence" in green color, it is controversial whether or not aliasing is depicted instead.

In most patients, the color flow examination of the cardiac chamber for abnormal flow signals can be performed simply by turning the color flow on and off as each of the standard two-dimensional echocardiographic views is imaged (see next section). Since the mean velocity of blood flow is displayed by color Doppler, aliasing of the flow signal occurs with pathologic cardiac flows and conveniently highlights cardiac shunts, valvular stenosis, and regurgitation. The major advantage provided by color flow imaging is the immediate spatial information on cardiac flows; the major disadvantages include loss of temporal resolution and inability to measure high velocities. For accurate resolution of the timing of valve flow relative to valve motion and electrocardiography, color flow can also be overlayed on an M-mode cardiac image. Color flow can also be used in conjunction with spectral Doppler either to align the continuous wave cursor with stenotic or regurgitant jets or to correct for angulation. In adults, color sensitivity is optimal at relatively low frequencies (i.e., 2.5 MHz).

The appearance of color flow is influenced by numerous parameters, including loading conditions, color frame rates, pulse repetition frequency, transducer frequency, gain settings, color map algorithms, and machine electronics.[2] In vitro studies have suggested that color jet areas are proportional to flow rates, and that jet kinetic energies are closely related to driving pressure.[3] In human subjects, reproducibility in the mapping of regurgitant color flow jets is greater for large than for small jets and also greater for aortic than for mitral regurgitant jets; there is a minimum variability of 15%.[4–6]

Color flow Doppler is most useful in the rapid detection and semiquantitation of valvular regurgitation and intracardiac shunts. Although color flow mitral, tricuspid, and pulmonary regurgitation are present in a high proportion of healthy subjects of all ages, aortic regurgitation is considered to be a pathologic finding.[7] Successful grading scales of the severity of valvular regurgitation by color flow Doppler have been developed using the depth of penetration of the jet into the receiving chamber, the area of the jet relative to that of the receiving chamber, and the width of the regurgitant jet at its origin. Although color flow is a semiquantitative technique, it is a major advance in cardiac imaging because it detects pathologic jets anywhere in the heart with great sensitivity and because it reduces the time required to preform comprehensive Doppler examinations.

Performing the Echocardiographic Examination

Positioning the Patient

Before the echocardiographic examination begins, patient height and weight should be recorded, blood pressure should be checked in the supine position, and electrocardiographic leads should be connected. At the University of California, San Francisco, the examination bed is made horizontal and subjects are positioned at 90° left lateral decubitus with the left hand tucked under the head. Technicians seat themselves at the subject's left side. A specially designed wedge-shaped section of the mattress is removed for transducer accessibility and placed behind the patient for support. During the study, the gains are optimized to enhance the endocardial image, chamber sizes are maximized, and respiration suspended at midexpiration before recording ten beats in each view.

Echocardiographic Views

The typical echocardiographic examination involves the placement of the transducer on the chest and abdomen to image the heart in various standard views, including the left parasternal, apical, subcostal, and suprasternal views.

The parasternal view is generally obtained from the second to the fifth intercostal spaces about 3 to 5 cm lateral to the left sternal border. This is the position employed for the standard complete M-mode echocardiographic examination and the first view used for two-dimensional echocardiographic evaluation. The M-mode "sweep" from cardiac base to apex allows for visualization of aortic and mitral valve opening, chamber sizes, and wall thickness.

Unlike M-mode echocardiography, two-dimensional echocardiography permits anatomic imaging from multiple viewing planes; the parasternal long- and short-axis and apical four-chamber views form three orthogonal viewing planes. The parasternal long-axis view is obtained by aligning the transducer with the right shoulder, and is useful for imaging the right ventricular free wall, interventricular septum, left ventricular posterior wall, and mitral and aortic valves (Fig. 12-1). The parasternal short-axis view can be obtained by rotating the transducer 90°, so that it is aligned with the left shoulder. By angling the transducer, cross-sectional short-axis views can be obtained at various levels through the heart from apex to base, and are useful for displaying the size and thickness of the left ventricle, the curvature of the septum, and the anatomy and motion of the mitral and aortic valves (Figs. 12-2A,B). At the level of the base, the aortic valve can be seen surrounded by the left and right atria, right ventricular outflow tract, and pulmonary artery (Fig. 12-3). The apical four-chamber view, obtained by placing the transducer over the point of maximal impulse and angling upward to maximize chamber dimensions, nicely displays the ventricles, atria, and atrioventricular valves (Fig. 12-4). The standard orientation for this view places the apex at the top of the screen and the left ventricle on the right side of the screen. Posterior angulation from this position demonstrates the coronary sinus, whereas anterior angulation reveals the so-called "five-chamber" view, which shows the aortic valve in addition to the other four chambers. A 90° counterclockwise rotation

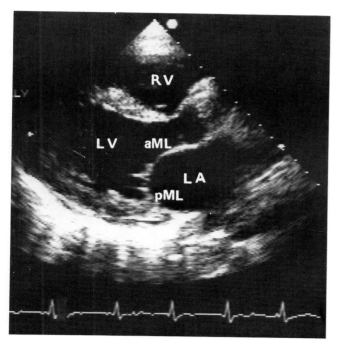

Figure 12-1. Normal parasternal long-axis view. (aML, anterior mitral leaflet; LA, left atrium; LV, left ventricle; pML, posterior mitral leaflet; RV, right ventricle.)

from this position permits imaging of the apical two-chamber view, which demonstrates the left ventricle (anterior and inferior walls) and left atrium (Fig. 12-5). Other cardiac views are obtained from the suprasternal notch, featuring images of the aortic arch and left pulmonary artery, and from the subcostal position, providing views of the heart (Fig. 12-6) as well as the liver, hepatic veins, inferior vena cava (Fig. 12-7), and descending aorta.

Quantitative Echocardiographic Measurement

M-Mode Echocardiography. Quantitative M-mode echocardiographic assessment of cardiac chamber sizes, wall thickness, and valve excursions is widely performed in clinical practice. Off-line analysis of "hard-copy" M-mode printout affords measurement of diameters of the left and right ventricular chambers, septal and posterior left ventricular walls, aortic root, left atrium, and aortic and mitral valve openings. Top normal and mean values for these parameters in healthy subjects are listed in Table 12-1. The so-called "mitral–septal separation," the perpendicular distance between the E point (most anterior deflection of the anterior leaflet of the mitral valve in early diastole) and a tangent drawn to the

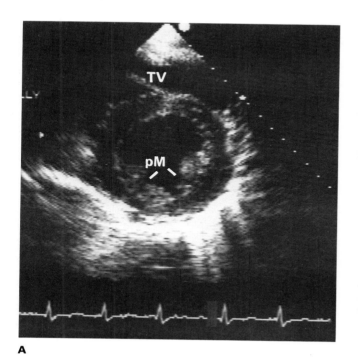

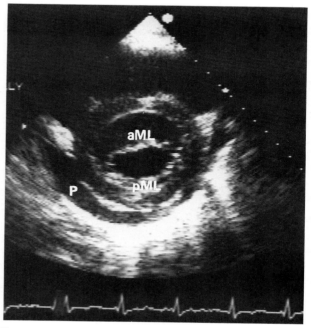

A   **B**

Figure 12-2. *A:* Normal parasternal short-axis view at the level of the papillary muscles. (pM, papillary muscles; TV, tricuspid valve.) *B:* Parasternal short-axis view at the level of the mitral valve. (aML, anterior mitral leaflet; pML, posterior mitral leaflet; P, small pericardial effusion.)

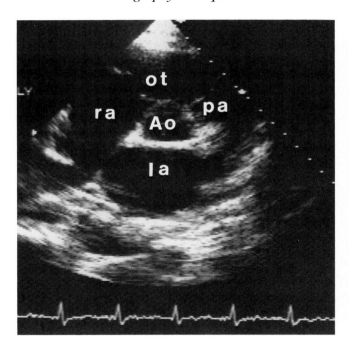

Figure 12-3. Normal parasternal short-axis view at the level of the aortic valve. (Ao, aortic valve; la, left atrium; ot, right ventricular outflow tract; pa, pulmonary artery; ra, right atrium.)

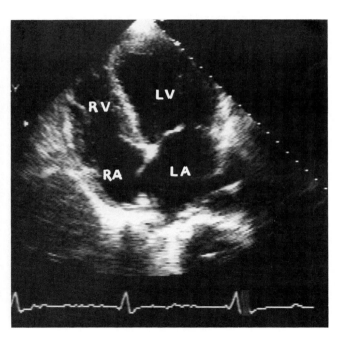

Figure 12-4. Normal apical four-chamber view. (LA, left atrium; LV, left ventricle; RA, right atrium; RV, right ventricle.)

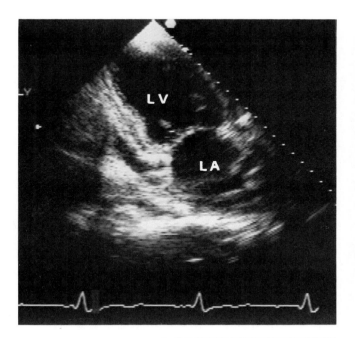

Figure 12-5. Normal apical two-chamber view. (LA, left atrium; LV, left ventricle.)

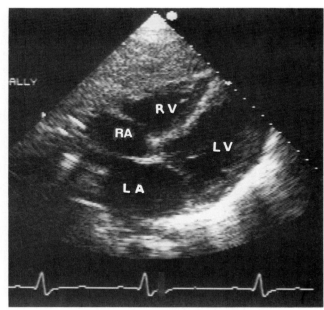

Figure 12-6. Normal subcostal view. (LA, left atrium; LV, left ventricle; RA, right atrium; RV, right ventricle.)

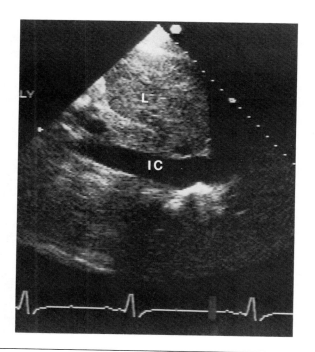

Figure 12-7. Inferior vena cava (IC) in the subcostal view. The liver (L) is at the top of the fan.

Table 12-1

Normal Cardiac Measurements by M-Mode Echocardiography

	Top Normal (cm)	Mean (cm)
Right ventricular dimension	2.6	1.7
Left ventricular dimension	5.7	4.7
Posterior left ventricular wall thickness	1.1	0.9
Ventricular septal wall thickness	1.1	0.9
Left atrial dimension	4.0	2.9
Aortic root dimension	3.7	2.7
Aortic cusp separation	2.6	1.9
Left ventricular shortening fraction	28%–44%	37%

left ventricle moves from its maximum end-diastolic to its minimum end-systolic dimension. End diastole can be marked at the peak of the R wave of the electrocardiogram of the video frame immediately after mitral valve closure; end systole can be marked at the end of the T wave or the video frame immediately before mitral valve opening.

Advantages of M-mode echocardiographic measurements include simplicity, rapidity, reproducibility, and the presence of copious published data on healthy and unhealthy subjects. M-mode quantitation can be performed by the technician or physician after every study, and diagnoses of left or right ventricular enlargement, left ventricular hypertrophy, asymmetric septal hypertrophy, left atrial enlargement, and left ventricular dysfunction can be made. Follow-up studies allow for long-term evaluation of the progression of cardiac disease processes or the effect of therapeutic interventions. For example, regression of left ventricular hypertrophy after the initiation of antihypertensive medication can be observed.

The main disadvantages of M-mode quantitation are blinded interrogation and single-dimension imaging. With the development of guided M-mode (cursor directed by the two-dimensional echocardiographic image), it is now easier to measure the largest diameter or thickness of a cardiac chamber. Even guided M-mode measurements do not reflect the variations in regional cardiac function and size that are demonstrated on a two-dimensional echocardiographic image, however. For example, a patient who has coronary artery disease and an apical aneurysm or a lateral wall motion abnormality might have normal M-mode values for left ventricular diameter and shortening fraction, since these parameters are measured near the cardiac base in an anteroposterior direction.

Two-Dimensional Echocardiography. Two-dimensional images, especially the apical views, have a lot of appeal, since the contracting heart appears similar to a left ventricular cineangiogram. In fact, left ventricular ejection fraction, volumes, and mass determined by two-dimensional echocardiography have been shown to correlate closely with simultaneous cineangiographic techniques, radionuclide methods, and autopsy.[9–16] Although echocardiography underestimates left ventricular volumes determined by angiography (due in part to exclusion of intertrabecular volume), this effect has been minimized with improvements in ultrasonic beam width, tracing methods, transducer position, and scan plane orientation within the ventricle.[15]

Two-dimensional echocardiography has become the procedure of choice to study cardiac morphology in patients with a variety of heart diseases. Although ana-

most posterior point reached by the interventricular septum within the same cycle, is a simple and useful indicator of left ventricular function.[8] In the absence of significant aortic insufficiency, a measured value for mitral–septal separation that exceeds 1.0 cm reliably indicates significant global left ventricular systolic dysfunction, with an ejection fraction below 40%. Another M-mode echocardiographic index of left ventricular systolic function is the shortening fraction of the left ventricular minor axis, which indicates the fractional distance that the tomic imaging provides a more accurate and comprehensive assessment of left ventricular geometry than M-mode, the measurement techniques are newer and less well established. Commercially available light-pen digitizing systems are employed for planimetry.

A truncated ellipsoid formula is used to estimate left ventricular mass.[17,18] This method determines myocardial wall volume by subtracting concentric truncated ellipsoids; volume is then multiplied by the density of myocardium (1.05 g/mL) to yield left ventricular mass. Total left ventricular length is measured in the four-chamber view from the middle of the atrioventricular groove to the apex. For the truncated ellipsoid formula, this length is the sum of the lengths of the semimajor axis of the inner ellipsoid and the truncated semimajor axis of the inner ellipsoid. Left ventricular length is taken as the maximum measured length in either the two- or four-chamber view. Average wall thickness is determined by the geometric subtraction of left ventricular short axis epicardial area and endocardial area at the tips of the papillary muscles. Papillary muscles are excluded from the planimetered left ventricular chamber.

Left ventricular volumes are measured using an application of the biplane Simpson's Rule.[9,19–22] Left ventricular end-diastolic volume, end-systolic volume, stroke volume, and ejection fraction are calculated from the apical two and four chamber views. Left atrial volume at end systole is also measured from these views. End-diastolic volumes are traced at the peak of the R wave of the electrocardiogram, or just after mitral valve closure. End-systolic volumes are traced at the frame preceding mitral valve opening.

The truncated ellipsoid formula for left ventricular mass has been validated in litter-matched dogs after aortic banding and in a healthy population.[17,18] The biplane Simpson's rule method for left ventricular volumes has been shown to be superior to M-mode, single-plane area-length, and biplane area-length methods by correlation with angiography.[11] The Simpson's rule technique for determination of left ventricular and left atrial volumes has also been studied in healthy populations.[19–21]

Quantitative two-dimensional echocardiography can be used to determine whether observed changes in cardiac morphology over time are significant. Angiographic studies of reproducibility of left ventricular volumes have shown a variation of 3% to 15% from beat to beat and a variation of 10% to 37% between sequential ventriculograms.[22–26] Serial radionuclide studies have shown a similar range of variability for ejection fraction, especially in patients with normal hearts.[27–29] Strict adherence to quantitative two-dimensional echocardiographic imaging and tracing techniques can produce measurements of volumes and mass in healthy subjects that are comparable to nuclear and angiographic methods in reproducibility.

Using the interobserver variability and 95% confidence limits for a given laboratory, a significant change in two-dimensional echocardiographic morphology for a given patient can be determined. Previous echocardiographic investigators have demonstrated an interobserver variability of 23% for left ventricular end-diastolic volume, 33% to 62% for end-systolic volume, 12% to 45% for ejection fraction, and 49 g for left ventricular mass.[6,30–32] Gordon and associated found 95% confidence limits of 10% for ejection fraction, 15% for left ventricular end-diastolic volume, and 25% for end-systolic volume.[31] *Group* data showed that mean population changes of 2% for end-diastolic volume and 5% for end-systolic volume would be significant. Computer-assisted endocardial surface identification may improve reproducibility of volume measurements.[33] This is important, since errors due to quantitative planimetry tend to exceed those due to image acquisition, especially in technically suboptimal studies.[32–35] Thus relatively little echocardiographic variability can be attributed to technicians. Ejection fraction, left ventricular mass, and average wall thickness tend to be the most reproducible two-dimensional echocardiographic measurements, whereas volume measurements (left ventricular end-diastolic and end-systolic volume, stroke volume, and left atrial volume) show the most variability.

Abnormalities of Left Ventricular Diastolic Function

Symptoms of congestive heart failure are usually attributed to left ventricular systolic dysfunction. It has become apparent in the last decade, however, that left ventricular diastolic dysfunction may also account for dyspnea on exertion or "flash pulmonary edema." Patients with diabetes, hypertension, aortic stenosis, and other forms of pathologic left ventricular hypertrophy often demonstrate noncompliant left ventricular pressure–volume relationships, such that small increases in left ventricular volume lead to marked increases in left ventricular filling pressure. A notable exception is the physiologic left ventricular hypertrophy acquired by highly trained athletes that has normal compliance characteristics.

Several echocardiographic findings have been found to correlate fairly well with invasively determined criteria for left ventricular diastolic dysfunction, although none are specific for this disorder. M-mode markers include abnormal posterior aortic root motion and mitral valve motion. The motion of the posterior aortic root mirrors changes in left atrial volume.[36,37] In the normal compliant left ventricle, the aortic root moves rapidly posteriorly in early diastole, reflecting vigorous passive filling. In noncompliant hearts, early posterior diastolic motion occurs slowly, but late diastolic motion is more prominent, reflecting dependence of left ventricular filling on atrial kick. Mitral valve motion by M-mode echocardiography shows a similar exaggerated atrial filling wave in patients with stiff ventricles. Other echocardiographic signs of abnormal diastolic function include flattened mitral E–F slope, abnormal diastolic left ventricular posterior wall motion, and enlarged left atrium in sinus rhythm.[35]

Currently, the most commonly used echocardiographic technique for the evaluation of left ventricular diastolic function is the Doppler analysis of mitral inflow.[39–42] The healthy young adult in sinus rhythm has a dominant or large early mitral peak flow velocity (E wave), a smaller late mitral peak flow velocity (A wave), an E:A ratio exceeding unity, and a short E wave deceleration time (Fig. 12-8). In patients with left ventricular diastolic dysfunction, a reversal of this normal pattern occurs, with a small E wave, a large A wave (so-called "A wave dominant mitral inflow pattern"), an E:A ratio less than unity, and a long E wave deceleration time (Fig. 12-9). In patients with hypertension, serial studies have shown that the development of this Doppler pattern occurs early, and may precede echocardiographic evidence of left ventricular hypertrophy.[43]

There are several important limitations in the application of these echocardiographic findings to the diagnosis of left ventricular dysfunction. First, the normal heart shows an increasing tendency to display these findings with age.[44] At 30 years of age, only a small percentage of healthy subjects demonstrate A wave dominant mitral inflow, whereas at 70 years of age, most healthy subjects show this phenomenon. Also Doppler parameters of mitral inflow depend on many other factors, including heart rate, loading conditions, left ventricular contractility, and presence or absence of mitral regurgitation.[45–47] Despite these problems, clinically useful information on left ventricular diastolic function can be provided in young patients in appropriate clinical settings. For example, in a 25-year-old patient with diabetes and hypertension, a prominent A wave dominant mitral inflow pattern and a prolonged deceleration time are suggestive of left ventricular diastolic dysfunction. Although loading conditions may affect the Doppler pattern of filling, simple changes in venous return do not appear to "normalize" an abnormal pattern, nor do they "abnormalize" a normal pattern.[48] Left ventricular filling in patients with diastolic abnormalities depends on atrial kick, so that hemodynamic deterioration might be predicted to occur with loss of atrial synchrony, such as atrial fibrillation or ventricular pacing. Also, patients with noncompliant hearts tolerate large fluid loads poorly. For example, patients undergoing renal transplantation who have A wave dominant mitral inflow patterns are subject to perioperative pulmonary edema.[49]

Coronary Artery Disease

Two-dimensional echocardiography permits real-time assessment of left ventricular wall motion and wall thickening that is useful in the diagnosis of myocardial infarction and ischemia. The area of the wall motion and thickening abnormality correlates with the vascular distribution of the coronary arteries.

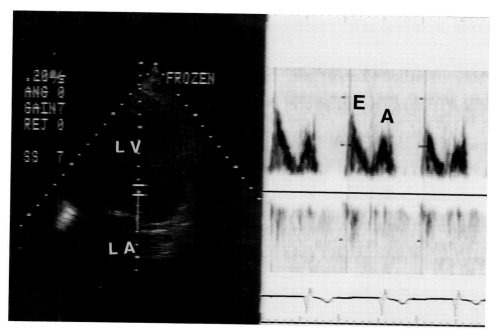

Figure 12-8. Normal mitral inflow pattern by pulsed-wave Doppler, obtained in the apical four-chamber view in the left ventricle just above the mitral leaflets. Sampling site for the Doppler recording is shown on the inset. (A, mitral A wave [active filling or atrial kick]; E, mitral E wave [passive filling].)

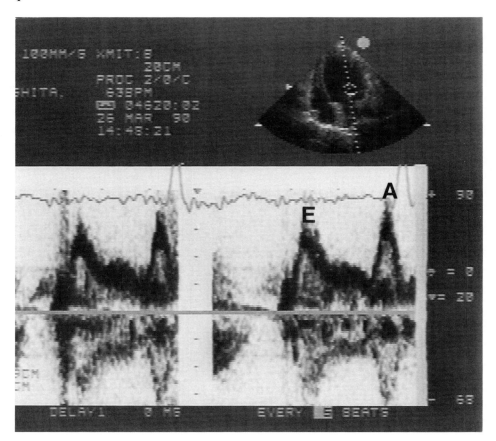

Figure 12-9. A wave dominant mitral inflow pattern, with the size of the A wave exceeding that of the E wave. Site at which Doppler recording was obtained is shown by the cursor on the inset. (A, mitral A wave [active filling or atrial kick]; E, mitral E wave [passive filling].)

Patterns of Wall Motion Asynergy in Myocardial Infarction

Transmural or Q wave myocardial infarctions are usually associated with left ventricular regional wall motion abnormalities, whereas subendocardial or non–Q wave infarctions may not always demonstrate clear, echocardiographic abnormalities.

Transmural anterior myocardial infarctions (due to acute occlusion in the distribution of the left anterior descending coronary artery) appear as a hypokinetic, akinetic, or dyskinetic region wall motion abnormality in the septum, anterior, anteroseptal, anterolateral, or apical walls. Occlusion of the septal perforators generally leads to septal asynergy, whereas occlusion of the diagonal branches leads to anterolateral and lateral wall asynergy. In acute thrombosis of a so-called "wrap-around" left anterior anterior descending coronary artery, dysfunction of the left ventricular apex and distal inferior wall may also occur. The interventricular septum can be imaged in multiple views, including parasternal short- and long-axis, apical four-chamber, and subcostal. The anterior wall of the left ventricle is best displayed in the parasternal short-axis and apical two-chamber views.

Transmural inferior myocardial infarctions (due to acute occlusion of the right or circumflex coronary artery) demonstrate wall motion abnormalities of the inferior or posterior segments. These segments are best imaged in the parasternal short-axis and apical two-chamber views. Lateral wall infarctions seem to be less common on echocardiography than anterior or inferior infarctions, and are secondary to acute occlusion in the distribution of the circumflex or diagonal branch of the left anterior descending coronary arteries. The lateral wall can be demonstrated in the parasternal short-axis and apical two-chamber views.

Diagnostic Efficacy of Echocardiography in Acute Myocardial Infarction

Two-dimensional echocardiography has been used successfully in the emergency room or intensive care unit to aid in the rapid diagnosis of acute myocardial infarction.[50] In selected patients with acute chest pain in whom thrombolytic therapy is being considered, the technique may be helpful in differentiating acute coronary occlusion from pericarditis or pulmonary embolism. In this regard, echocardiography is most useful in detecting and localizing a patient's *first* transmural myocardial infarction. Unless previous wall motion information is available, the diagnostic efficacy of the technique decreases in patients with previous infarctions. In technically excellent echocardiograms, *acute* myocardial infarctions usually demonstrate asynergy with preserved wall thickness and gray-scale intensity, whereas *chronic* infarctions tend to show focal myocardial thinning and high gray-scale intensity, consistent with scar. In the patient with bundle-branch block, paced rhythm, or severe ischemic cardiomyopathy with left ventricular dilation, wall motion analysis for diagnosis and localization of acute or chronic infarction may be difficult.

In distal coronary occlusions, the portions of the left ventricular wall supplied by branches of the proximal vessel are often spared. Thus, the base of the heart can have normal wall motion, whereas the middle or apical portions of the ventricle can demonstrate asynergy. The reverse of this usual trend may be noted after coronary artery bypass grafting, where proximal coronary artery occlusion may occur in the absence of distal vessel occlusion. This type of patient can demonstrate basal left ventricular asynergy with normal apical wall motion.

Complications of Myocardial Infarction

Echocardiography with Doppler has assumed a leading role in the detection or confirmation of complications of myocardial infarction (Table 12-2). If readily available, this noninvasive test can provide invaluable diagnostic information in patients with infarction-associated hypotension, new systolic murmur, or pulmonary edema. For example, in a patient with acute anterior infarction, a prominent decrease in blood pressure might be secondary to hypovolemia, cardiogenic shock, cardiac rupture with tamponade, papillary muscle dysfunction, or right

Table 12-2

Complications of Acute Myocardial Infarction That Can Be Diagnosed or Confirmed by Echocardiography

Right ventricular infarction
Cardiogenic shock
Left ventricular thrombus
Pericardial effusion
Ventricular septal rupture
Papillary muscle dysfunction or rupture
Left ventricular free wall rupture
Infarct expansion
Left ventricular aneurysm
Left ventricular pseudoaneurysm

ventricular infarction. By allowing a complete evaluation of the size and contractility of both ventricles, the presence or absence of pericardial effusion, the respiratory behavior of the inferior vena cava, and the presence and degree of mitral regurgitation, echocardiography usually permits the diagnosis of any of these entities.

Right ventricular infarction complicates approximately one third of inferior myocardial infarctions, and often manifests on echocardiography as right ventricular free-wall asynergy on the parasternal short- and long-axis, apical four-chamber, and subcostal views. However, the presence of a right ventricular free-wall motion abnormality does not correlate with the hemodynamic importance of a right ventricular infarction (i.e., presence of hypotension or jugular venous distention). Two-dimensional echocardiographic findings that are indicative of hemodynamically significant right ventricular infarction include plethora of the inferior vena cava with blunted respiratory response (indicating elevated right atrial pressure), poor descent of the right ventricular base (indicating decreased right ventricular contractile function), and right ventricular enlargement.[51]

In the acute myocardial infarction patient with a new systolic murmur, two-dimensional echocardiography used together with Doppler and an intravenous injection of agitated saline ("bubble study") can differentiate ventricular septal rupture from acute mitral regurgitation. In patients who have the former, the ventricular septal defect can often be directly imaged and shunt flow confirmed by transseptal passage of air bubbles or detection of high-velocity blood flow by continuous-wave Doppler.[52] In patients who have the latter, the cause and severity of mitral regurgitation can be investigated. Mitral regurgitation in this setting is usually due to left ventricular dilation or ischemia or infarction of the wall supporting a papillary muscle. Rarely, rupture of a papillary muscle itself may be detected; this lesion requires urgent surgery.

In the patient who has an acute myocardial infarction complicated by pulmonary edema, echocardiography is useful to assess regional left ventricular function in the infarct and noninfarct zone, global left ventricular function, and the presence or absence of other associated cardiac problems. Severe wall motion abnormalities outside the infarct zone can predict the development of cardiogenic shock and death.[53]

Left ventricular thrombus formation complicates about 30% to 40% of anterior myocardial infarctions and less than 5% of inferior infarctions.[54–56] To decrease the incidence of systemic emboli, most cardiologists recommend anticoagulation for treatment of left ventricular thrombi. Two-dimensional echocardiography is the leading modality for the diagnosis and follow-up of this lesion. Although anticoagulation appears to provide protec-

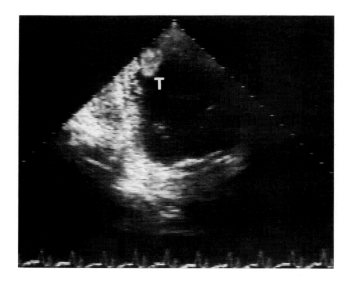

Figure 12-10. Apical two-chamber view showing an apical thrombus (T).

tion against embolic events, resolution of left ventricular thrombi does not always occur on this therapy.[56] Thrombi usually appear as apical structures that have a "gray" texture similar to liver, and must be distinguished from left ventricular trabeculae, false tendons, and chest wall artifacts (Fig. 12-10). To appreciate the full size of an apical thrombus, anterior and posterior angulation of the transducer may be helpful (Fig. 12-11). Echocardiographic features that are associated with a risk for thrombus formation after myocardial infarction include left-ventricular apical aneurysm, spontaneous contrast (indicating slow flow in the ventricle), and reverse or circular diastolic flow in the cardiac apex by pulsed-mode Doppler.[57,58] When thrombi are already present, serial studies have shown that the embolic potential is highest for protruding or freely mobile thrombi.[59] Spontaneous variations in shape and mobility patterns are common in left ventricular thrombi complicating acute anterior myocardial infarction, however.[60]

Pericardial effusion is not uncommon in acute transmural myocardial infarction, and can occur early (peri-infarction pericarditis) or late in the course of recovery (Dressler's syndrome). By demonstrating a small pericardial effusion, echocardiography may help in confirming the cause of pleuritic or atypical chest pain that occurs after infarction. Rarely, acute cardiac rupture associated with cardiac tamponade has been rapidly diagnosed and successfully repaired with the help of echocardiography.[61]

Finally, two-dimensional echocardiographic imaging is helpful in the detection of left ventricular myocardial infarct expansion, aneurysm, and pseudoaneu-

rysm.[62–64] The true aneurysm is characterized by dyskinetic wall motion (usually at the apex), a wide neck, and a low risk of cardiac rupture. In contrast, the pseudoaneurysm has a narrow neck (often located at the inferior wall) and a relatively high risk of rupture.

Color-flow Doppler imaging is also useful in the diagnosis of complications of acute myocardial infarction. In patients who develop new murmurs after myocardial infarction, the technique can readily distinguish interventricular shunting due to septal perforation from mitral regurgitation due to papillary muscle rupture or dysfunction.[65,66] In addition, color flow can highlight the presence of aneurysm, apical thrombus, and pseudoaneurysm.[67,68]

Coronary Artery Imaging

With the development of more sophisticated two-dimensional imaging systems, some progress has been made in directly imaging the coronary arteries from the precordium. Using a 3 MHz transducer and a strobe freeze-frame display, high-grade stenoses of the left main coronary artery have been reliably detected in the parasternal short-axis view.[69] Angiographic atherosclerotic stenoses correlate with the presence of obstructing high-intensity echoes in the wall of the vessel. Likewise, modifications of standard precordial echocardiographic views have been devised that permit the technician to follow the course of the proximal left anterior descending, circumflex, and right coronary arteries.[70] The circumflex coro-

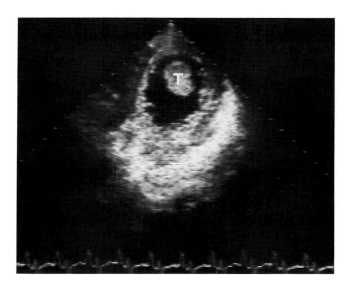

Figure 12-11. Same patient as in Figure 12-10. Angulation of the transducer reveals the full size of the apical thrombus (T).

nary artery is the most difficult to image. Highly echogenic structures in the aortic root (such as a prosthesis or calcified valve) can limit resolution of the coronary ostia.[70] Transesophageal echocardiography can circumvent this problem, howewver, and appears even more promising.

Myocardial Disease

Two-dimensional echocardiography with Doppler plays a valuable role in the diagnosis and morphologic classification of cardiomyopathy. Classically, there are three general forms of cardiomyopathy—hypertrophic, restrictive, and dilated.

Hypertrophic Cardiomyopathy

Hypertrophic cardiomyopathy is an inherited cardiac disorder characterized by myocardial fiber disarray, left ventricular diastolic dysfunction, dynamic left ventricular outflow tract obstruction, and ventricular arrhythmias. Several echocardiographic findings are characteristic. Asymmetric septal hypertrophy is a hallmark feature that is defined as a ratio of septal to posterior wall thickness exceeding 1.3:1, and can be measured on M-mode or two-dimensional studies.[71] Although typical patients with hypertrophic cardiomyopathy manifest septal hypertrophy near the base of the septum, left ventricular hypertrophy may be symmetric and diffuse, localized to the distal septum or the apex, or minimal.[72–74] Also, patients who have hypertension, uremia, coronary artery disease with inferior myocardial infarction, and aortic stenosis may occasionally demonstrate asymmetric hypertrophy.[75–78]

Dynamic left ventricular outflow tract obstruction is another feature that is characteristic but not pathognomonic of hypertrophic cardiomyopathy. Abnormal systolic anterior motion (SAM) of the mitral valve into the left ventricular outflow tract can often be demonstrated (Fig. 12-12), and provides a possible explanation for the cause of the subaortic pressure gradient. When the leaflet actually makes contact with the septum, a significant pressure gradient is likely to be present.[79,80] Like the outflow tract gradient, SAM may be dynamic and intermittent, and may be demonstrated only after premature ventricular contractions, Valsalva maneuver, or amyl nitrite administration. After successful therapeutic interventions, such as beta blocker medication or surgical myectomy, SAM may no longer be provocable. Other conditions that have been reported to display SAM include concentric hypertrophy, high cardiac output states, anemia, hypovolemia, and pericardial effusion.[81–84] Two-dimensional echocardiography can sometimes localize the part of the mitral apparatus that is involved in SAM, that is, mitral leaflet versus chordal structures.

Continous-wave Doppler evaluation of the left ventricular outflow tract allows measurement of the resting gradient. After inhaling amyl nitrite, the patient may develop a significant increase in outflow tract gradient, with a characteristic high-pitched whistling audio signal and a "horse's-tail" spectral configuration. Other echocardiographic signs of hypertrophic cardiomyoapthy include systolic left ventricular cavity obliteration, "crowding," transient midsystolic closure of the aortic valve (Fig. 12-13), and mitral annular calcification. Other Doppler evidence includes the presence of mitral regurgitation and a prominent "A wave dominant" mitral inflow pattern. As noted in an earlier section, the latter finding is suggestive of left ventricular diastolic dysfunction, especially in young patients.

Restrictive Cardiomyopathy

Since restrictive cardiomyopathy is less common and more difficult to diagnose than other types of cardiomyopathy, echocardiographic experience is limited in this disorder. On two-dimensional echocardiography, restrictive hearts may demonstrate small or normal-sized ventricles, normal or thick chamber walls, enlarged atria, and normal or decreased left ventricular contractile function. However, an abnormal echocardiographic appearance may only be evident late in the clinical course of the dis-

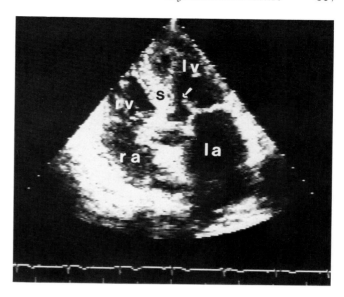

Figure 12-12. Apical four-chamber view showing systolic anterior motion of the mitral valve (*arrow*) toward the septum (s). (la, left atrium; lv, left ventricle; ra, right atrium; rv, right ventricle.)

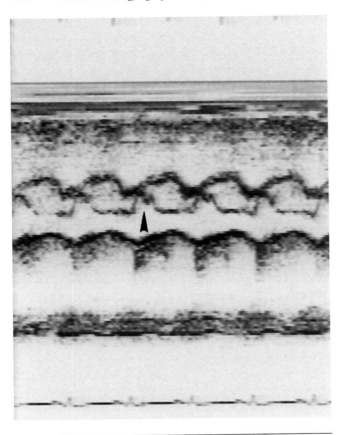

Figure 12-13. M-mode echocardiogram through the aortic valve demonstrating transient midsystolic closure of the aortic valve (*arrow*).

ease. Since the clinical evaluation may not be able to distinguish between restrictive cardiomyopathy and constrictive pericarditis, the pericardium, interventricular septum, and inferior vena cava should be carefully imaged (see section on constrictive pericarditis). In restrictive cardiomyopathy, Doppler evaluation of mitral inflow characteristically shows an elevated early diastolic velocity, a short deceleration time, and a relatively low and abbreviated atrial flow velocity.[85]

Other echocardiographic features of restrictive cardiomyopathy may reflect the cause and site of involvement of the underlying disease process. Patients with amyloidosis may have selective left or right ventricular involvement, thick atrial as well as ventricular walls, a "scintillating appearance" of the myocardium, and small pericardial effusions (Fig. 12-14A). Unlike the case with left ventricular hypertrophy due to hypertension, electrocardiographic R wave voltage displayed on the screen may be notably quite small. Radiation-induced cardiac disease may occur with restrictive cardiomyopathy, constrictive pericarditis, advanced heart block, or left ventricular aneurysms. Endomyocardial fibrosis displays "cement-filled" ventricles due to apical obliteration by fibrosis (Fig. 12-14B), thickening of the posterior leaflet of the mitral valve and surrounding structures, and mitral regurgitation.

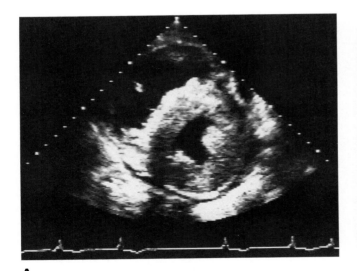

A

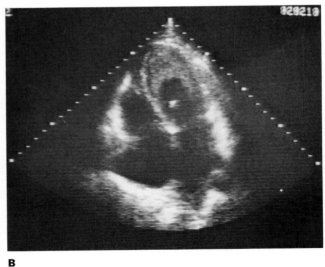

B

Figure 12-14. *A:* Parasternal short axis view of the left ventricle in a patient with amyloidosis showing severe concentric hypertrophy, "scintillating appearance" of the myocardium, and a small posterior pericardial effusion. *B:* Apical four-chamber view in a patient with endomyocardial fibrosis showing "cement-filled" right and left ventricles.

Dilated Cardiomyopathy

Using M-mode echocardiography, patients who have idiopathic dilated cardiomyopathy demonstrate prominent left ventricular and left atrial enlargement (often four-chamber enlargement) with hypokinesis of the left ventricular walls, marked mitral–septal separation, decreased mitral valve opening, and gradual closure of the aortic valve. The degree of left ventricular chamber enlargement is generally out of proportion to the degree of hypertrophy; in fact, wall thickness is usually normal.

Two-dimensional echocardiography allows better appreciation of global left ventricular dysfunction in multiple views. In advanced dilated cardiomyopathy, the shape of the left ventricle changes from elliptical to spherical (Fig. 12-15A,B). The ratio of left ventricular transverse to longitudinal diameter correlates fairly well with ejection fraction. The shape, size, and function of the left ventricle can be followed after therapeutic interventions, such as afterload reduction or cessation of alcohol abuse. The presence of left ventricular thrombus can also be determined. In patients who are undergoing treatment with Adriamycin, echocardiography with quantitative planimetry is a convenient method for the early detection of left ventricular dysfunction. Regional wall motion abnormalities, especially anteroapical and apical, are not uncommon in dilated cardiomyopathy, and do not necessarily indicate that coronary artery disease is the underlying cause.[86]

In patients with dilated cardiomyopathy, Doppler echocardiography usually shows decreased forward flow velocities across all four valves. Therefore, in the event that high-velocity forward aortic valve flow is demonstrated, aortic stenosis should be excluded as the cause of left ventricular dysfunction. Due to dilation of the annuli of the atrioventricular valves, mild or moderate mitral and tricuspid insufficiency are common in dilated cardiomyopathy. In the setting of severe mitral regurgitation, however, left ventricular dilation and dysfunction may be secondary, and consideration should be given to mitral valve replacement or repair. Unlike patients with hypertension associated with concentric left ventricular hypertrophy and A wave dominant mitral inflow patterns, those with dilated cardiomyopathy show E wave dominant mitral inflow patterns. Finally, significant left ventricular dysfunction and dilation should be associated with elevated resting pulmonary artery pressures. The pulmonary artery systolic pressure can be estimated by the peak velocity of the tricuspid insufficiency jet and the respiratory behavior of the inferior vena cava (see section on hemodynamics).

Pericardial Disease

Pericardial Effusion

Echocardiography is the major clinical tool available for the evaluation of pericardial effusions. Although the role of this noninvasive technique in the diagnosis and demonstration of the size of a pericardial effusion has been well established, the determination of the hemodynamic

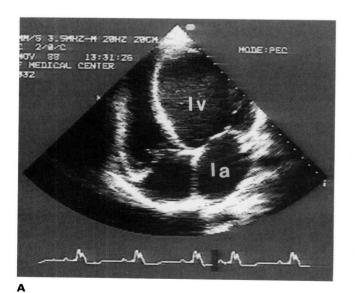

A

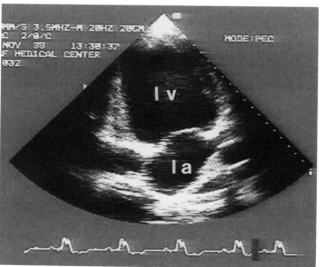

B

Figure 12-15. *A, B:* Apical four- (*left*) and two-chamber (*right*) views in a patient with dilated cardiomyopathy demonstrating the spherical shape of the left ventricle. (la, left atrium; lv, left ventricle.)

significance of an effusion remains difficult. Various M-mode, two-dimensional, and Doppler echocardiographic signs have been studied as early markers of cardiac tamponade.

The pericardium consists of a thick fibrous parietal layer and a thin serosal visceral layer. The superimposition of the epicardium and these normal pericardial layers produces one of the most sonoreflective areas of the heart. When pericardial fluid accumulates in this potential space, a sonolucent space develops.

Feigenbaum and associates first described the sonographic diagnosis of pericardial effusion in 1965 using an A scan.[87] Cardiac ultrasound represented a significant clinical advance, because the operator could distinguish a dilated heart from a large pericardial effusion without resorting to hazardous invasive studies. The diagnostic evaluation of pericardial effusion was further tested and refined with M-mode echocardiography. Horowitz and associates found that in the normal state there is no more than 20 mL of serous fluid in the pericardial sac, and that even this small amount of fluid can cause trivial separation between the layers of the pericardium.[88] For an M-mode echocardiogram to suggest an abnormal fluid accumulation, complete separation of the posterior pericardial layers throughout the cardiac cycle is required.

The differential diagnosis of pericardial effusion by M-mode echocardiography includes pericardial fat, pleural effusion, ascites, and vascular structures.[89] Pericardial fat appears as a sonolucent space that is anterior to the heart in the long-axis parasternal and subcostal views. The best clues to its identification are its absence posteriorly and above the right atrium in the apical four-chamber view, and the presence of low-level echoes within the space. Left pleural effusion can be distinguished from pericardial fluid by the absence of fluid accumulation between the pericardial layers and location anterior to the right ventricle. Likewise, ascitic fluid accumulates in the peritoneal cavity below the diaphragm on the subcostal view. Occasionally other structures, such as the descending thoracic aorta, lower pulmonary veins, and coronary sinus can be confused with pericardial effusions on M-mode echocardiography.

When attempting to distinguish pericardial effusion from other structures, two-dimensional echocardiography can clarify the anatomy, because it permits real-time imaging of the pericardium and cardiac chambers in a variety of tomographic planes. Advantages of this technique included assessment of the geographic distribution of pericardial fluid around the heart and improved imaging of pericardial thickening, pericardial masses, loculations, and cardiac chamber collapse in cardiac tamponade.

Quantification of the Size of a Pericardial Effusion by Echocardiography. Many echocardiographers use the diameter of the pericardial effusion on M-mode echocardiography as an index of effusion size. For example, a small effusion is generally less than 2 mm in diameter, a moderate effusion less than 5 mm, and a large effusion greater than 5 mm. In a study of patients undergoing cardiac surgery, Horowitz and associates compared the volume of pericardial fluid recovered intraoperatively with the preoperative M-mode echocardiogram.[88] These investigators estimated the size of the effusions by subtracting the volume of the heart (estimated as the cube of the epicardial radius by M-mode echocardiography) from the total volume (heart plus pericardial effusion) within the pericardial sac. Although this method generally works well for small or moderately sized pericardial effusions, in large effusions the distribution of fluid is often predominantly apical, so that the calculations may underestimate effusion size.[90]

A simple two-dimensional echocardiographic approach can be employed in the estimation of the volume of a pericardial effusion.[91] A small effusion (generally less than 100 mL in volume) appears as a sonolucent anterior and posterior space that does not circumvent the ventricles. A moderately-sized effusion (approximately 100 to 500 mL in volume) demonstrates circumventricular pericardial fluid that does not permit contact between the visceral and parietal pericardial layers in any view. A large effusion (greater than 500 mL in volume) generally extends beyond the viewing screen, preventing the visualization of both the visceral and parietal pericardial layers in certain views. Large effusions may also be associated with swinging of the heart.

Evaluation of the Hemodynamic Significance of a Pericardial Effusion

M-Mode Echocardiography. Early markers of tamponade proposed by investigators in M-mode echocardiography have included reciprocal respiratory variation in right and left ventricular size, inspiratory reductions in mitral D–E excursion and E–F slope, systolic notching of the right ventricular wall, and right ventricular expiratory end-diastolic compression.[92–96] None of these echocardiographic signs has proven to be optimally sensitive or specific in the diagnosis of cardiac tamponade.

Two-Dimensional Echocardiography. With the advent of two-dimensional echocardiography, dynamic collapse or inversion of the right atrial and right ventricular free walls has become the favored signpost of tamponade (Table 12-3).[97–105] Right atrial collapse is defined by two-dimensional echocardiography as dynamic inversion of the anterosuperior right atrial free wall that occurs during late diastole or early systole and varies with respiration (Fig. 12-16). Right ventricular collapse is defined as early diastolic inversion of the right ventricular free wall that varies with respiration (Fig. 12-17).

In experimental studies where graded acute cardiac

Table 12-3

Sensitivity and Specificity of Two-Dimensional Echocardiographic Signs for Cardiac Tamponade and Pericardial Constriction

	Sensitivity (%)	Specificity (%)
Cardiac Tamponade		
Inferior vena cava plethora	97	40
Right atrial collapse	55	68
Right ventricular collapse	48	84
Pericardial Constriction		
Inferior vena cava plethora	79	80
Pericardial adhesion	79	90
Early diastolic septal bounce	62	93

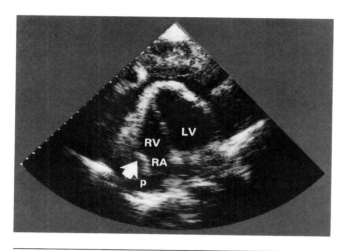

Figure 12-16. Apical four-chamber view in a patient with a large pericardial effusion, showing systolic right atrial collapse (*arrow*). (LV, left ventricle; p, pericardial effusion; RA, right atrium; RV, right ventricle.)

hemodynamic significance of pericardial effusion or constriction. Plethora of the inferior vena cava is defined as a decrease in proximal vena caval diameter by less than 50% after deep inspiration. Using the trailing-edge to leading-edge technique, maximum inferior vena cava diameters before inspiration and minimum diameters after inspiration are measured in the subcostal view within the first 2 cm of the entrance to the right atrium. The vena cava is differentiated from the descending aorta in the subcostal view by its right-sided location and lack of systolic pulsations.

The "caval respiratory index" is defined as the percentage decrease in inferior vena cava diameter after inspiration or sniff. This index has been previously correlated with catheter measurement of central venous pressure. In a study of 175 patients, Moreno and coworkers first reported that this index correlated well with right atrial pressure ($r = 0.71$), but that the absolute diameter of the inferior cava did not correlate well.[106] In critically ill patients, there is a similar correlation ($r = 0.73$).[107] For a caval respiratory index less than 50%, the predictive value for a right atrial pressure greater than or equal to 10 mm Hg is 87%. For an index greater than or equal to 50%, the predictive value for a right atrial pressure less than 10 mm Hg is 82%.

A retrospective study of 115 patients with moderate or large pericardial effusions, demonstrated that plethora is often the first two-dimensional echocardiographic sign to appear during the course of tamponade and the last to resolve after pericardial drainage.[91] Compared with patients who had responsive vena cavae, those with plethora have higher heart rates, lower systolic blood pressures, larger pericardial effusions, and more severe hemodynamic abnormalities. As an echocardiographic marker of cardiac tamponade, plethora is far more sen-

tamponade is induced by saline infusion through a pericardial catheter, these signs correlate with hemodynamically significant effusions.[101,102] Since the right atrium is a thinner and more compliant structure than the right ventricle, collapse of the former structure generally occurs earlier than the latter structure in the course of cardiac tamponade. In most clinical studies, however, both right atrial and right ventricular collapse have been found to indicate "incipient" tamponade, that may precede hemodynamic evidence of tamponade.[97,98,104,105]

Plethora of the Inferior Vena Cava. Subcostal imaging of the inferior vena cava during passive and deep respiration should be a routine part of the echocardiographic examination, especially in patients with pericardial disease. The respiratory behavior of this structure is useful in the estimation of right atrial pressure and the

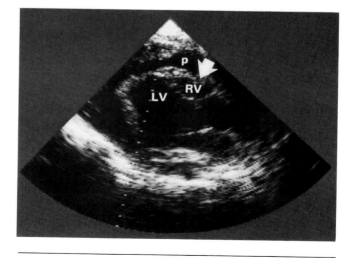

Figure 12-17. Parasternal long-axis view in the same patient as in Figure 12-16, indicating early diastolic right ventricular collapse (*arrow*). Abbreviations as in Figure 12-16.

sitive, but less specific than right-sided chamber collapse (see Table 12-3).

Other conditions associated with plethora of the inferior vena cava include right ventricular failure (secondary to left ventricular dysfunction, right ventricular myocardial infarction, pulmonary hypertension, or tricuspid insufficiency) and inability to inspire deeply because of decreased mentation, respiratory muscle weakness, severe breathlessness, or pleuritic chest pain. The latter problem can occasionally be alleviated by having patients "sniff" while imaging the inferior vena cava. In cooperative patients a hand-held manometer can be used to measure the force of graded sustained inspirations.[110] Positive-pressure ventilation also causes dilation of the inferior vena cava; certain stable patients who are mechanically ventilated may be transiently removed from the ventilator (generally for less than 30 seconds) to allow vena cava imaging during spontaneous breathing.

Since plethora is a nonspecific marker of elevated central venous pressure, this sign should be identified in an appropriate clinical setting (i.e., presence of moderate or large pericardial effusion without right ventricular failure). The caval respiratory index may be *most useful to exclude cardiac tamponade,* however, since the absence of this sensitive echocardiographic sign effectively rules out a hemodynamically significant effusion that requires immediate pericardial drainage.

Doppler Echocardiography. Other useful signs of cardiac tamponade by spectral or color Doppler echocardiography include exaggerated respiratory variation in transvalvular flow velocities and isovolumic relaxation time, and abolished or reversed blood flow in the hepatic veins and vena cavae during the first expiratory cardiac cycle.[109–113] For example, in healthy subjects or patients who have pericardial effusions without tamponade, mitral time velocity integrals and peak early diastolic velocities (E wave) vary by no more than 10% over the respiratory cycle. In patients who have cardiac tamponade, however, these parameters are significantly lower and show decreases of more than 30% during inspiration. Early diastolic velocities tend to vary more than late diastolic velocities (A waves) throughout the respiratory cycle.

The accurate measurement of Doppler indices requires that a respiratory monitor be displayed on the echocardiography screen. In patients with cardiac tamponade, the mechanism of change in these indices appears related to respiratory variation in cardiac preload.[114] False-positive results can also occur in other conditions associated with pulsus paradoxus, including acute pulmonary embolism, obstructive pulmonary disease, acute left ventricular volume overload, right ventricular infarction, and constrictive or effusive–constrictive pericardial disease.[115] In the presence of tachycardia

or arrhythmias, Doppler signals may be technically difficult to record. Furthermore, the operator must ensure that the ultrasound beam does not translocate during inspiration, causing a shift in the site or angle of interrogation. Continuous-wave Doppler is preferred over pulsed-wave Doppler to help avoid this problem.

Echocardiography is also helpful in assessing the hemodynamic significance of pericardial effusions in patients with atypical presentations of cardiac tamponade, such as low-pressure tamponade, loculated effusion, effusive–constrictive disease, elevated diastolic filling pressures, and postcardiac surgery. These patients may not demonstrate typical clinical features of cardiac tamponade and can present diagnostic problems.

Low-Pressure Cardiac Tamponade. Clinical, hemodynamic, and echocardiographic evidence of cardiac tamponade has been reported in patients with right atrial pressures that are less than 10 mm Hg, often in the setting of dehydration or trauma.[116–120] Thus, jugular venous distention or pulsus paradoxus may be absent in the presence of a large pericardial effusion that causes equalization of diastolic filling pressures. On two-dimensional echocardiography these patients may manifest right heart collapse in the absence of plethora of the inferior vena cava.[119] Although in one preliminary report 30% of patients with right atrial collapse had right atrial pressures less than 12 mm Hg, low-pressure tamponade is probably much more unusual.[120]

Loculated Pericardial Effusion. Loculations are commonly noted after pericardiotomy or purulent pericarditis.[121] In animal models, the combination of mild serosal injury and spilled blood consistently lead to the formation of extensive postoperative pericardial adhesions within days to weeks.[122] Loculations cause compartmentation of pericardial fluid, which may allow for selective compression of cardiac chambers. Loculations may also have a "tethering effect" between the pericardial layers, such that chamber inversion may be less likely to occur in the setting of cardiac tamponade. In a series of dog studies, Fowler and Gabel surgically constructed pockets of pericardium overlying the atria and ventricles such that fluid could be introduced into each pocket selectively.[123–125] They found that the hemodynamics of tamponade could be produced by localized compression of either the atria or the ventricles, with compression of the atria and the right side of the heart showing the most prominent effects. In agreement with these experimental observations, two-dimensional echocardiography in humans has shown that when a significant amount of loculated pericardial fluid abuts any one of the four cardiac chambers, chamber collapse and clinical evidence of tamponade may be present.

Effusive–Constrictive Pericardial Disease. A transient constrictive phase is not uncommon in the resolution period of effusive pericarditis.[126] As the pericardial effusion resolves, the thickened inflamed pericardium may compress the heart and cause constrictive physiology. Depending on the phase of illness, patients may manifest clinical features of either pericardial constriction or cardiac tamponade. Echocardiography may be helpful in the evaluation of this condition. Echocardiographic features of effusive–constrictive disease include pericardial thickening with a small to moderate pericardial effusion (often loculated), early diastolic septal bounce, adhesion of the pericardial layers, and plethora of the inferior vena cava.[127] Since all features of constriction usually resolve with anti-inflammatory medication alone, pericardiectomy is rarely required.

Conditions Associated with Elevated Right Heart Filling Pressures. In patients who have chronically elevated right heart intracavitary pressures and thus decreased wall compliance, the right atrium and ventricle may be relatively resistant to collapse in the setting of cardiac tamponade. Lack of right heart chamber collapse and pulsus paradoxus has been described during tamponade of hearts with right or left ventricular hypertrophy, pulmonary hypertension, atrial septal defect, or severe valvular disease.[91,96,98,100,128] In severe pulmonary hypertension, left ventricular diastolic collapse in the setting of a nonloculated pericardial effusion has been described as the only echocardiographic marker of cardiac tamponade.[129]

Therapy Guided by Echocardiography. Two-dimensional echocardiography may also be useful before pericardial drainage to localize the fluid and determine the approach most likely to achieve safe drainage (i.e., subcostal or parasternal pericardiocentesis versus open pericardiotomy). During the procedure iteself, echocardiography may be used to confirm the location of the catheter within the pericardial space, determine if and when cardiac chamber collapse resolves, and assess the size of the remaining effusion. When the pericardiocentesis needle approaches the parietal pericardium, a "dimpling" phenomenon is observed on the echocardiographic image. With puncture of the parietal pericardium, this dimpling disappears. Correct placement of the catheter can be confirmed echocardiographically either by visualization of the catheter tip or by injection of 1 mL of agitated saline into the pericardial effusion. Echocardiographically guided pericardiocentesis has been found to be a safe and reliable technique.[130] After drainage has been performed, follow-up imaging on a daily basis is useful to detect early reaccumulation of fluid. The persistence or recurrence of plethora after pericardiocentesis suggests pericardial constriction, effusive–constrictive disease, or a hemodynamically significant residual effusion.

Pericardial Constriction

The diagnosis of constrictive pericarditis and its differentiation from restrictive cardiomyopathy can pose a difficult clinical problem.[131,132] Since clinical signs of constriction are often subtle and pericardial calcification on chest radiography is now rare, echocardiography has become the preeminent noninvasive diagnostic tool. Similar to the situation with cardiac tamponade, M-mode echocardiographic signs of pericardial constriction, such as premature opening of the pulmonary valve, abnormal diastolic flattening of the left ventricular posterior wall, and abnormal diastolic ventricular or atrial septal motion, have not proven to be optimally sensitive or specific.[133–138] For example, rapid early diastolic filling of the ventricles, which is a physiologic hallmark of constriction, may cause premature opening of the pulmonic valve and abnormalities in left ventricular posterior wall and posterior aortic root motion. Other conditions with rapid early diastolic ventricular filling, such as severe valvular regurgitation, may also demonstrate these findings on the echocardiogram, however. Furthermore, several investigators contend that no single M-mode echocardiographic abnormality is specific for constrictive pericarditis.[139,140]

Two-dimensional echocardiography appears to improve the diagnostic efficacy for constriction.[127,141] Early diastolic septal bounce, plethora of the inferior vena cava with blunted respiratory response, and pericardial adhesion with lack of sliding of the visceral over the parietal pericardium are useful two-dimensional echocardiographic features in the diagnosis of pericardial constriction.[127] Early diastolic septal bounce is defined as the presence of a rapid early diastolic septal motion abnormality. The bounce occurs just after mitral valve opening on the echocardiogram or just after the end of the T wave on the electrocardiogram. Although the bounce is best illustrated in real time, on frame-by-frame video analysis it appears as a to-and-fro motion of the interventricular septum caused by transient rapid reversal of transseptal pressure gradients.[135–137] Inferior vena cava plethora reflects elevated right atrial pressures, and can be viewed as the echocardiographic analog of the Kussmaul's sign. Pericardial adhesion is defined as a lack of the normal sliding motion of the visceral over the parietal pericardium in any view or location in the pericardial layers. This sign manifests as thickened, parallel, adherent pericardial layers that pull together during systole and probably denotes chronic pericardial inflammation, loculation, and fibrosis.

Of these three two-dimensional echocardiographic signs of pericardial constriction, pericardial adhesion and plethora of the inferior vena cava are the most sensitive, whereas early diastolic septal bounce is the most specific (see Table 12-3). The presence of *either* pericardial adhesion or vena cava plethora increases sensitivity at the expense of specificity, whereas the presence of *both* of these echocardiographic signs improves specificity at the expense of sensitivity. Interobserver reproducibility is highest for early diastolic septal bounce and lowest for pericardial adhesion. After pericardiectomy or medical therapy that lead to resolution of clinical evidence of pericardial constriction, these two-dimensional echocardiographic signs of constriction usually resolve.

For these two-dimensional echocardiographic signs of constriction, false positives are often explained by other abnormalities of septal motion (left bundle-branch block or right ventricular pacing), other causes of elevated right heart filling pressures (right heart failure), and pericardial adhesion localized to the anterior chest (anterior pericardiotomy or radiation therapy). False negatives are usually due to technical problems with imaging.

Valvular Heart Disease

For more than 20 years, echocardiography has been successfully applied to the evaluation of valvular heart disease. This technique has been widely employed to determine the location of murmurs detected on auscultation, the cause of valve disease, and the severity of valvular stenosis or regurgitation. Each advance in echocardiography, including M-mode and two-dimensional imaging, Doppler, color-flow, and transesophageal echocardiography, has provided useful insights into the pathology and hemodynamic significance of valve lesions (Table 12-4). Echocardiographic imaging provides an anatomic evaluation of the appearance and motion of the cardiac valves and the enlargement or hypertrophy of affected cardiac chambers. Doppler contributes hemodynamic information on cardiac blood flow, including pressure gradients, flow directions, and flow volumes. Color-flow Doppler imaging immediately detects pathologic jets anywhere in the heart and reduces the time required to map the direction and extent of regurgitant flows. In stenotic valve lesions, the size of the orifice can often be measured fairly accurately by M-mode or two-dimensional imaging. In regurgitant lesions, however, the determination of hemodynamic significance is more dependent on Doppler and color flow echocardiography. The application of all of these echocardiographic techniques in combination has replaced cardiac catheterization as the most useful diagnostic test in valvular heart disease.

Table 12-4

Evaluation of the Hemodynamic Significance of Valve Lesions by Echocardiography and Doppler

M-Mode and Two-Dimensional Imaging

Valve appearance—thickness, calcification, bicuspid, vegetation, redundancy
Valve motion—opening and closing characteristics, fluttering, abnormal leaflet coaptation, prolapse, doming, mitral E to F slope
Effect of valve lesion on adjacent valve or chamber motion—early closure of mitral or aortic valve, increased atrial or septal motion
Hypertrophy or enlargement of affected chambers—ventricular or atrial enlargement, left or right ventricular hypertrophy, poststenotic dilation of the aorta or pulmonary artery
Direct measurement of stenotic orifice area

Spectral Doppler

Characteristics of pathologic jet—peak velocity, acceleration, area and penetration of regurgitant signal, signal intensity, "V-wave cutoff" sign
Peak velocity of inflow signal (regurgitant lesions)
Presence or absence of pulmonary hypertension
Calculation of stenotic valve area—continuity equation, modified Gorlin equation, pressure half-time

Color Flow Doppler Imaging

Depth, width, and area of regurgitant jet
Width of stenotic jet

Mitral Stenosis

M-mode echocardiography first established the value of cardiac ultrasound in the investigation of mitral valve motion.[142] The normal anterior mitral valve M-mode echogram shows a bifid, or "M shape," with an initial opening to the E point and a rapid initial diastolic closure (steep E-to-F slope) (Fig. 12-18). Normal posterior mitral leaflet motion mirrors the anterior leaflet, and thus moves posteriorly during mitral valve opening. In contrast, stenotic mitral valves show characteristic M-mode patterns, with slow initial closure (diminished E-to-F slope), anterior motion of the posterior leaflet during diastole (due to fusion of the commissures), limited leaflet separation, and leaflet thickening (Fig. 12-19).

Two-dimensional echocardiography improves the ability to recognize distinctive pathologic mitral valve patterns, localize lesions to specific valves or leaflets, assess secondary cardiac hypertrophy or dilation, and directly measure valve areas. The major cause of mitral stenosis in the United States is still rheumatic heart disease. Mitral stenosis may occur alone or in association with aortic and tricuspid valve disease. Rheumatic mitral stenosis demonstrates limited leaflet motion with a "bent-knee" sign of the anterior mitral valve leaflet (see Fig. 12-19), "doming" of the mitral valve, and chordal foreshortening and

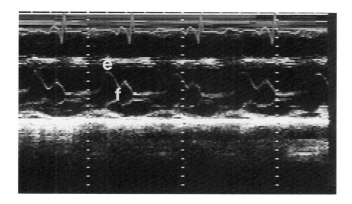

Figure 12-18. Normal M-mode echocardiogram of the mitral valve. e and f on the anterior mitral leaflet tracing indicate the mitral E-to-F slope.

thickening (Fig. 12-20). The valve leaflets are most thickened and immobile at the leaflet tips, and least mobile at the leaflet bodies. Extensive calcification of the valvular and subvalvular apparatus may be present (Fig. 12-21); these findings have been associated with a poor response to surgical commissurotomy or percutaneous balloon valvuloplasty. Other less common causes of obstruction to mitral inflow include congenital malformations, mitral annular calcification, endocarditis, and left atrial myxoma.

Two-dimensional echocardiography permits a reliable and reproducible direct measurement of the stenotic mitral valve orifice area.[143,144] In fact, the measurement of mitral valve orifice area by this technique may be more accurate than cardiac catheterization in patients in whom concomitant valvular regurgitation alters measurements of forward cardiac output.[145,146] The best image of the mitral valve orifice can be obtained in a parasternal short-axis view. Completing a slow sweep from the level of the aorta and left atrium to the ventricle at the papillary muscles allows the true mitral valve orifice to be located at the commissural tips of the mitral valve leaflets. Receiver gain settings must be set appropriately; low gain settings lead to image dropout and high gain settings lead to image saturation and a false impression of a narrowed orifice.[144] The area of this orifice can be planimetered in early diastole on-line or off-line with the use of video analysis systems.

The normal Doppler mitral inflow pattern has two peaks, the first indicating passive early diastolic filling (E wave) and the second signifying active filling (A wave or "atrial kick"). The normal peak mitral inflow velocity is less than 1.3 m/sec. In mitral stenosis, the peak rate of inflow is generally elevated to 1.5 to 3.0 m/sec; using the modified Bernoulli formula this velocity correlates with a peak pressure gradient of 9 to 36 mm Hg. Also, the rate

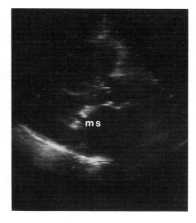

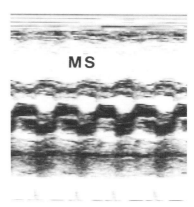

Figure 12-19. Two-dimensional and M-mode echocardiography in a patient with severe rheumatic mitral stenosis. Findings include diminished E-to-F slope, anterior motion of the posterior leaflet during diastole, limited leaflet separation, and leaflet thickening.

of left ventricular filling is reduced in mitral stenosis, so that the downslope of the E wave is reduced. Unlike the E to F slope of M-mode echocardiography, the downslope of the mitral inflow E wave by Doppler correlates with the mitral valve area.[147] Quantitation of the Doppler pattern has been accomplished with the "pressure half-time," that is, the time (in milliseconds) needed for the initial diastolic gradient to decrease by one half. The corresponding mitral flow velocity at the pressure half-time can be expressed as

$$V_{1/2} = V_{max} \times 1.414$$

A normal pressure half-time is less than 60 msec. As mitral stenosis becomes more severe, the E wave deceleration becomes flatter and the pressure half-time longer. Empirically, a pressure half-time of 220 msec has been found to correlate with a mitral valve area of 1.0 cm^2; therefore mitral valve area can be estimated as 220 divided by the pressure half-time.[148,149] In addition to mitral valve area, the pressure half-time is influenced by

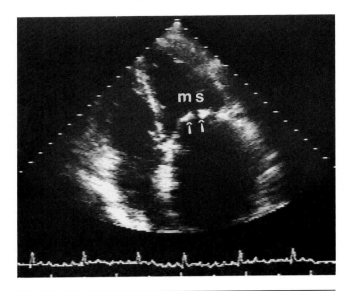

Figure 12-20. Apical four-chamber view in the same patient as in Figure 12-19 showing "doming" of the mitral valve in diastole (*arrows*), thickening of the mitral valve leaflets, and severe left atrial enlargement. (ms, mitral stenosis.)

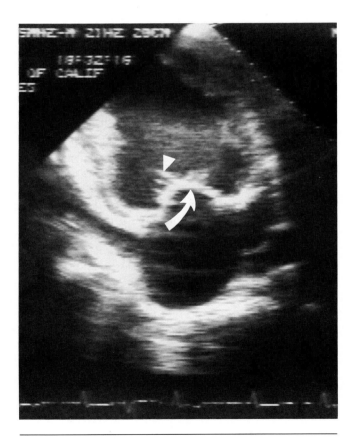

Figure 12-21. Apical two-chamber view in another patient with rheumatic mitral stenosis, demonstrating extensive calcification and thickening of the valvular (*curved arrow*) and subvalvular (*arrowhead*) apparatus.

flow, left atrial pressure, and compliance of left heart chambers. Erroneous results can be obtained in patients with atrial tachycardia or atrial fibrillation with rapid ventricular responses or varying cycle lengths, curvilinear decay patterns, and first-degree block.[150] In addition, in the presence of significant aortic regurgitation or cardiomyopathy, use of the pressure half-time method may lead to underestimation of the severity of mitral stenosis, because of marked increases in early diastolic left ventricular pressure and subsequent rapid fall in Doppler velocity.[151] Color-flow Doppler imaging has also found application in the detection of mitral stenosis (Plate 1); preliminary reports suggest that the width of the color flow mitral inflow jet may correlate with mitral valve area.[152–154]

Overall, the best determination of the severity of mitral stenosis should not depend on the results of any one measurement. Data on the M-mode appearance of the mitral valve apparatus and left atrium, two-dimensional echocardiographic planimetry of the mitral orifice area, and Doppler pressure half-time and peak mitral flow velocity should be combined to enhance clinical decision making.

Other Diseases of the Mitral Valve. Although several other diseases that involve the mitral valve apparatus have distinctive echocardiographic findings, none of these findings are pathognomonic. Myxomatous mitral valve disease may show redundant, thickened leaflets with systolic prolapse of either the mitral coaptation point or leaflets into the left atrium (Fig. 12-22).[155] Generally there is no restriction of valvular motion. The tricuspid valve may show prolapse as well. In the mitral valve prolapse syndrome, echocardiographic risk factors for endocarditis, stroke, sudden death, and progression to severe mitral regurgitation include mitral valve thickening with redundant leaflets and increased left ventricular size.[156] In reports of patients with isolated severe mitral regurgitation in industrialized nations, mitral valve prolapse has been the most common underlying cause, occurring in 38% to 64% of patients.[157,158] One group of investigators has proposed that since the normal human mitral annulus has a saddle-shaped configuration, with high points located anteriorly and posteriorly, leaflet displacement above the annular hinge points should be used as a criterion for mitral valve prolapse only in echocardiographic views that are oriented anteroposteriorly (i.e., parasternal long-axis and apical two-chamber view, not apical four-chamber view).[159] Using Doppler echocardiography, mitral valve prolapse may be associated with a characteristic late systolic mitral regurgitation signal.

Endocarditis often presents with vibratory or whip-like vegetations on the cardiac valves (see next section). Flail mitral valve leaflet due to ruptured chordae tendineae may complicate mitral valve prolapse or endocar-

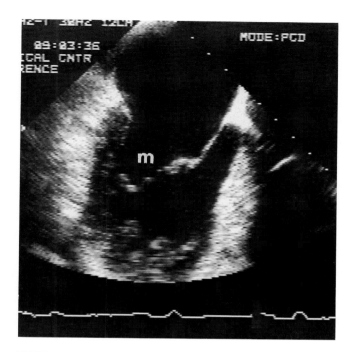

Figure 12-22. Transesophageal echocardiogram of a myxomatous mitral valve (m) demonstrating redundant leaflets.

ditis, and displays noncoaptation of the leaflets and erratic systolic motion into the left atrium. The poorly supported leaflet can be identified as the one that moves into the left atrium. Mitral annular calcification shows high-intensity echoes in the mitral annulus, and may be associated with aging, chronic renal failure, hypertrophic cardiomyopathy, chronic severe mitral regurgitation, and other states. Mitral valve involvement in systemic lupus erythematosus may demonstrate either Libman-Sachs endocarditis or diffuse thickening of the leaflets with decreased mobility.[160] The former entity has a verrucous echocardiographic appearance and a fairly benign prognosis, whereas the latter complication is prone to hemodynamic deterioration and progression to valve surgery. Finally, congenital abnormalities of the mitral valve, such as parachute and cleft valves, may be diagnosed by two-dimensional echocardiography (see Chapter 13).

Mitral Regurgitation

As suggested above, visualization of abnormal mitral leaflet closure patterns, such as incomplete closure in rheumatic disease, severe prolapse, ruptured chordae tendineae, or flail pattern often suggest significant mitral regurgitation.[161] Several secondary M-mode and two-dimensional echocardiographic findings have also been described in association with hemodynamically significant mitral regurgitation. These signs include increased

atrial emptying volume, exaggerated interventricular septal motion, and gradual closure of the aortic valve during systole.[162–164] The presence of both exaggerated atrial or septal motion and early closure of the aortic valve increases specificity for severe mitral regurgitation. Since these signs are not especially sensitive for mitral regurgitation, however, Doppler and color flow imaging have become the mainstays of diagnosis.

In patients with chronic mitral regurgitation, echocardiography has also been used to follow left ventricular size and function to appropriately plan mitral valve surgery. Schuler and associates found that patients with moderate left ventricular dilation and normal ejection fraction preoperatively have regression of myocardial hypertrophy and only minimal decrease in left ventricular shortening fraction after mitral valve replacement.[165] In patients with severe left ventricular dilation (preoperative end-diastolic diameters over 7 cm or end-systolic diameters over 5 cm) and low normal or decreased ejection fraction, however, left ventricular ejection fraction becomes markedly improved and chamber dilation and myocardial hypertrophy persist after surgery. In these patients, preoperative left ventricular systolic function was partially dependent on the afterload reducing effects of mitral regurgitation. Borow and associates found that preoperative end-systolic volume (over 60 mL/m²), which reflects myocardial contractility and is independent of preload, was better than end-diastolic volume or ejection fraction for predicting perioperative cardiac death.[166] Another group has used left ventricular end-systolic wall stress to provide preoperative prognostic information.[167]

On pulsed-wave Doppler examination, mitral regurgitation appears as a turbulent systolic signal within the left atrium that is directed away from the transducer. The detection of mitral regurgitation by this method is extremely sensitive; in fact, pulsed-wave Doppler evidence of mitral regurgitation may be detected in healthy patients or those with no murmur of mitral regurgitation.

The extent of penetration and the area of the mitral regurgitation jet relative to the left atrium can be mapped by moving the pulsed-wave Doppler cursor from the valve leaflets backward throughout the atrium.[168–170] Mapping of the jet is usually accomplished in the parasternal long-axis or apical views. When mitral regurgitation can only be detected close to the mitral leaflets, the severity of the leak is generally trivial or mild. When the pulsed-wave signal can be tracked to the most posterior portions of the left atrium or into the pulmonary veins or left atrial appendage, however, mitral regurgitation is usually moderate to severe. Likewise, the greater the area or volume of the left atrium that is encompassed by the mitral regurgitation signal, the more severe the lesion. In patients with poor left ventricular function, very large atria, or eccentric jets (as in flail mitral valve leaflet), mapping systems may underestimate the significance of the leak. Other pulsed-Doppler findings of hemodynamically significant mitral regurgitation include a high *intensity* regurgitant signal relative to mitral inflow (large regurgitant volumes have more moving red blood cells) and a high velocity mitral *inflow* signal (forward inflow must increase to accommodate a large regurgitant volume) (see Table 12-4).[171]

Continuous-wave Doppler is almost as sensitive as pulsed-wave Doppler in the detection of mitral regurgitation. When mitral regurgitation is demonstrated in the apical position by this mode, the spectral signal generally appears as a high-velocity, parabolic, holosystolic envelope that appears below the baseline (Fig. 12-23). The velocity of the signal is generally greater than or equal to 4 m/sec because the normal systolic gradient between the left ventricle and left atrium is high. Low-velocity mitral regurgitation jets (around 3 m/sec) are usually due to either technical deficiency in aligning the transducer parallel to the jet or severe left ventricular dysfunction. The presence of an asymmetric spectral signal that truncates in late systole correlates hemodynamically with the presence of a left atrial "V wave"; this finding results from early equalization of pressures across the mitral valve and often indicates severe mitral regurgitation.[171]

In patients with normal aortic valves, a mitral valve regurgitant fraction can be calculated from a combination of M-mode, two-dimensional, and Doppler information.[172] Total left ventricular stroke volume can be measured by planimetry, forward stroke volume as the product of aortic valve area (from M-mode diameter) and forward aortic flow (integral of aortic Doppler flow signal), and regurgitant volume as the difference of these two stroke volumes. Mild mitral regurgitation generally

has a regurgitant fraction of about 20%; severe mitral regurgitation may show values of 60% or more. This method can be used to follow patients quantitatively over time or after therapeutic interventions; however, the reproducibility of the calculations may be difficult in suboptimal studies.

Color-flow Doppler provides a near real-time flow map of the origin and direction of mitral regurgitation in the left atrium.[173] Although this information can also be obtained by interrogating the entire left atrium by pulsed-wave Doppler as noted above, the latter method may be tedious, technically difficult, and unreliable, especially in patients with eccentric jets. Color flow can be used to align the continuous-wave Doppler cursor for maximizing spectral Doppler signals. By color flow, mitral regurgitation in the apical view usually appears as a systolic flame-shaped stream of blue color flowing retrograde from the left ventricle to the left atrium. Color-flow Doppler approaches ventriculography in its sensitivity to detect mitral regurgitation and its ability to grade the severity of regurgitation.[174] Although about 40% of healthy subjects have mitral regurgitant color-flow jets that emulate from the posteromedial commissure, these jets are generally small in area.[175] Small jets that penetrate less than 2 cm into the left atrium generally signify mild mitral regurgitation. Large jets that fill more than half of the left atrium, extend to the posterior portion of the left atrium, or penetrate into the left atrial appendage or pulmonary veins indicate significant mitral regurgitation (Plates 2 and 3). In patients with very large left atria, loss of color sensitivity at maximum depths may occasionally result in the erroneous impression that mitral regurgitation is mild. The size of the jet as it forms at the valve and the convergence of the jet as it forms on the atrial (do-

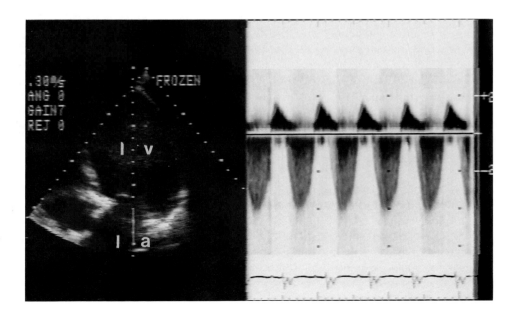

Figure 12-23. Continuous-wave Doppler of the mitral valve in the apical view. The parabolic jets exceed 4 m/sec in peak velocity. (la, left atrium; lv, left ventricle.)

nor) side of the valve are newer indicators of the severity of mitral regurgitation.

Aortic Stenosis

On M-mode echocardiography, the normal aortic valve opens as a "box" within the aortic root (Fig. 12-24). In aortic stenosis, characteristic M-mode findings include thickening of the valve leaflets and limited opening diameter. In patients with bicuspid aortic valves, an eccentric valve opening pattern has been described.[176] Although in some patients M-mode echocardiography permits a fair assessment of the severity of aortic stenosis, the method can be unreliable in patients with congenital or calcific aortic stenosis, in whom systolic doming or severe calcification of the aortic valve may mimic or obscure leaflet motion.[177] On M-mode echocardiography, most adult patients with critical aortic stenosis have calcified aortic valves or left ventricular hypertrophy. Thus, in patients with noncalcified valves, good aortic leaflet motion, and normal left ventricular wall thickness, critical aortic stenosis is extremely unlikely.

Because it offers a wider field of vision and spatial orientation, two-dimensional echocardiography permits the entire aortic valve to be imaged throughout the cardiac cycle and increases the ability to measure the true aortic valve orifice diameter (Fig. 12-25).[177] Patients who have supravalvular or subvalvular stenosis, or thickening and immobility confined to one aortic cusp with normal motion of another leaflet can be more easily recognized. The maximal aortic intercusp distance visualized in any standard two-dimensional view has been used to assess the severity of stenosis. Although this distance is generally greater than 15 mm in healthy subjects and less than 11 mm in patients with critical aortic stenosis, the specificity of the intercusp distance in distinguishing critical from noncritical aortic stenosis is limited.[178] Similar to M-mode echocardiography, a drawback of measuring valve opening diameter is that patients with left ventricular dysfunction may demonstrate poor aortic leaflet opening due to decreased stroke volume.

With the development of continuous-wave Doppler techniques, a more direct method for noninvasively measuring the pressure gradient across the aortic valve during systole became available.[179–182] The rate of progression of aortic stenosis can be easily followed over time by using serial studies for pressure gradient.[183] Correlations of the pressure drop across stenotic aortic valves by Doppler and cardiac catheterization are extremely close. One must be aware that the peak pressure gradient measured by Doppler is a true maximum gradient, however, whereas the peak gradient measured by catheter is actually a "peak-to-peak" pressure gradient.

Since the direction of stenotic aortic jet flows may

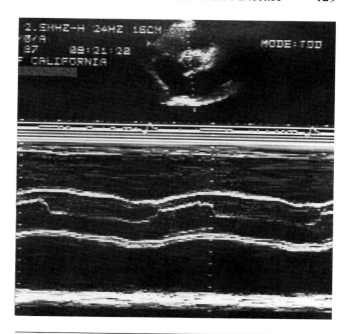

Figure 12-24. Normal aortic valve opening (rectangular box) by M-mode echocardiography.

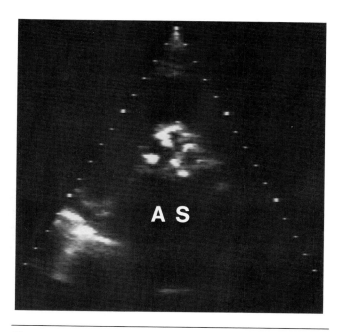

Figure 12-25. Parasternal short-axis view of calcific aortic stenosis (AS).

vary with valvular anatomy, peak aortic flow velocity should be carefully sought in several views, including the parasternal, apical, right parasternal, subcostal, and suprasternal.[184] A small nonimaging transducer (Pedoff transducer) may be best suited for this purpose. The normal peak aortic flow velocity is less than 1.2 m/sec (Fig.

12-26). In patients with high cardiac output states or significant aortic insufficiency, peak aortic flow velocity may increase up to 1.5 to 2.0 m/sec without evidence of anatomic stenosis. When peak flow velocities exceed 2.0 m/sec, some degree of stenosis is generally present. Using the modified Bernoulli equation, the pressure gradient across the stenotic valve can be calculated. In general, peak aortic velocities greater than 4.0 m/sec indicate critical aortic stenosis (Fig. 12-27), whereas peak velocities less than 3.0 m/sec indicate noncritical stenosis.[185] For peak velocities between 3.0 and 4.0 m/sec, the assessment of aortic valve area, left ventricular function, and the degree of aortic insufficiency should also be considered in evaluating the severity of the lesion. The acceleration of aortic flow or the time to peak flow can also be used as guides to the severity of aortic stenosis. Similar to the delayed carotid upstrokes noted on physical examination in patients with severe aortic stenosis, the aortic Doppler signal may show a delay in the upstroke to peak velocity in these patients (Fig. 12-28).

Aortic valve area can be calculated using the "continuity formula," based on the principle of conservation of mass, that is, laminar blood flow volume is the product of cross-sectional area and the spatial–temporal mean flow velocity.[186] The volume of blood flow across the left ventricular outflow tract is the same as the volume of blood flow across the aortic valve. To determine aortic valve area, this formula calls for the measurement of mean left ventricular outflow tract velocity, left ventricular outflow tract diameter and area, and mean aortic flow velocity. These simple measurements can be performed during the echocardiographic evaluation. Precise determination of left ventricular outflow tract area can be difficult in some patients, however, and may limit the accuracy and reproducibility of the technique.

Color-flow Doppler imaging is also useful in the identification of aortic stenosis; the technique can be helpful in the differentiation of native aortic valvular, supravalvular, and various forms of subaortic stenosis.[187–190] In addition, preliminary investigation suggests that the severity of stenosis may be estimated by the width of the color flow jet.

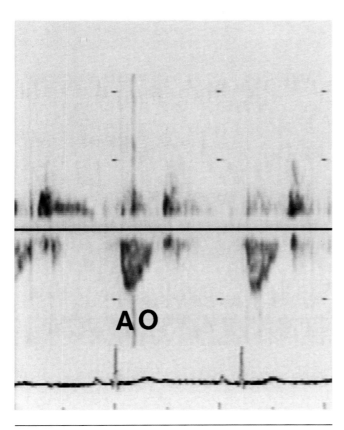

Figure 12-26. Normal aortic valve flow by continuous-wave Doppler (AO); peak velocity is 0.8 m/sec. Calibration marks indicate 1 m/sec.

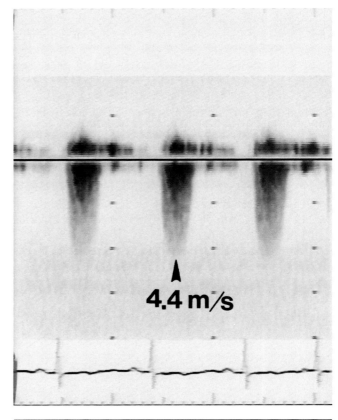

Figure 12-27. Continuous-wave Doppler through the aortic valve (Ao) obtained from the apex in a patient with critical aortic stenosis. Peak velocity is 4.4 m/sec corresponding to a pressure gradient of 77 mm Hg. Calibration marks indicate 2 m/sec.

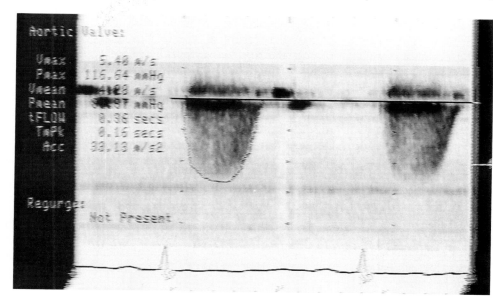

Aortic Valve:

Vmax   5.48 m/s
Pmax   115.64 mmHg
Vmean   ....
Pmean   ....
tFLOW   0.36 secs
TnPk   0.16 secs
Acc   33.13 m/s2

Regurg:

Not Present

Figure 12-28. Severe aortic stenosis by continuous-wave Doppler. The aortic Doppler signal displays a delay in the upstroke to peak velocity, with a prolonged acceleration time of 33 m/sec^2.

Aortic Regurgitation

The ability to evaluate the progression and severity of aortic regurgitation by echocardiography has improved significantly over the years. As is the case with chronic mitral regurgitation, M-mode and two-dimensional imaging methods are most useful to evaluate the long-term effect of volume loading on left ventricular size and function. Doppler echocardiography and color-flow imaging permit a direct assessment of the severity of the regurgitant jet itself, however.

On M-mode echocardiography, the presence of aortic regurgitation has been identified by the presence of fluttering of the anterior leaflet of the mitral valve or the interventricular septum in diastole.[191,192] Although these signs are not helpful in determining the severity of the leak, the oscillating structure indicates the direction of the regurgitant jet flow. Conversely, early closure of the mitral valve by M-mode echocardiography (prior to the onset of the electrocardiographic QRS complex) is a reliable sign of acute severe aortic regurgitation in infective endocarditis (Fig. 12-29).[193]

In significant aortic regurgitation, two-dimensional echocardiography of the anterior mitral valve leaflet may demonstrate a concave deformity as well as fluttering when the regurgitant jet impinges on this structure. Two-dimensional echocardiography is also useful to clearly illustrate anatomic abnormalities of the aortic valve and neighboring structures that are associated with aortic regurgitation, such as bicuspid valve, vegetations, subvalvular membrane, supracristal ventricular septal defect, aortic valve prolapse, and aortic dissection, ectasia or aneurysm.

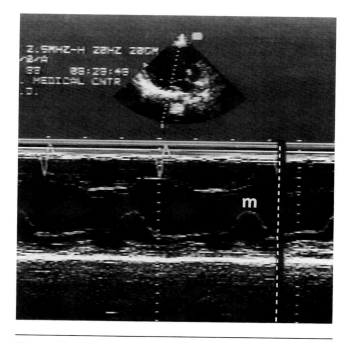

Figure 12-29. M-mode echocardiogram of the mitral valve (m) in a patient with severe aortic regurgitation. The mitral valve closes early, before the onset of the QRS complex (*dotted line*).

Considerable research has been devoted to the use of M-mode and two-dimensional echocardiography in determining the timing of aortic valve replacement. Studies have examined numerous parameters, including left ventricular size, function, and wall stress.[194–198] Although early reports suggested that a preoperative left ventricular systolic diameter exceeding 55 mm or a shortening fraction less than 25% correlated with left ventricular decompensation and adverse surgical outcome, subsequent studies have not been confirmatory.[194,195] Thus, the decision to perform aortic valve replacement should not be based on any one echocardiographic measurement; rather the echocardiogram is most useful to follow left ventricular size, function, and degree of aortic insufficiency over time and confirm the clinical impression of stability or progressive deterioration.

Doppler and color-flow imaging are now considered the most reliable echocardiographic techniques for evaluating the severity of aortic regurgitation. By pulsed-wave Doppler, aortic regurgitation appears as a harsh-sounding, high-velocity, aliasing pandiastolic signal in the left ventricular outflow tract. The sensitivity of pulsed-wave Doppler for the detection of aortic regurgitation is significantly greater than for auscultation, but similar to aortic root angiography.[199] The signal can be detected and mapped back into the left ventricle in the parasternal long- and short-axis, apical, and suprasternal views. The area of signal turbulence relative to the area of the left ventricular outflow tract correlates with the severity of aortic regurgitation.[200] In addition, the velocity and extent of retrograde diastolic flow in the aorta and other large proximal arteries correlates with the severity of the lesion by angiography (Fig. 12-30).[201–203]

Continuous-wave Doppler allows for determination of the gradient across the aortic valve throughout diastole. In severe aortic insufficiency this gradient decreases rapidly, whereas in mild regurgitation the transvalvular gradient decreases slowly. The pressure half-time measurement, obtained the same way as in mitral stenosis, is useful to quantitate the rate of decrease in the diastolic transvalvular gradient. Unlike mitral stenosis, a relatively flat slope indicates mild aortic regurgitation (Fig. 12-31), and a relatively steep slope indicates significant aortic regurgitation (Fig. 12-32). The pressure half-time is inversely related to regurgitant fraction and angiographic severity of aortic regurgitation. A Doppler half-time value of 400 msec reliably separates mild from significant aortic regurgitation; a value below 200 msec indicates severe aortic regurgitation.[204] The Doppler half-time has also been shown to depend on aortic and left ventricular compliance, so that misleading half-time measurements may occasionally be recorded.[205] The Doppler signal of aortic regurgitation can be differentiated from that of mitral stenosis by the peak velocity (typically about 4 m/sec in the former and 2 m/sec in the latter); the Doppler half-time method is still useful when both valvular lesions are present.[206] Before measuring the pressure half-time of aortic regurgitation, one must ensure that the jet has not been truncated. As noted above, a typical peak aortic regurgitation velocity should be greater than 4 m/sec, reflecting the high pressure gradient across the aortic valve in diastole.

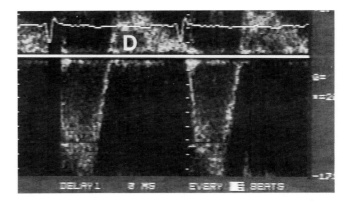

Figure 12-30. Pulsed-wave Doppler reveals abnormal reverse flow (above the baseline, D) in the descending aorta (a), signifying aortic regurgitation.

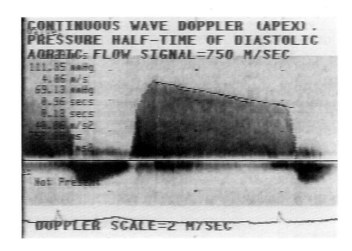

Figure 12-31. Continuous-wave Doppler in a patient with mild aortic regurgitation. Note the flat slope, with a pressure half-time of 750 m/sec.

By color-flow, aortic insufficiency appears as an abnormal mosaic of diastolic flow originating from the aortic valve and penetrating into the left ventricle (Plate 4). Aortic insufficiency flow can be differentiated from mitral stenosis flow by its origin from the aortic valve in several views and its presence early in diastole during isovolumic relaxation, before the mitral valve opens. Unlike mitral regurgitation, the maximal length and long-axis area of aortic insufficiency jets do not correlate with the angiographic grade of severity.[207] The thickness of the aortic regurgitant jet in the long-axis and area of the origin of the jet in the short-axis relative to the size of the left ventricular outflow tract are better predictors of severity. Also, the maximal mosaic pattern of diastolic flow in the left ventricle has a fair correlation with left ventricular end-diastolic and end-systolic volumes measured by

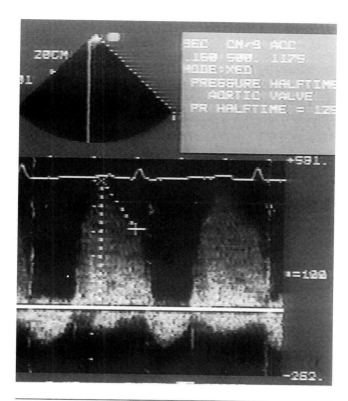

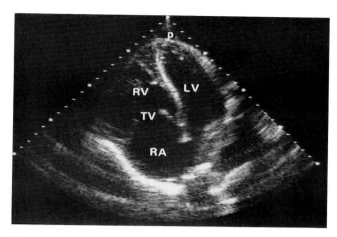

Figure 12-33. Systolic apical four-chamber view in a patient with carcinoid heart disease. The tricuspid valve (TV) leaflets are thickened, retracted and fixed in a partially open position. The right ventricle (RV) and right atrium (RA) are enlarged and there is a small pericardial effusion (p). (LV, left ventricle.) (Reproduced with permission from the American Journal of Cardiology.)

Figure 12-32. Continuous-wave Doppler in a patient with moderate to severe aortic regurgitation. Compared with Figure 12-31, note the relatively steep slope, with a pressure half-time of 125 m/sec.

scintigraphy.[208] The size of the jet as it crosses the valve and the size of the convergence jet on the donor side of the valve are being investigated as further indicators of severity. Reverse flow in the descending aorta can be seen as a color change in the same way that pulsed-wave Doppler shows reversed diastolic flow.

Tricuspid Stenosis

Tricuspid stenosis is a fairly uncommon acquired valve lesion, but may be secondary to rheumatic (usually in association with mitral and aortic valve involvement) or carcinoid (usually in association with pulmonary valve involvement) heart disease. The assessment of leaflet thickening and limited leaflet motion can be made by M-mode or two-dimensional echocardiography, whereas the transvascular gradient can be determined by pulsed- or continuous-wave Doppler.

In advanced cases of carcinoid heart disease, the apical four-chamber view characteristically shows thickened, retracted tricuspid valve leaflets that are fixed in a partially open position (Fig. 12-33). Although mild or moderate tricuspid stenosis may be present in these valves, the dominant cardiac lesion is usually severe tri-

cuspid insufficiency with right ventricular volume overload.[209] The acquired combination of tricuspid and pulmonary stenosis and insufficiency is nearly pathognomonic of this disorder. The development of cardiac lesions is related to chronic exposure of the right heart endocardium to high levels of circulating serotonin and other vasoactive substances.[210] Carcinoid heart disease is progressive and often fatal.

Tricuspid Regurgitation

Unlike tricuspid stenosis, acquired tricuspid regurgitation is common in echocardiography. The lesion may be caused by a primary valve disorder or secondary to pulmonary hypertension or right ventricular failure. Helpful imaging findings associated with tricuspid regurgitation include incomplete closure of the tricuspid valve, tricuspid vegetations, tricuspid valve prolapse, and retrograde movement of bubbles across the tricuspid valve after injection of agitated saline into an arm vein.

By pulsed-Doppler, tricuspid regurgitation appears as a pansystolic turbulent signal in the right atrium. Doppler interrogation of the tricuspid valve is usually performed in the parasternal short-axis and apical four-chamber views, but tricuspid regurgitation can also be appraised in the inferior vena cava. Pulsed- and continuous-wave Doppler are so sensitive in the detection of tricuspid regurgitation that the clinical significance of the signal has been questioned.[211] The presence of Doppler-detectable tricuspid insufficiency in most patients with heart disease is a fortunate situation for the echocardiographer, however, since it permits an estimation of right ventricular systolic pressure by the modified Bernoulli formula. Thus, the Doppler signal not only allows for an assessment of the severity of tricuspid regurgitation, but also enhances the ability to evaluate the hemodynamic effect of left heart valvular and myocardial lesions. For example, clinically important mitral stenosis, aortic insufficiency, or left ventricular dysfunction should all be associated with some degree of pulmonary hypertension. In patients who have technically suboptimal tricuspid insufficiency Doppler signals, the intravenous injection of agitated saline can enhance the quality of the jets and permit more accurate measurement of the peak velocity.

Although the peak velocity of tricuspid regurgitation is useful in calculating the peak right ventricular systolic pressure, it is not as helpful in the assessment of the severity of tricuspid regurgitation itself. In this regard, important Doppler parameters are analagous to mitral regurgitation, and include the area and penetration of the jet relative to the right atrium, intensity of the jet relative to tricuspid inflow, velocity of tricuspid inflow (in the absence of tricuspid stenosis), and presence of the "V wave" cutoff sign due to early equalization of the pressure gradient across the tricuspid valve.[212] In severe cases the usual parabolic shape of the tricuspid regurgitation signal is replaced by a dark, sharply contoured signal that resembles aortic flow.

Color-flow Doppler also has been applied to the detection and grading of tricuspid regurgitation.[213,214] Similar to mitral regurgitation, tricuspid regurgitation in the apical four-chamber view appears as a blue jet that penetrates the right atrium in a retrograde fashion (Plate 5). Tricuspid regurgitant jets can be oriented in a variety of directions, and thus should be imaged in multiple views, including apical, four-chamber, right ventricular inlet, short-axis parasternal through the cardiac base, and subcostal. The angle of the color flow jet can be used to align the continuous-wave Doppler cursor to accurately measure the peak tricuspid regurgitation velocity. Tricuspid regurgitation is found with the same frequency with color-flow Doppler as with conventional Doppler or right ventriculography and is more sensitive and specific than contrast two-dimensional echocardiography.[213] Similar to mitral or aortic regurgitation, semiquantitative grading scales are based on the depth and area of penetration into the receiving chamber, the right atrium. In addition, systolic reversal of flow in the inferior vena cava or hepatic veins indicates significant tricuspid regurgitation.

Pulmonary Valve Disease

Acquired pulmonary valve disease is uncommon, but may occur in association with indwelling pulmonary artery catheters, endocarditis, and pulmonary hypertension.

Pulmonary stenosis is usually congenital, but can also be due to carcinoid heart disease. M-mode and two-dimensional imaging are helpful to demonstrate valve thickening, limited mobility, doming, and poststenotic dilation of the pulmonary artery. Pulsed- or continuous-wave Doppler can be used to interrogate the valve in the parasternal short-axis view and measure the transvalvular pressure gradient.

Similar to tricuspid regurgitation, the presence of pulmonary regurgitation is common on Doppler studies

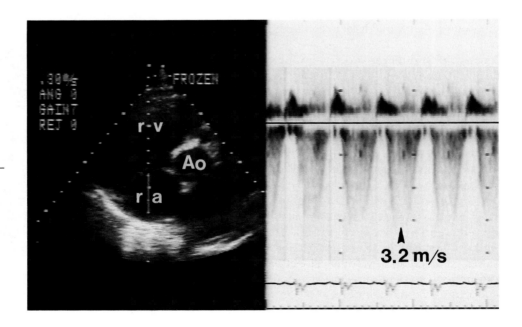

Figure 12-34. Continuous-wave Doppler of tricuspid regurgitation in the parasternal short-axis view. Peak tricuspid regurgitation velocity is 3.2 m/sec, correlating with a transtricuspid pressure gradient of 41 mm Hg, and a right ventricular systolic pressure of 41 + right atrial pressure. (Ao, aortic valve; ra, right atrium; rv, right ventricle. Doppler scale, 1.0 m/sec.)

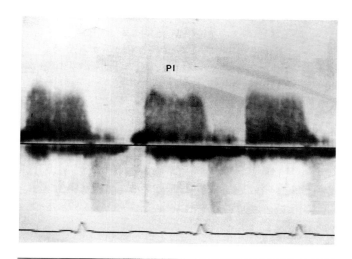

Figure 12-35. Pulmonary insufficiency (PI) by continuous-wave Doppler of the pulmonary valve. (Doppler scale, 1 m/sec.)

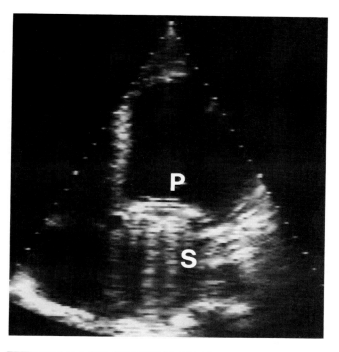

Figure 12-36. Apical four-chamber view of a mitral valve prosthesis (P) that causes ultrasound reverberations (S) and adjacent shadowing of the left atrium; this creates difficulty in the detection of mitral regurgitation in the left atrium.

in patients with and without heart disease (Fig. 12-35). Because of the lack of a standard for comparison, quantitation of pulmonary regurgitation by Doppler has not been possible; however, applying the modified Bernoulli formula to the jet does allow for the estimation of right ventricular end-diastolic pressure. Color-flow Doppler imaging can be used to detect and map pulmonary regurgitation (Plate 6).

Prosthetic Valves

Unlike native heart valves, prosthetic valves are composed of highly echoreflective materials that can cause ultrasound shadowing distal to and in the central portion of the valves (Fig. 12-36). Despite this limitation, echocardiography with Doppler has become increasingly useful in the evaluation of both metallic and bioprosthetic valves (Fig. 12-37). It is now standard practice to obtain a baseline echocardiogram with Doppler soon after prosthetic valve implantation and obtain annual follow-up studies thereafter. For bioprosthetic valves, the frequency of follow-up studies should be increased after 7 or 8 years because of the high rate of valve failure after this time.

Because of the wide variety of prosthetic valve types, positions, and sizes, considerable experience may be required to recognize pathologic imaging and Doppler flow patterns. In patients with ball-cage or tilting disc valves, M-mode and two-dimensional echocardiography can be used to determine the opening and closing excursions of the moving portion of the valve.[215,216] When thrombosis or endocarditis occurs on or around the

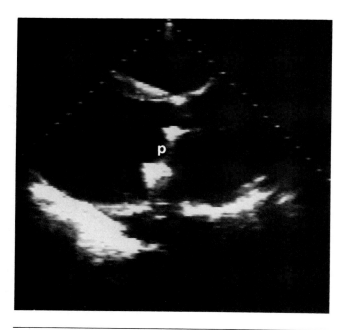

Figure 12-37. Parasternal long-axis view of a Bjork-Shiley prosthesis (p) in the mitral position; the valve sewing ring is imaged.

valve, the motion of the ball, disc, or leaflets can be impaired. Occasionally, the thrombus or vegetation can be imaged by two-dimensional echocardiography.[217-220] In bioprosthetic valves, thickening of the leaflets, flail or prolapse of the leaflets, and "stent creep" (inward angulation of the distal portion of the stents over time) are echocardiographic markers of valve degeneration.[221,222] Dehisced prosthetic valves may show a characteristic rocking motion in diastole.

Similar to native valve disease, Doppler echocardiography can be used to investigate the presence and severity of prosthetic valve regurgitation or stenosis. The pressure half-time measurement has been applied to the evaluation of prosthetic aortic insufficiency. Because of shadowing of the left atrium by mitral valve prostheses, prosthetic mitral regurgitation may be difficult to detect or quantify. Transesophageal echocardiography is useful in these patients to detect, localize, and map prosthetic mitral regurgitant jets (Plate 7) (see section on transesophageal echocardiography).

The diagnosis of prosthetic valve stenosis by Doppler examination is limited by the fact that all prosthetic valves are mildly stenotic relative to normal native valves, especially in the smaller sizes. Furthermore, transvalvular gradients can be transiently elevated in high cardiac output states, such as fever or severe anemia. Normal ranges for peak and mean Doppler-derived gradients across mitral and aortic valve prostheses of various types and sizes have been published.[223-227] When a transvalvular gradient is more than two standard deviations above the normal mean value for that valve size and type, prosthetic valvular stenosis should be considered. A trend showing significant increase in transvalvular gradients over time by serial echocardiograms is a more reliable index of obstruction, however. The pressure half-time method is also useful in prosthetic mitral stenosis.

Color-flow Doppler is also useful for the assessment of prosthetic mitral valve dysfunction, especially in conjunction with transesophageal imaging. The different prostheses show specific jet patterns, which are helpful in differentiating normal from pathologic backflow.[228-231] Color flow can often distinguish paravalvular and transvalvular prosthetic regurgitation and assess the severity of the leak (see Plate 7).

Cardiac Masses

Echocardiography has assumed a prominent role in the detection, diagnosis, and follow-up of various types of intracardiac and extracardiac masses. Cardiac masses may be discovered incidentally on routine echocardiography, or sought in the investigation of systemic or pulmonary emboli, valvular obstruction, or other symptoms.

Thrombi

Left ventricular thrombi have been discussed previously, and can occur in patients who have coronary artery disease with apical aneurysms, dilated cardiomyopathy, or endomyocardial fibrosis.

Similar to left ventricular thrombi, left atrial thrombi may cause systemic emboli. Atrial thrombi develop in conditions associated with slow atrial blood flow, such as atrial fibrillation, mitral stenosis, or prosthetic mitral valve. The presence of left atrial thrombus is often associated with the echocardiographic appearance of spontaneous contrast within that chamber (Fig. 12-38). Significant mitral regurgitation can prevent the development of left atrial thrombi by a "sweeping" action in that chamber. Thrombi may occur in the left atrial appendage (Fig. 12-39) or around the perimeter of the atrial chamber (Fig. 12-40). Unlike ventricular thrombi, atrial thrombi often are undetected by precordial echocardiography because of decreased resolution at the greater depths of field required for atrial imaging. Transesophageal echocardiography has become the imaging modality of choice for the detection and follow-up of these lesions.

Right atrial or ventricular thrombi are uncommon, but have occasionally been reported in association with right ventricular infarction or contusion, pulmonary emboli, or indwelling cardiac catheters. Pulmonary emboli usually arise from venous clots in the lower extremities. Rarely, so-called "emboli in transit" may be imaged in the

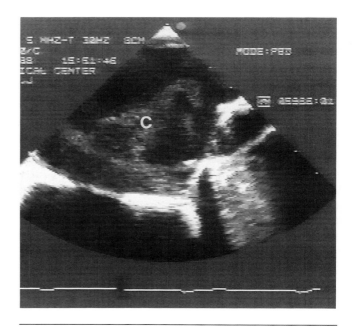

Figure 12-38. Transesophageal echocardiogram demonstrating spontaneous contrast (C) in the left atrium of a patient with a mitral valve prosthesis.

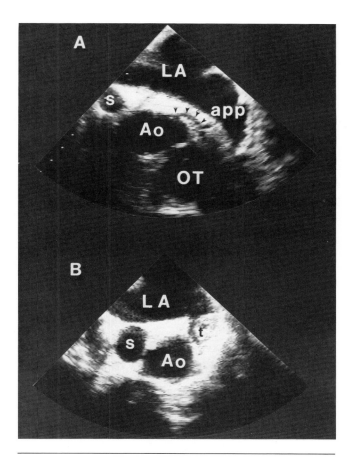

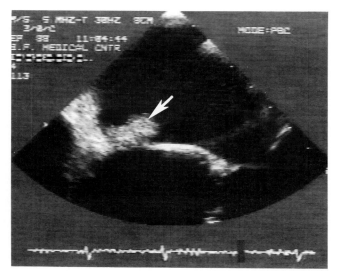

Figure 12-40. Transesophageal echocardiogram of a left atrial thrombus (t) on the wall of the left atrium.

Figure 12-39. *A:* Transesophageal echocardiogram of a normal left atrial appendage (LA, app) that is free of thrombus. (Ao, aortic valve; OT, right ventricular outflow tract; s, superior vena cava.) The left main coronary artery (*black arrows*) and its bifurcation into the left anterior descending and circumflex coronary arteries is also noted. *B:* Transesophageal echocardiogram in a patient who has a left atrial appendage thrombus (t).

right atrium on the way to the lungs. Due to the "sticky" nature of these venous clots, they may adhere to the mouth of the inferior vena cava, the eustachian valve, tricuspid valve, or other structures. Indwelling catheters in the right heart, such as pacemaker leads, Hickman catheters, or Swan-Ganz catheters, have also been implicated in the development of adherent thrombi. Thrombolytic therapy has been used to successfully dissolve these thrombi, and may be delivered through the catheter itself. Surgical resection of other large clots may occasionally be indicated to prevent massive pulmonary embolism.

Tumors

The most common primary cardiac neoplasm is the myxoma. Although 90% of cardiac myxomas are located

in the left atrium attached to the interatrial septum, myxomas may also occur in the right atrium or the ventricles. These tumors often have characteristic echocardiographic features, including pedunculated attachment to the interatrial septum near the foramen ovale and multicystic internal architecture (Fig. 12-41). Emboli may be caused by dislodgement of pieces of tumor or adherent thrombi. Large left atrial myxomas can prolapse through the mitral valve and obstruct mitral inflow causing a murmur and a Doppler signal that resembles mitral stenosis. Myxomas can also occur in multiple or atypical sites, especially in familial cases, or have a wide-based attachment to the atrial wall (Fig. 12-42).

Other tumors that may involve the heart include lymphoma, rhabdomyoma, rhabdomyosarcoma, Kaposi's sarcoma, and metastases of solid tumors, such as malignant melanoma, lung cancer, and breast cancer. Extracardiac tumors may invade the heart from adjacent structures (such as lung, lymph nodes, pericardium, or pleura), or travel up the inferior vena cava into the right atrium (renal cell carcinoma or hepatoma). Compression of the right ventricle by expanding anterior mediastinal masses may mimic cardiac tamponade, and has been reported secondary to abscess, hematoma, and tumor. High parasternal views may be useful in differentiating pericardial from mediastinal disease, and in elucidating the cause of the mass.[232]

Vegetations

On two-dimensional echocardiography, valvular vegetations are a useful marker of endocarditis. Vegetations

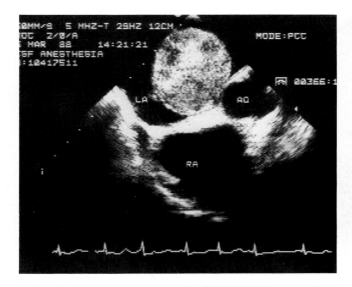

Figure 12-41. Transesophageal echocardiogram demonstrating a large left atrial (LA) myxoma that is attached to the interatrial septum near the aortic valve (AO). (RA, right atrium.) Note the multicystic internal architecture and the small protruding section of the tumor (adjacent to the LA label).

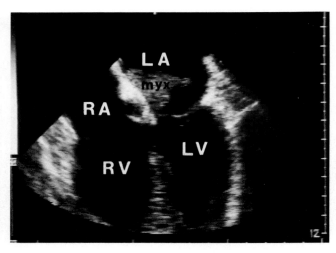

Figure 12-42. Transesophageal echocardiogram of another left atrial (LA) myxoma (myx) that has a broad-based attachment to the interatrial septum and a nonspherical shape. (LV, left ventricle; RA, right atrium; RV, right ventricle.)

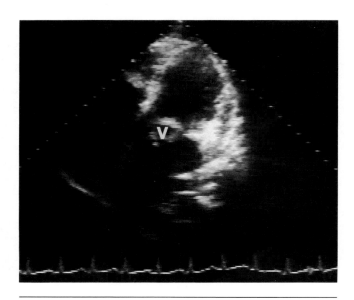

Figure 12-43. Apical four-chamber view showing a bulky vegetation (V) on the mitral valve. The patient had *Staphylococcus aureus* endocarditis.

usually appear as shaggy, echogenic, vibrating masses on the cardiac valves that respond to valvular motion. Bulky vegetations are suggestive of *Staphylococcus aureus* or fungal organisms (Fig. 12-43). Intravenous drug addicts who have endocarditis often have vegetations on the tricuspid valve; nondrug-abusers more often demonstrate mitral and aortic valve vegetations.

Although vegetations can be detected by echocardiography in 50% to 90% of patients, the diagnosis of endocarditis should still be primarily based on clinical evaluation and results of blood cultures.[233–236] Screening patients with bacteremia for vegetations is a low-yield procedure unless the patient has significant risk factors for endocarditis.[237] Because of previous treatment with antibiotics or fastidious organisms, some patients with endocarditis may have persistently negative blood cultures. Echocardiography assumes a more important diagnostic role in these patients with culture-negative endocarditis, since the demonstration of vegetations dictates a prolonged course of antibiotic therapy.[238] After resolution of endocarditis, valvular vegetations may remain present for years without change. In patients with previous endocarditis or calcified, flail, prolapsing, thickened, or prosthetic valves, the echocardiographic diagnosis of new vegetations can be exceedingly difficult. Transesophageal echocardiography may improve resolution and diagnostic efficacy in these cases (Fig. 12-44). Other entities that may mimic infected vegetations include Libman-Sachs endocarditis in systemic lupus, marantic endocarditis, and Lambl's excrescence.

Echocardiography and spectral Doppler studies are also useful in detecting complications of endocarditis. Acute bacterial endocarditis may lead to valvular destruction and insufficiency, whereas subacute bacterial endocarditis is usually more benign. Vegetations can cause val-

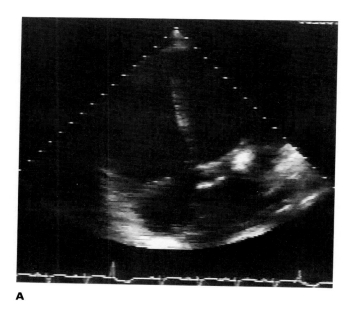
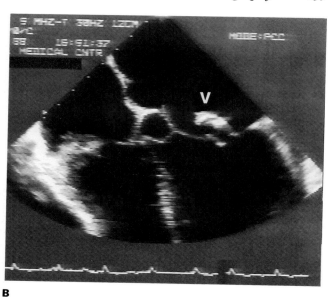

A   **B**

Figure 12-44. *A:* Apical four-chamber view indicating a poorly resolved mass on the mitral valve. *B:* Transesophageal echocardiogram in the same patient clearly shows a vegetation (V) on the posterior mitral leaflet.

vular insufficiency by interfering with closure of the valve or by causing disruption of leaflet or chordal continuity. Flail mitral valve due to ruptured chordae tendineae has a characteristic echocardiographic pattern with lack of co-aptation of the mitral leaflets and abnormal movement of the affected leaflet into the left atrium (Plate 8).[239–242] Cardiac abscess is a severe complication that has a poor prognosis, especially in association with prosthetic valve endocarditis. Abscesses usually appear as masslike lesions with necrotic, echo-free centers and are located near the aortic or mitral annulus (Fig. 12-45). Cardiac abscesses may present with bacteremia refractory to antibiotic therapy, prosthetic valve dehiscence, and high-degree atrioventricular block. Other complications of endocarditis that can be detected by two-dimensional echocardiography include purulent pericarditis and satellite lesions.

Color-flow Doppler can help confirm these and other complications of bacterial endocarditis, such as mitral valve perforation, ruptured sinus of Valsalva aneurysm, and cardiac fistulae.[243,244] In patients who develop flail mitral valve leaflet due to ruptured chordae tendineae, color flow demonstrates eccentric, turbulent mitral regurgitation jets that closely adhere to the periphery of the left atrium and move away from the damaged leaflet in a circular fashion. In flail *anterior* leaflet mitral regurgitant jets are directed toward the posterolateral atrial wall, whereas in flail *posterior* leaflet jets are directed toward the interatrial septum (see Plate 8).

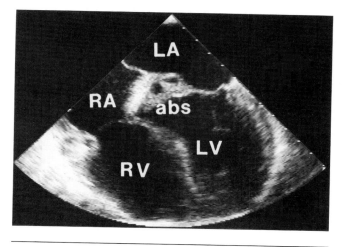

Figure 12-45. Transesophageal echocardiogram showing a bacterial abscess (abs) adjacent to the aortic valve. The necrotic spaces in the abscess are evident and can potentially rupture into adjacent chambers (LA, left atrium; RA, right atrium; RV, right ventricle) to form a fistula. (LV, left ventricle.)

New Developments in Echocardiography

Functional Evaluation with Stress Testing

Although many patients with heart disease complain only of symptoms during exertion, cardiac investigations are usually performed at rest. Since echocardiography allows for dynamic evaluaton of cardiac function during exercise, exercise echocardiography has rapidly become a useful diagnostic tool. Exercise two-dimensional imaging is used primarily to detect the presence and extent of coronary artery disease, whereas exercise Doppler of aortic, mitral, and tricuspid valves is used to evaluate global left ventricular systolic and diastolic function, valvular function, transvalvular gradients, and pulmonary artery pressure.

Exercise Two-Dimensional Echocardiography

The goal of exercise two-dimensional echocardiography is to detect changes in left ventricular function and wall motion by comparing cardiac images at rest and at peak exercise. The detection of segmental left ventricular dysfunction is useful in the diagnosis and localization of obstructive coronary artery disease. Since the normal left ventricle becomes hypercontractile during exercise, the development of reversible asynergy, decreased wall thickening, decreased left ventricular ejection fraction, or increased left ventricular end-systolic volume during exercise can indicate hemodynamically significant atherosclerotic coronary disease supplying the abnormal segments.

Because of improvements in two-dimensional echocardiographic equipment, the technical quality and popularity of exercise echocardiography has increased over the past decade.[245–249] Technically satisfactory studies can now usually be obtained in at least 75% to 90% of patients. The use of slow-motion bidirectional video playback units and digitized cine-loop display systems has helped to improve offline analysis and detection of endocardial motion (Fig. 12-46). Successful studies have been performed using upright treadmill, upright bicycle, or supine bicycle exercise; continuous or immediate post exercise echocardiographic monitoring; and a variety of standard echocardiographic views, including apical, parasternal, and subcostal. Because tachypnea and tachycardia develop at peak exercise, the heart may be visible for only one or two beats at end-expiration. The ischemic wall motion abnormalities induced by exercise usually persist for some time after peak exercise, however. The apical views have often been noted to produce a better image at peak exercise than at rest.

Advantages of exercise echocardiography include lack of exposure to contrast or radiation, portability, multiple viewing planes, ability to assess wall thickening, usage after therapeutic interventions (such as coronary angioplasty), immediate results, and evaluation of a large number of cycles in real time throughout exercise. The widespread availability of echocardiography makes the technique accessible to small hospitals or clinics where

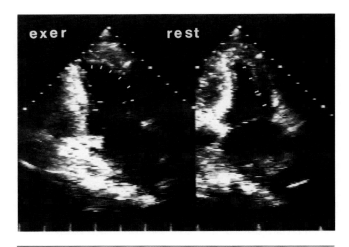

Figure 12-46. Exercise echocardiography: apical two-chamber views of the left ventricle at rest and at peak exercise (exer) demonstrate anterior akinesis and left ventricular dilatation at peak exercise (*white markers*). The electrocardiograms at the bottom indicate the difference in heart rates.

nuclear medicine facilities may not be established. Disadvantages of the technique include the need for a skilled operator, lack of detection of all ischemic beds in multivessel coronary artery disease, and technical difficulties in muscular, obese, or emphysematous patients.

Exercise two-dimensional echocardiography has been validated by comparison with coronary angiography and other noninvasive techniques. Reversible areas of segmental left ventricular asynergy by exercise two-dimensional imaging correlate with reversible perfusion defects by exercise thallium 201 perfusion scanning.[245] In addition, the sensitivity and specificity of exercise echocardiography for the diagnosis of coronary artery disease compares favorably with exercise electrocardiography, thallium 201 perfusion scanning, and radionuclide ventriculography.[247–249] Exercise echocardiography can also be helpful in predicting the occurrence of adverse cardiac events after myocardial infarction.[250] The test should be considered in patients with an abnormal baseline electrocardiogram, orthostatic or hyperventilation-induced electrocardiographic changes, nonspecific ST-segment and T wave abnormalities due to drug effect or ventricular hypertrophy, or a previous nondiagnostic routine treadmill test.[247] To apply this diagnostic method to patients who cannot exercise, pharmacologic interventions using dipyridamole, dobutamine, or adenosine infusions have been developed.

Exercise Doppler

Unlike two-dimensional echocardiographic imaging, Doppler echocardiography is widely used to assess flows and pressure gradients across heart valves. Because Doppler displays instantaneous changes in these parameters, it is an excellent technique for the study of physiologic and therapeutic interventions, including exercise. Since the diameter of the aortic valve increases only minimally during exercise, integration of the continuous-wave aortic Doppler signal (flow-velocity integral) throughout exercise allows for a beat-to-beat estimation of forward left ventricular stroke volume; cardiac output can be estimated as the product of heart rate and flow velocity integral.[251–255] Peak acceleration of the aortic Doppler signal correlates with left ventricular ejection fraction and has been used as an index of global left ventricular performance.[251,252] In some patients who have technically inadequate two-dimensional echocardiographic images, satisfactory aortic Doppler tracings may still be obtained from the suprasternal notch.[253]

In young healthy subjects, aortic flow velocity and aortic acceleration increase progressively with exercise. In patients with multivessel coronary artery disease, the increase in these parameters is often blunted and correlates with exaggerated increases in pulmonary artery wedge pressure.[254] Blunted increases in peak aortic velocity and acceleration during exercise are also common in healthy elderly patients or in those treated with propranolol, however.[255,256] In children with valvar aortic stenosis, a prominent increase in peak transaortic velocity by continuous-wave Doppler during exercise suggests a critical valvular lesion.[257]

Doppler analysis of mitral valve flow during exercise may also be helpful in evaluating patients with ischemic and valvular heart disease. Similar to aortic valve flow, a blunted increase in mean mitral flow velocity during exercise occurs in patients with stress-induced ischemia; this phenomenon may be secondary to changes in left ventricular compliance.[258] The development of mitral regurgitation by color Doppler during exercise also suggests multivessel coronary artery disease.[259] In patients with mitral stenosis, a marked and early rise in the transmitral gradient during exercise by continuous-wave Doppler echocardiography indicates hemodynamically significant stenosis. Since the transmitral pressure gradient partly depends on left ventricular function, patients with low cardiac outputs generally have low resting gradients. In these patients, calculation of mitral valve area during exercise may be less subject to error than calculation during rest. After successful mitral commissurotomy or balloon valvuloplasty, decreases in transmitral pressure gradient at rest and at peak exercise can be demonstrated by continuous-wave Doppler.[260]

Continuous-wave Doppler echocardiography also permits the calculation of pulmonary artery systolic pressure at rest and during exercise by evaluation of tricuspid regurgitation.[261] In patients with chronic parenchymal pulmonary disease, a rapid and exaggerated rise in pulmonary artery systolic pressure during exercise suggests associated pulmonary vascular disease.

Finally, one of the greatest advantages of exercise echocardiography is versatility. A skilled exercise technician may combine the two-dimensional imaging and the Doppler evaluations in one or more views to follow ventricular function, cardiac output, valvular gradients, and pulmonary artery systolic pressure throughout graded exercise. For example, in the presence of reversible left ventricular dyssynergy by two-dimensional echocardiography, the development of mitral regurgitation at peak exercise or the lack of increase in peak Doppler aortic flow velocity during exercise suggests left main or multivessel coronary artery disease. Also, in the investigation of dyspnea on exertion in a 60-year-old patient with known rheumatic mitral stenosis, rapid increases in transmitral and pulmonary artery systolic pressures during exercise indicates hemodynamically significant mitral valve disease, whereas reversible dyssynergy would indicate associated atherosclerotic coronary disease.

Transesophageal Echocardiography

The esophagus provides an airless posterior ultrasonic window to the heart from directly behind the left atrium. To circumvent the chest wall, ribs, and lungs, a miniature phased-array transducer is placed at the tip of the housing of a flexible gastroscope that has had its optics removed.[262–264] The ultrasound beam is steerable in that the scope can be advanced, withdrawn, or rotated within the esophagus and the angle that the transducer makes with the esophagus can be altered slightly by manipulation of the anteroposterior and lateral flexion controls. Commercially available transesophageal echocardiography systems provide high resolution M-mode and two-dimensional imaging, pulsed-wave Doppler, and color-flow Doppler; newer features may include biplane imaging and continuous-wave Doppler.

Transesophageal echocardiography can be performed easily and quickly in a variety of clinical settings, including the ambulatory clinic, the operating room, and the intensive care unit. The test has an excellent safety record with no known deaths or esophageal perforations; the only major complications reported have been transient recurrent laryngeal nerve paralysis and subacute bacterial endocarditis.[265] Minor complications have included atrial and ventricular arrhythmias, vasovagal reactions, transient bronchospasm and hypoxemia, and insignificant bleeding. Relative contraindications include a history of dysphagia, previous mediastinal irradiation, esophageal pathology or surgery, coagulopathy, or active upper gastrointestinal bleeding.

In the anesthetized patient, the unlocked esophageal probe is introduced into the esophagus after endotracheal intubation and systemic sedation. For ambulatory studies, patients should be instructed to fast for at least 4 hours. Systemic sedation can often be avoided, but is used selectively. Local anesthesia of the hypopharynx is achieved by having the patient gargle and swallow dilute viscous lidocaine. After the gag reflex is suppressed, the patient is placed in the left lateral recumbent position, the unlocked esophageal probe introduced and a bite block placed to protect both the probe and the teeth. Intermittent suctioning of secretions is performed as needed and vital signs and rhythm are monitored throughout the procedure. In unstable patients or those with respiratory problems, oxygen saturation is also monitored by oximeter and resuscitation equipment is made immediately available.

Standard transesophageal views include the four-chamber view through the left atrium (usually obtained at about 35 to 40 cm from the incisors), short-axis views of the cardiac base through the left atrium (allows imaging of the aortic valve and surrounding structures), and short-axis view of the left ventricle (usually obtained at about 40 to 45 cm, just beyond the gastroesophageal junction). Short- and long-axis views of the aorta can also be performed. The standard orientation (Fig. 12-47) displays the four-chamber view of the heart with the left atrium at the top of the fan and the left ventricle to the viewer's right.[266,267]

The most common indications for transesophageal echocardiography are listed in Table 12-5. Since the data obtained from transthoracic and transesophageal imaging are complementary, it is customary to perform trans-

Table 12-5

Indications for Transesophageal Echocardiography

Inadequate transthoracic echocardiographic image—obesity, emphysema, mechanical ventilation, chest wounds or tubes
Intraoperative monitoring—left ventricular function, wall motion, adequacy of surgical repair of mitral regurgitation or congenital heart lesion
Aortic pathology—dissection, aneurysm
Left atrial thombi and tumors
Prosthetic valve disease—stenosis, regurgitation, endocarditis, ring abscess
Native valve disease—endocarditis, flail mitral valve, ruptured chordae tendineae
Congenital heart disease—detection of atrial or ventricular shunts

thoracic imaging before transesophageal imaging. Transesophageal echocardiography is useful in the cardiac evaluation of patients who have technically inadequate transthoracic echocardiograms. Such patients are often obese, mechanically ventilated, or recovering from cardiothoracic surgery in the intensive care unit. For example, it may be difficult to perform precordial imaging in a patient who develops hypotension after coronary artery bypass surgery because of the presence of mediastinal blood and air, chest bandages, drainage tubes, positive-pressure ventilation, and decreased patient mobility. Transesophageal echocardiography can be performed at the bedside in these patients to identify cardiac tamponade, hypovolemia, or left ventricular dysfunction.[268,269]

Transesophageal echocardiography is also an important tool for the intraoperative assessment of left ventricular size, function, and wall motion in high-risk cardiac patients, including elderly patients and those with coronary artery disease or depressed left ventricular function.[270–278] In our institution, intraoperative transesophageal monitoring has been most useful for patients undergoing coronary artery bypass or major peripheral vascular surgery. Advantages of this relatively noninvasive technique for intraoperative monitoring include rapidity of preparation, continuous evaluation, high resolution, removal from the operative field, and ease of interpretation. The short-axis view of the left ventricle at the papillary muscle level provides a stable image that is convenient for long-term monitoring. Off-line digitized cine-loop display systems permit comparisons of ventricular size and segmental wall motion before and after various anesthetic and surgical procedures (i.e., induction of anesthesia, skin incision, pericardial incision, cross-clamp of the aorta, coronary artery grafting, and valve replacement) and allow for timely therapeutic interventions (i.e., administration of fluids for hypovolemia, intravenous nitroglycerine for ischemic wall motion abnormalities) (Fig. 12-48). Moreover, transesophageal echocardiography is more sensitive than elecrocardiog-

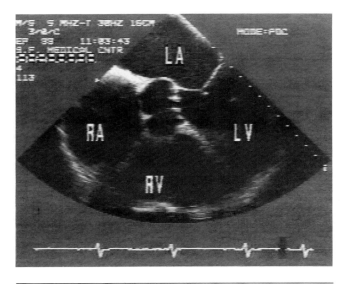

Figure 12-47. Standard orientation of the transesophageal echocardiographic four-chamber view. The left atrium (LA) is at the top of the screen, and the left ventricle (LV) is to the viewer's right. The aortic valve is clearly seen. (RA, right atrium; RV, right ventricle.)

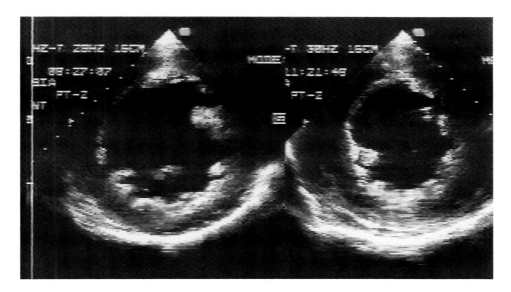

Figure 12-48. Intraoperative transesophageal echocardiograms of the left ventricle at the level of the papillary muscles at the beginning (*left*) and the end (*right*) of vascular surgery, when the patient was hypotensive. Based on the small size and vigorous contraction of the ventricle at the end of surgery, a diagnosis of hypovolemia was made. Fluids were administered and the blood pressure responded appropriately.

raphy for the detection of ischemia, may be superior to the pulmonary artery wedge pressure as a guide to pre-load, and readily detects intracardiac air embolism during upright neurosurgical procedures or open heart surgery.[273,275,278,279]

Transesophageal echocardiography is rapidly emerging as one of the diagnostic methods of choice for the evaluation of aortic dissection. Transesophageal imaging can be performed rapidly in the intensive care unit or emergency room to detect the extent of dissection, the site of intimal flaps, and complications such as aortic insufficiency and pericardial tamponade.[280,281] Because of technical factors, there may be difficulty in visualizing pathology at the top of the aortic arch; the recent introduction of biplane instruments promises to improve the access to this area. Despite this problem, the sensitivity and specificity of the technique compare favorably with angiography, computed tomography, and magnetic resonance imaging.

Because of the location of the transducer directly behind the left atrium, transesophageal imaging is far more powerful than transthoracic imaging for the detection of left atrial thrombus and tumor (see Figs. 12-39 to 12-42). This technique has become useful in the evaluation of patients who have emboli of unknown origin; the finding of thrombus in the body or appendage of the left atrium is an indication for long-term anticoagulation.[282,283] On transesophageal echocardiography, patients with severe mitral stenosis often have markedly enlarged left atria, atrial fibrillation, spontaneous contrast, and a tendency to form left atrial thrombus. Since atrial thrombus can be fragmented or dislodged during catheter manipulations, we choose to refer patients with severe mitral stenosis associated with atrial thrombus for surgical therapy (open commissurotomy or valve replacement)

rather than balloon valvuloplasty. For patients with atrial myxomas and other cardiac tumors, transesophageal echocardiography can be helpful in the determination of the site of attachment, size, internal architecture, and friability.[284]

Because of ultrasound shadowing that occurs behind mitral and aortic valve prostheses during transthoracic echocardiography, it is often difficult to adequately evaluate for prosthetic valve dysfunction. Transesophageal echocardiography provides a posterior approach to these structures, however, and thus allows for detection, localization, and semiquantitation of prosthetic regurgitation. In patients with prosthetic mitral valves, transesophageal echocardiography with color-flow Doppler permits the differentiation between a normal "seating-puff" and pathologic regurgitation, and between valvular and perivalvular leaks.[285,286] This technique also helps to determine the severity of mitral regurgitation; jets that occupy a large volume of the left atrium and penetrate into the left atrial appendage or pulmonary veins are usually hemodynamically severe. Note that it is our practice to administer prophylactic intravenous antibiotics to all patients with prosthetic valves and to patients with other major indications for prophylaxis who undergo this procedure.[287]

Transesophageal echocardiography is also useful in the evaluation of native heart valve dysfunction. In patients with endocarditis this technique is more sensitive than transthoracic echocardiography in the detection of vegetations, ring abscesses, and fistulae (see Figs. 12-44 and 12-45).[288–289] The demonstration of ruptured chordae tendineae (see Plate 8) or perforated valve leaflets makes mitral valve repair an excellent possibility for the cardiac surgeon, whereas the presence of subvalvular calcification or significant anterior mitral leaflet disease suggests that valve replacement would be more appropriate.[290–292] Furthermore, after valve repair is attempted, intraoperative transesophageal color-flow imaging provides information on the amount of residual mitral regurgitation.

Finally, because of the high-resolution imaging of the aortic root provided by this technique, transesophageal echocardiography permits identification of the proximal left and right coronary arteries in nearly all patients (see Fig. 12-39). Preliminary research suggests a possible role in the detection or exclusion of stenoses in the left main, proximal left anterior descending, and left circumflex coronary arteries by direct visualization of the lesion or detection of abnormal color flow signals arising from such stenoses.[293–295]

References

1. Feigenbaum H. Echocardiography. Philadelphia: Lea & Febiger, 1976:1.

2. Sahn DJ. Instrumentation and physical factors related to visualization of stenotic and regurgitant jets by Doppler color flow mapping. J Am Coll Cardiol 1988;12:1354.

3. Simpson IA, Valdes-Cruz LM, Sahn DJ, Murillo A, Tamura T, Chung DJ. Doppler color flow mapping of simulated in vitro regurgitant jets: evaluation of the effects of orifice size and hemodynamic variables. J Am Coll Cardiol 1989;13:1195.

4. Wong M, Matsumura M, Suzuki K, Omoto R. Technical and biologic sources of variability in the mapping of aortic, mitral and tricuspid color flow jets. Am J Cardiol 1987;60:847.

5. Hoit BD, Jones M, Eidbo EE, Elias W, Sahn DJ. Sources of variability for Doppler color flow mapping of regurgitant jets in an animal model of mitral regurgitation. J Am Coll Cardiol 1989;13:1631.

6. Smith MD, Grayburn PA, Spain MG, DeMaria AN. Observer variability in the quantitation of Doppler color flow jet areas for mitral and aortic regurgitation. J Am Coll Cardiol 1988;11:579.

7. Yoshida K, Yoshikawa J, Shakudo M, et al. Color Doppler evaluation of valvular regurgitation in normal subjects. Circulation 1988;78:840.

8. Massie BM, Schiller NB, Ratshin RA, Parmley WM. Mitral-septal separation: new echocardiographic index of left ventricular function. Am J Cardiol 1977;39:1008.

9. Schiller NB, Acquatella H, Ports TA, et al. Left ventricular volume from paired biplane two-dimensional echocardiographs. Circulation 1979;60:547.

10. Goerke RJ, Carlsson E. Calculations of right and left cardiac ventricular volumes. Method using standard computer equipment and biplane angiocardiograms. Invest Radiol 1967;2:360.

11. Silverman NH, Ports TA, Snider AR, Schiller NB, Carlsson E, Heilbron DC. Determination of left ventricular volume in children: echocardiographic and angiographic comparisons. Circulation 1980;62:548.

12. Reichek N, Helak J, Plappert T, et al. Anatomic validation of left ventricular mass estimates from clinical two dimensional echocardiography: initial results. Circulation 1983;67:348.

13. Helak JW, Reichek N. Quantitation of human left ventricular mass and volume by two dimensional echocardiography: in vitro anatomic validation. Circulation 1981;63:1398.

14. Erbel R, Schweizer P, Lambertz H, et al. Echoventriculography—a simultaneous analysis of two-dimensional echocardiography and cineventriculography. Circulation 1983;67:205.

15. Schnittger I, Fitzgerald PJ, Daughters GT, et al. Limitations of comparing left ventricular volumes by two dimensional echocardiography, myocardial markers and cineangiography. Am J Cardiol 1982;50:512.

16. Ren JF, Dotler MN, DePace NL, et al. Comparison of left ventricular ejection fraction and volumes by two-dimensional echocardiography, radionuclide angiography, and cineangiography. J Cardiol Ultrason 1983;2:213.

17. Schiller NB, Skiodebrand C, Schiller E, et al. In vivo assessment of left ventricular mass by two dimensional echocardiography. Circulation 1983;68:210.

18. Byrd BF III, Wahr DW, Wang YS, Bouchard A, Schiller NB. Left ventricular mass and volume/mass ratio determined by two-dimensional echocardiography in normal adults. J Am Coll Cardiol 1985;6:1021.

19. Wahr D, Wang Y, Schiller N. Clinical quantitative echocardiography. II. Left ventricular volume in a normal adult population. J Am Coll Cardiol 1983;1:863.

20. Schabelman S, Schiller NB, Silverman NH, Ports TA. Left atrial volume estimation by two-dimensional echocardiography. Cathet Cardiovasc Diagn 1981;7:165.

21. Wang Y, Heilbron D, Gutman J, Wahr D, Schiller N. Clinical quantitative echocardiography. I. End systolic atrial volume in a normal adult population. Chest 1984;86:595.

22. Cohn PF, Levine JA, Bergeron FA, Gorlin R. Reproducibility of the angiographic left ventricular ejection fraction in patients with coronary artery disease. Am Heart J 1974;88:713.

23. Carleton RA. Change in left ventricular volume during angiocardiography. Am J Cardiol 1971;27:460.

24. Hammermeister KE, Warbasse JR. Immediate hemodynamic effects of cardiac angiography in man. Am J Cardiol 1973;31:307.

25. McAnulty JH, Kremkau EL, Rosch J, Hattenbauer MT, Rahimtoola SH. Sponatenous changes in left ventricular function between sequential studies. Am J Cardiol 1974;34:23.

26. Jeppson GM, Clayton PD, Blair TJ, Liddle HV, Jensen RL, Klausner SC. Changes in left ventricular wall motion after coronary bypass surgery: signal or noise? Circulation 1981;64:945.

27. Wackers FJ, Berger HJ, Johnstone DE, et al. Multiple gated cardiac blood pool imaging for left ventricular ejection fraction: validation of the technique and assessment of variability. Am J Cardiol 1979;43:1159.

28. Marshall RC, Berger HJ, Reduto LA, Gottschalk A, Zaret B. Variability in sequential measures of left ventricular performance assessed with radionuclide angiocardiography. Am J Cardiol 1978;41:531.

29. Berger HJ, Davies RA, Batsford WP, Hoffer PB, Gottschalk A, Zaret BL. Beat-to-beat left ventricular performance assessed from the equilibrium cardiac blood pool using a computerized nuclear probe. Circulation 1981;63:133.

30. Tortoledo FA, Quinones MA, Fernandez GC, et al. Quantification of left ventricular volumes by two-dimensional echocardiography: a simplified and accurate approach. Circulation 1983;67:579.

31. Gordon EP, Schnittger I, Fitzgerald PJ, Williams P, Popp RL. Reproducibility of left ventricular volumes by two-dimensional echocardiography. J Am Coll Cardiol 1983;2:506.

32. Himelman RB, Cassidy MM, Landzberg JS, Schiller NB. Reproducibility of quantitative two-dimensional echocardiography. Am Heart J 1988;115:425.

33. Conetta DA, Geiser EA, Oliver LH, Miller AB, Conti CR. Reproducibility of left ventricular area and volume measurements using a computer endocardial edge-detection algorithm in normal subjects. Am J Cardiol 1985;56:947.

34. Felner JM, Blumenstein BA, Schlant RC, et al. Sources of variability in echocardiographic measurements. Am J Cardiol 1980;45:995.

35. Wallerson DC, Devereux RB. Reproducibility of quantitative echocardiography: factors affecting variability of imaging and Doppler measurements. Echocardiography 1986;3:219.

36. Strunk BL, Fitzgerald JW, Lipton M, Popp RL, Barry WH. The posterior aortic wall echocardiogram: its relationship to left atrial volume change. Circulation 1976;54:744.

37. Djalaly A, Schiller NB, Poehlmann HW, Arnold S, Gertz EW. Diastolic aortic root motion in left ventricular hypertrophy. Chest 1981;79:442.

38. Kramer PH, Djalaly A, Poehlmann MS, Schiller NB. Abnormal diastolic left ventricular posterior wall motion in left ventricular hypertrophy. Am Heart J 1983;106:1066.

39. Danford DA, Huhta JC, Murphy DJ. Doppler echocardiographic approaches to ventricular diastolic function. Echocardiography 1986;3:33.

40. Rokey R, Kuo LC, Zoghbi WA, Limacher MC, Quinones MA. Determination of parameters of left ventricular diastolic filling with pulsed Doppler echocardiography: comparison with cineangiography. Circulation 1985;71:543.

41. Friedman BJ, Drinkovic N, Miles H, Shih WJ, Mazzoleni A, DeMaria AN. Assessment of left ventricular diastolic function: comparison of Doppler echocardiography and gated blood pool scintigraphy. J Am Coll Cardiol 1986;8:1348.

42. Spirito P, Maron BJ, Bonow RO. Noninvasive assessment of left ventricular diastolic function: comparative analysis of Doppler echocardiographic and radionuclide angiographic techniques. J Am Coll Cardiol 1986;7:518.

43. Phillips RA, Coplan NL, Krakoff LR, et al. Doppler echocardiographic analysis of left ventricular filling in treated hypertensive patients. J Am Coll Cardiol 1987;9:317.

44. Bryg RJ, Williams GA, Labovitz AJ. Effect of aging on left ventricular diastolic filling in normal subjects. Am J Cardiol 1987;59:971.

45. Nishimura RA, Abel MD, Hatle LK, Tajik AJ. Assessment of diastolic function of the heart: background and current applications of Doppler echocardiography. II. Clinical studies. Mayo Clin Proc 1989;64:181.

46. Choong CY, Herrmann HC, Weyman AE, Fifer MA. Preload dependence of Doppler-derived indexes of left ventricular diastolic function in humans. J Am Coll Cardiol 1987;10:800.

47. Ishida Y, Meisner JS, Tsujioka K, et al. Left ventricular filling dynamics: influence of left ventricular relaxation and left atrial pressure. Circulation 1986;74:187.

48. Downes TR, Nomeir AM, Stewart K, Mumma M, Kerensky R, Little WC. Effect of alteration in loading conditions on both normal and abnormal patterns of left ventricular filling in healthy individuals. Am J Cardiol 1990;65:377.

49. Himelman RB, Landzberg JS, Amend W, et al. Cardiac consequences of renal transplantation: changes in left ventricular morphology and function. J Am Coll Cardiol 1988;12:915.

50. Horowitz RS, Morganroth J, Parrotto C, Chen CC, Soffer J, Pauletto FJ. Immediate diagnosis of acute myocardial infarction by two-dimensional echocardiography. Circulation 1982;65:323.

51. Goldberger JJ, Himelman RB, Wolfe CL, Schiller NB. Right ventricular infarction: recognition and hemodynamic significance by two-dimensional echocardiography. J Am Soc Echo 1991;4:140.

52. Farcot JC, Boisante L, Rigaud M, Bardet J, Bourdarias JP. Two-dimensional echocardiographic visualization of ventricular septal rupture after acute anterior myocardial infarction. Am J Cardiol 1980;45:370.

53. Gibson RS, Bishop HL, Stamm RB, Crampton RS, Beller GA, Martin RP. Value of early two-dimensional echocardiography in patients with acute myocardial infarction. Am J Cardiol 1982;49:1110.

54. Asinger RW, Mikell FL, Elsperger J, Hodges M. Incidence of left-ventricular thrombosis after acute transmural myocardial infarction. N Engl J Med 1981;305:297.

55. Keating EC, Gross SA, Schlamowitz RA, et al. Mural thrombi in myocardial infarctions: prospective evaluation by two-dimensional echocardiography. Am J Med 1983;74:989.

56. Weinreich DJ, Burke JF, Pauletto FJ. Left ventricular mural thrombi complicating acute myocardial infarction: long-term follow-up with serial echocardiography. Ann Intern Med 1984;100:789.

57. Maze SS, Kotler MN, Parry WR. Flow characteristics in the dilated left ventricle with thrombus: qualitative and quantitative Doppler analysis. J Am Coll Cardiol 1989;13:873.

58. Delemarre BJ, Visser CA, Bot H, Dunning AJ. Prediction of apical thrombus formation in acute myocardial infarction based on left ventricular spatial flow pattern. J Am Coll Cardiol 1990;15:355.

59. Visser CA, Kan G, Meltzer RS, Dunning AJ, Roelandt J. Embolic potential of left ventricular thrombus after myocardial infarction: a two-dimensional echocardiographic study of 119 patients. J Am Coll Cardiol 1985;5:1275.

60. Domenicucci S, Bellotti P, Chiarella F, Lupi G, Vecchio C. Spontaneous morphologic changes in left ventricular thrombi: a prospective two-dimensional echocardiographic study. Circulation 1987;75:737.

61. Desoutter P, Halphen C, Haiat R. Two dimensional echocardiographic visualization of free ventricular wall rupture in acute anterior myocardial infarction. Am Heart J 1984;108:1360.

62. Erlebacher JA, Weiss JL, Eaton LW, Kallman C, Weisfeldt ML, Bulkley BH. Late effects of acute infarct dilation of heart size: a two-dimensional echocardiographic study. Am J Cardiol 1982;49:1120.

63. Weyman AE, Peskoe SM, Williams ES, Dillon JC, Feigenbaum H. Detection of left ventricular aneurysms by cross-sectional echocardiography. Circulation 1976;54:936.

64. Davidson KH, Parisi AF, Harrington JJ, Barsamian EM, Fishbein MC. Pseudoaneurysm of the left ventricle: an unusual echocardiographic presentation. Ann Intern Med 1977;86:430.

65. Messner-Pellenc P, Leclercq F, Krebs R, et al. Doppler color echocardiography in the diagnosis of 4 septal perforations complicating anterior myocardial infarction. Arch Mal Coeur 1988;81:1243.

66. Izumi S, Miyatake K, Beppu S, et al. Mechanism of mitral regurgitation in patients with myocardial infarction: a study using real-time two-dimensional Doppler flow imaging and echocardiography. Circulation 1987;76:777.

67. Natello GW, Nanda NC, Zachariah ZP. Color Doppler recognition of left ventricular pseudoaneurysm. Am J Med 1988;85:432.

68. Roelandt JR, Sutherland GR, Yoshida K, Yoshikawa J. Improved diagnosis and characterization of left ventricular pseudoaneurysm by Doppler color flow imaging. J Am Coll Cardiol 1988;12:807.

69. Rink LD, Feigenbaum H, Godley RW, et al. Echocardiographic detection of left main coronary artery obstruction. Circulation 1982;65:719.

70. Douglas PS, Fiolkoski J, Berko B, Reichek N. Echocardiographic visualization of coronary artery anatomy in the adult. J Am Coll Cardiol 1988;11:565.

71. Henry WL, Clark CE, Epstein SE. Asymmetric septal hypertrophy (ASH): echocardiographic identification of the pathognomonic anatomic abnormality of IHSS. Circulation 1973;47:225.

72. Shapiro LM, McKenna WJ. Distribution of left ventricular hypertrophy in hypertrophic cardiomyopathy: a two-dimensional echocardiographic study. J Am Coll Cardiol 1983;2:437.

73. Kereiakes DJ, Anderson DJ, Crouse L, Chatterjee K. Apical hypertrophic cardiomyopathy. Am Heart J 1983;106:855.

74. Maron BJ, Epstein SE, Bonow RO, Wyngaarden MK, Wesley YE. Obstructive hypertrophic cardiomyopathy associated with minimal left ventricular hypertrophy. Am J Cardiol 1984; 53:377.

75. Smolenskii AV. Asymmetric hypertrophy of the myocardium in patients with hypertension (echocardiographic data). Kardiologiia 1983;23:69.

76. Abbasi AS, Slaughter JC, Allen MW. Asymmetric septal hypertrophy in patients on long-term hemodialysis. Chest 1978;74:548.

77. Stern A, Kessler KM, Hammer WJ, Kreulen TH, Spann JF. Septal-free wall disproportion in inferior infarction: the echocardiographic differentiation from hypertrophic cardiomyopathy. Circulation 1978;58:700.

78. Hess OM, Schneider J, Turina M, Carroll JD, Rothlin M, Krayenbuehl HP. Asymmetric septal hypertrophy in patients with aortic stenosis: an adaptive mechanism or a coexistence of hypertrophic cardiomyopathy? J Am Coll Cardiol 1983;1:783.

79. Gustavson A, Liedholm H, Tylen U. Hypertrophic cardiomyopathy: a correlation between echocardiography, angiographic, and hemodynamic findings. Ann Radiol (Paris) 1977;20:419.

80. Pollick C, Rakowski H, Wigle ED. Muscular subaortic stenosis: the quantitative relationship between systolic anterior motion and the pressure gradient. Circulation 1984;69:43.

81. Maron BJ, Gottdiener JS, Perry LW. Specificity of systolic anterior motion of anterior mitral leaflet for hypertrophic cardiomyopathy. Br Heart J 1981;45:206.

82. Maron BJ, Gottdiener JS, Roberts WC, Henry WL, Savage DD, Epstein SE. Left ventricular outflow tract obstruction due to systolic anterior motion of the anterior mitral valve leaflet in patients with concentric left ventricular hypertrophy. Circulation 1978;57:527.

83. Levisman JA. Systolic anterior motion of the mitral valve due to hypovolemia and anemia. Chest 1976;70:687.

84. Schulman P, Come PC, Isaacs R, Radvany P. Left ventricular outflow obstruction induced by tamponade in hypertrophic cardiomyopathy. Chest 1981;80:110.

85. Appleton CP, Hatle LK, Popp RL. Demonstration of restrictive ventricular physiology by Doppler echocardiography. J Am Coll Cardiol 1988;11:757.

86. Sunnerhagen KS, Bhargava V, Shabetai R. Regional left ventricular wall motion abnormalities in idiopathic dilated cardiomyopathy. Am J Cardiol 1990;65:364.

87. Feigenbaum H, Waldhausen JA, Hyde LP. Ultrasound diagnosis of pericardial effusion. JAMA 1965;191:711.

88. Horowitz MS, Schultz CS, Stinson EB, Harrison DC, Popp RL. Sensitivity and specificity of echocardiographic diagnosis of pericardial effusion. Circulation 1974;50:239.

89. Schiller NB. Echocardiography in pericardial disease. Med Clin N Am 1980;64:253.

90. Parameswaran R, Goldberg H. Echocardiographic quantitation of pericardial effusion. Chest 1983;83:767.

91. Himelman RB, Kircher B, Rockey DC, Schiller NB. Inferior vena cava plethora with blunted respiratory response: a sensitive echocardiographic sign of cardiac tamponade. J Am Coll Cardiol 1988;12:1470.

92. D'Cruz IA, Cohen HC, Prabhu R, Glick G. Diagnosis of cardiac tamponade by echocardiography: changes in mitral valve motion and ventricular dimensions, with special reference to paradoxical pulse. Circulation 1974;52:460.

93. Settle HP, Adolph RJ, Fowler NO, Engel P, Agruss NS, Levenson NI. Echocardiographic study of cardiac tamponade. Circulation 1977;56:951.

94. Shiina A, Yaginuma T, Kondo K, et al. Echocardiographic evaluation of impending cardiac tamponade. J Cardiogr 1979;9: 555.

95. Vignola PA, Pohost GM, Curfman GD, Myers GS. Correlation of echocardiographic and clinical findings in patients with pericardial effusion. Am J Cardiol 1976;37:701.

96. Schiller NB, Botvinick EH. Right ventricular compression as a sign of cardiac tamponade: an analysis of echocardiographic ventricular dimensions and their clinical implications. Circulation 1977;56:774.

97. Kronzon I, Cohen ML, Winer HE. Diastolic atrial compression: a sensitive echocardiographic sign of cardiac tamponade. J Am Coll Cardiol 1983;2:770.

98. Gillam LD, Guyer DE, Gibson TC, Etta King M, Marshall JE, Weyman AE. Hemodynamic compression of the right atrium: a new echocardiographic sign of cardiac tamponade. Circulation 1983;68:294.

99. Engel PH, Hon H, Fowler ND, Plummer S. Echocardiographic study of right ventricular wall motion in cardiac tamponade. Am J Cardiol 1982;50:1018.

100. Leimgruber PP, Klopfenstein HS, Wann LS, Brooks HL. The hemodynamic derangement associated with right ventricular diastolic collapse in cardiac tamponade: an experimental echocardiographic study. Circulation 1983;68:612.

101. Armstrong WF, Schilt BF, Helper DJ, Dillon JC, Feigenbaum H. Diastolic collapse of the right ventricle with tamponade: an echocardiographic study. Circulation 1982;65:1491.

102. Rifkin RD, Pandian NG, Funai JT, et al. Sensitivity of right atrial collapse and right ventricular diastolic collapse in the diagnosis of graded cardiac tamponade. Am J Noninvas Cardiol 1987;1:73.

103. Sagar KB, Wann LS, Klopfenstein HS. Echocardiography in the diagnosis of cardiac tamponade. Echocardiography 1987; 4:29.

104. Singh S, Wann LS, Schuchard GH, et al. Right ventricular and right atrial collapse in patients with cardiac tamponade—a combined echocardiographic and hemodynamic study. Circulation 1984;6:966.

105. Shono H, Yoskikawa J, Yoshida K, et al. Value of right ventricular and right atrial collapse in identifying tamponade. J Cardiogr 1986;16:627.

106. Moreno FLL, Hagan AD, Holmen JR, Pryor TA, Stickland RD, Castle CH. Evaluation of size and dynamics of the inferior vena cava as an index of right-sided cardiac function. Am J Cardiol 1984;53:579.

107. Kircher B, Himelman RB, Schiller NB. Estimation of right atrial pressure by two-dimensional echocardiography of the respiratory behavior of the inferior vena cava (Abstract). Circulation (Suppl II) 1988;78:550.

108. Simonson JS, Schiller NB. Sonospirometry: a new method for non-invasive estimation of mean right atrial pressure based on two-dimensional echographic measurements of the inferior vena cava during measured inspiration. J Am Coll Cardiol 1988;11:557.

109. Burstow DJ, Oh JK, Bailey KR, Seward JB, Tajik AJ. Cardiac tamponade: characteristic Doppler observations. Mayo Clin Proc 1989;64:312.

110. Leeman DE, Levine MJ, Come PC. Doppler echocardiography in cardiac tamponade: exaggerated respiratory variation in transvalvular blood flow velocity integrals. J Am Coll Cardiol 1988;11:572.

111. Appleton CP, Hatle LK, Popp RL. Cardiac tamponade and pericardial effusion: respiratory variation in transvalvular flow ve-

locities studied by Doppler echocardiography. J Am Coll Cardiol 1988;11:1020.

112. Appleton CP, Hatle LK, Popp RL. Superior vena cava flow velocity patterns can diagnose cardiac tamponade in patients with pericardial effusions (Abstract). J Am Coll Cardiol (Suppl) 1987;9:118A.

113. Linden RW, Byrd BF. Superior vena cava Doppler flow patterns in cardiac tamponade and pericardial constriction. Clin Res 1987;36:105A.

114. Choong CY, Herrmann HC, Weyman AE, Fifer MA. Preload dependence of Doppler-derived indexes of left ventricular diastolic function in humans. J Am Coll Cardiol 1987;10:800.

115. Hoit B, Sahn DJ, Shabetai R. Doppler-detected paradoxus of mitral and tricuspid valve flows in chronic lung disease. J Am Coll Cardiol 1986;8:706.

116. Antman EM, Cargill V, Grossman W. Low pressure cardiac tamponade. Ann Intern Med 1979;91:403.

117. Tassi AA, Davies AL. Pericardial tamponade due to penetrating fragment wounds of the heart. Am J Surg 1969;118:535.

118. Labib SB, Udelson JE, Pandian NG. Echocardiography in low pressure cardiac tamponade. Am J Cardiol 1989;63:1156.

119. Fowler NO. Inferior vena cava plethora as an echocardiographic sign of cardiac tamponade (Editorial). J Am Coll Cardiol 1988;12:1478.

120. Levine MJ, Lorell BH, Diver DJ, Come PC. Low-pressure tamponade identified by echocardiography: hemodynamic results and outcome after pericardiocentesis (Abstract). Circulation 1988;78:II-472.

121. D'Cruz I, Kensey K, Campbell C, Replogle R, Jain M. Two-dimensional echocardiography in cardiac tamponade occurring after cardiac surgery. J Am Coll Cardiol 1985;5:1250.

122. Cliff WJ, Grobety J, Ryan GE. Postoperative pericardial adhesions: the role of mild serosal injury and spilled blood. J Thorac Cardiovasc Surg 1973;65:744.

123. Fowler NO, Gabel M. The hemodynamic effects of cardiac tamponade: mainly the result of atrial, not ventricular compression. Circulation 1985;71:154.

124. Fowler, NO, Gabel M. Regional cardiac tamponade: a hemodynamic study. J Am Coll Cardiol 1987;10:164.

125. Fowler NO, Gabel M, Buncher B. Cardiac tamponade: a comparison of right versus left heart compression. J Am Coll Cardiol 1988;12:187.

126. Sagrista-Sauleda J, Permanyer Mirald G, Candell-Riera J, Angel J, Soler-Soler J. Transient cardiac constriction: an unrecognized pattern of evolution in effusive acute idiopathic pericarditis. Am J Cardiol 1987;59:961.

127. Himelman RB, Lee E, Schiller NB. Septal bounce, vena cava plethora, and pericardial adhesion: informative two-dimensional echocardiographic signs in the diagnosis of pericardial constriction. J Am Soc Echo 1988;1:333.

128. Gaffney FA, Keller AM, Peshock RM, Lin J, Firth BG. Pathophysiologic mechanisms of cardiac tamponade and pulsus alternans shown by echocardiography. Am J Cardiol 1984;53:1662.

129. Frey MJ, Berko B, Palevsky H, Hirshfeld JW, Herrmann HC. Recognition of cardiac tamponade in the presence of severe pulmonary hypertension. Ann Intern Med 1989;111:615.

130. Callahan JA, Seward JB, Nishimura RA, et al. Two-dimensional echocardiographically guided pericardiocentesis: experiment in 117 consecutive patients. Am J Cardiol 1985;55:476.

131. Meaney E, Shabetai R, Bhargava V, et al. Cardiac amyloidosis, constrictive pericarditis, and restrictive cardiomyopathy. Am J Cardiol 1976;38:547.

132. Benotti JR, Grossman W, Cohn PF. Clinical profile of restrictive cardiomyopathy. Circulation 1980;61:1206.

133. Wann LS, Weyman AE, Dillon JC, Feigenbaum H. Premature pulmonary valve opening. Circulation 1977;55:128.

134. Voelkel AG, Pietro DA, Folland ED, Fisher ML, Parisi AF. Echocardiographic features of constrictive pericarditis. Circulation 1978;58:871.

135. Pool PE, Seagren SC, Abbasi AS, Chariszi Y, Kraus R. Echocardiographic manifestations of constrictive pericarditis. Chest 1975;68:684.

136. Gibson TC, Grossman W, McLaurin LP, Moos S, Craige E. An echocardiographic study of the interventricular septum in constrictive pericarditis. Br Heart J 1976;38:738.

137. Candel-Riera J, Del Castillo HG, Permanyer-Miraldo G, Soler-Soler J. Echocardiographic features of the interventricular septum in chronic constrictive pericarditis. Circulation 1978;57:1154.

138. Tei C, Child JS, Hiromitsu T, Shah PM. Atrial systolic notch on the interventricular septal echogram: an echocardiographic sign of constrictive pericarditis. J Am Coll Cardiol 1983;1:907.

139. Chandaratna PAN. Uses and limitations of echocardiography in the evaluation of pericardial disease. Echocardiography 1984; 1:55.

140. Engel PJ, Fowler NO, Tei C, et al. M-Mode echocardiography in constrictive pericarditis. J Am Coll Cardiol 1985;6:471.

141. Lewis BS. Real time two dimensional echocardiography in constrictive pericarditis. Am J Cardiol 1982;49:1789.

142. Zaky A, Nasser WK, Feigenbaum H. Study of mitral valve action recorded by reflected ultrasound and its application in the diagnosis of mitral stenosis. Circulation 1968;37:789.

143. Nichol PM, Gilbert BW, Kisslo JA. Two-dimensional echocardiographic assessment of mitral stenosis. Circulation 1977; 55:120.

144. Martin RP, Rakowski H, Kleiman JH, Beaver W, London E, Popp RL. Reliability and reproducibility of two dimensional echocardiographic measuresment of the stenotic mitral valve orifice area. Am J Cardiol 1979;43:560.

145. Wann LS, Weyman AE, Feigenbaum H, Dillon JC, Hohnston KW, Eggleton RC. Determination of mitral valve area by cross-sectional echocardiography. Ann Intern Med 1978;88:337.

146. Henry WL, Griffith JM, Michaelis LL, McIntosh CL, Morrow AG, Epstein SE. Measurement of mitral orifice area in patients with mitral valve disease by real-time two-dimensional echocardiography. Circulation 1975;51:827.

147. Hatle L, Brubakk A, Tromsdal A, Angelsen B. Noninvasive assessment of pressure drop in mitral stenosis by Doppler ultrasound. Br Heart J 1978;40:131.

148. Hatle L, Angelsen B, Tromsdal A. Noninvasive assessment of atrioventricular pressure half-time by Doppler ultrasound. Circulation 1979;60:1096.

149. Holen J, Aaslid R, Landmark K, Simonsen S, Ostrem T. Determination of effective orifice area in mitral stenosis from non-invasive ultrasound Doppler data and mitral flow rate. Acta Med Scand 1977;201:83.

150. Nishimura RA, Miller FA, Callahan MJ, Benassi RC, Seward JB, Tajik AJ. Doppler echocardiography: theory, instrumentation, technique, and application. Mayo Clin Proc 1985;60:321.

151. Nakatani S, Masuyama T, Kodama K, et al. Value and limitations of Doppler echocardiography in the quantification of stenotic mitral valve area: comparison of the pressure half-time and the continuity equation methods. Circulation 1988;77:78.

152. Khandheria BK, Tajik AJ, Reeder GS, et al. Doppler color flow imaging: a new technique for visualization and characterization of the blood flow jet in mitral stenosis. Mayo Clin Proc 1986;61:623.

153. Kawahara T, Tamai J, Mitani M, Seo H, Yamagishi M, Miyatake K. A new method for determination of mitral valve area in

mitral stenosis by color Doppler flow imaging technique (Abstract). Circulation 1989;80:II-669.

154. Rodriguez L, Levine RA, Monterroso VH, et al. Validation of valve area calculation using the proximal isovelocity surface area in patients with mitral stenosis: a color Doppler study (Abstract). Circulation 1989;80:II-677.

155. Kerber RE, Isaeff DM, Hancock EW. Echocardiographic patterns in patients with the syndrome of systolic click and late systolic murmur. N Engl J Med 1971;284:691.

156. Nishimura RA, McGoon MD, Shub C, Miller FA, Ilstrup DM, Tajik AJ. Echocardiographically documented mitral-valve prolapse: long-term follow-up of 237 patients. N Engl J Med 1985; 313:1305.

157. Waller BF, Morrow AG, Maron BJ, et al. Etiology of clinically isolated, severe, chronic, pure mitral regurgitation: analysis of 97 patients over 30 years of age having mitral valve replacement. Am Heart J 1982;104:276.

158. Olson LJ, Subramanian R, Ackermann DM, Orszulak TA, Edwards WD. Surgical pathology of the mitral valve: a study of 712 cases spanning 21 years. Mayo Clin Proc 1987;62:22.

159. Levine RA, Triulzi MO, Harrigan P, Weyman AE. The relationship of mitral annular shape to the diagnosis of mitral valve prolapse. Circulation 1987;75:756.

160. Galve E, Candell-Riera J, Pigrau C, et al. Prevalence, morphologic types, and evolution of cardiac valvular disease in systemic lupus erythematosus. N Engl J Med 1988;319:817.

161. Wann LS, Feigenbaum H, Weyman AE, Dillon JC. Crosssectional echocardiographic detection of rheumatic mitral regurgitation. Am J Cardiol 1978;41:1258.

162. Ren JF, Kotler MN, DePace NL, et al. Two-dimensional echocardiographic determination of left atrial emptying volume: a non-invasive index in quantifying the degree of nonrheumatic mitral regurgitation. J Am Coll Cardiol 1983;2:729.

163. Gehl LG, Mintz GS, Kotler MN, Segal BL. Left atrial volume overload in mitral regurgitation: a two-dimensional echocardiographic study. Am J Cardiol 1982;49:33.

164. Fujino T, Ito M, Kanaya S, et al. Echocardiographic abnormal motion of interventricular septum in mitral insufficiency. J Cardiogr 1976;6:613.

165. Schuler G, Peterson KL, Johnson A, et al. Temporal response of left ventricular performance to mitral valve surgery. Circulation 1979;59:1218.

166. Borow KM, Green LH, Mann T, et al. End-systolic volume as a predictor of postoperative left ventricular performance in volume overload from valvular regurgitation. Am J Med 1980; 68:665.

167. Zile MR, Gaasch WH, Carrol JD, Levine HJ. Chronic mitral regurgitation: predictive value of preoperative echocardiographic indices of left ventricular function and wall stress. J Am Coll Cardiol 1984;3:235.

168. Kalmanson D, Veyrat C, Bouchareine F, Degroote A. Noninvasive recording of mitral valve flow velocity patterns using pulsed Doppler echocardiography: application to diagnosis and evaluation of mitral valve disease. Br Heart J 1977;39:517.

169. Baker DW, Rubenstein SA, Lorch GS. Pulse Doppler echocardiography: principles and applications. Am J Med 1977;63:69.

170. Miyatake K, Kinoshita N, Nagata S, et al. Intracardiac flow pattern in mitral regurgitation studied with combined use of the ultrasonic pulsed Doppler technique and cross-sectional echocardiography. Am J Cardiol 1980;45:155.

171. Hatle L, Angelsen B. Doppler ultrasound in cardiology: physical principles and clinical applications. 2nd ed. Philadelphia: Lea & Febiger, 1985:176.

172. Blumlein S, Bouchard A, Schiller NB, et al. Quantitation of mitral regurgitation by Doppler echocardiography. Circulation 1986;74:306.

173. Helmcke F, Nanda NC, Hsiung MC, et al. Color Doppler assessment of mitral regurgitation using orthogonal planes. Circulation 1987;75:175.

174. Miyatake K, Izumi S, Okamoto M, et al. Semiquantitative grading of severity of mitral regurgitation by real-time two-dimensional Doppler flow imaging technique. J Am Coll Cardiol 1986;7:82.

175. Yoshida K, Yoshikawa J, Shakudo M, et al. Color Doppler evaluation of valvular regurgitation in normal subjects. Circulation 1988;78:840.

176. Kececioglu-Draelos Z, Goldberg SJ. Role of M-mode echocardiography in congenital aortic stenosis. Am J Cardiol 1981;47: 1267.

177. Weyman AE, Feigenbaum H, Dillon JC, Chang S. Crosssectional echocardiography in assessing the severity of valvular aortic stenosis. Circulation 1975;52:828.

178. DeMaria AN, Bommer W, Joye J, Lee G, Bouteller J, Mason DT. Value and limitations of cross-sectional echocardiography of the aortic valve in the diagnosis and quantification of the valvular aortic stenosis. Circulation 1980;62:304.

179. Hatle L, Angelsen BA, Tromsdal A. Noninvasive assessment of aortic stenosis by Doppler ultrasound. Br Heart J 1980;43:284.

180. Stamm RB, Martin RP. Quantification of pressure gradients across stenotic valves by Doppler ultrasound. J Am Coll Cardiol 1983;2:707.

181. Nishumura R, Miller F, Callahan M, et al. Doppler echocardiography: theory, instrumentation, technique, and application. Mayo Clin Proc 1985;60:321.

182. Teirstein P, Yock P, Popp R. The accuracy of Doppler ultrasound measurement of pressure gradients across irregular, dual, and tunnel like obstructions to blood flow. Circulation 1985; 72:557.

183. Nitta M, Nakamura TO, Hultgren HN, Bilisoly J, Tovey DA. Progression of aortic stenosis in adult men: detection by noninvasive methods. Chest 1987;92:40.

184. Williams G, Labovitz A, Nelson J, Kennedy H. Value of multiple echocardiographic views in the evaluation of aortic stenosis in adults by continuous-wave Doppler. Am J Cardiol 1985;55: 445.

185. Otto CM, Pearlman AS. Doppler echocardiography in adults with symptomatic aortic stenosis: diagnostic utility and cost-effectiveness. Arch Intern Med 1988;148:2553.

186. Otto CM, Pearlman AS, Comess KA, et al. Determination of the stenotic aortic valve area in adults using Doppler echocardiography. J Am Coll Cardiol 1986;7:509.

187. Fan PH, Kapur KK, Nanda NC. Color-guided echocardiographic assessment of aortic valve stenosis. J Am Coll Cardiol 1988; 12:441.

188. Nishimura RA, Tajik AJ, Reeder GS, Seward JB. Evaluation of hypertrophic cardiomyopathy by Doppler color flow imaging: initial observations. Mayo Clin Proc 1986;61:631.

189. Blazer D, Kotler MN, Parry WR, Wertheimer J, Nakhjavan FK. Noninvasive evaluation of mid-left ventricular obstruction by two-dimensional and Doppler echocardiography and color flow Doppler echocardiography. Am Heart J 1987;114:1162.

190. Friedman DM, Schmer V, Rutkowski M. Two-dimensional color Doppler in discrete membranous subaortic stenosis. Am Heart J 1988;115:686.

191. D'Cruz I, Cohen HC, Prabhu R, Ayabe T, Click G. Flutter of left ventricular structures in patients with aortic regurgitation, with special reference to patients with aortic regurgitation. Am Heart J 1976;9:684.

192. Skorton DJ, Child JS, Perloff JK. Accuracy of the echocardiographic diagnosis of aortic regurgitation. Am J Med 1980; 69:377.

193. Mann T, McLaurin L, Grossman W, Craige E. Assessing the

hemodynamic severity of acute aortic regurgitation due to infective endocarditis. N Engl J Med 1975;293:108.

194. Henry WL, Bonow RO, Borer JS, et al. Observations on the optimum time for operative intervention for aortic regurgitation. I. Evaluation of the results of aortic valve replacement in symptomatic patients. Circulation 1980;61:471.

195. Henry WL, Bonow RO, Rosing DR, Epstein SE. Observations on the optimum time for operative intervention for aortic regurgitation. II. Serial echocardiographic evaluation of asymptomatic patients. Circulation 1980;61:484.

196. Schuler G, Peterson KL, Johnson AD, et al. Serial noninvasive assessment of left ventricular hypertrophy and function after surgical correction of aortic regurgitation. Am J Cardiol 1979;44:585.

197. Stone PH, Clark RD, Goldschlager N, Selzer A, Cohn K. Determinants of prognosis of patients with aortic regurgitation who undergo aortic valve replacement. J Am Coll Cardiol 1984;3:1118.

198. McDonald IG, Jelinek VM. Serial M-mode echocardiography in severe chronic aortic regurgitation. Circulation 1980;62:1291.

199. Richards KL, Cannon SR, Crawford MH, Sorensen SG. Noninvasive diagnosis of aortic and mitral valve disease with pulsed-Doppler spectral analysis. Am J Cardiol 1983;51:1122.

200. Ciobanu M, Abbasi AS, Allen M, Hermer A, Spellberg R. Pulsed Doppler echocardiography in the diagnosis and estimation of severity of aortic insufficiency. Am J Cardiol 1982;49:339.

201. Quinones MA, Young JB, Waggoner AD, Ostojic MC, Ribeiro LGT, Miller RR. Assessment of pulsed Dopper echocardiography in detection and quantification of aortic and mitral regurgitation. Br Heart J 1980;44:612.

202. Veyrat C, Cholot N, Abitbol G, Kalmanson D. Non-invasive diagnosis and assessment of aortic valve disease and evaluation of aortic prosthesis function using echo pulsed Doppler velocimetry. Br Heart J 1980;43:393.

203. Diebold B, Peronneau P, Blanchard D, et al. Non-invasive quantification of aortic regurgitation by Doppler echocardiography. Br Heart J 1983;49:1667.

204. Teague SM, Heinsimer JA, Anderson JL, et al. Quantification of aortic regurgitation utilizing continuous wave Doppler ultrasound. J Am Coll Cardiol 1986;8:592.

205. Teague SM, Marty W, Saadatmanesh V, et al. The effect of mean pressure gradient, chamber compliance, and orifice size upon the Doppler halftime method (Abstract). J Am Coll Cardiol 1988;11:204A.

206. Masuyama T, Kitabatake A, Kodama K, Uematsu M, Nakatani S, Kamada T. Semiquantitative evaluation of aortic regurgitation by Doppler echocardiography: effects of associated mitral stenosis. Am Heart J 1989;117:133.

207. Perry GJ, Helmcke F, Nanda NC, Byard C, Soto B. Evaluation of aortic insufficiency by Doppler color flow mapping. J Am Coll Cardiol 1987;9:952.

208. Bouchard A, Yock P, Schiller NB, et al. Value of color Doppler estimation of regurgitant volume in patients with chronic aortic insufficiency. Am Heart J 1989;117:1099.

209. Himelman RB, Schiller NB. Clinical and echocardiographic comparison of patients with the carcinoid syndrome with and without carcinoid heart diseae. Am J Cardiol 1989;63:347.

210. Lundin L, Norheim I, Landelius J, Oberg K, Theodorsson-Norheim E. Carcinoid heart disease: relationship of circulating vasoactive substances to ultrasound-detectable cardiac abnormalities. Circulation 1988;77:264.

211. Waggoner AD, Quinones MA, Young JB, et al. Pulsed Dopper echocardiographic detection of right-sided valve regurgitation: experimental results and clinical significance. Am J Cardiol 1981;47:279.

212. Miyatake K, Okamoto M, Kinoshita N, et al. Evaluation of tricuspid regurgitation by pulsed Doppler and two-dimensional echocardiography. Circulation 1982;66:777.

213. Suzuki Y, Kambara H, Kadota K, et al. Detection and evaluation of tricuspid regurgitation using a real-time, two-dimensional, color-coded Doppler flow imaging system: comparison with contrast two-dimensional echocardiography and right ventriculography. Am J Cardiol 1986;57:811.

214. Fisher EA, Goldman ME. Simple, rapid method for quantification of tricuspid regurgitation by two-dimensional echocardiography. Am J Cardiol 1989;63:1375.

215. Johnson ML, Holmes JH, Paton BC. Echocardiographic determination of mitral disc valve excursion. Circulation 1973;47:1274.

216. Siggers DC, Srivongse SA, Deuchar D. Analysis of dynamics of mitral Starr-Edward valve prosthesis using reflected ultrasound. Br Heart J 1971;33:401.

217. Ben-Zvi J, Hildner FJ, Chandraratna PA, Samet P. Thrombosis on Bjork-Shiley aortic valve prosthesis: clinical, arteriographic, echocardiographic, and therapeutic observation in seven cases. Am J Cardiol 1974;34:538.

218. Copans H, Lakier JB, Kinsley RH, Colsen PR, Fritz VU, Barlow JB. Thrombosed Bjork-Shiley mitral prostheses. Circulation 1980;61:169.

219. Nagata S, Park YD, Nagae K, et al. Echocardiographic features of bioprosthetic endocarditis. Br Heart J 1984;51:263.

220. Effron MK, Popp RL, Filly K, Pittman M, Briskin G. Two-dimensional echocardiographic assessment of bioprosthetic valve dysfunction and infective endocarditis. J Am Coll Cardiol 1983;2:597.

221. Alam M, Goldstein S, Lakier JB. Echocardiographic changes in the thickness of porcine valves with time. Chest 1981;79:663.

222. Bansal RC, Morrisson DL, Jacobsen JG. Echocardiography of porcine aortic prostheses with flail leaflets due to degeneration and calcification. Am Herat J 1984;107:591.

223. Holen J, Simonsen S, Froysaker T. An ultrasound technique for the noninvasive determination of the pressure gradient in the Bjork-Shiley mitral valve. Circulation 1979;59:436.

224. Ramirez ML, Wong M, Sadler N, Shahu PM. Doppler evaluation of bioprosthetic and mechanical aortic valves: data from four models in 107 stable, ambulatory patients. Am Heart J 1988;115:418.

225. Wilkins GT, Gillam LD, Kritzer GL, Levine RA, Palacios IF, Weyman AE. Validation of continuous-wave Doppler echocardiographic measurements of mitral and tricuspid prosthetic valve gradients: a simultaneous Doppler-catheter study. Circulation 1986;74:786.

226. Weinstein IR, Marbarger P, Perez JE. Ultrasonic assessment of the St. Jude prosthetic valve: M mode, two-dimensional, and Doppler echocardiography. Circulation 1983;68:897.

227. Panidis IP, Ross J, Mintz GS. Normal and abnormal prosthetic valve function as assessed by Doppler echocardiography. J Am Coll Cardiol 1986;8:317.

228. Vandenberg BF, Dellsperger KC, Chandran KB, Kerber RE. Detection, localization, and quantitation of bioprosthetic mitral valve regurgitation: an in vitro two-dimensional color-Doppler flow-mapping study. Circulation 1988;78:529.

229. Kapur F, Fan P, Nanda NC, Yoganathan AP, Goyal RG. Doppler color flow mapping in the evaluation of prosthetic mitral and aortic valve function. J Am Coll Cardiol 1989;13:1561.

230. Jones M, Eidbo EE. Doppler color flow evaluation of prosthetic mitral valves: experimental epicardial studies. J Am Coll Cardiol 1989;13:234.

231. Nellessen U, Schnittger I, Appleton CP, et al. Transesophageal two-dimensional echocardiography and color Doppler velocity mapping in the evaluation of cardiac valve prostheses. Circulation 1988;78:848.

232. Himelman RB, Abbott JA, Schiller NB. Diagnosis of mediastinal lesions by two-dimensional echocardiography. Echocardiography 1988;5:219.

233. Martin RP, Meltzer RS, Chia BL, Stinson EB, Rakowski H, Popp RL. Clinical utility of two-dimensional echocardiography in infective endocarditis. Am J Cardiol 1980;46:379.

234. Hickey AJ, Wolfer J, Wilcken DEL. Reliability and clinical relevance of detection of vegetations by echocardiography in bacterial endocarditis. Br Heart J 1981;46:624.

235. Wann LS, Dillon JC, Weyman AE, Feigenbaum H. Echocardiography in bacterial endocarditis. N Engl J Med 1976;295:135.

236. Thompson KR, Nanda NC, Gramiak R. The reliability of echocardiography in the diagnosis of infective endocarditis. Radiology 1977;125:373.

237. Stratton JR, Werner JA, Pearlman AS, Janko CL, Kliman S, Jackson MC. Bacteremia and the heart: serial echocardiographic findings in 80 patients with documented or suspected bacteremia. Am J Med 1983;73:851.

238. Rubenson DS, Tucker CR, Stinson EB, et al. The use of echocardiography in diagnosing culture-negative endocarditis. Circulation 1981;64:641.

239. Sweatmen T, Selzer A, Kamagaki M, Cohn K. Echocardiographic diagnosis of mitral regurgitation due to ruptured chordae tendineae. Circulation 1972;46:580.

240. Mintz GS, Kotler MN, Segal BL, Parry WR. Two-dimensional echocardiographic recognition of ruptured chordae tendineae. Circulation 1978;57:244.

241. Child JS, Skorton DJ, Taylor RD, et al. M-mode and cross-sectional echocardiographic features of flail posterior mitral leaflets. Am J Cardiol 1979;44:1383.

242. Ballester M, Foale R, Presbitero P, Yacoub M, Rickards A, McDonald L. Cross-sectional echocardiographic features of ruptured chordae tendineae. Eur Heart J 1983;4:795.

243. Miyatake K, Yamamoto K, Park YD, et al. Diagnosis of mitral valve perforation by real-time two-dimensional Doppler flow imaging technique. J Am Coll Cardiol 1986;8:1235.

244. Chow LC, Dittrich HC, Dembitsky WP, Nicod PH. Accurate localization of ruptured sinus of valsalva aneurysm by real-time two-dimensional Doppler flow imaging. Chest 1988;94:462.

245. Wann LS, Faris JV, Childress RH, Dillon JC, Weyman AE, Feigenbaum H. Exercise cross-sectional echocardiography in ischemic heart disease. Circulation 1979;60:1300.

246. Crawford MH, Amon KW, Vance WS. Exercise 2-dimensional echocardiography: quantitation of left ventricular performance in patients with severe angina pectoris. Am J Cardiol 1983;51:1.

247. Armstrong WF, O'Donnel J, Dillon JC, McHenry PL, Morris SN, Feigenbaum H. Complementary value of two-dimensional exercise echocardiography to routine treadmill exercise testing. Ann Intern Med 1986;105:829.

248. Limacher MC, Quinones MA, Poliner LR, Nelson JG, Winters WL Jr, Waggoner AD. Detection of coronary artery disease with exercise two-dimensional echocardiography: description of a clinically applicable method and comparison with radionuclide ventriculography. Circulation 1983;67:1211.

249. Ryan T, Vasey CG, Presti CF, et al. Exercise echocardiography: detection of coronary artery disease in patients with normal left ventricular wall motion at rest. J Am Coll Cardiol 1988;11:993.

250. Ryan T, Armstrong WF, O'Donnell JA, Feigenbaum H. Risk stratification after acute myocardial infarction by means of exercise two-dimensional echocardiography. Am Heart J 1987;114:1305

251. Harrison MR, Smith MD, Friedman BJ, DeMaria AN. Uses and limitations of exercise Doppler echocardiography in the diagnosis of ischemic heart disease. J Am Coll Cardiol 1987;10:809.

252. Mehta N, Boyle G, Bennett D, et al. Hemodynamic response to treadmill exercise in normal volunteers: an assessment by Doppler ultrasonic measurement of ascending aortic blood velocity and acceleration. Am Heart J 1988;116:1298.

253. Mehdirad AA, Williams GA, Labovitz AJ, Bryg RJ, Chaitman BR. Evaluation of left ventricular function during upright exercise: correlation of exercise Doppler with postexercise two-dimensional echocardiographic results. Circulation 1987;75:413.

254. Maeda M, Yokota M, Iwase M, Miyahara T, Hayashi H, Sotobata I. Accuracy of cardiac output measured by continuous wave Doppler echocardiography during dynamic exercise testing in the supine position in patients with coronary artery disease. J Am Coll Cardiol 1989;13:76.

255. Lazarus M, Dang TY, Gardin JM, Allfie A, Henry WL. Evaluation of age, gender, heart rate and blood pressure changes and exercise conditioning on Doppler measured aortic blood flow, acceleration, and velocity during upright treadmill testing. Am J Cardiol 1988;62:439.

256. Harrison MR, Smith MD, Nissen SE, Grayburn PA, DeMaria AN. Use of exercise Doppler echocardiography to evaluate cardiac drugs: effects of propranolol and verapamil on aortic blood flow velocity and acceleration. J Am Coll Cardiol 1988;11:1002.

257. Martin GR, Soifer SJ, Silverman NH, Dae MW, Stanger P. Effects of activity on ascending aortic velocity in children with valvar aortic stenosis. Am J Cardiol 1987;59:1386.

258. Mitchell GD, Brunken RC, Schwaiger M, Donohue BC, Krivokapich J, Child JS. Assessment of mitral flow velocity with exercise by an index of stress-induced left ventricular ischemia in coronary artery disease. Am J Cardiol 1988;61:536.

259. Zachariah ZP, Hsiung MC, Nanda NC, Kan M, Gatewood RP. Color Doppler assessment of mitral regurgitation induced by supine exercise in patients with coronary artery disease. Am J Cardiol 1987;59:1266.

260. Tamai J, Nagata S, Akaike M, et al. Improvement in mitral flow dynamics using exercise after percutaneous transvenous mitral commissurotomy: noninvasive evaluation using continuous wave Doppler technique. Circulation 1990;81:46.

261. Himelman RB, Stulbarg MS, Kircher B, et al. Noninvasive evaluation of pulmonary pressure during exercise by saline-enhanced Doppler echocardiography in chronic pulmonary disease. Circulation 1989;79:863.

262. Schluter M, Hanrath P. Transesophageal echocardiography: potential advantages and initial clinical results. Pract Cardiol 1983;9:149.

263. Hisanaga K, Hisanaga A, Nagata K, Ichi Y. Transesophageal cross-sectional echocardiography. Am Heart J 1980;100:605.

264. Schluter M, Langenstein BA, Polster J, et al. Transesophageal cross-sectional echocardiography with phased array transducer system: technique and initial clinical results. Br Heart J 1982;48:67.

265. Schiller NB, Maurer G, Ritter SB, et al. American Society of Echocardiography Committee on Special Procedures: statement on transesophageal echocardiography. J Am Soc Echo 1989;2:354.

266. Schluter M, Hinrichs A, Their W, et al. Transesophageal two-dimensional echocardiography: comparison of ultrasonic and anatomic sections. Am J Cardiol 1984;53:1173.

267. Beppu S, Nakatani S, Tanaka N, et al. Transesophageal echocardiographic diagnosis of localized pericardial coagula: a special cause of cardiac tamponade (Abstract). Circulation (Suppl II) 1988;78:299.

268. Chan KL. Transesophageal echocardiography in the management of intubated cardiac patients (Abstract). Circulation (Suppl II) 1988;78:299.

269. Cucchiara RF, Nugent M, Seward JB, Messick JM. Air embolism in upright neurosurgical patients: detection and localization by

two-dimensional transesophageal echocardiography. Anesthesiology 1984;60:353.

270. Matsumoto M, Oka Y, Strom J, et al. Application of transesophageal echocardiography to continuous intraoperative monitoring of left ventricular performance. Am J Cardiol 1980; 46:95.

271. Cahalan MK, Kremer PF, Beaupre PN, et al. Intraoperative myocardial ischemia detected by transesophageal 2-dimensional echocardiography. Anesthesiology 1983;59:3.

272. Beaupre PN, Cahalan MK, Kremer PF, et al. Does pulmonary artery occlusion pressure adequately reflect left ventricular filling during anesthesia and surgery? Anesthesiology 1983; 59:3.

273. Beaupre PN, Roizen MF, Cahalan MK, et al. Hemodynamic and two-dimensional echocardiographic analysis of an anaphylactic reaction in a human. Anesthesiology 1984;60:482.

274. Beaupre PN, Kremer PF, Cahalan MK, et al. Intraoperative detection of changes in left ventricular segmental wall motion by transesophageal echocardiography (Abstract). Am Heart J 1984;107(I):1081.

275. Smith JS, Cahalan MK, Benefiel DJ, et al. Intraoperative detection of myocardial ischemia in high risk patients: electrocardiography vs two-dimensional transesophageal echocardiography. Circulation 1985;72:1015.

276. Shively B, Watters T, Benefiel D, et al. The intraoperative detection of myocardial infarction by transesophageal echocardiography (Abstract). J Am Coll Cardiol 1986;7A:2.

277. Topol EJ, Humphrey LS, Blanck TJJ, et al. Characterization of post-cardiopulmonary bypass hypotension with intraoperative transesophageal echocardiography. Anesthesiology 1983;59:3.

278. Martin RW, Colley PS. Evaluation of transesophageal Doppler detection of air embolism in dogs. Anesthesiology 1983;59:3.

279. Furuya H, Suzuki T, Okumura F, et al. Detection of air embolism by transesophageal echocardiography. Anesthesiology 1983;58:124.

280. Mohr-Kahaly S, Erbel R, Rennollet H, et al. Ambulatory follow-up of aortic dissection by transesophageal two-dimensional and color-coded Doppler echocardiography. Circulation 1989; 80:24.

281. Borner N, Erbel R, Braun B, Henkel B, Meyer J, Rumpelt J. Diagnosis of aortic dissection by transesophageal echocardiography. Am J Cardiol 1984;54:1157.

282. Aschenberg W, Schlüter M, Kremer P, Schroder E, Siglow V, Bleifeld W. Transesophageal two-dimensional echocardiography for the detection of left atrial appendage thrombus. J Am Coll Cardiol 1986;7:163.

283. Zenker G, Erbel R, Dramer G, et al. Transesophageal two-dimensional echocardiography in young patients with cerebral ischemic events. Stroke 1988;19:345.

284. Obeid AI, Marvasti M, Parker F, Rosenberg J. Comparison of transthoracic and transesophageal echocardiography in diagnosis of left atrial myxoma. Am J Cardiol 1989;63:1006.

285. Taams MA, Gussenhoven EJ, Cahalan MK, et al. Transesophageal Doppler color flow imaging in the detection of native and Bjork-Shiley mitral valve regurgitation. J Am Coll Cardiol 1989;13:95.

286. Lee E, Kee L, Schiler NB. Transesophageal echocardiography and color flow imaging assessment of prosthetic and native valve dysfunction (Abstract). Circulation (Suppl II) 1988; 78:607.

287. Shylman ST, Amren DP, Bisno AL, et al. Prevention of bacterial endocarditis: a statement for health professionals by the Committee on Rheumatic Fever and Infective Endocarditis of the Council on Cardiovascular Disease in the Young. Circulation 1984;70:1123A.

288. Daniel WG, Schroder E, Mugge A, Licthen PR. Transesophageal echocardiography in infective endocarditis. Am J Cardiac Imaging 1988;2:78.

289. Erbel R, Rohmann S, Drexel M, et al. Improved diagnostic value of echocardiography in patients with infective endocarditis by transesophageal approach: a prospective study. Eur Heart J 1988;9:43.

290. Schluter M, Kremer P, Hanrath P. Transesophageal 2-D echocardiographic feature of flail mitral leaflet due to ruptured chordae tendineae. Am Heart J 1984;108:609.

291. Czer LSC, Maurer G, Bolger AF, et al. Intraoperative evaluation of mitral regurgitation by Doppler color flow mapping. Circulation (Suppl III) 1987;76:III108.

292. Maurer G, Czer LSC, Chaux A, et al. Intraoperative Doppler color flow mapping for assessment of valve repair for mitral regurgitation. Am J Cardiol 1987;60:333.

293. Taams MA, Gussenhoven EJ, Cornel JH, et al. Detection of left coronary artery stenosis by transesophageal echocardiography. Eur Heart J 1988;9:1162.

294. Zwicky P, Daniel WG, Mugge A, Lichtlen PR. Imaging of coronaries by color-coded transesophageal Doppler echocardiography. Am J Cardiol 1988;62:639.

295. Yamagishi M, Miyatake K, Beppu S, et al. Assessment of coronary blood flow by transesophageal two-dimensional pulsed Doppler echocardiography. Am J Cardiol 1988;62:641.

Chapter 13

Echocardiography of Congenital Heart Disease

Christian E. Hardy

James G. Sullivan

Over the past decade, improvements in two-dimensional echocardiography, Doppler echocardiography, and color Doppler technology have dramatically advanced the non-invasive approach to the diagnosis and management of congenital and acquired heart disease. In many cases these noninvasive studies eliminate the need for invasive cardiac catheterization. Two-dimensional echocardiography can define cardiac anatomy and evaluate regional wall motion and ventricular function. Doppler echocardiography detects abnormal flows resulting from valve stenosis and, using the Bernoulli principle, estimates peak instantaneous gradients across these valves, determines the presence and severity of valve regurgitation, and estimates pulmonary-to-systemic flow ratios in left-to-right shunting lesions. Color-flow Doppler echocardiography combines the principles of both two-dimensional and Doppler echocardiography.

This chapter reviews basic echocardiography and Doppler echocardiography and examines the approach to the pediatric patient. Emphasis is initially on the normal examination and is followed by several examples of abnormal cardiac anatomy.

Basic Principles

A two-dimensional echocardiographic picture is made of multiple separate planes of ultrasound reflected from the heart. Early two-dimensional echocardiography employed a single large piezoelectric crystal that was rocked from side to side through the multiple planes of a sector by mechanical means. As the crystal passed through these planes it was electrically stimulated to generate individual ultrasound waves and receive the reflected waves from the cardiac structures.

Newer technology of phased and annular array employ the use of multiple stationary crystals. Each plane of the sector is the function of an individual piezoelectric crystal. Multiple crystals are electrically stimulated with a short burst of electricity, causing them to oscillate and send off ultrasound waves. This stimulation occurs in a sequential or phased order with a slight time delay between firings.

After each crystal emits an ultrasound wave it becomes a receiver for the reflected sound waves. These reflected waves stimulate the (now receiving) crystal. The crystal transforms the information from reflected waves to electrical impulses. The processing circuitry then sends these individual lines of information to the scan converter, which assembles them into a predetermined position on the video display. These assembled lines of information collectively make up a frame of the two-dimensional echocardiographic picture. Multiple frames of information displayed in rapid succession allows the two-dimensional images to be displayed in real time.

Technique

Two-dimensional echocardiography in children is performed from multiple acoustic windows, including the subcostal, apical, parasternal, and suprasternal. The subcostal window has the advantage of using the liver as an echo window, which allows for finer resolution and detail. This window also allows the entire heart to be visualized in contrast to parasternal windows, which are hindered by overlying lung tissue. Subxyphoid imaging may not be possible in the older patient because of the depth the echo beam must travel, resulting in poor picture resolution.

Two-dimensional echo is best done using sweeps of the transducer rather than single tomographic views. This allows precise anterior/posterior, superior/inferior, and left/right orientation of normal and abnormal anatomy. All sweeps are performed from one cardiac border to the other and then back again. The entire heart is therefore interrogated. The use of multiple echocardiographic windows and sweeps allows the echocardiographer to assemble a three-dimensional mental picture of the cardiac anatomy and the relationships of different structures. This three-dimensional approach is far superior to any single tomogram. All views are displayed in the anatomic orientation with the base of the heart at the top of the screen and the apex of the heart at the bottom. The right side of the heart is displayed on the left side of the screen and the left side of the heart on the right side of the screen, as on a chest radiograph. This orientation also facilitates the comparison of echo images with those obtained at the time of cardiac catheterization.

Choice of transducers is very important. Typical transducers in pediatrics are 3.5 MHz and 5 MHz. In tiny premature infants the 7 MHz transducer is often used. High-frequency transducers give good resolution and detail, whereas low-frequency transducers provide the best penetration. Always use the highest-frequency transducer that gives adequate penetration of the patient and therefore the best image resolution. Sweeps are initially performed with the short or medium focal length transducers to evaluate intracardiac anatomy. Repeat sweeps using long-focal-length transducers allow better visualization of more distant structures, including extracardiac anatomy. Just as with echocardiographic windows, not all information can be obtained with a single transducer. Care must be exercised to avoid excessive pressure on the patient with the transducer, particularly in small or premature infants. The echocardiographic examination should not be painful to the child. Good penetration is a function of the frequency of the transducer, not the pressure applied to it.

Sedation

Echocardiography in children, unlike that of adults, poses the unique problem of patient agitation and movement. Because echocardiography may be quite frightening to children there may be crying and movement, necessitating sedation for an accurate study. This is particularly important in the patient with extremely complex anatomy, or in whom detailed physiologic evaluation is imperative. Some caution must be used in interpretation of physiologic data in the sedated patient, since gradients may be significantly different from those in the awake state. Often, children less than 1 month of age can be studied without sedation. We use chloral hydrate in doses of 60 mg/kg for children 1 to 18 months old, and 75 mg/kg for children 18 months to three years old. Caution should be used when sedating patients with known pulmonary disease, and all patients should be closely monitored with pulse oximetry by trained personnel. In the awake patient natural separation anxiety is decreased if a parent is allowed to stay with the child during the study. Warming the echocardiography gel, dimming the lights, or distracting with a video or cartoon may help to establish calm in the laboratory.

Two-Dimensional Echocardiography

Imaging Planes

Subcostal Approach

Transverse Plane. Once the ECG is attached to the patient and a clear signal appears on the screen showing both a p wave and a QRS complex, the transducer is placed perpendicular to the abdomen in the subxyphoid region. You must first determine if your displayed image is anatomically correct with respect to right/left orientation. With the plane of the transducer directed transversely, approximately 3 cm of liver is visualized. If the transducer is rocked to the patient's right, the structures on the right side of the patient are seen to move leftward on the screen. If it is rocked to the patient's left, the structures on the left side of the patient move rightward on the screen. If this does not happen the image should be reversed and the process repeated. This places the image in an anatomic orientation on the screen.

The first image from this position demonstrates the spine seen as a bright reflection medial and posterior (Fig. 13-1). In the patient with normal abdominal situs, immediately anterior and to the left of the spine is the descending aorta, which pulsates with each heart beat. To the left of the aorta is the stomach (which may be filled with fluid or gas), and anterior and to the right of the spine is the inferior vena cava. The inferior vena cava may pulsate as a result of inspiration and expiration. The inferior vena cava is usually elliptical, differentiating it from the round descending aorta. Determination of the abdominal situs is important, since many forms of congenital heart disease are associated with abnormal visceral-atrial situs.

With the plane of the transducer aligned transversely, perpendicular to the abdomen, the sweep begins

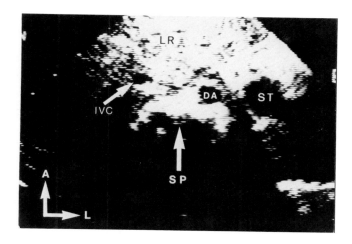

Figure 13-1. Normal abdominal transverse plane used to determine visceral and abdominal situs from the subcostal window. (SP, spine; DA, descending aorta; ST, stomach; IVC, inferior vena cava; LR, liver; A, anterior; L, left.)

posterior and then fans slowly anteriorly and superiorly. The side-to-side orientation of the transducer is maintained at all times. This is called the subcostal frontal sweep (Fig. 13-2).

As the sweep proceeds, the inferior vena cava is seen entering the posterior portion of the right atrium. As the transducer sweeps superiorly, the interatrial septum and the right and left lower pulmonary veins are seen entering the left atrium. At this point the left ventricle and mitral valve are visible (Fig. 13-3).

Continuing still more anteriorly and superiorly, the right ventricular inflow valve, tricuspid valve, and anterior right atrium are seen. At this time the left ventricle, left ventricular outflow tract, aortic valve, and proximal ascending aorta are seen (Fig. 13-4).

As the transducer proceeds further, the right ventricular outflow tract and pulmonary valve are seen. At this point the frontal scan is complete and the reverse scan begins.

Long Axial Oblique. For the long axial oblique sweep the transducer is again placed in the subcostal region, its plane being aligned at a 45° angle to the midline between the right shoulder and left hip (Fig. 13-5). The sweep proceeds from a posterior/inferior direction to a superior/lateral direction toward the left shoulder. The plane of the transducer is maintained throughout the sweep.

Early in the sweep, the superior vena cava is seen entering the right atrium. The atrial septum is seen in its entirety from the superior vena cava to the crux of the heart. A patent foramen ovale may be present in the midsection (Fig. 13-6).

This is one of the best views for examining the atrial septum for secundum atrial septal defects. Pulmonary veins enter the posterior aspect of the left atrium. The left atrium, mitral valve, and left ventricle are present. As the sweep continues, the tricuspid valve comes into view often in cross-section. The left ventricle is seen from the apex to the aortic valve.

Still further, the ascending aorta and transverse aortic arch are seen (Fig. 13-7). Occasionally in small babies some of the brachiocephalic vessels and the entire aortic arch are visible. The anterior right atrium, tricuspid valve, and inlet right ventricle are present. The right pulmonary artery appears in oblique cross-section under the aortic arch. As the sweep continues toward the left shoulder, the left ventricle appears in a modified cross section. Toward the right are a portion of the right ventricle, foreshortened right ventricular outflow tract, pulmonary valve, and proximal portion of the main pulmonary artery. Occasionally, the proximal portion of the left pulmonary artery is also present.

(*Text continues on page 458*)

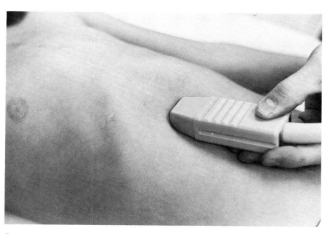

A

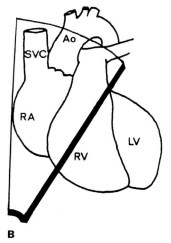

B

Figure 13-2. *A:* Subcostal frontal plane; *B:* subcostal frontal plane.

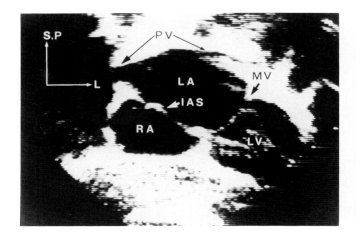

Figure 13-3. Normal subcostal frontal view with posterior angulation. (PV, pulmonary vein; LA, left atrium; RA, right atrium; IAS, interatrial septum; LV, left ventricle; MV, mitral valve; S, superior; P, posterior; L, left.)

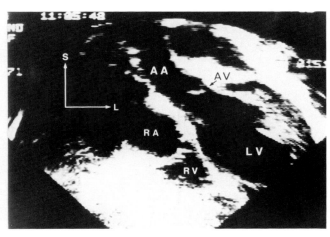

Figure 13-4. Normal subcostal frontal view with superior angulation. (LV, left ventricle; AV, aortic valve; AA, ascending aorta; RA, right atrium; RV, right ventricle; S, superior; L, left.)

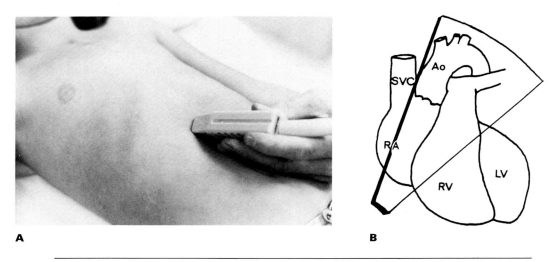

A   B

Figure 13-5. Subcostal long axial oblique planes.

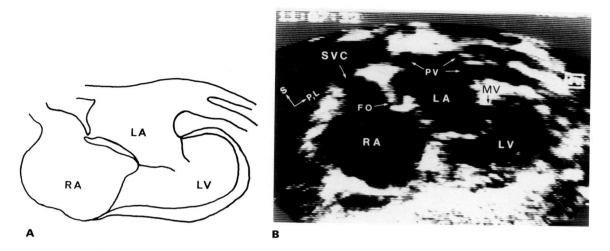

Figure 13-6. *A:* Subcostal long axial oblique plane; *B:* normal subcostal long axial oblique view with posterolateral angulation. (SVC, superior vena cava; FO, foramen ovale; PV, pulmonary veins; LA, left atrium; LV, left ventricle; MV, mitral valve; RA, right atrium; S, superior; P, posterior; L, left.)

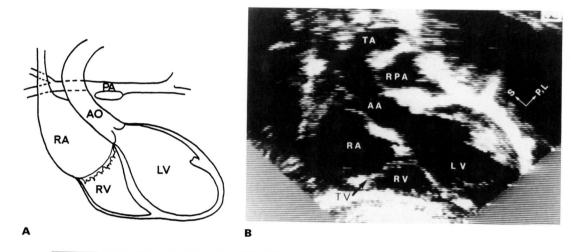

Figure 13-7. *A:* Subcostal long axial oblique plane; *B:* normal subcostal long axial oblique view with anterolateral angulation. (LV, left ventricle; AA, ascending aorta; TA, transverse aortic arch; RA, right atrium; TV, tricuspid valve; RV, right ventricle; RPA, right pulmonary artery; S, superior; P, posterior; L, lateral.)

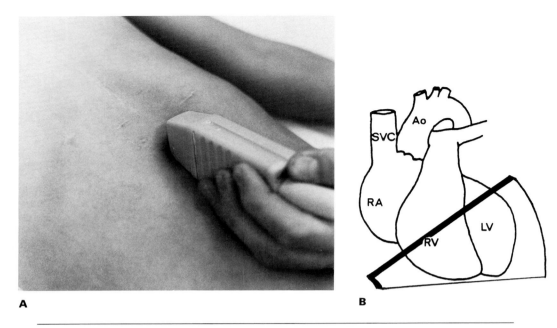

Figure 13-8. Subcostal sagittal planes.

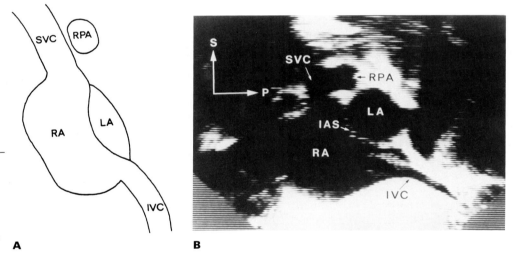

Figure 13-9. *A:* Subcostal sagittal plane; *B:* normal subcostal sagittal view. (SVC, superior vena cava; IVC, inferior vena cava; RA, right atrium; RPA, right pulmonary artery; LA, left atrium; IAS, interatrial septum; S, superior; P, posterior.)

Sagittal Plane. In this sweep the transducer is directly cephalocaudal and parallel to the midline of the patient (Fig. 13-8). Beginning to the right of the midline the sweep proceeds toward the patient's left side; the plane of the transducer remains constant.

The first images are those of the inferior vena cava and superior vena cava entering the right atrium simultaneously. The interatrial septum is seen between the right and left atria. The right pulmonary artery is posterior to the superior vena cava and superior to the interatrial septum (Fig. 13-9). As the transducer sweeps toward the patient's left side, the tricuspid valve, right

ventricular inflow and outflow tracts, pulmonary valve, proximal portion of the main pulmonary artery, and proximal portion of the left pulmonary artery are easily seen (Fig. 13-10).

In this plane, the right ventricular outflow tract is parallel to the beam of the transducer, making this ideal for Doppler interrogation of the right ventricular outflow tract and main pulmonary artery. The right ventricle is seen as a crescent around the cross-section of the left ventricle and mitral valve. A short axis of the left ventricle allows analysis of left ventricular free wall and septal motion. Defects in the interventricular septum are com-

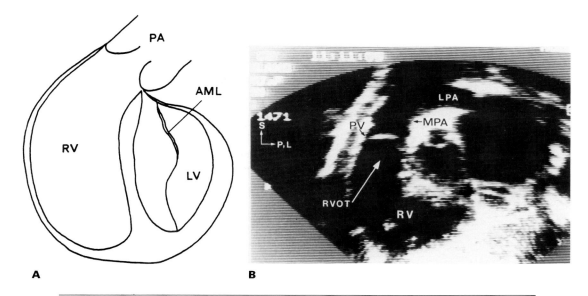

Figure 13-10. *A:* Subcostal sagittal (superolateral) plane; *B:* normal subcostal sagittal view with leftward angulation. (RV, right ventricle; RVOT, right ventricular outflow tract; PV, pulmonary valve; MPA, main pulmonary artery; LPA, left pulmonary artery; S, superior; P, posterior; L, left.)

monly visible during this sweep. The sweep is completed by moving farther to the patient's left and toward the left ventricular apex.

Right Anterior Oblique View. Unlike the previous sweeps, this is a single tomographic view. Some angulation may be required for optimal visualization. This view is similar to the right anterior oblique angiographic view. The plane of the transducer is aligned to a 45° angle to the midline between the right hip and left shoulder. The angle of the transducer is superior and lateral (Figs. 13-11, 13-12).

This view is particularly helpful in analyzing the entire right side of the heart. The left and right atria, interatrial septum, tricuspid valve, right ventricular outflow, pulmonary valve, and main pulmonary artery are all seen clearly. The right pulmonary artery branches off toward the patient's right. The left pulmonary artery is out of view, posteriorly into the screen. This view is helpful in evaluating right-sided obstructive lesions such as tetralogy of Fallot.

Apical Approach

Four-Chamber View and Long Axis. Both the apical four-chamber view and the apical long axis view are achieved by placing the transducer on the left anterolateral chest wall at the point of maximal impulse. The plane of the transducer for the four-chamber view is between the patient's right hip and left shoulder with the transducer pointing toward the patient's right shoulder (Fig.

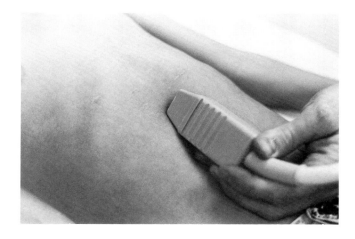

Figure 13-11. Subcostal right anterior oblique view.

13-13). All four cardiac chambers, the tricuspid valve, and the mitral valve are visualized (Fig. 13-14).

The tricuspid valve inserts into the ventricular septum slightly more apically than the mitral valve. The right ventricle has coarser septal trabeculations than the left. The muscular interventricular septum separating the right and left ventricles is parallel to the plane of the transducer and is easily scanned. There are also chordal septal attachments to the right ventricular side of the interventricular septum from the tricuspid valve. There are

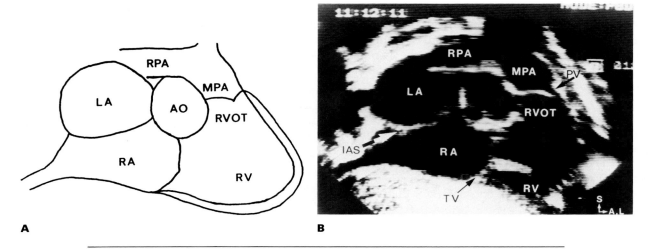

A   **B**

Figure 13-12. *A:* Subcostal right anterior oblique view; *B:* normal right anterior oblique view. (LA, left atrium; RA, right atrium; IAS, interatrial septum; TV, tricuspid valve; RV, right ventricle; RVOT, right ventricular outflow tract; MPA, main pulmonary artery; PV, pulmonary valve; RPA, right pulmonary artery; S, superior; A, anterior; L, left.

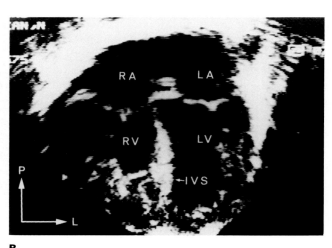

Figure 13-13. Apical four-chamber view.

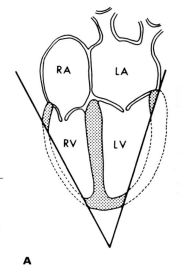

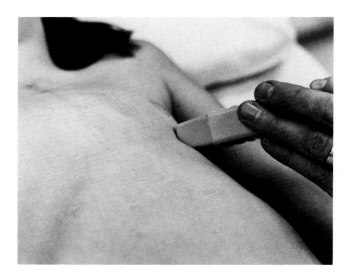

Figure 13-14. *A:* Apical four-chamber view; *B:* normal apical four-chamber view. (RA, right atrium; RV, right ventricle; LA, left atrium; LV, left ventricle; IVS, interventricular septum; P, posterior; L, left.)

A   **B**

normally no mitral valve chordal attachments to the interventricular septum on the left ventricle. The interatrial septum, being thinner and farther from the transducer is commonly not well visualized in its entirety. Therefore, caution should be taken not to misdiagnose atrial septal defects from this view.

For the apical long axis view, the transducer remains in the same position on the anterolateral chest wall as the apical four-chamber view but is rotated clockwise, aligning the plane of the transducer between the right shoulder and left hip. The transducer remains pointed posteriorly toward the right shoulder. The apical long axis view nicely demonstrates the left atrium, mitral valve, left ventricle, and left ventricular outflow tract (Figs. 13-15, 13-16). The entire left ventricular outflow tract is imaged to the aortic valve and the proximal ascending aorta.

Continuity between the aortic and mitral valves, the aortic root, and the ventricular septum are confirmed.

Parasternal Views

Long Axis. To perform the parasternal long axis view, the transducer is placed on the left chest in approximately the third or fourth intercostal space, to the left of the sternum perpendicular to the chest wall. Aligning the plane of the transducer between the right shoulder and left hip, the most anterior chamber is the right ventricle, separated from the left ventricle by the interventricular septum (Figs. 13-17, 13-18). The aorta and aortic valve are seen anterior to the left atrium. The anterior and posterior leaflets of the mitral valve are demonstrated. The left ventricular outflow is nicely evaluated in this view.

Positioning the transducer rightward in the long axis view as described previously displays the right ventricular inflow and tricuspid valve anatomy (Fig. 13-19). This view is helpful for evaluation of tricuspid regurgitation, as well as displacement of the septal tricuspid valve leaflet seen in Ebstein's anomaly.

Short Axis. The parasternal short axis view is achieved by placing the transducer on the patient's left chest in the left third or fourth intercostal space to the left of the sternum. The plane of the transducer is aligned between the left shoulder and right hip with the transducer pointing perpendicular to the chest wall (Fig. 13-20). The short axis plane can also be achieved by turning the transducer 90° clockwise from the parasternal long axis plane. The sweep is performed from the ventricular apex to the base of the heart and back again. When the transducer is angled inferiorly and laterally the anterior right and posterior left ventricles are seen in cross-sec-

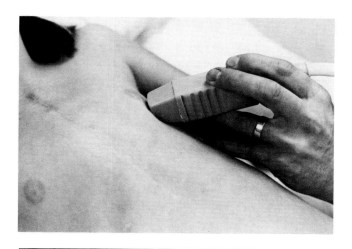

Figure 13-15. Apical long axis view.

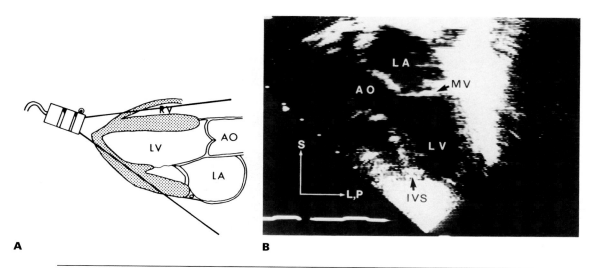

A   **B**

Figure 13-16. *A:* Apical long axis view; *B:* normal apical long axis view. (LA, left atrium; LV, left ventricle; MV, mitral valve; AO, aorta; IVS, interventricular septum; S, superior; L, left; P, posterior.)

tion. In this view the right ventricle appears as a crescent shape anterior and to the right of the spherical left ventricle (Fig. 13-21).

When the transducer sweeps through the left ventricle from the apex toward the base of the heart the two papillary muscles—the anterolateral and the posteromedial—are identified. The left ventricular borders include the ventricular septum and, posteriorly and laterally, the left ventricular free wall. Sweeping more superiorly and medially the great vessels come into view. This is an ex-

cellent view for confirming the orientation of the aorta to the pulmonary artery. In the patient with normal anatomy, the pulmonary valve is anterior and to the left of the aortic valve (Fig. 13-22). This allows good visualization of the right ventricular outflow tract, pulmonary valve, main pulmonary artery, and proximal right and left branch pulmonary arteries. These structures wrap around the aortic valve in cross-section. All three leaflets of the aortic valve should be visible and uniform in size (Fig. 13-23).

Suprasternal Views

Aortic Arch and Patent Ductus Arteriosus. The suprasternal approach to the aorta and the brachiocephalic vessels is particularly useful in young children. The transducer is placed in the suprasternal notch and angled posteriorly and inferiorly (Figs. 13-24 and 13-25). The plane of the transducer is between the right hip and the left shoulder. Occasionally some clockwise rotation of the transducer is necessary to elongate the full aortic arch. A high right parasternal view often shows the aorta in neonates and small children. Also from this view the arch vessels are examined and the sidedness of the aortic arch is determined. A high left parasternal view with the plane of the transducer parallel to the spine is often used for imaging the patent ductus arteriosus (Fig. 13-26).

Specific Lesions

The following examples show two-dimensional images of multiple types of congenital and acquired heart disease as seen from different views.

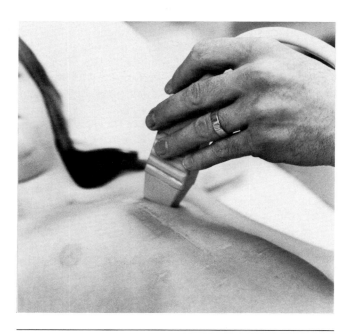

Figure 13-17. Parasternal long axis view.

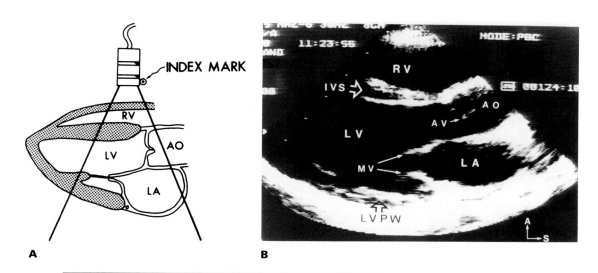

Figure 13-18. *A:* Parasternal long axis view; *B:* normal parasternal long axis view. (AO, aorta; AV, aortic valve; LA, left atrium; MV, mitral valve; LV, left ventricle; IVS, interventricular septum; RV, right ventricle; LVPW, left ventricular posterior wall; S, superior; A, anterior.)

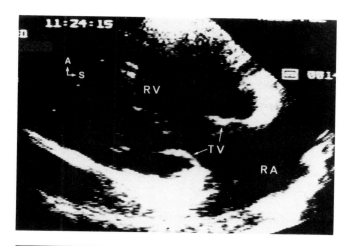

Figure 13-19. Parasternal long axis view with rightward angulation. (RV, right ventricle; RA, right atrium; TV, tricuspid valve; A, anterior; S, superior.)

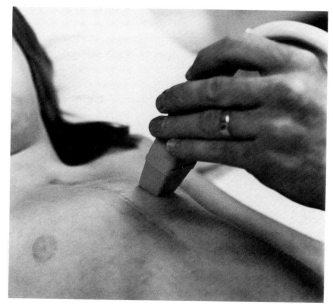

Figure 13-20. Parasternal short axis.

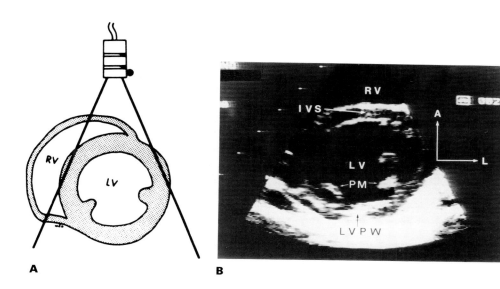

Figure 13-21. *A:* Parasternal short axis; *B:* normal parasternal short axis view of the ventricles. (RV, right ventricle; LV, left ventricle; IVS, interventricular septum; PM, papillary muscle; LVPW, left ventricular posterior wall; A, anterior; L, left.)

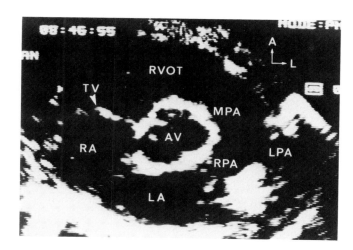

Figure 13-22. Parasternal short axis view at the level of the aortic valve. (AV, aortic valve; RVOT, right ventricular outflow tract; TV, tricuspid valve; RA, right atrium; LA, left atrium; LPA, left pulmonary artery; MPA, main pulmonary artery; RPA, right pulmonary artery; A, anterior; L, left.)

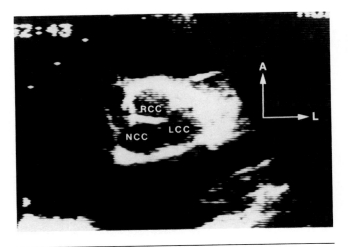

Figure 13-23. Normal trileaflet aortic valve from a parasternal short axis view. (RCC, right coronary cusp; NCC, noncoronary cusp; LCC, left coronary cusp; A, anterior; L, left.)

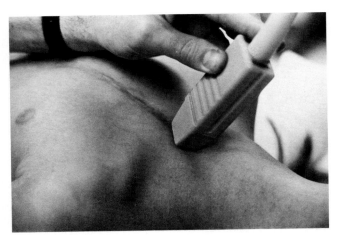

Figure 13-24. Suprasternal notch view.

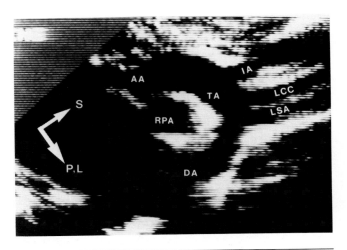

Figure 13-25. Aortic arch view from suprasternal notch. The ascending aorta (AA), transverse aortic arch (TA) and upper descending aorta (DA) are well seen. All three arch vessels are seen. The right pulmonary artery (RPA) is seen in cross-section under the aortic arch. (IA, innominate artery; LCC, left common carotid artery; LSA, left subclavian artery; S, superior; P, posterior; L, left.)

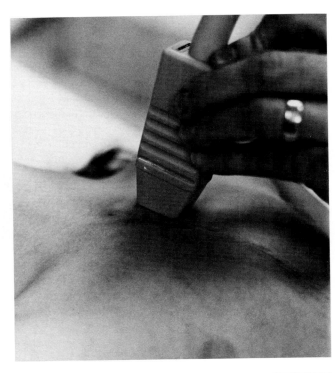

Figure 13-26. High parasternal view.

Atrial Septal Defects. Secundum atrial septal defect is caused by a failure of the septum primum to form properly. This results in a defect in the centralmost portion of the atrial septum (Fig. 13-27). The atrial septal defect may be any size or shape. A patent foramen ovale results from a failure of the septum primum to close properly against the septum secundum, and should not be confused with a true secundum atrial septal defect. In lesions resulting in increased left atrial or right atrial volume or pressure, the septum is bowed away from the chamber with elevated pressure or volume, which pro-

duces either left-to-right or right-to-left shunting through the patent foramen ovale. Care should be taken to view the atrial septum in multiple orthogonal planes, since false drop outs may appear from certain windows, particularly the apical four-chamber view. Common associated findings with atrial septal defects include volume overload of the right ventricle, resulting in a dilated chamber, ventricular septal bowing toward the left ventricle, and paradoxical motion of the septum during systole.

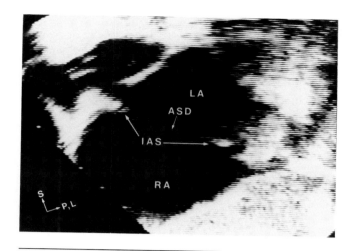

Figure 13-27. Subcostal long axial oblique view of a large secundum atrial septal defect. (ASD, atrial septal defect; IAS, interatrial septum; RA, right atrium; LA, left atrium; S, superior; P, posterior; L, left.)

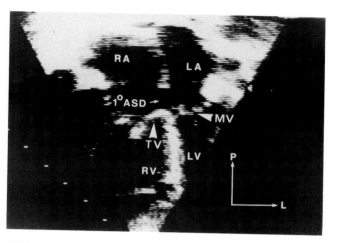

Figure 13-28. Apical four-chamber view of primum atrial septal defect. The mitral (MV) and tricuspid valve (TV) components of the common atrioventricular valve insert into the interventricular septum at the same level. No ventricular septal defect is seen. (RA, right atrium; LA, left atrium; RV, right ventricle; LV, left ventricle; P, posterior; L, left.)

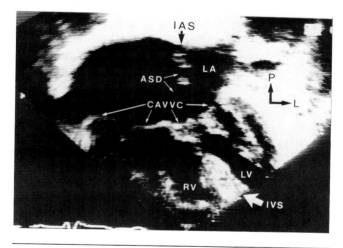

Figure 13-29. Apical four-chamber view of a complete atrioventricular septal defect (common atrioventricular canal) with the valve in the closed position during systole (CAVVC). There are chordal attachments present within the left (LV) and right (RV) ventricles, and attachments to the interventricular septal crest (IVS) across a large ventricular septal defect. A large primum atrial septal defect (ASD) and a small secundum atrial septal defect are present. The right atrium is larger than the left atrium (LA) due to malalignment of the interatrial septum (IAS). (P, posterior; L, left.)

Primum atrial septal defect is caused by a failure of the endocardial cushions to complete the lower portion of the atrial septum (Fig. 13-28). This defect is often associated with a cleft in the mitral valve, which is seen best on a parasternal short axis sweep of the left ventricle from either the parasternal or subcostal sagittal view. Mitral regurgitation is common within this cleft, and careful Doppler interrogation of the left atrium is important. A large coronary sinus ostium secondary to increased flow from a left superior vena cava should not be confused with an atrial septal defect.

Sinus venosus atrial septal defects are located either at the inferior vena cava–right atrial junction or the superior vena cava–right atrial junction. Because these defects are usually associated with partial anomalous pulmonary venous drainage, the site of connection of all pulmonary veins should be determined. Most commonly, the right upper pulmonary vein enters to the right of the atrial septum in a sinus venosus atrial septal defect of the superior vena caval type.

Complete Atrioventricular Canal. Complete atrioventricular septal (atrioventricular canal) defect results from a failure of the endocardial cushions to complete the septation of the atria, ventricles, and common atrioventricular valve. This results in a primum atrial septal defect, an inlet type of ventricular septal defect, and a single, large common atrioventricular valve (Figs. 13-29, 13-30).

Complete defects are classified by Rastelli according to the morphology and attachments of the atrioventricular valve. This valve morphology is critically important to the surgical approach. Type A has a superior bridging leaflet with chordal attachments to the ventricular septal crest. This superior bridging leaflet may or may not be divided. It is the most common type. In type B, the bridging leaflet is divided but not attached to the ventricular septal crest, and in type C, the superior leaflet is not divided or attached to the septal crest. The valve is often incompetent and careful Doppler interrogation of the left atrium is essential for determining the presence and severity of regurgitation. In addition, the position of

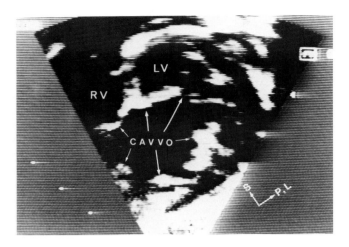

Figure 13-30. Subcostal long axial oblique view of an open common atrioventricular valve (CAVVO) in a patient with complete atrioventricular septal defect (common atrioventricular canal). (S, superior; P, posterior; L, left; LV, left ventricle; RV, right ventricle.)

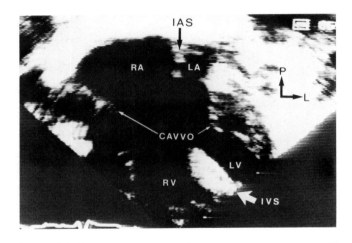

Figure 13-31. Apical four-chamber view of a complete atrioventricular septal defect (common atrioventricular canal) with the valve in the open position during diastole (CAVVO). The common atrioventricular valve is malaligned toward the right ventricle (RV), which is larger than the left ventricle (LV). The right atrium (RA) is larger than the left atrium (LA). (IAS, interatrial septum; IVS, interventricular septum; P, posterior; L, left.)

the valve over the ventricular septum is crucial. If the common atrioventricular valve is malaligned towards the right, the right ventricle is large and the left ventricle is hypoplastic (Fig. 13-31). Similarly, if the valve is malaligned towards the left ventricle, the right ventricle will be hypoplastic. The valve leaflets are often evaluated best in a short axis sweep of the ventricles. This may necessitate a change in surgical approach, since the ventricular sizes may not allow for a biventricular repair.

Ventricular Septal Defect. Ventricular septal defects are the most common form of congenital structural

heart defects. The defect may be in any portion of the ventricular septum; therefore, all portions of the septum should be scanned from multiple approaches, since no single view shows the entire ventricular septum. The exact location of the defect is important to the surgical approach, since high defects beneath the pulmonary valve are difficult to visualize from the transatrial approach, and inlet VSDs are difficult to visualize from the transpulmonary approach.

Muscular ventricular septal defects may be anterior, posterior, in the midportion of the septum, or toward the ventricular apex. Apical muscular defects are often best visualized with the apical four-chamber view (Fig. 13-32).

The superior and inferior margins are typically well defined in large muscular defects; however, small defects may be hidden in the coarse trabeculae of the right ventricle and visible only with color flow Doppler. In patients with large malalignment or conoventricular defects, the entire septum should be scanned, since smaller muscular defects are often present and may need to be closed at the time of surgical repair.

Perimembranous (conoventricular) defects involve both the membranous portion of the ventricular septum and the septum immediately around the membranous septum. This is located between the aortic annulus and the tricuspid annulus (Fig. 13-33). These defects may be associated with aneurysm formation around the defect creating a wind sock appearance (Fig. 13-34). This aneurysmal tissue is of tricuspid valve origin and often significantly decreases the effective size of the ventricular septal defect and reduces the left-to-right shunt. At the time of surgery, when this aneurysm is removed, the defect may be quite large.

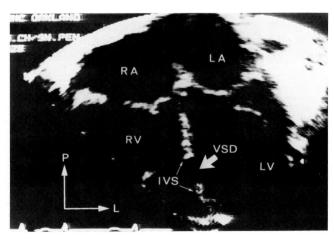

Figure 13-32. Apical four-chamber view of a large muscular ventricular septal defect (VSD). (RA, right atrium; LA, left atrium; RV, right ventricle; LV, left ventricle; IVS, interventricular septum; P, posterior; L, left.)

Patent Ductus Arteriosus. The transducer is placed in the high left parasternal region in order to identify a patent ductus arteriosus. The transducer is angled posteriorly in a sagittal plane to the left of the midline. In this "ductus view" the main pulmonary artery, left pulmonary artery, and descending aorta are seen. The main pulmonary artery can be seen giving rise to the patent ductus with the left pulmonary artery separated from the ductus. This view shows the ductus originating from the descending aorta at the inferior edge of the left subclavian artery and connecting to the pulmonary artery just to the left of the bifurcation (Figs. 13-35, 13-36). A Doppler sample volume placed in the pulmonary artery demonstrates continuous turbulent flow coming into the main pulmonary artery from the descending aorta. Color flow Doppler is particularly helpful for the localization of the flow in very small or eccentric jets.

Coarctation of the Aorta. Aortic coarctation is typically located just distal to the left subclavian artery in the juxtaductal region. There is often associated poststenotic dilatation of the descending aorta (Fig. 13-37). The transverse arch should also be examined carefully, since there may be diffuse tubular hypoplasia. The entire aortic arch should be visualized and interrogated closely with Doppler to avoid either false-positive or false-negative results. A segmental approach is necessary to examine the entire aortic arch, since it is not well seen in a single view.

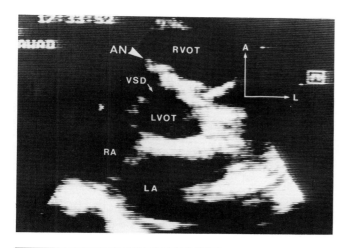

Figure 13-33. Parasternal short axis view of a conoventricular (perimembranous) septal defect (VSD). There is early aneurysm formation (AN) from the tricuspid valve tissue. (RVOT, right ventricular outflow tract; LVOT, left ventricular outflow tract; RA, right atrium; LA, left atrium; A, anterior; L, left.)

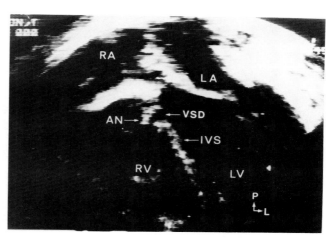

Figure 13-34. Apical long axis view of a conoventricular septal defect (VSD) with partial closure by an aneurysm formation (AN). (RA, right atrium; LA, left atrium; RV, right ventricle; LV, left ventricle; IVS, interventricular septum; P, posterior; L, left.)

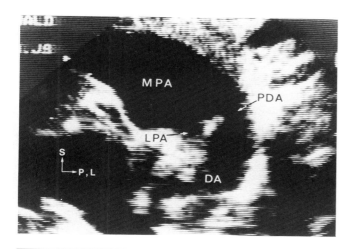

Figure 13-35. Suprasternal sagittal view of a patent ductus arteriosus (PDA). The left pulmonary artery (LPA) origin is seen. (MPA, main pulmonary artery; DA, descending aorta; S, superior; P, posterior; L, left.)

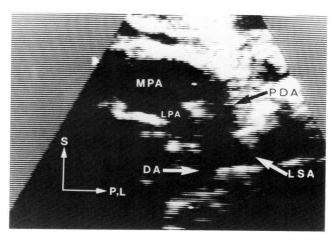

Figure 13-36. Suprasternal sagittal view showing a patent ductus arteriosus (PDA) connecting the main pulmonary artery (MPA) to the descending aorta (DA). The left subclavian artery (LSA) arises directly across from the aortic end of the patent ductus. (LPA, left pulmonary artery; S, superior; P, posterior; L, left.)

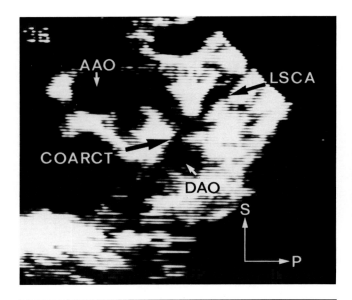

Figure 13-37. Aortic arch view of a discrete coarctation of the thoracic aorta (COARCT) immediately distal to the take-off of the left subclavian artery (LSCA). Poststenotic dilatation of the descending aorta (DAO) is present immediately distal to the coarctation. (AAO, ascending aorta; S, superior; P, posterior.)

Mitral Stenosis. When evaluating the mitral valve, all components should be viewed from the apical and parasternal views (Fig. 13-38). Mitral stenosis is often caused by shortened or thickened chordae. A parachute mitral valve results when all chordae insert into a single papillary muscle. Ventricular septal defects and other left-sided obstructive lesions such as coarctation of the aorta and aortic stenosis are often associated.

Ebstein's Anomaly. Ebstein's anomaly results from a displacement of the septal and posterior leaflets of the tricuspid valve toward the right ventricular apex (Fig. 13-39). The portion of the right ventricle proximal to this displacement becomes "atrialized" and often has thin walls and poor contractility. The tricuspid valve displacement may be only mild and result in few or no symptoms. However, if the valve leaflets are thickened and irregular and the displacement is severe, there is moderate to severe tricuspid regurgitation, right ventricular dysfunction, and right ventricular outflow tract obstruction. This results in cyanosis secondary to inadequate pulmonary blood flow and right-to-left shunting at the atrial level.

Bicuspid Aortic Valve. The normal aortic valve has three cusps. Bicuspid aortic valve is quite common and results from an absence or partial fusion of one commissure (Fig. 13-40). The valve may be stenotic and there may be poststenotic dilatation of the ascending aorta.

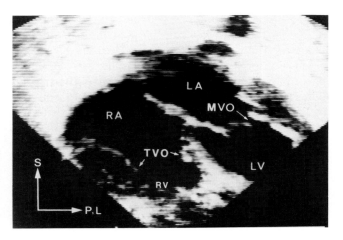

Figure 13-38. Modified apical four-chamber view showing a small mitral valve opening (MVO) compared to the tricuspid valve opening (TVO) in a patient with mitral stenosis. (RA, right atrium; LA, left atrium; RV, right ventricle; LV, left ventricle; S, superior; P, posterior; L, left.)

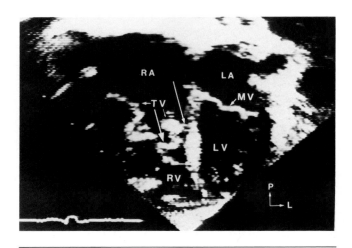

Figure 13-39. Apical four-chamber view of a patient with Ebstein's anomaly. The tricuspid valve (TV) leaflets are irregular and thickened, and the septal leaflet (*arrows*) is displaced well into the right ventricle (RV). (RA, right atrium; LA, left atrium; MV, mitral valve; LV, left ventricle; P, posterior; L, left.)

Tricuspid Atresia. Tricuspid atresia results from a failure of genesis of the tricuspid valve. There may be no valve tissue at all or a poorly formed imperforate membrane (Figs. 13-41, 13-42).

Since the only egress of blood from the right atrium occurs through an atrial communication, the interatrial septum bows from right to left. There should be nonrestrictive flow through a foramen ovale or atrial septal defect. It is essential for the patient to demonstrate laminar flow and should be checked carefully on all patients. If there is any evidence of a restrictive communication the patient should undergo a balloon atrial septostomy. The size of the right ventricle is a function of the size of

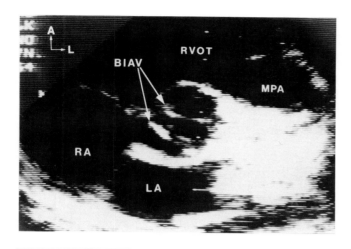

Figure 13-40. Parasternal short axis view of a bicuspid aortic valve (BIAV). Two distinct aortic valve leaflets (*arrows*) are present instead of three. (RA, right atrium; LA, left atrium; RVOT, right ventricular outflow tract; MPA, main pulmonary artery; A, anterior; L, left.)

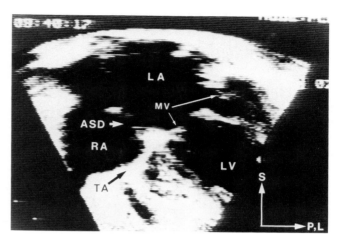

Figure 13-41. Subcostal long axial oblique view of tricuspid atresia (TA). A secundum atrial septal defect (ASD) allows systemic venous return to flow from the right atrium (RA) to the left atrium (LA). Pulmonary blood flow is through a ventricular septal defect or a patent ductus arteriosus. (MV, mitral valve; LV, left ventricle; S, superior; L, left; P, posterior.)

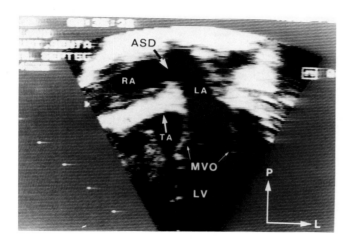

Figure 13-42. Apical four-chamber view of tricuspid atresia (TA). (RA, right atrium; ASD, atrial septal defect; LA, left atrium; MVO, mitral view in an open position; LV, left ventricle; P, posterior; L, left.)

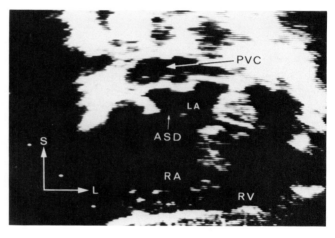

Figure 13-43. Subcostal frontal view of the pulmonary venous confluence (PVC) behind the left atrium (LA) in a patient with total anomalous pulmonary venous return. No pulmonary veins are seen entering the left atrium. A secundum atrial septal defect (ASD) is present. The right atrium (RA) and right ventricle (RV) are enlarged, suggesting volume overload to the right heart. (S, superior; L, left.)

the ventricular septal defect. In tricuspid atresia with pulmonary atresia, the right ventricle is severely hypoplastic.

Total Anomalous Pulmonary Venous Connection. Total anomalous pulmonary venous connection can be of several types. Initial examination will show that the pulmonary venous confluence does not drain directly into the left atrium (Fig. 13-43).

In the supradiaphragmatic type, the confluence typically drains into a vertical vein, which then drains into the innominate vein which in turn drains into the right atrium by way of the superior vena cava. In this type there

is usually no obstruction to pulmonary blood flow (Fig. 13-44).

The increase in venous return through the superior vena cava results in an increased velocity in the Doppler flow pattern into the right atrium. Care should be taken to evaluate the coronary sinus, since the pulmonary veins may connect to the coronary sinus. This results in an enlarged coronary sinus and accelerated and disturbed flow by Doppler at the mouth of the coronary sinus.

In the infradiaphragmatic type, the vertical vein courses inferiorly, piercing the diaphragm, and typically

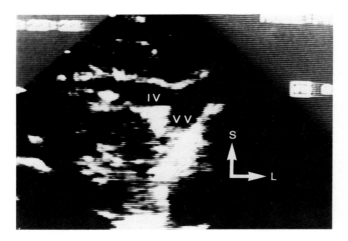

Figure 13-44. Suprasternal frontal view of an enlarged vertical vein (VV) arising from a pulmonary venous confluence in a patient with total anomalous pulmonary venous return above the diaphragm. The vertical vein connects to the innominate vein (IV), which in turn drains to the superior vena cava and the right atrium. (S, superior; L, left.)

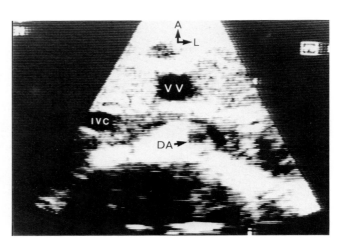

Figure 13-45. Subcostal transverse view of the abdomen showing a large vertical vein (VV) arising from a pulmonary venous confluence in a patient with total anomalous pulmonary venous connection below the diaphragm. The vertical vein descends into the liver. The descending aorta (DA) and the inferior vena cava (IVC) are seen in their normal locations. (A, anterior; L, left.)

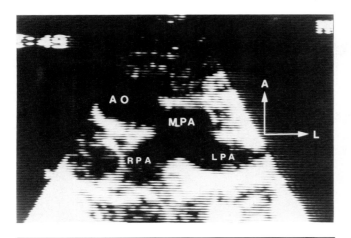

Figure 13-46. Parasternal short axis view of a patient with *d*-transposition of the great arteries. The aorta (AO) is located anterior and to the right of the main pulmonary artery (MPA). The main pulmonary artery gives rise to a normal-sized right pulmonary artery (RPA) and left pulmonary artery (LPA). (A, anterior; L, left.)

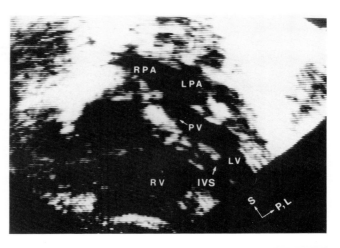

Figure 13-47. Subcostal long axial oblique view of a *d*-transposition of the great arteries. The pulmonary artery arises from the left ventricle (LV) and gives rise to the right (RPA) and left (LPA) pulmonary arteries. The left ventricle is smaller than the right ventricle (RV) and there is bowing of the interventricular septum (IVS) toward the left ventricle. (PV, pulmonary valve; S, superior; P, posterior; L, left.)

connects to the portal vein. Less commonly, it may connect to the ductus venosus, hepatic veins, or inferior vena cava (Fig. 13-45). Turbulent flow may be seen in the inferior vena cava. Usually in the infradiaphragmatic type there is obstruction to pulmonary venous return.

All types of anomalous pulmonary venous connections may result in a small left atrium because of decreased flow. With careful echo and Doppler evaluation, most patients do not require cardiac catheterization prior to surgical correction.

Dextro-Transposition of the Great Arteries.
Transposition of the great arteries results from a reversal of the normal anteroposterior relationship of the great vessels. In transposition, usually the aortic valve is anterior and to the right of the pulmonary valve (Fig. 13-46). This results in the aorta arising from the right ventricle and the pulmonary artery arising from the left ventricle (Fig. 13-47).

The interventricular septum often bows from right

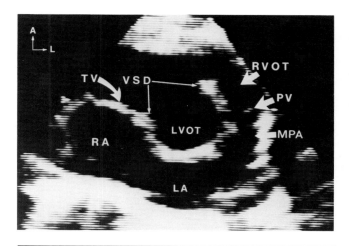

Figure 13-48. Parasternal short axis view of a patient with tetralogy of Fallot. A large nonrestrictive malalignment type ventricular septal defect (VSD) is present. The right ventricular outflow tract (RVOT), pulmonary valve (PV), and main pulmonary artery (MPA) are small. (LVOT, left ventricular outflow tract; TV, tricuspid valve; RA, right atrium; LA, left atrium; A, anterior; L, left.)

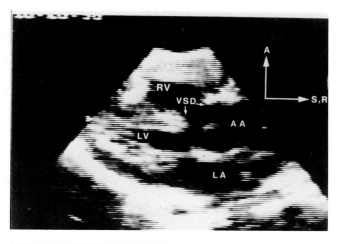

Figure 13-49. Parasternal long axis view showing a malalignment type ventricular septal defect (VSD) and overriding aorta in a patient with tetralogy of Fallot. (RV, right ventricle; LV, left ventricle; LA, left atrium; AA, ascending aorta; A, anterior; S, superior; R, right.)

to left because the right ventricle has pressure at the systemic level. Associated lesions include ventricular septal defects, valvular and/or subvalvular pulmonic stenosis, and occasionally coarctation of the aorta. When possible, the coronary arteries should be checked carefully since their position is critical for the arterial switch operation.

Tetralogy of Fallot. In tetralogy, the parietal band is displaced anterior, superior, and to the left. This results in right ventricular outflow tract obstruction (infundibular stenosis) overriding of the aorta, a malalignment ventricular septal defect, and right ventricular hypertrophy (Figs. 13-48, 13-49).

Varying degrees of outflow tract obstruction from very minimal pulmonic stenosis to pulmonary atresia may be present. Careful inspection of the outflow and pulmonary arteries is crucial in determining whether the patient needs urgent surgery. The subcostal right anterior oblique and sagittal views demonstrate this region well. Options in the newborn period include palliation with an aorticopulmonary shunt and full repair. If the pulmonary arteries are very small, palliation may allow for improved growth of the pulmonary arteries and ultimately a better corrective operation.

Truncus Arteriosus. Truncus arteriosus results from failure of septation of the embryonic truncus. There is a large malalignment ventricular septal defect located beneath the common truncal valve (Fig. 13-50). Truncus is classified into four types. In type I truncus, the most common kind, the main pulmonary artery arises as a single vessel either laterally or posteriorly from the trunk. This vessel then bifurcates into the right and left pulmo-

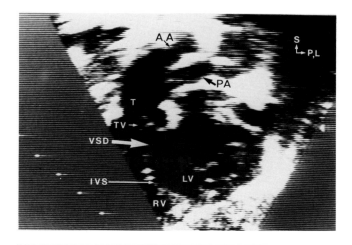

Figure 13-50. Subcostal sagittal view of a truncus arteriosus. A malalignment ventricular septal defect (VSD) is located beneath the common trunk (T). Immediately above the truncal valve (TV) sinuses, the pulmonary artery (PA) arises posteriorly. The ascending aorta (AA) is seen to continue on its normal superior course. (IVS, interventricular septum; LV, left ventricle; RV, right ventricle; S, superior; P, posterior; L, left.)

nary arteries (Fig. 13-51). In type II, the pulmonary arteries originate separately but very close together from the posterior aspect of the trunk. In type III only one pulmonary artery arises from the trunk and the other arises from a ductus arteriosus. In type IV, there is an associated small ascending aorta and an interrupted aortic arch. The truncal valve should be interrogated with Doppler to determine possible associated truncal valve stenosis or regurgitation.

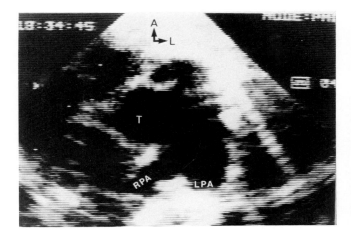

Figure 13-51. Parasternal short axis view of a patient with truncus arteriosus. The pulmonary artery arises posterolateral from the common trunk (T) and then bifurcates into the right pulmonary artery (RPA) and the left pulmonary artery (LPA). (A, anterior; L, left.)

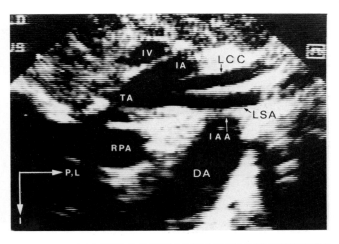

Figure 13-52. Suprasternal aortic arch view of type A interruption of the aortic arch (IAA). The innominate artery (IA), left common carotid artery (LCC) and left subclavian artery (LSA) all arise from the transverse arch (TA) prior to the interruption. Blood flow to the descending aorta (DA) is supplied from a large patent ductus arteriosus (not shown). (IV, innominate vein; RPA, right pulmonary artery; I, inferior; P, posterior; L, left.)

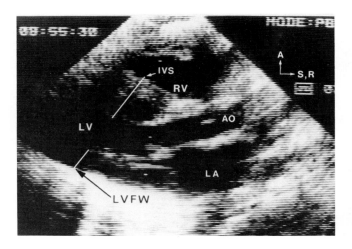

Figure 13-53. Parasternal long axis view of a patient with hypertrophic cardiomyopathy. The ventricular septum (IVS) is thickened when compared with the left ventricular free wall (LVFW). The left ventricular outflow tract is prone to obstruction from the interventricular septal hypertrophy. (LV, left ventricle; LA, left atrium; AO, aorta; RV, right ventricle; A, anterior; S, superior; R, right.)

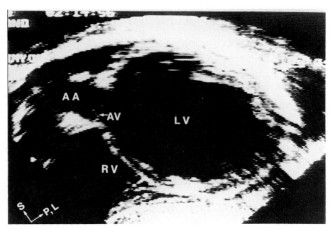

Figure 13-54. Subcostal long axial oblique view of a patient with dilated congestive cardiomyopathy. The left ventricle (LV) is grossly dilated with very poor contractility. (RV, right ventricle; AV, aortic valve; AA, ascending aorta; S, superior; P, posterior; L, left.)

Interrupted Aortic Arch. The aortic arch is best viewed from the suprasternal notch. The interruption of the aortic arch may occur in several different locations. In type A, the interruption is distal to the left subclavian (Fig. 13-52). In type B, the most common, the interruption is between the left subclavian and the left common carotid, and in type C the interruption is proximal to the origin of the left common carotid.

Cardiomyopathy. Cardiomyopathy occurs in children in either hypertrophic or dilated forms. In hyper-

trophic cardiomyopathy, the interventricular septum is thickened when compared to the left ventricular free wall. This is best visualized from the long and short axis views (Fig. 13-53). The left ventricular outflow is prone to obstruction from dynamic compression. In addition, there is often systolic anterior motion of anterior mitral leaflet valve, which can contribute to outflow obstruction.

In congestive cardiomyopathy, the left ventricle is seen as a dilated, poorly functioning chamber. In children, this type of ventricle is often observed as a consequence of viral myocarditis (Figs. 13-54, 13-55). Congestive cardiomyopathy can cause dilation or distortion of

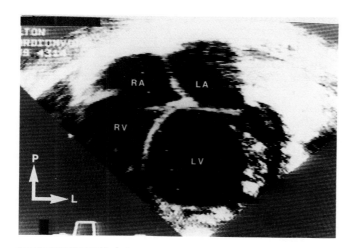

Figure 13-55. Apical four-chamber view of a dilated congestive cardiomyopathy. Gross left ventricular (LV) dilation is often accompanied by distortion of the aortic and mitral valve coaptation with associated insufficiency. Excessively bright reflectance of the left ventricular endocardium is associated with endocardial fibroelastosis. (RV, right ventricle; RA, right atrium; LA, left atrium; P, posterior; L, left.)

the aortic valve or mitral valve and may result in insufficiency.

Doppler Echocardiography

Doppler echocardiography and color-flow Doppler are two of the most dramatic advances in noninvasive assessment of cardiac function. In this application the Doppler equation is used to calculate the velocity of blood flow. The frequency shift measures the blood velocity if the speed of sound in tissue and the angle between the ultrasound beam and the blood flow are known:

$$v = \Delta f \times (c / 2 f_0 \cos \Theta)$$

where

Δf = the frequency shift

c = the speed of sound in tissue (1560 m/sec)

f_0 = transmitted (transducer) frequency

$\cos \Theta$ = cosine of the angle between the blood flow and the transducer

Doppler peak velocity accuracy and strength of signal require that the transmitted sound wave be as parallel as possible to the direction of the blood flow (Fig. 13-56).

The Doppler probe emits a sound pulse toward the cardiac structures. As the reflected impulse is received by the transducer, the signal is processed. The information processed is a function of the red blood cell motion within the volume sampled. The computer does a fast Fourier transformation, which determines the fre-

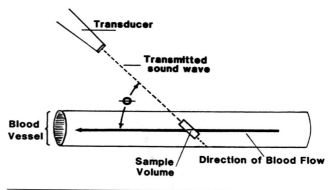

Figure 13-56.

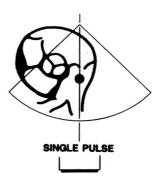

SINGLE PULSE

Figure 13-57. Pulsed Doppler.

quency shifts present and their prevalence. Unlike two-dimensional echocardiography, Doppler requires low-frequency transducers for optimal interrogation.

Two types of conventional Doppler are available: pulsed Doppler and continuous-wave Doppler. Pulsed Doppler interrogation uses a pulsed mode of transmission to evaluate a specific region of blood flow. Establishing a temporal gate allows determination of Doppler shift within a specific axial area at a known distance from the transducer. This area is known as the sample volume. In pulsed Doppler the transducer waits for the return of the signal and then emits another sound wave (Fig. 13-57). Since pulsed Doppler must wait for the return of the sig-

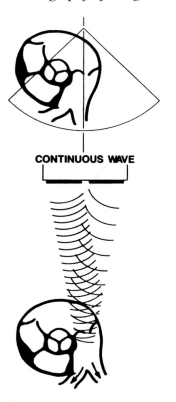

Figure 13-58. Continuous-wave Doppler.

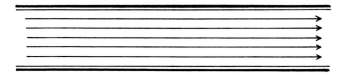

Figure 13-59. Laminar flow.

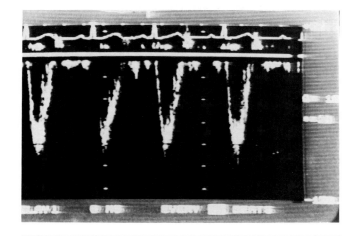

Figure 13-60. Normal pulsed Doppler display of great vessel showing laminar systolic flow.

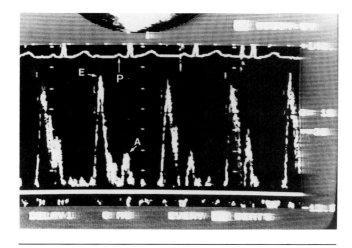

Figure 13-61. Normal pulsed Doppler display of an atrioventricular valve inflow. (E, A, P, see text.)

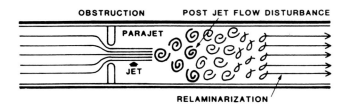

Figure 13-62. Disturbed-turbulent flow.

nal, it is not good for interrogating at significant depths because of the time delay of impulse return. This form of Doppler is also limited by its inability to evaluate high flow velocities accurately.

In continuous-wave Doppler there is interrogation using a wave of almost constant amplitude that persists for a large number of cycles and is used for sampling Doppler shift regardless of the distance from the transducer (Fig. 13-58). This technique analyzes the entire line of blood flow along its path. Continuous-wave Doppler allows unambiguous determination of high-velocity flow; however, the range is ambiguous, since information is obtained along an entire line instead of a single confined location. Laminar flow results when direction and velocity of all blood flow in a specific region are uniform (Fig. 13-59). Doppler interrogation of this laminar flow results in a musical audio signal and flamelike or laminar envelope (Fig. 13-60). Flow begins at the opening of the semilunar valve and stops with closure. By convention, the flow away from the transducer is displayed below the baseline and flow toward the transducer is displayed above the baseline. Fig. 13-61 demonstrates normal Doppler flow of an atrioventricular valve inflow. The e wave corresponds to the passive phase of ventricular filling immediately after ventricular systole. The A wave corresponds to the active phase of ventricular filling as the atria contract immediately after the p wave. Again, the Doppler signal is seen to be flamelike and laminar.

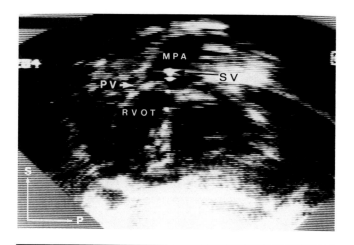

Figure 13-63. Pulsed Doppler sample volume placement in the main pulmonary artery. (SV, sample volume; MPA, main pulmonary artery; PV, pulmonary valve; RVOT, right ventricular outflow tract; S, superior; P, posterior.)

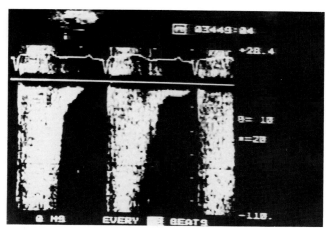

Figure 13-64. Pulsed Doppler of the main pulmonary artery in a patient with pulmonary valve stenosis demonstrating systolic high-velocity turbulent flow.

When flow through an obstructed or insufficient valve is disturbed, there is a random array of red cell velocities in multiple directions and in a very disorganized fashion (Fig. 13-62). This turbulent flow is seen as a filled-in Doppler signal and has a harsh audible component. Figure 13-63 shows the Doppler sample volume placed in the main pulmonary artery just distal to a thickened pulmonary valve. The pulsed Doppler display from this sample volume shows systolic turbulent flow with increased velocity (Fig. 13-64). Because the flow velocity is high, there is aliasing of the spectral display with pulsed Doppler. The peak velocity is therefore not resolved. Continuous-wave spectral display demonstrates resolution of the spectral envelope at 3.6 m/sec (Fig. 13-65).

Using a simplified Bernoulli equation,

$$\text{pressure gradient (mm Hg)} = 4 \times V^2$$

where

$$v = \text{peak Doppler velocity in m/sec}$$

the calculated gradient from the right ventricle to the main pulmonary artery is 52 mm Hg. It is imperative to sample above and below the valve of concern and to evaluate from multiple locations distal to the obstruction to determine the highest velocity. This calculated gradient is a peak instantaneous gradient, which differs from a peak-to-peak gradient as measured in the cardiac catheterization laboratory. The Doppler-calculated gradients usually are no more than 10 to 15 mm Hg different from each other, the instantaneous peak being slightly higher.

Figure 13-66 demonstrates the pulsed Doppler sample volume located in the right atrium just proximal to the tricuspid valve. The spectral display from the sample volume shows systolic turbulent flow with an in-

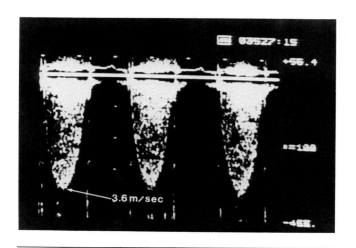

Figure 13-65. Continuous-wave Doppler of the pulmonary artery in a patient with pulmonary valve stenosis.

creased, unresolved peak flow (Fig. 13-67). With continuous wave Doppler there is resolution of the peak flow at 3.3 m/sec, giving a calculated right ventricular pressure 44 mm Hg greater than the right atrial v wave (Fig. 13-68).

Using Doppler, regurgitation can be semiquantitatively estimated. Regurgitation to the valve level only is considered mild, while regurgitant jets that extend to fill an entire chamber are considered severe.

Color-flow Doppler has recently become an indispensable part of the noninvasive evaluation of the heart and great vessels. Color-flow allows the examiner to have two-dimensional and Doppler data superimposed continuously. This eliminates the need for switching back and forth between two-dimensional and Doppler images.

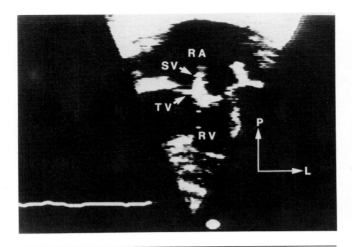

Figure 13-66. Pulsed Doppler sample volume placement behind the tricuspid valve in a patient with tricuspid regurgitation. (SV, sample volume; RA, right atrium; TV, tricuspid valve; RV, right ventricle; P, posterior; L, left.)

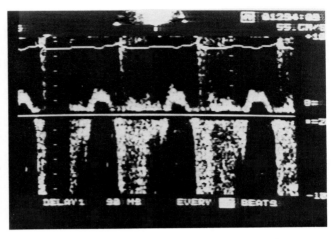

Figure 13-67. Pulsed Doppler display in a patient with tricuspid regurgitation showing systolic high-velocity turbulent flow.

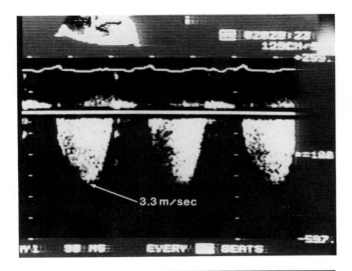

Figure 13-68. Continuous-wave Doppler spectral display in a patient with tricuspid regurgitation.

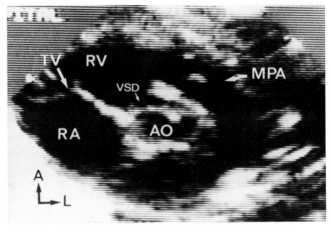

Figure 13-69. Parasternal short axis view of a conoventricular septal defect. (TV, tricuspid valve; RV, right ventricle; VSD, ventricular septal defect; RA, right atrium; AO, aorta; MPA, main pulmonary artery; A, anterior; L, left.)

Doppler flow is translated into shades of blue and red, blue being flow directed away from the transducer and red flow toward the transducer. Shades of red or blue correspond to different velocities. This technique allows the user to evaluate multiple areas of the heart and great vessels simultaneously. In addition, the pulsed Doppler sample volume can be much more accurately placed into the region of maximal velocity, allowing the best estimation of peak flow velocities. Color-flow is extremely sensitive and allows visualization of very small defects, such as patent ductus arteriosus or small muscular ventricular septal defects otherwise difficult to see with conventional two-dimensional echo.

Figure 13-69 demonstrates a parasternal short axis view of a conoventricular septal defect using standard two-dimensional echocardiography. The ventricular septal defect is visible. When color-flow data are added, the Doppler depiction of the turbulent flow is seen. Left-to-right shunting is displayed by yellow color-flow (arrows) (Plate 9).

Figure 13-70 demonstrates a patent ductus arteriosus observed from the suprasternal notch. The patent ductus can be seen. When color flow is added, the ductal jet of flow can be seen shunting left to right toward the main pulmonary artery as displayed by the yellow and red Doppler flow area (arrows) (Plate 10).

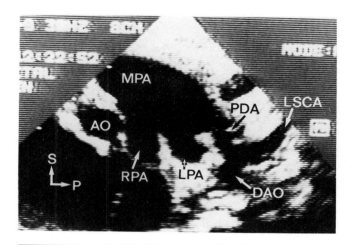

Figure 13-70. Patent ductus arteriosus (PDA) view with two-dimensional echocardiography. (MPA, main pulmonary artery; AO, aorta; RPA, right pulmonary artery; LPA, left pulmonary artery; LSCA, left subclavian artery; DAO, descending aorta; S, superior; P, posterior.)

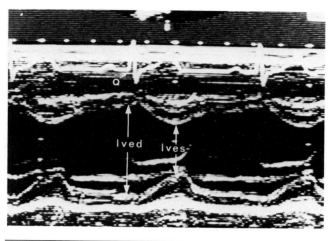

Figure 13-71. Normal left ventricular M-mode display for calculation of left ventricular shortening fraction. (LVED, left ventricular end-diastolic dimension; LVES, left ventricular end-systolic dimension.)

M-Mode Echocardiography

M-mode echocardiography is being used less and less with the advances in two-dimensional echo and Doppler. M-mode is still used for the assessment of ventricular function and for quantification of chamber and vessel dimensions. Figure 13-71 demonstrates a normal left ventricular M-mode display used for the calculation of the left ventricular shortening fraction. The M-mode tracing is recorded through the left ventricle at the level of the mitral valve chordae. The left ventricular end-diastolic measurement (LVED) is measured at the onset of the Q-wave from the posterior side of the interventricular septum to the endocardial margin of the posterior left ventricular wall. The left ventricular end-systolic measurement (LVES) is performed at peak systolic contraction of the left ventricular free wall. The shortening fraction is then calculated as

$$\frac{\text{LVED} - \text{LVES}}{\text{LVED}} = \text{shortening fraction percent}$$

and is expressed as a percentage. The normal range for left ventricular shortening is 30% to 45%. This calculation must be carefully scrutinized, however, since it is extremely sensitive to changes in both preload and afterload.

Fetal Echocardiography

Recent advances in fetal echocardiography allow for prenatal diagnosis of congenital heart defects and rhythm disturbances. The incidence of structural congenital heart disease is approximately 0.7% to 0.8%. The recurrence risk given one sibling with congenital heart disease is 1% to 4% and as high as 10% to 12% in certain lesions, and offspring of parents with congenital heart disease also have an increased risk of 2% to 4%. Therefore, fetal echocardiography may be helpful in those patients with a strong family history of congenital heart disease. Other reasons for referral include suspected cardiac malformations on obstetric ultrasound; known fetal chromosomal abnormalities; maternal drug ingestion (lithium, amphetamines, alcohol, anticonvulsants, chemotherapy); maternal diabetes or collagen vascular disease; sustained fetal tachycardia or bradycardia; or irregular cardiac rhythms.

Cardiac movement can be detected by ultrasound at 6 weeks' gestation. Cardiac imaging is possible usually after 14 to 16 weeks and becomes more optimal from 18 to 35 weeks. Optimal imaging should be done through the fetal abdomen. If an adequate acoustic window cannot be found, the mother may be repositioned to either right or left lateral decubitus. The fetal heart should be scanned in multiple sweeps. All the valves and chambers are identified, the normal relation of the great arteries is confirmed, and the systemic and pulmonary veins are identified.

The four-chamber view is usually easily obtained (Fig. 13-72). This demonstrates the two atria, which are usually similar in size, as are the two ventricles. The right ventricle may be slightly larger. The mitral and tricuspid valves can easily be seen, and flow across the valve can be interrogated using Doppler echocardiography. A normal four-chamber view usually indicates no structural heart disease.

Figure 13-73 is a four chamber view in a fetus at 33

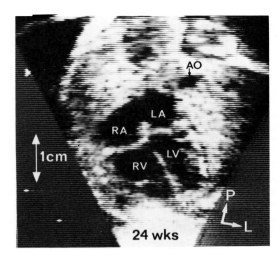

Figure 13-72. Transverse echocardiographic view of a fetus at 24 weeks' gestation. A normal four-chamber view is demonstrated. (RA, right atrium; LA, left atrium; LV, left ventricle; RV, right ventricle; AO, descending aorta; P, posterior; L, left.)

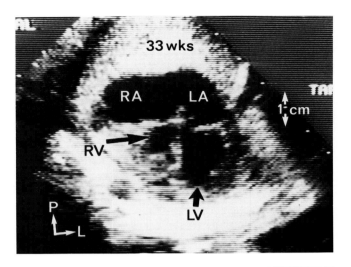

Figure 13-73. Transverse echocardiographic frame demonstrating the four-chamber view of a fetus at 33 weeks' gestation with hypoplastic right ventricle. (RV, right ventricle; RA, right atrium; LA, left atrium; LV, left ventricle; P, posterior; L, left.)

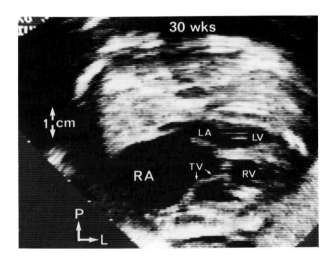

Figure 13-74. Transverse echocardiographic view of a fetus at 30 weeks' gestation with Ebstein's anomaly. (RA, right atrium; TV, tricuspid valve; RV, right ventricle; LA, left atrium; LV, left ventricle; P, posterior; L, left.)

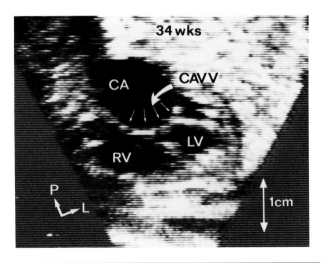

Figure 13-75. Transverse echocardiographic view of a fetus at 34 weeks' gestation in the four-chamber view. A common atrioventricular valve (CAVV) is demonstrated. (CA, common atrium; RV, right ventricle; LV, left ventricle; P, posterior; L, left.)

weeks' gestation showing a normal left atrium and left ventricle. The right ventricle is hypoplastic.

Figure 13-74 demonstrates massive cardiomegaly in a fetus at 30 weeks gestation. The right atrium and right ventricle are markedly dilated. The tricuspid valve is abnormal and displaced toward the right ventricular apex. Tricuspid regurgitation is demonstrated with Doppler. This was felt to be consistent with Ebstein's anomaly.

Figure 13-75 shows an example of a four-chamber view in a fetus at 34 weeks' gestation with a complete common atrioventricular canal. A single common atrio-

ventricular valve is present. There is a primum atrial septal defect and a canal-type ventricular septal defect.

Acknowledgments. Doppler diagrams are used by permission of the American Society of Echocardiography (ASE). Reprinted from "Recommendations for Terminology and Display for Doppler Echocardiography" as established by "The Doppler Standards and Nomenclature Committee" of the ASE. Echo diagrams are used by permission from the "Report of the ASE on Nomenclature and Standards in Two-dimensional Echocardiography" as established by the "Committee on Nomenclature and Standards in Two-Dimensional Echocardiography."

Grateful appreciation is expressed to Dr. J. Gregg Helton for his invaluable assistance with this manuscript.

References

1. Berman W. Pulsed Doppler ultrasound in clinical pediatrics. Mount Kisco, NY: Futura Publishing Co., 1983.
2. Feigenbaum H. Echocardiography. London: Lea and Febiger.
3. Goldberg S, Allen H, Marx G, Flinn C. Doppler echocardiography. Philadelphia: Lea and Febiger, 1985.
4. Goldberg S, Hugh A, Sahn D. Pediatric and adolescent echocardiography. Chicago: YearBook Medical Publishers, 1980.
5. Hatle L, Angelsen B. Doppler ultrasound in cardiology. Philadelphia: Lea and Febiger, 1985.
6. Huhta J. Pediatric imaging/Doppler ultrasound of the chest: extracardiac diagnosis. Philadelphia: Lea and Febiger, 1986.
7. Kisslo J, Adams D, Belkin R. Doppler color flow imaging. New York: Churchill Livingstone, 1988.
8. Ludomirsky A, Huhta J. Color Doppler of congenital heart disease in the child and adult. Mount Kisco, NY: Futura Publishing Co, 1987.
9. Reed K, Anderson C, Shenker L: Fetal echocardiography: an atlas. New York: Alan R. Liss, 1988.
10. Salcedo E. Atlas of echocardiography. Philadelphia: WB Saunders, 1985.
11. Seward JB, Takij AH, Edwards WS, Hagler DJ. Two-dimensional echocardiographic atlas. New York: Springer-Verlag, 1988.
12. Snider R, Serwer G. Echocardiography in pediatric heart disease. Chicago: YearBook Medical Publishers, 1990.
13. Williams R, Bierman F, Sanders S. Echocardiographic diagnosis of cardiac malformations. Boston: Little, Brown, 1986.

Index

The letter *f* following a page number indicates a figure; the letter *t* indicates a table.

ISBN 0-397-51107-8

90000
9 780397 511075